Self-Instruction
in
Mental Health Nursing

Second Edition

N. Okon Ironbar,
RMN, RGN, DipN (Lond), BTA Cert, RNT, Cert Ed (Leeds);
*Director of Studies, In service Education (Nursing) Consultancy Service;
Formerly Senior Nurse Tutor/Course Manager, Continuing Education and
Training, East Berkshire Nursing and Midwifery Education Centre, Wexham
Park Hospital, Slough.*

Alan Hooper,
MSc, RMN, SRN, DipN, DANS, RNT;
*Head of Studies, Mental Health, Learning Disabilities and Child Branch
Programmes, Tor Faculty of Tor, South West College of Health, Exeter.*

Baillière Tindall
*London   Philadelphia   Toronto
Sydney   Tokyo*

Baillière Tindall   24–28 Oval Road
London NW1 7DX, England

The Curtis Center, Independence Square West,
Philadelphia, PA 19106–3399, USA

Harcourt Brace & Company
55 Horner Avenue
Toronto, Ontario M8Z 4X6, Canada

Harcourt Brace & Company, Australia
32–52 Smidmore Street, Marrickville, NSW 2204,
Australia

Harcourt Brace & Company, Japan
Ichibancho Central Building, 22-1 Ichibancho
Chiyoda-ku, Tokyo 102, Japan

First edition published 1983
Second edition published 1989
Fifth printing 1997

British Library Cataloguing in Publication Data

Ironbar, N. Okon
   Self-instruction in mental health
   nursing.—2nd ed.
   1. Psychiatric patients. Nursing –
   Questions & answers
   I. Title   II. Hooper, Alan   III. Self-
   instruction in psychiatric nursing
   610.73´68´076

ISBN 0-7020-1327-7

Typeset by Photo-Graphics, Honiton, Devon
Printed and bound in Great Britain by
Mackays of Chatham PLC, Chatham, Kent

Introduction

This is a period of significant change for mental health care services. Changes in the pattern of care, organization of services, professional education and clinical practice are likely to have profound consequences for both service users and providers. While the outcomes are uncertain, it is very likely that the nature of the services offered and the roles of those who work within them will undergo radical revision.

As with all major transitions, these changes can create situations of challenge and opportunity or of uncertainty and stress. In order to take advantage of these developments mental health nurses will need to be politically aware and professionally assertive. Of fundamental importance is the nursing profession's own belief in the value and validity of their own role. Professional self-esteem and a sound research base are basic requisites of credible and effective nursing practice.

Commitment to ongoing professional development and education is an essential part of the process of being able to determine and lead these changes rather than merely reacting to them. Within such an environment nurses need to accept that the skills and knowledge base of today have a limited "half-life" and require constant renewal. Never has "learning how to learn", as a basis for professional practice, been more important. The extensive revision of this edition is intended to reflect many of the changes in mental health services and practice. The underlying philosophy and contents of this book should help all learners (using the term in its widest sense) to develop a sound understanding of major mental health problems and appropriate therapeutic interventions.

Particular emphasis has been placed upon the key role of the mental health nurse in assessing, planning, implementing and evaluating care. A certain degree of overlap and repetition is intentional in reinforcing these core skills of mental health nursing practice.

The retitling of the book as "mental health" rather than "psychiatric" nursing and the use of the word "client" or "person" in preference to "patient" are both indications of the way that practice and perceptions are changing. Likewise, the place of care – residential or community – has not been specified in the nursing interventions. This is intended to take into account the increasing diversity of settings in which mental health care is provided.

Acknowledgements

Thanks are due to the many people who have helped to prepare this revised edition: Diana Hammond and Sam for their continued support; Sarah V. Smith, Associate Nursing Editor, Baillière Tindall, for her guidance and encouragement; Chris Gibson for his technical advice; Edith Vardy, typist; and Rosemary Morris and David Inglis, formerly of Baillière Tindall.

The professional stimulation and influence of many others should also be acknowledged: the teachers and learners of Exeter School of Nursing, Mental Health; the staff of Exeter Mental Health Unit; Fred Waite; and Carolyn Jones.

Promoting Personal Learning

"Self-instruction in Mental Health Nursing" is designed to facilitate and support a programme of self-directed learning. The book is divided into a number of topics which can be worked through systematically. In each section the unit objectives, concise information, useful references and opportunities for self-evaluation provide a framework for the progressive development of a sound knowledge base.

In addition to the use of this book as a study guide, students can also considerably enhance their learning potential by reviewing and developing their own educational strategy and philosophy.

1. *Accept and take responsibility for your own learning.* This involves commitment, self-discipline, determining personal priorities, meeting challenges, acknowledging your own successes and failures.
2. *Develop your learning skills.* Learning involves a wide range of cognitive, emotional and behavioural skills. Like all skills they can be developed and improved. Basic skills include planning and organizing your studies, making effective use of time, pacing yourself, reading quickly and comprehensively, making concise notes, extending your vocabulary, creating a conducive personal learning environment, understanding how references are stated and used, being able to follow up references, keeping an index of useful books and journal articles.
3. *Exercise your rights.* As a learner you have the right to:
    (i)   detailed information about course structure, instructional strategies and attainment criteria;
    (ii)   be allowed to take responsibility for your own learning;
    (iii)   be treated with respect as an intelligent, capable and equal human being;
    (iv)   ask questions and be given informed answers;
    (v)   express your own opinions and values;
    (vi)   receive instruction from competent teachers and practitioners;
    (vii)   challenge and question educational methods and clinical practice;
    (viii) access to adequate and appropriate learning resources;
    (ix)   be given honest, regular and accurate feedback on your progress and attainment;

(x)   participate in educational planning and evaluation of clinical and classroom experiences.

4. *Identify potential learning resources*:
   (i)   people:– practitioners, fellow learners, instructors and teachers, librarians, clients;
   (ii) services:– local, national and professional libraries; voluntary, statutory and professional organizations.

5. *Learn how to use a library*. Ask the staff what resources and facilities are available, e.g. inter-library loans, literature searches, photocopying. Familiarize yourself with the layout of books and journals. Find out how to use catalogue cards, microfiches, indexes and bibliographies.

6. *Read professional journals regularly*. Journals have a special role in professional development, communication and practice. They serve as a forum for the dissemination of current ideas, opinions, information and research. Consider forming or joining a journal club.

7. *Use this volume as a workbook*. For example: underline and highlight particularly relevant or significant information; make your own note in the margin alongside the text; where appropriate, add in further assessment details, desired outcomes and interventions from your own experience; use the book to develop your own personal practice database.

8. *Learn how to identify, create and use learning opportunities*. All situations have some learning potential in them. The optimum use of learning opportunities requires careful planning, assertiveness and using initiative. Relate your learning to your practical experience. The most powerful learning opportunities arise as part of everyday experience. Analyse your current work environment for learning opportunities.

Suggested References

Barrass, R. (1984). *Study!* Chapman and Hall, London.

Bligh, D. (1978). What's the Use of Lectures?, revised edition. D. A. and B. Bligh.

Dickson, A. (1982). *A Woman in Your Own Right! Assertiveness and You*. Quartet Books, London.

Gibbs, G. (1981). *Teaching Students to Learn*. Open University Press, Milton Keynes.

Good, M. and South, C. (1988). *In the Know. 8 Keys to Successful Learning*. BBC Books, London.

Marshall, L. and Rowland, F. (1981). *A Guide to Learning Independently*. Open University Press, Milton Keynes.

Royal College of Nursing (1987). *Nursing Students Bill of Rights*. Royal College of Nursing, London.

Contents

TOPIC 1

The Practice of Mental Health Nursing

At the end of this Topic the learner should aim to:

1. Understand how human needs influence the role of the mental health nurse.
2. Describe the factors involved in developing therapeutic relationships.
3. Specify the purposes of nurse-client communication.
4. Outline the application of "primary nursing" to mental health nursing practice.

Human Needs and the Role of the Mental Health Nurse

Unit Objectives

At the end of this Unit the learner should be able to:

1. Define the term "need".
2. List the needs for healthy living.
3. Describe the role of the mental nurse in enabling people to meet their mental and physical health needs.

Human Needs

In order to maintain their physical and mental health people have certain essential requirements or needs that must be met. All human activity can in fact be viewed as being directed by the individual towards the attainment of these physical, social and emotional needs. If an individual experiences a deficit in their basic needs then they are usually motivated to take some course of action towards meeting this deficiency and to restore their equilibrium.

When people have mental health problems, however, their ability to meet their needs independently can be adversely affected. The nature of their problems may be such that their ability to recognize this deficiency is limited or they are unable to initiate and co-ordinate their efforts effectively. This can result in frustration, conflict or deprivation for the person. Depending upon the nature and extent of the person's inability to meet their needs they may experience increased tension and stress or be placed in a life-threatening situation.

One of the fundamental roles of the mental health nurse, therefore, is to enable people with mental health problems to meet their basic needs and to restore the individual's well-being as far as possible. This may involve the nurse in giving direct care or in facilitating the development of the individual's ability to meet their own health care needs.

Although the experience and requirement of needs is universal, the way an individual strives and makes choices about their needs is an expression of their uniqueness. People's needs are an expression of:

1. The culture that they live in, i.e. values of the society, religion, social class, ethnic group.
2. Their own upbringing, i.e. the influence of their parents and peer group, their education and life experiences.
3. Their personal identity, i.e. personality, attitudes, self-awareness, relationships, occupation, personal goals.

One requirement of skilled and effective mental health nursing practice is to be able to identify accurately the unique care needs of each individual and to select interventions designed to meet them. The effectiveness of nursing care is an indication of the extent that it actually meets personal needs.

A Hierarchy of Human Needs

There are many ways of considering human needs. One of the most common models used is that proposed by Maslow (1970; see Exhibit 1.1.1). It has the merit of being logical, understandable and also applicable to health care

Exhibit 1.1.1—Maslow's hierarchy of needs

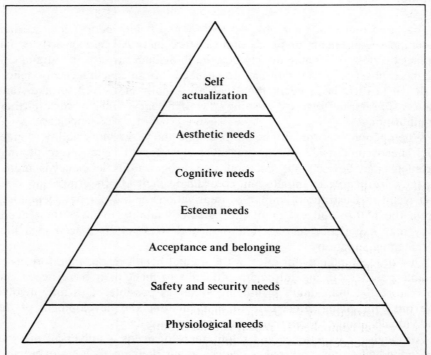

situations. It is described as a "hierarchy" because it is presented as a structure of ascending needs. Each successive level of needs, starting at the bottom, has to be met before a person is able to direct their attention to the next level. In many situations found in mental health practice, individuals may invert their priorities, become over-concerned with certain needs or demonstrate a lack of insight in regard to meeting their needs.

Physiological needs

Exhibit 1.1.2 Physiological needs

Specific requirements	For the person having difficulty in meeting their needs this may be experienced as:
Nutrition and fluids	Hunger, thirst, discomfort, excessive intake, anorexia, physical difficulty, nausea, anxiety
Oxygen	Breathlessness, dizziness, hyperventilation
Warmth	Coldness and shivering, perspiration
Rest	Tiredness, lethargy, drowsiness, exhaustion
Environmental stimulation	Boredom, stress, confusion, monotony
Cleanliness	Body odour, skin irritation
Elimination	Discomfort, excessive, inability
Physical activity	Stiffness, loss of muscle tone, exhaustion
Sex	Frustration, conflict, stress, impotence, frigidity, loss of libido

People with mental health problems may be unwilling, unable, not aware or have a distorted awareness of their physiological needs. They may be:

- confused,
- anxious,
- frightened,
- feeling threatened,
- misperceiving reality,
- distracted by persistent thoughts,
- feel compelled to repeat certain actions,
- dependent upon certain drugs,
- lacking in information.

Nurse's role:

- to assess the person's ability to meet their physical needs;
- to provide direct care, if required;
- to facilitate the ability of the person to meet their own needs.

Mental health nursing interventions may include:

- forming a therapeutic relationship,
- reassurance and explanation,
- counselling,
- guidance and demonstration,
- prompting,
- encouragement,
- providing information,
- teaching new skills,
- environmental control,
- supervision and monitoring,
- direct intervention,
- habit training,
- observation,
- organizing physical activities,
- reality orientation,
- health education.

Safety and security needs

Exhibit 1.1.3 Safety and security needs

Specific requirements	For the person having difficulty in meeting their needs this may be experienced as:
Feeling safe	Anxiety, tension, threat, fear
Security	Insecurity, doubt, uncertainty
Protection from harm	Fear of harm from others or unable to control own behaviour
Predictability and order	Disorder and chaos
Knowing what is going to happen	Worry, uncertainty, doubt, indecisiveness, not knowing
Trust and reliance on others	Mistrust of others, suspiciousness, doubting the intention or integrity of others

| Being in control | Unpredictability, loss of choice, feeling trapped |
| Maintain identity | Fear of stigma, guilt, shame, change of role and personal identity |

People with mental health problems may experience a variety of situations in which their needs for security can be threatened. These include:

1. Anxiety upon requiring care, either at home or in hospital. In both situations there is a loss of autonomy and a fear of the unknown. There may also be feelings of guilt and shame about being labelled "mentally ill".
2. Anxiety is a common symptom of mental health problems. It may be disproportionate, unpleasant and out of personal control. It significantly adds to the stress that the person experiences.
3. Risk to self and others from loss of insight, loss of control or fear.

The person may be:

- confused,
- frightened,
- feeling threatened,
- over-active,
- lacking in energy and motivation,
- uninhibited,
- misperceiving reality,
- driven by persistent and intrusive thoughts,
- feeling trapped, hopeless and suicidal,
- hostile and intolerant,
- craving alcohol or drugs.

Nurse's role:

- to assess the degree of threat to the person's security needs;
- to provide physical and emotional protection;
- to facilitate the ability of the person to meet their security needs.

Mental health nursing interventions may include:

- forming a therapeutic relationship,
- observation,
- reassurance,
- counselling,
- providing information,
- health education,

- teaching new skills,
- anxiety management,
- encouragement,
- modelling calm behaviour,
- setting limits on potentially self-injurious behaviour,
- removing environmental risks,
- direct intervention.

Acceptance and belonging

Exhibit 1.1.4 Acceptance and belonging

Specific requirements	For the person having difficulty in meeting their needs this may be experienced as:
Acceptance	Rejection, feeling distanced, aloofness, detachment
Love and affection	Feeling unloved, difficulty in expressing emotions, lack of emotions, sadness, unpredictable mood swings
Warm communicating relationships	Hostility, conflict, inability to communicate, lack of social and life skills, isolation, distrust, stressful and demanding relationships, insecurity
Group companionship	Feeling stigmatized, alone, threatened by others, social withdrawal, low self-esteem, lacking in confidence, alienation

Difficulties in relationships and feelings of rejection and isolation feature prominently with people who are having mental health problems. These may indicate a change in their own perception, the effect of their behaviour on their close relationships or reflect their social experience. Resolving these problems and enabling people to meet their needs for acceptance and belonging are key areas of mental health nursing practice.

Nurse's role:

- to assess the person's ability to meet their social needs;
- to facilitate the ability of the prson to meet their social needs.

Mental health nursing interventions may include:

- forming a therapeutic relationship,
- observation,
- reassurance,
- providing information,
- health education,
- teaching new skills,
- social skills training,
- promoting self-esteem,
- group work,
- counselling,
- organizing group activities with the emphasis on cooperation and communication,
- encouraging contact with relatives and friends.

Esteem needs

Exhibit 1.1.5 Esteem needs

Specific requirements	For the person having difficulty in meeting their needs this may be experienced as:
Positive self-worth	Low self-esteem, worthlessness, valuelessness, thoughts of self-harm
Autonomy and control	Over-dependence, lack of choice and control, over-regulation, helplessness, hopelessness, passivity
Sense of mastery and competence	Lack of control, lack of skills, inability, handicap, uselessness
Recognition from others	Lack of recognition as an individual, depersonalization, loss of identity, being ignored, ridiculed
Appreciation by others	Being devalued, derided, hostility, rejection
Personal status	Stigma, guilt, shame, disinhibited

People have a powerful need to be acknowledged as individuals in their own right and as a person of worth to others. The self-esteem that a person has is a key factor in the way that a person relates to others and the priority that they give to meeting their own needs. High self-esteem is associated with confident and assertive behaviour, low self-esteem with insecurity and self-deprecation.

A person's self-esteem develops from the feedback they are given from their relationships and life experiences. Early parental influences are particularly significant in developing self-worth. Successful life experiences and rewarding relationships with others do much to promote high self-esteem. Experiences of failure and rejection damage and devalue a person's self-esteem. It is significant that people with mental health problems frequently complain of low or loss of self-esteem.

The personal identity of people with mental ill-health is also often insecure. People complain of loss of identity, personal uncertainty about their role and image and at times of even feeling unreal. Occasionally, the way that a person wishes to express their identity and uniqueness may bring them into conflict with more generally held views about appearance, social behaviour and sexuality.

Nurse's role:

- to assess the person's self-esteem,
- to facilitate personal autonomy,
- to enable the person to regain a positive self-image.

Mental health nursing interventions may include:

- forming a therapeutic relationship,
- reinforcing self-esteem,
- reassurance,
- providing a safe environment,
- encouragement
- counselling,
- providing information,
- teaching new life-skills,
- assertiveness training,
- social skills training,
- facilitating choice,
- teaching decision-making skills,
- teaching problem-solving skills,
- encouraging personal responsibility,
- personalized care,
- personalized possessions,
- personalized space,
- personal recognition
- taking risks,
- health education,
- promoting social and family contacts,
- group work.

Cognitive needs

Exhibit 1.1.6 Cognitive needs

Specific requirements	For the person experiencing difficulty in meeting their needs this may be experienced as:
Knowledge	Lack of information, misinformation, forgetfulness, additional stress
Curiosity	Loss of interests, indifference, apathy, narrowed interests, morbid interest
Understanding	Puzzlement, bewilderment, incomprehension, poor or partial understanding, poor judgement, difficulty solving problems
Self-awareness and insight	Poor insight, loss of self-awareness, blaming others, not recognizing that they have problems, inappropriate behavioural and emotional responses, communication difficulties
Orientation	Confusion, unable to anticipate events, reduced alertness
Problem solving	Helplessness, feeling trapped, indecisiveness, hopelessness, poor concentration

People have an innate curiosity about the world and relationships between things. An understanding of and orientation to our immediate environment are important in contributing towards our feelings of security and our ability to relate towards others. People in health care need to have accurate information about their difficulties, the resources available to them and the roles of the various agencies. They also need the opportunity to use the experience of ill-health to increase their self-understanding and ability to cope.

Nurse's role:

- to assess the person's insight, orientation and understanding of their health care needs,
- to facilitate the development of the person's knowledge base and coping skills.

Mental health nursing interventions may include:

- forming a therapeutic relationship,
- counselling,
- reassurance,
- encouragement,
- providing information,
- teaching new life skills,
- health education,
- social skills training,
- giving feedback,
- teaching decision-making skills,
- teaching problem-solving skills,
- reality orientation,
- counselling,
- role play,
- drama and music therapy,
- group work.

Aesthetic needs

Exhibit 1.1.7 Aesthetic needs

Specific requirements	*For the person having difficulty in meeting their needs this may be experienced as*:
Creativity	Loss of imagination, lack of spontaneity, poverty of ideas, thought blocking, agitation
Personal expression	Frustration, difficulty in expressing themselves, inhibition, thought difficulties
Recreational interests	Loss of interest, boredom, physical limitations, hopelessness, helplessness, passivity, lack of control
Meaningful activity	Pointlessness, stress, unrewarding, undemanding, poor concentration, distraction
Beauty	Drabness, dullness, ugliness
Spiritual needs	Guilt, loss of faith

Aesthetic needs cover a wide range of activities and feelings that relate to the uniqueness of every individual. Each person strives to project themselves through their activities, hobbies, clothing and "territory". The needs are important for personal expression, personal identity, beliefs, diversion, reward and pleasure. People make large psychological and social "investments" in aesthetic needs. They participate in activities or buy ornaments or pictures, which to others may seem wasteful or pointless. However, to that person these things are crucial to their enjoyment, pleasure and meaning of life. Opportunities need to be provided for people to continue and participate in expressive outlets. The activities can be diversional, intrinsically pleasing, provide an outlet for feelings that might not be easily expressed in other ways, and give feedback on the person's recovery.

Nurse's role:

- to identify the person's unique recreational and expressive needs;
- to facilitate the ability of the person to meet their aesthetic needs.

Mental health nursing interventions may include:

- forming a therapeutic relationship,
- reassurance,
- encouragement,
- identifying potential resources,
- identifying potential outlets,
- organizing activities,
- participating in activities,
- helping to personalize the environment,
- helping to brighten the environment,
- drama and music,
- role play
- providing information,
- teaching new skills,
- facilitating choice,
- sense of humour,
- facilitating the practice and compliance with spiritual beliefs.

Self-actualization needs

Exhibit 1.1.8 Self-actualization needs

Specific requirements	*For the person having difficulty in meeting their needs this may be experienced as:*
Drive for self-improvement	Hopelessness, helplessness, unrealistic expectations, goals too low, lack of information, apathy

Personal growth	Lack of insight, lack of awareness, lack of opportunity, immaturity
Potential for change	Rigidity, insecurity, unadaptability, resistance, conservatism, denial

The drive for self-improvement is a powerful motivator. In many direct and indirect ways people are striving continually to better understand themselves and to develop their potential. Time is invested in many educational and learning activities. People try to analyse their own motivation and the subtleties of their relationships. The product of these endeavours is a personal feeling of maturity and mastery over life and that one is living life to the full. Many psychotherapeutic techniques have as their objective the improvement of the person's insight, their ability to relate to others, the development of coping skills and a sense of mastery.

Nurse's role:

- to assess the individual's potential for personal growth;
- to facilitate the development of the individual's potential.

Mental health nursing interventions may include:

- forming a therapeutic relationship,
- counselling,
- providing information,
- health education,
- support and guidance,
- encouragement,
- setting goals,
- teaching problem solving,
- teaching coping skills,
- promoting insight,
- giving feedback,
- social skills training,
- group work,
- taking risks,
- promoting change.

Unit Instructions

When you have researched the suggested references, have mastered the Unit Objectives and successfully answered the Self-assessment Questions, proceed with the Unit Written Test.

Suggested References

Campbell, C. (1978). *Nursing Diagnosis and Intervention in Nursing Practice*. John Wiley, New York.

Darcy, P. T. (1985). *Mental Health Nursing Source Book*. Baillière Tindall, London and San Diego.

Dexter, G. and Wash, M. (1986). *Psychiatric Nursing Skills: A Patient-centred Approach*. Croom Helm, London.

French, P. (1983). *Social Skills for Nursing Practice*. Croom Helm, London.

Goffman, E. (1963). *Stigma*. Pelican, London.

Hayter, J. (1981). Territoriality as a universal need. *Journal of Advanced Nursing*, Vol. 6, No. 2, pp. 79–85.

Hase, S. and Douglas, A. (1986). *Human Dynamics and Nursing*. Churchill Livingstone, Melbourne.

Irving, S. (1983). *Basic Psychiatric Nursing*, 3rd edition. W. B. Saunders, Philadelphia.

Lyttle, J. (1986). *Mental Disorder: Its Care and Treatment*. Baillière Tindall, London and San Diego.

Martin, P. (Ed.) (1987). *Psychiatric Nursing: A Therapeutic Approach*. Macmillan, London.

Robinson, L. (1983). *Psychiatric Nursing as a Human Experience*, 3rd edition. W. B. Saunders, Philadelphia.

Watkins, P. N. and Goodchild, J. L. (1980). *The Care of Distressed and Disturbed People*. Heinemann Medical, London.

Wilson, H. and Kneisl, C. (1988). *Psychosocial Nursing Concepts: An Activity Book*, 3rd edition. Addison-Wesley, New York.

Self-assessment Questions

SAQ 1. Define the term "need".

SAQ 2. List six human needs as described by Maslow.

SAQ 3. Describe briefly four interventions that can improve a person's self-esteem.

SAQ 4. Identify six interventions that can promote a person's needs for acceptance and belonging.

Unit 1.1: Written Test

1. In what ways can a person experience difficulty in meeting their needs for safety and security?

2. What interventions by a mental health nurse can help a person to meet their security needs?

UNIT 1.2

Therapeutic Relationships

Unit Objectives

At the end of this Unit the learner should be able to:

1. Describe the stages of development of a therapeutic relationship.
2. Outline the characteristics of a therapeutic relationship.
3. Identify behaviours that indicate trust in a therapeutic relationship.

Therapeutic Relationships

In their occupational role mental health nurses are involved with numerous relationships with a wide range of people. These include members of the mental health care team, support workers, clients and their families. A basic requirement of successful mental health nursing practice is the ability to form effective relationships with each of these groups and, in particular, with clients and their families.

In practice, mental health nurses are in contact with clients for far longer periods than are any other members of the health care team. Nurses are the only occupational group to offer continuous direct contact. This time factor provides mental health nurses with a unique opportunity to develop very close relationships with clients. Clients value their relationships with mental health nurses and nurses need to recognize that in this relationship they have the potential to utilize a powerful therapeutic resource.

A therapeutic relationship does not happen automatically and nurses need to realize that it is only achieved as the end result of skilled and goal-directed interventions. They need to understand both the stages of development of a therapeutic relationship and also the qualities that distinguish it from other relationships.

Phases of the Nurse–Client Relationship

Initial phase or introductory phase

At their first contacts, both parties are strangers to each other and need to become acquainted. Often people are anxious, worry about how they appear and wonder what the other person thinks of them. People may feel awkward, ill at ease and restrict the amount that they are prepared to disclose.

Basically, at this stage both parties *assess* and *appraise* each other. The key points are:

- names – what both prefer to be called;
- appearance – physical characteristics, clothes;
- personality – what they imagine the other person to be like;
- manner – how the other person presents themself.

From these factors the two parties, consciously and unconsciously, form their initial impressions of each other. Whether accurate or not, these first impressions will form the basis of their relationship. Misunderstandings at this stage will take a considerable effort to modify later on.

Nurses, therefore, need to be particularly sensitive to their introductions to clients and their families and to give this essential groundwork a high priority. Nurses need to consider how they present to other people and to demonstrate:

- confidence – through their posture, tone of voice, competence, organization;
- warmth – to show genuine concern, personal recognition, respect, support.

The goals and purposes of the relationship should be discussed with the person and, if known, the duration of the relationship. The nurse should state how she intends to work with the client from the beginning.

Development of the relationship: working phase

The quality of the relationship determines how effective the nurse can be in helping the person. The goal, which will take skill and time to achieve, is a therapeutic nurse–client relationship, i.e. one in which the client is enabled to work through his problems, maintain his individuality and to learn from his experiences. The nurse's role is to use his/her skills to facilitate this process and to ensure that the client's needs are respected and met.

The resources and skills that are required to facilitate the development of therapeutic relationships with clients include:

1. *Time*. Nurses should give a high priority to spending uninterrupted time with their clients. Time should be specifically allocated in advance for client contact.
2. *Responsiveness*. Nurses need to be alert and responsive to communications from clients. They should acknowledge all statements positively.

They need to be aware of both the content of the statements made and also the underlying emotion.

3. *Promoting self-esteem*. People with mental health problems frequently feel devalued and rejected. Often they feel a sense of shame and guilt about their problems and the need to seek help. The nurse needs to help the person work through these feelings and to use their relationship to restore the person's self-esteem and dignity.

4. *Acknowledging the uniqueness of the relationship*. Throughout their careers, mental health nurses will have therapeutic relationships with numerous people. Each one of these relationships will reflect the distinct individuality of both the nurse and the client. Through the recognition and acceptance of a client's uniqueness, nurses show the value that they put upon the person and the need to seek individual solutions.

5. *Confidentiality*. People may be talking about very intimate details of their lives. People are more prepared to disclose such information if they are sure that it will be treated confidentially. Nurses need to emphasize that the information is confidential to the health care team and is used to help the clients resolve their difficulties.

6. *Non-judgemental responses*. Nurses need to be aware of their own values and beliefs and to ensure that they do not interfere with the development of the relationship. Nurses should not consciously or unconsciously criticize the person or devalue their beliefs.

7. *Encouragement, support and hope*. Mental health problems can be very demoralizing and frequently people feel trapped and helpless. Overcoming problems can be a very stressful process with uncertain progress. Nurses need to offer positive feedback and to reinforce hope.

8. *Pacing*. The nurse needs to pace the development of the relationship to the person's ability to copy with intimacy. For some people this will be rapid and smooth, for others it may be a slow and halting process. The nurse needs to be alert to the person's responses and not to exert undue pressure, as this will only be counterproductive.

9. *Consistency*. Nurses may be working with people who are insecure, changeable and emotionally disturbed. In order to work effectively with people, nurses need to operate from a position of personal stability and consistency of approach. It requires nurses to have effective coping skills for their own stresses and to feel confident in their clinical skills.

10. *Empathy*. The ability to identify and interpret accurately the underlying emotional message in a person's communications. From this basis the nurse can then increase his/her understanding of the person's needs and respond more appropriately.

11. *Trust*. From an ability to meet the client's needs the nurse can work towards the development of trust in the relationship. This is not easily achieved and people vary considerably in their ability to trust others. When mutual trust has been achieved within the relationship, then clients are far more likely to be responsive to the nurse's efforts to facilitate change and personal growth (see Exhibit 1.2.1).

Exhibit 1.2.1 Trust

Trust is shown by:	*A lack of trust is shown by:*
Honesty and openness	A reluctance to disclose
Confidence in the helper	Lack of confidence in helper
Cooperation	Frequently uncooperative
A willingness to share	Suspicious
An openness to new experiences	Resistance to change
Increased awareness	Defensiveness
Increased closeness	Distance and aloofness
Feeling safe	Feel threatened by others
Punctuality and attendance	Lateness and non-attendance

Termination phase

Depending upon the client's response to therapeutic interventions, the relationship with the nurse will have to end at some stage. What is important within a therapeutic relationship is to use this experience constructively and to work through the stress of ending a relationship.

Ideally, from their initial contact with a client, nurses should state the boundaries within which their relationship exists; that the nurse has a professional commitment to work with the client during his need for care and that part of this process is to work towards the client regaining autonomy and control over his own life.

In this way termination can offer valuable feedback to the client on his progress and be seen as a positive rather than negative step to take. The issue of termination and its anxieties should be realistically presented and the problems openly discussed with a view to facilitating the client's ability to cope.

Therapeutic and Social Relationships

Therapeutic relationships can be very stressful. Working closely with people who are under stress can be a very demanding and emotionally draining experience. Nurses need to be aware of the effect that such relationships can have on them. This requires insight, self-awareness and an ability to cope effectively with stress.

In social relationships the range of options and alternatives open to individuals in how they relate, communicate and deal with stress is virtually infinite.

In therapeutic relationships the nurse has definite legal and professional responsibilities that set limits or boundaries on her actions. For the nurse it should be a facilitating or enabling relationship in which the client is helped to meet his needs. The needs of the client remain paramount throughout within the framework of established therapeutic and professional practice. Periodically, the client may attempt to draw the nurse outside these boundaries in order to meet needs that the nurse can never legitimately fulfil. These are commonly concerned with fulfilling the person's social and sexual needs. The nurse needs to ensure that the process and time boundaries are clearly stated, understood and periodically reinforced. The limits that are set should be seen both as a guide and a support to the nurse in developing therapeutic relationships.

Some contrasting elements of social and therapeutic relationships are shown in Exhibit 1.2.2.

Exhibit 1.2.2 Contrasting elements of social and therapeutic relationships

Social	*Therapeutic*
Open-ended time period	Restricted to period of care
Personal choice	Restricted choice
Both partners' needs considered	Client's needs predominant
Multi-purpose	Primary purpose of care
Sympathy	Empathy
Confiding	Confidential
Tolerant to personal limit	Professional tolerance
Inconsistent	Consistent
Judgemental	Non-judgemental
Unstructured	Structured
Emotional and social basis	Professional basis
Personal responsibility	Professional responsibility
Personal boundaries	Professional boundaries

Unit Instructions

When you have researched the suggested references, have mastered the
Unit Objectives and successfully answered the Self-assessment Questions,
proceed with the Unit Written Test.

Suggested References

Altschul, A. and McGovern, M. (1985). *Psychiatric Nursing*, 6th edition. Baillière
 Tindall, London and San Diego.
Chilton, S. (1982). The nurse–patient relationship I. *Nursing Times*, 10 March, Vol.
 78, No. 10, pp. 420–422.
Chilton, S. (1982). The nurse–patient relationship 2. *Nursing Times*, 17 March, Vol.
 78, No. 11, pp. 448–450.
Copp, L. A. (1986). The nurse as advocate for vulnerable persons. *Journal of
 Advanced Nursing*, Vol. 11, No. 3, pp. 253–263.
Darcy, P. T. (1985). *Mental Health Nursing Source Book*. Baillière Tindall, London
 and San Diego.
Dexter, G. and Wash, M. (1986). *Psychiatric Nursing Skills: A Patient-centred
 Approach*. Croom Helm, London.
Doona, M. E. (1979). *Travelbee's Intervention in Psychiatric Nursing*, 2nd edition.
 F. A. Davis, Philadelphia.
Hase, S. and Douglas, A. (1986). *Human Dynamics and Nursing*. Churchill
 Livingstone, Melbourne.
Irving, S. (1983). *Basic Psychiatric Nursing*, 3rd edition. W. B. Saunders, Philadelphia.
Kagan, C., Evans, T. and Kay, B. (1986). *A Manual of Interpersonal Skills for
 Nurses: An Experiential Approach*. Harper and Row, London.
Kingston, B. (1987). *Psychological Approaches in Psychiatric Nursing*. Croom Helm,
 London.
Lancaster, J. (1980). *Adult Psychiatric Nursing*. Henry Kimpton, London.
Lyttle, J. (1986). *Mental Disorder: Its Care and Treatment*. Baillière Tindall, London
 and San Diego.
Martin, P. (Ed.) (1987). *Psychiatric Nursing: A Therapeutic Approach*. Macmillan,
 London.
Murgatroyd, S. (1985). *Counselling and Helping*. British Psychological Society and
 Methuen, London.
Nelson-Jones, R. (1983). *Practical Counselling and Helping Skills*. 2nd edition.
 Cassell, London.
Nelson-Jones, R. (1986). *Human Relationship Skills*. Holt, Rinehart and Winston,
 London.
Robinson, L. (1983). *Psychiatric Nursing as a Human Experience*, 3rd edition. W.
 B. Saunders, Philadelphia.
Sundeen, S. *et al.* (1981). *Nurse–Client Interaction*, 2nd edition. C. V. Mosby,
 St. Louis.
Wilson, H. and Kneisl, C. (1988). *Psychosocial Nursing Concepts: An Activity Book*,
 3rd edition. Addison-Wesley, New York.

Yuen, F. K. H. (1986). The nurse–client relationship: a mutual learning experience. *Journal of Advanced Nursing*, Vol. 11, No. 5, pp. 529–533.

Self-assessment Questions

SAQ 5. Describe the stages through which a therapeutic relationship progresses.

SAQ 6. List five characteristics that a nurse needs to demonstrate in order to develop a therapeutic relationship.

SAQ 7. Differentiate between five behaviours that indicate trust and distrust in a therapeutic relationship.

SAQ 8. Identify four differences between a social and a therapeutic relationship.

Unit 1.2: Written Test

1. What do you understand by the term "therapeutic relationship?"
2. Which stages of development does a therapeutic relationship progress through.

UNIT 1.3

Therapeutic Communication

Unit Objectives

At the end of this Unit the learner should be able to:

1. Describe the purposes of therapeutic communications.
2. Differentiate between verbal and non-verbal communications.
3. Identify the main characteristics of therapeutic communication.
4. Outline strategies for overcoming common communication difficulties.

Communication Skills

The ability to communicate is a basic requirement of effective mental health nursing practice. Nurses spend a great deal of their time communicating in order to meet clients' needs and also to co-ordinate and plan the activities of the health care team. It is essential, therefore, that nurses have an awareness of the processes and skills of communication in order to be competent practitioners.

Objectives of nurse–client communication

1. To initiate, develop and maintain a therapeutic relationship.
2. (a) To assess the client's care needs.
   (b) To plan with the person and his family an individualized care programme.
   (c) To implement specific goal-directed nursing interventions with the client.
   (d) To evaluate with the client his individualized care programme.
3. To exchange information.
4. To meet the social needs of the client.
5. To monitor and evaluate the client's progress and response to clinical treatment programmes.

Verbal and Non-verbal Communication

Studies of human communication show that it is a complex process of verbal and non-verbal skills. For the purposes of everyday communication, these tend to be used in an automatic way and are rarely given much conscious consideration. Within therapeutic relationships, however, the use of these communication skills is very important if the nurse is to achieve her desired objectives. They need to be used, therefore, in a conscious and structured way to be fully effective. Like all skills they have to be used appropriately, selectively and with sensitivity.

Verbal Communication

The words we use to communicate say as much about the speaker as they do about the message they wish to communicate. They can indicate the speaker's mood, perception, attitudes, values, belief system, education and upbringing. The expectation is that the words chosen will also be appropriate to the content and objectives of the current conversation. However, the nature of language is such that much of the meaning behind words is conveyed in the way that they are spoken. We have a degree of control over what we say but much less control of the way that we speak. The verbal presentation or "para-language" can give emphasis to the intended meaning or can even contradict the message if it is said in such a way as to invalidate the original intention. Inherently, when we listen to the words of a message we are also listening to how it is said. Significant elements of verbal communication include:

- clarity – is it clear or indecipherable;
- volume – inaudible or loud;
- rate – slow, medium-paced or fast;
- tone – appropriate, soft, sarcastic, hostile;
- intonation and stress put on particular words;
- silences, pauses and hesitation;
- respiration and sighing.

Non-verbal Communication

Every time we communicate verbally our bodies complement the message with a complex repertoire of movements and gestures. For effective communication we do not just need to listen to what someone has to say, we also have to be in a position to observe their non-verbal behaviour. These movements and gestures add emphasis to the intended meaning and can often communicate messages to others – physically – that we are not aware of. Generally, it is expected that there will be a degree of congruence or matching between the verbal statements and the accompanying non-verbal behaviour. However, there are times when the verbal and non-verbal communications are not in harmony and may be sending out conflicting messages. Often the sender is not aware of this difference.

These non-verbal signals are also important in maintaining the flow of communications between people and to synchronize what they say. Subtle indications are given by tone of voice, posture and expression, that a person has finished speaking and when they expect others to reply. The non-verbal signals also offer a source of feedback to the speaker as to other people's response to what they are saying. Observations are made of other people's facial expressions and postures to see if they are interested, in agreement or are hostile to what we have to say. The signals given also indicate the nature and state of the relationship with the others present. Non-verbal behaviour can be used to show trust, genuineness, confidence, warmth and intimacy with the speaker. They can also be used to show hostility, anger, indifference and mistrust in the speaker. The primary non-verbal behaviours include:

- eye contact and looking,
- facial expressions,
- posture,
- body movements,
- head movements,
- hand gestures,
- touch.

Therapeutic Communication

Used with sensitivity and understanding, communication can be a very potent therapeutic tool. For example, it can be used to:

- develop therapeutic relationships,
- increase insight and self-awareness,
- promote learning and the acquisition of new skills,
- raise self-esteem and confidence,
- facilitate autonomy and independence,
- set limits on potentially self-harmful behaviour,
- offer feedback to a person on his progress,
- give positive feedback to encourage desired changes,
- reinforce orientation to time, place and person,
- reduce anxiety.

However, in order to achieve these objectives the nurse has to learn to communicate from a sound knowledge and skills base. Current research evidence would seem to indicate that nurses interact in a haphazard and unstructured way with clients and do not use the therapeutic potential inherent in these contacts. There is, though, other research evidence that shows that nurses can learn to develop and improve their communication skills and to use these to better effect in client care. Mental health nurses have a unique care role and potential for facilitating therapeutic change if they are prepared to use their contacts constructively.

The fundamental objectives of the educational process in psychiatric nursing are to facilitate the development of the practitioner's self-awareness, understanding and communication skills. The effectiveness of this process is a crucial factor in determining the ability of the nurse to meet other people's needs.

There is currently a vast literature available on all aspects of human communication and a wide variety of theoretical and methodological perspectives. While there are some differences of terminology and approach there are certain features of communication that appear to be particularly relevant in a therapeutic context. Some of these are as follows.

Self-awareness and insight

In order to be in a position to help other people to deal objectively with their problems, nurses needs considerable self-awareness and insight. They need to be clear about their own needs and their motivation for wanting to help others, and they need insight into their own attitudes, beliefs and values and how these influence the way in which they develop relationships. This is particularly important, because nurses have to be able to cope with and feel comfortable with a wide range of sensitive issues.

There needs to be congruity between the nurses' self-image and the way that they are seen by others. Helpers have to be confident about what they are doing and must be reasonably well-adjusted in terms of having control over their own lives. They also need to be able to evaluate periodically their own life circumstances and to set themselves realistic goals. A degree of maturity is required in order to give perspective to both the nurse's and the client's needs.

It is important to be positive about the helping process and to retain belief in the value of personal support, in order to be able to communicate hope and to remain personally motivated. Helping others work through their problems is a very demanding and responsible activity and requires the nurse to be able to cope with the stresses that can be generated.

Working consistently with people who have chronic and seemingly intractable problems can drain even the most enthusiastic helper. Professional "burn out", characterized by insensitivity, cynicism, low motivation, indifference and disinterest, are very real problems for carers. Nurses need to have the opportunity within their work role to take time out periodically for personal and professional evaluation. Sources of on-going support should be identified and each nurse should have access to a support network for dealing with stress.

Motivation towards development of own skills and knowledge

All helpers have an obligation towards clients to improve their skills and knowledge. They need to be actively motivated towards personal and professional growth and to be flexible and open about their own practice. This requires a commitment to undertake further study through reading, peer group support, attending workshops and courses and using other opportunities to increase learning. Experience is of value in personal development, but it needs to be used as part of a structured programme in which it is analysed and external feedback is available to validate the practitioners' judgements (see "Clinical Supervision", pp. 36).

The nature of the relationship

The nurse and the client have two very distinct roles. Within a helping setting the nurse should be working towards the development of a therapeutic relationship (see Unit 1.2). This is attained through the skilful use of communication to develop their relationship and to meet the client's needs. Trust can be reinforced by the content of what the nurse has to say and through the use of non-verbal communication. In communication terms the objective is to establish a rapport between the two parties so that there is a harmonious feeling of mutual respect and understanding. The nurse needs to give clear guidelines and to explain the therapeutic purpose of communicating from the commencement of their meetings. This should include an overview of the strategies and approaches that will be used. Each contact with the client should be used to facilitate the attainment of their health care needs. This necessitates the nurse working within a structured and goal-orientated programme where contacts are pre-planned as part of a comprehensive therapeutic strategy.

Environmental control and proximity

Communication is facilitated if it takes place in an environment which is private and free from interruption and distraction. This includes the level of background noise, temperature, light, ventilation, cleanliness and the appropriateness of the place. Inappropriate environmental conditions can seriously inhibit communication because people will focus on these factors rather than attending to the conversation. Although nurses may be in situations where they have little environmental control they should, as far as possible, try to minimize the influence of such factors. The nurse may have the choice of where and when the communication takes place and be able to position chairs, desks, tables, etc., to the best effect. Furniture should be moved aside or a place chosen in which there is a clear space between the participants.

In communication, both the distance between the participants and their proximity can influence the interation. Generally, the nearer the nurse is to the client the more involved they will be perceived to be. However, people vary in how close they like to be in relation to others, and whether they interpret this as supportive or threatening. Physical closeness, if the other person is comfortable with this, facilitates the use of touch, which can be very comforting and reassuring. The angle at which the nurse faces the other person is also significant. Being face to face tends to be interpreted as confrontational and threatening. People are generally more comfortable if they are positioned at an angle to each other, such that they are able to gain eye contact easily and yet they are able to look away periodically without significant body movements being involved.

Interventions to promote communication

All approaches to counselling, psychotherapy and group work stress the need to make interventions that will facilitate the client's communication. For a variety of reasons, both personal and clinical, the person may have difficulty or be reluctant to communicate. The nurse's role through her use of verbal and non-verbal skills is to create an environment in which the person is enabled to express himself.

In order to promote communication from others nurses must first use and demonstrate good communication skills themselves. These are a prerequisite for using more advanced specific counselling and group work interventions. Effective basic verbal and non-verbal skills include:

1. Speaking clearly, avoiding jargon, checking that the other person has understood.
2. Making sure that what you say is relevant.
3. Giving specific details and avoiding vagueness.
4. Being concise and not overloading the other person with excessive detail.
5. Knowing what you want to say.
6. Choosing the best place and moment to say it.
7. Expressing the message in an appropriate way.
8. Looking approachable, reducing barriers, responding to approaches.
9. Adopting an open and non-defensive posture, i.e. arms open, looking relaxed, calm, mirroring the other person's posture.
10. Speaking at the same physical height as the other person.
11. Facing the other person and adopting a posture that indicates involvement, periodically leaning forward.
12. Identifying and maintaining the social distance and proximity that the other person feels comfortable with.
13. Establishing good eye contact and gaze, i.e. periodically making and breaking eye contact, looking at the other person.
14. Using touch where appropriate to indicate support and intimacy.

15. Attending to the other person, looking interested and involved.
16. Asking questions.
17. Giving affirmative gestures and head nods.

Specific aspects of questioning and other responding techniques are considered in more detail in Unit 5:1 on "Counselling Skills".

Active listening

In everyday communication listening tends to be a fairly passive process. People do not normally concentrate very much, their minds wander, they think out what they are going to say next, jump from topic to topic and interrupt the other speaker. How much effort they put into listening will also depend upon their relationship with the speaker, the attractiveness of the speaker to them, their mood and whether they are tired or not. Listening is also a very selective process and much sensory information is filtered out as not being significant or too much for the listener to cope with. As a consequence, much of the verbal and non-verbal communication between people can be misperceived, missed or distorted.

Active listening is a very deliberate and conscious focussing of attention upon what the other person is communicating. It requires a listener to clear their mind of their own concerns and concentrate specifically upon the other person. It involves astute observation of:

- the other person's verbal and non-verbal communication, i.e. what they say, how they say it, what they leave out, listening for themes;
- the listener's own behaviour, thoughts and feelings;
- the nature of the interaction and relationship between the participants.

To be fully effective the listener also has to signal to the speaker through his non-verbal behaviour that he is alert and responsive to the communication. This is achieved through selective use of eye contact, head nods and verbal prompting.

Providing support and promoting insight

Many people with mental health problems are experiencing a degree of stress. The therapeutic process itself can be stressful – the need to change behaviour, perceptions or attitudes, the gradual awakening of insight, reviewing sensitive and painful issues in a person's life. These can be experienced as very threatening and such stress should be acknowledged and seen as a positive sign of development. Issues should be dealt with in such a way that they are non-threatening beyond the ability of the person to cope with them with guidance and support. This may require the nurse to proceed gradually in the demands and expectations that she/he has of the client.

Throughout the therapeutic process it is important to maintain the person's self-esteem and respect and to impart hope. Hope is a very powerful motivator and can be used constructively to help the person regain a sense of control over his own life. A wide variety of therapeutic techniques may be used to promote understanding and insight. These can include information, health education, guidance, listening and reflecting, giving feedback, role play and experiential methods.

An ability to cope with silence

Silence is a very prominent feature of human communication. It may be an absence of verbal communication but not of non-verbal communication. Through their eye movements, posture, gestures, facial expressions and other body movements, people can still be communicating a considerable amount of relevant messages.

The difficulty for the nurse in dealing with silence is that there is a strong social expectation to communicate verbally and silence is taken to indicate indifference, hostility or rejection. In situations of silence nurses may experience considerable anxiety and try to talk themselves to fill the void. It has to be accepted that silence has an important role to play in communication and that it requires skill and experience for the nurse to remain relaxed and to focus on the possible meaning of the silence.

Silence may indicate a period of reflection and thinking through on the part of the client or it may indicate that the person feels pressured and is unable to respond. In this way silence serves a useful purpose by reducing the pace of the communication. It also gives both parties time to review and to introduce a more meaningful topic, if appropriate. Silence also allows the person to discover that he can be accepted even though he remains silent. Even in situations where the person is unable to communicate he can derive comfort and security from the accepting presence of the nurse.

Communication problems

There are many barriers to effective communication. Misunderstandings and misperceptions are common in everyday life. They may represent simple inattention or distractions, or the influence of more profound factors. People who are unwell or in distress may also experience additional difficulties in communicating. Hence it is important that the nurse is aware of these barriers and possible ways of overcoming them (see Exhibit 1.3.1).

Exhibit 1.3.1 Communication problems

Common communication barriers	Overcoming barriers
1. Verbal	
Not speaking clearly, mumbling	Speaking clearly
Being vague	Being specific
Talking too much	Setting a limit on how much you speak
Talking too little	Encouraging the other person to talk
Too much detail	Moderate amount of information given
Use of slang, dialect, jargon	Awareness of own linguistic code
Flat, monotonous voice Unvaried tone and pace Detached, disinterested tone	Using varied tone of voice and inflection
Words not match non-verbal messages	Ensure congruity of own verbal and non-verbal communication
Personal meaning to words	Seek clarification and mutual understanding
Limited vocabulary	Extend and develop own vocabulary Study video and audio transcriptions of self plus skilled role models Role play with feedback
2. Non-verbal	
Fidgeting	Relaxed posture, observe self on video
Distracting mannerisms	Attention to own mannerisms
Not observing or ignoring cues from the other person	Maintain observation of other person
Not looking at the other person Not maintaining eye contact	Maintain appropriate eye contact and demonstrate active listening
Too close to other person Too far away from other person	Identify and maintain appropriate proximity and social distance

3. *Attending and listening*

Not listening to the other person	Active listening and concentration
Preoccupied with own concerns	Keeping a clear mind
Thinking out what you are going to say rather than listening	Focussing on the here and now
Tiredness	Remaining alert
Switching off	Attending and concentrating
Anxious	Keeping calm and relaxed, analysing own anxieties
Distractability	Remaining focussed on conversation
Changing topic, failing to focus on other person's problems	Ensure topics are fully explored
Focussing on minor and irrelevant details and ignoring main points	Listen to what the person says and what they do not say. Identify underlying themes and concerns

4. *Sensitivity*

Similarity of own problems	Remaining objective
Assume other person understands	Check out understanding, ask for feedback
Pretending to understand. Failing to ask for clarification	Seek clarification
Misinterpreting	Give feedback to check out understanding
Jumping to conclusions	Pause and think carefully before speaking
Patterns of behaviour, mannerisms and expressed values that upset and offend other person – being defensive, distrustful, rigid, lack of empathy, patronizing, judgemental, stereotyping, cultural barriers, hostility to speaker	Develop awareness of own value system and communication skills through self-analysis, supervision, process recordings, analysing audio and visual transcripts. Professional and personal self-development. Participation in training events. Studying theory and practice of communication

Ignoring signs of
frustration, confusion
or disinterest in other
person

5. *Sensory deficits*
   Visual loss of varying   Speak clearly
   degrees

   Partial or full hearing   Face the person at same height
   loss

                                   Spend time, be patient

                                   Check for understanding

                                   Ensure aids are effective and working

                                   Provide written or audio record of
                                     significant information

6. *Communication skill
   deficits*
   Ineffective role models   Model-effective communication skills

   Lack of learning   Teach social and communication skills,
   opportunities   provide opportunities to role play
   Poor social skills   with feedback

   Social anxiety

   Low self-esteem   Promote self-esteem

   Lacking in confidence   Teach assertiveness skills
   Passivity

   Withdrawn and   Encourage interaction and give positive
   apathetic   reinforcement

   Disorientation   Promote reality orientation

   Social isolation   Identify potential social activities

7. *Environmental
   distractions*   Environmental control to create a
   Excessive or distracting   conducive environment and minimize
   background noise   distractions

   Too hot, cold or   Monitor and regulate temperature
   draughty

   Stuffy, smokey   Ensure adequate ventilation
   atmosphere

   Excessive sunlight or   Regulate lighting
   inadequate lighting

   Lack of privacy or   Ensure privacy and freedom from
   disruptions   interruption

Clinical Supervision

In order to develop effective communication and relationship skills a trainee needs very specific feedback and guidance on the way that they are working with other people's social and psychological difficulties. One method that is commonly used in interpersonal helping occupations is that of "supervision". In a clinical context it has a very different meaning than that associated with management practice.

In clinical supervision practitioners are expected to meet regularly with their supervisor for the purpose of examining in detail their clinical work. It is used for both novices and experienced working practitioners. The supervisor is ideally someone who has extensive clinical experience and training and is, therefore, in a position to provide expert support and guidance. A fundamental requirement of effective supervision is that the practitioner works with a supervisor that they can trust and respect and who will challenge them professionally. The objectives for supervision are to:

1. Discuss in detail specific aspects of the practitioner's case work.
2. Focus on the skills base of the interventions, the goals of the therapy and the nature of their relationship with their clients.
3. Encourage self-evaluation of the practitioner's approach.
4. Give guidance and advice on professional practice.
5. Offer support and validation for professional decisions.
6. Give feedback to individuals on their performance.
7. Promote professional self-development.
8. Help the practitioner cope with personal and professional stress,

Supervision may be given on an individual or a group basis. It requires a commitment from all involved to be as open and honest as possible and to work on self-development.

Process Recording/Diary

As part of a supervisory process practitioners may also be required to present detailed written summaries of their contacts with clients. (Audio-tape or video recordings may be used in certain settings if permission is given by the client and their use is appropriate.) These detailed summaries are known as "process recordings" or "a diary" and are used to:

- record the content and process of specific interactions;
- provide a basis for the analysis of such contacts.

The objectives of collecting information in this way are to:

- encourage the systematic development of the practitioner's communicating skills;

- integrate the theory and practice of communication skills;
- encourage self-evaluation of the practitioner's communication skills.

If process recordings are to be used in a therapeutic relationship, then they need to be used in a structured way:

1. Initially, the methodology and purpose need to be explained to any prospective users and significant others.
2. Guidance is given on the observations to make, suggested interviewing strategies, methods of recording and how the diary will be used.
3. Specific objectives are set for each practitioner in relation to his/her individual learning needs.
4. Process recordings may be used with either one or several of the practitioner's clients.
5. The client's cooperation is sought. The purpose of the diary needs to be explained and the confidentiality of the material guaranteed.
6. A verbal "contract" may be formed which states the timing, duration, frequency and location of contacts. Environmental conditions should be sought that ensure privacy and freedom from interruptions and facilitate communication.
7. Either during his/her meeting with the client or immediately afterwards the practitioner should record as many details as possible of their interaction. This should include:

   (a) what the practitioner said and observations of their own feelings and non-verbal behaviour;
   (b) what the client said and their observations of the client's behaviour and emotional reactions.

   The more accurate the transcript the more useful it will be. It might be verbatim or in note form. A particular format may be specified by the supervisor.
8. The recording is then analysed in detail by the practitioner who reviews their communication techniques, observation skills, feelings about the session and their relationship with the client and objectives for the session.

   The initial analysis helps to promote self-awareness and an understanding of communication skills.
9. The analysed recording is then discussed with their supervisor who can comment upon the practitioner's approach and self-analysis. They can offer feedback and validation of the interventions and also suggest ways of developing the practitioner's skills. In a group context the practitioners can discuss mutually their recordings with their peers.
10. The practitioner proceeds with the client work, utilizing the insights and objectives developed from supervision.

Unit Instructions

When you have researched the suggested references, have mastered the Unit Objectives and successfully answered the Self-assessment Questions, proceed with the Unit Written Test.

Suggested References

Altschul, A. (1972). *Patient–Nurse Interaction*. Churchill Livingstone, Edinburgh.

Altschul, A. and McGovorn, M. (1985). *Psychiatric Nursing*, 6th edition. Baillière Tindall, London and San Diego.

Argyle, M. (1983). *The Psychology of Interpersonal Behaviour*, 4th edition. Penguin, Harmondsworth.

Ashton, K. (1981). It's the way that you do it . . . *Nursing Times*, 23 April, Vol. 77, No. 16, pp. 718–720.

Barber, P. and Norman, I. (1987). Skills in supervision. *Nursing Times*, 14 January, Vol. 83, No. 2, pp. 56–57.

Bleazard, R. (1984). Knowing oneself. *Nursing Times*, 7 March, Vol. 80, No. 10, pp. 44–46.

Burnard, P. (1985a). Listening to people. *Nursing Mirror*, 17 July, Vol. 161, No. 3, pp. 28–29.

Burnard, P. (1985b). Learning to communicate. *Nursing Mirror*, 21 August, Vol. 161, No. 8, pp. 30–31.

Burnard, P. (1987). Meaningful dialogue. *Nursing Times*, 20 May, Vol. 83, No. 20, pp. 43–45.

Clark, J. M. (1981). Patient's needs and nurses' skills. *Nursing*, July, Vol. 1, No. 27, pp. 1164–1165.

Dexter, G. and Wash, M. (1986). *Psychiatric Nursing Skills: A Patient-centred Approach*. Croom Helm, London.

Doona, M. E. (1979). *Travelbee's Intervention in Psychiatric Nursing*, 2nd edition. F. A. Davis, Philadelphia.

Egan, G. (1986). *The Skilled Helper*, 3rd edition. Brooks/Cole. Monterey, California.

Faulkner, A. (1981a). Aye, there's the rub. *Nursing Times*, 19 February, Vol. 77, No. 8, pp. 332–336.

Faulkner, A. (1981b). The communicator as a person. *Nursing*, July, Vol. 1, No. 27, pp. 1162–1163.

Ford, K. and Jones, A. (1987). *Student Supervision*. Macmillan, London.

French, P. (1983). *Social Skills for Nursing Practice*. Croom Helm, London.

Hargie, O. (Ed.) (1986). *A Handbook of Communication Skills*. Croom Helm, London.

Hargie, O., Saunders, C. and Dickson, D. (1987). *Social Skills in Interpersonal Communication*, 2nd edition. Croom Helm, London.

Hewit, F. S. (1981). The nurse and the patient-communication skills. *Nursing Times*,

Hills, K. (1985). Gaining and giving insight. *Nursing Mirror*, 6 February, Vol. 160, No. 6, pp. 28–29.

Hopson, B. and Scally, M. (1980). *Lifeskills Teaching Programme No 1*. Lifeskills Associates, Leeds.

Hunt, G. and Eadie, W. (1987). Interviewing: A Communication Approach. Holt, Rinehart and Winston, New York.

Irving, S. (1983). *Basic Psychiatric Nursing*, 3rd edition. W. B. Saunders, Philadelphia.

Kagan, C., Evans, T. and Kay, B. (1986). *A Manual of Interpersonal Skills for Nurses: An Experiential Approach*. Harper and Row, London.

Lancaster, J. (1980). *Adult Psychiatric Nursing*. Medical Examination Publishing Co.,

Macilwaine, H. (1978a). Communication in the nurse/patient relationship. *Nursing Mirror*, 16 February, Vol. 146, No. 7, pp. 32–34.

Macilwaine, H. (1978b). Breaking through the communication barrier. *Nursing Mirror*, 7 December, Vol. 147, No. 23, pp. 19–21.

MacMillan, P. (1981). The bridge builders' guide – 1. *Nursing Times*, 22 January, Vol. 77, No. 4, pp. 151–152.

Marson, S. (1979). Nursing, a helping relationship. *Nursing Times*, 29 March, Vol. 75, No. 13, pp. 541–544.

Martin, P. (Ed.) (1987). *Psychiatric Nursing: A Therapeutic Approach*. Macmillan, London.

Munro, E. A., Mantuei, R. J. and Small, J. J. (1983). *Counselling a Skills Approach*, revised edition. Methuen, New Zealand.

Nelson-Jones, R. (1982). *The Theory and Practice of Counselling Psychology*. Holt, Rinehart and Winston, London.

Nelson-Jones, R. (1983). *Practical Counselling and Helping Skills*. 2nd edition. Cassell, London.

Nelson-Jones, R. (1986). *Human Relationship Skills*. Holt, Rinehart and Winston, London.

Nicol, E. (1981). Recorded patient–nurse interaction – an advance in psychiatric nursing. *Nursing Times*, 29 July, Vol. 77, No. 31, pp. 1351–1352.

Porritt, L. (1984). *Communication: Choices for Nurses*. Churchill Livingstone, Edinburgh.

Powell, D. (1982). *Learning to Relate*. Royal College of Nursing, London.

Priestley, P. and McGuire, J. (1983). *Learning to Help*. Tavistock, London.

Robinson, L. (1983). *Psychiatric Nursing as a Human Exprience*, 3rd edition. W. B. Saunders, Philadelphia.

Rowan, J. (1983). *The Reality Game*. Routledge and Kegan Paul, London.

Scammell, B. E. (1981). Communication? I've heard it all before. *Nursing*, July, Vol. 1, No. 27, pp. 1159–1161.

Smith, L. (1979). Communication Skills. *Nursing Times*, 31 May, Vol. 75, No. 22, pp. 926–929.

Stewart, W. (1983). *Counselling in Nursing*. Harper and Row, New York.

Sundeen, S. *et al.* (1981). *Nurse–client Interaction*, 2nd edition. C. V. Mosby, St. Louis.

Towell, D. (1975). *Understanding Psychiatric Nursing*. Royal College of Nursing, London.

Wilson, H. and Kneisl, C. (1988). *Psychosocial Nursing Concepts: An Activity Book*, 3rd edition. Addison-Wesley, New York.

Self-assessment Questions

SAQ 9. What is meant by the term "non-verbal behaviour"?
SAQ 10. Why is self-confidence important in therapeutic communication?
SAQ 11. List six behaviours that can facilitate communication.
SAQ 12. Describe four communication problems that can arise and ways of overcoming them.

Unit 1.3: Written Test

1. What are the characteristics of therapeutic communication?
2. What communication problems can arise in nurse-client interaction and what strategies may be used to overcome them?

Primary Nursing in Mental Health Care

Unit Objectives

At the end of this Unit the learner should be able to:

1. Define the term "primary nursing".
2. Outline the roles and responsibilities of the primary nurse.
3. Describe the advantages of working in a nursing team.
4. List the benefits of primary nursing for clients.

Primary Nursing

In order to work together effectively mental health nurses need to communicate with one another and to co-ordinate their activities. This requires a clear statement and understanding of each nurse's role and responsibilities for client care. A system of organizing nursing care at client-contact level – known as "primary nursing", or sometimes called "team nursing" – meets this criteria by providing a structural framework of specific roles and responsibilities. With the move away from task-centred to client-centred care, it is a system that has steadily gained ground. In primary or team nursing:

1. The nursing staff of a care area are divided into a number of smaller teams.
2. Each nursing team is headed by a trained nurse who is known as a "primary nurse" or "team leader".
3. Each nursing team is responsible for the nursing care of a specific group of clients throughout the period of their health care.
4. The primary nurse is responsible for ensuring that each client's nursing care needs are met and for organizing the activities of the nursing team to achieve this goal.

In practice this may mean that within a care environment there may be several teams of nurses working alongside each other, each caring for a different group of clients. There may be several nurses in each team who are responsible collectively for the nursing care of perhaps 6–10 people – numbers will vary depending upon the staffing levels and number of clients. Working times within the team are usually arranged so as to ensure that, as far as possible, someone from each team is available to their clients at all times.

The term "primary nurse" may also be used in situations where the mental health nurse works individually with his/her own clients in the community or in a special treatment centre.

Clients may be allocated to specific nursing teams in one of several different ways:

1. A nursing team may work alongside a specific psychiatrist and take responsibility for the nursing care of that psychiatrist's clients. This is particularly effective where there are several psychiatrists involved with the care area.
2. The nursing team may specialize in a certain aspect of care, e.g. assessment, rehabilitation.
3. To ensure that each team has an equal number of clients.

Whatever method is used it is important that the nurses are committed to this approach and that the method is followed consistently.

As soon as a person comes into contact with the health care services and requires mental health nursing care, then they should be introduced to both the primary nurse and the nursing team who will be looking after them. This may mean that even prior to admission the client and his family may be contacted by the primary nurse in order to introduce themselves, explain how the nursing team will care for them and to act as a reference point throughout their health care. Ideally, a member of the same nursing team should also receive the person into the care environment in order to start to develop their therapeutic relationship.

Aims of Primary Nursing

The aims of primary nursing are to ensure:

- individual client care,
- continuity and consistency of nursing care.

A team of psychiatric nurses working with a specific group of people achieves these aims through:

1. Closer contact between the nurses and clients.
2. The opportunity to develop closer relationships between the nurses and clients.
3. Closer relationships between the nurses who work as a small team.

4. Closer relationships between the members of the nursing team and the multidisciplinary care team.
5. More effective and economical use of time. The nurses can concentrate their skills on a particular group of clients and liaison with other health care workers is much more specific.

It is important to realize that working in a nursing team does not mean that all other people are ignored. The nursing staff still have professional responsibilities for the safety and welfare of everyone who is receiving care within their ward or hostel. In situations of potential conflict, self-harm, fire warnings, etc., the nurse still has obligations to ensure the safety of all concerned.

If approached by clients from other nursing care teams the nurse should still respond positively to requests and, if necessary, should redirect the person to a nurse from their own care team.

The Roles of the Primary Nurse

Primary nurses have three main work roles: these are managerial, clinical and educational.

Managerial

1. They are the manager of a team of nurses. The managerial responsibilities include:

   (a) Leadership of the nursing team, in particular creating a team identity.
   (b) Planning the activities of the team.
   (c) Decision making and identifying priorities.
   (d) Delegating work to members of the team.
   (e) Monitoring the work activities of team members.
   (f) Giving feedback and guidance to individuals and the team.
   (g) Communicating and co-ordinating within the team, with other nursing teams and with other health care workers. The range of activities include team meetings, care review meetings, ward meetings, written communications.
   (h) Personnel functions for the team, e.g. maintaining good relationships and morale, resolving conflicts and problems between people.

2. They also participate in management of the ward or care centre by:

   (a) Liaising and co-ordinating with the other nursing teams.
   (b) Assisting the other nursing teams if required.
   (c) Contributing to overall policy management.

(d) Maintaining the safety, hygiene and therapeutic atmosphere of the care environment.

(e) Acting up for the Charge Nurse if required.

Clinical

The primary nurse organizes the nursing care activities of their team by:

1. Ensuring that each client has an individualized care programme that is consistently implemented and regularly evaluated.
2. Participating directly in the care of clients through regular individual and group contact.
3. Offering a range of specific psychiatric nursing and clinical skills relevant to the client group. Possible areas of practice may include:
   - social skills training,
   - counselling,
   - reality orientation,
   - group work,
   - anxiety management,
   - behavioural programmes,
   - family therapy,
   - drama.

   A clinically skilled nurse may also act as a resource to the other nursing teams.
4. Allocating, if appropriate, specific nurses within the care team as "key workers" with certain clients. A key worker is expected to work very closely with their individual clients and to provide detailed feedback to the team.
5. Communicating with the client and their relatives.
6. Attending and contributing to clinical meetings with other members of the care team.

Educational

The primary nurse has educational responsibilities in terms of:

1. Their own continued professional self-development through personal study, in-service training, post-basic courses.
2. The education of the members of their nursing team, other professionals and the clients' needs for health education.
3. The educational needs of learners allocated to their nursing team for a specific clinical placement. Usually they would be responsible for:

   - the learners' clinical instruction,

- giving guidance and feedback to the learners,
- monitoring and evaluating the learners' progress.

The Role of the Charge Nurse in a Primary Nursing System

The introduction of a primary nursing system has considerable implications for the role of the Charge Nurse/Sister. Although a number of their previous functions are delegated to primary nurses they also assume a number of other responsibilities:

1. Ward or hostel manager. In many areas they now have 24-hour responsibility and are expected to take managerial decisions in respect of the personnel and resources they control.
2. To co-ordinate the functioning of the primary nursing teams.
3. To monitor the primary nursing teams.
4. As a resource for the nursing teams – clinical, managerial and educational.
5. Accountability for the actions of the nursing teams.
6. The development of care area policy.
7. To represent the staff and care area at meetings.
8. To act up for the Senior Nurse if required.
9. To act down/provide cover for primary nurses.

Professional Responsibility and Accountability

Professional groups of people are given considerable autonomy in the way that they carry out their work. However, they must also be able to validate the decisions that they make and to justify their actions. Generally, these actions should be seen to promote the welfare of their clients and should be part of a planned programme.

Accountability is the obligation to be answerable for one's actions to someone who is recognized as having the right to demand information and explanation. *Responsibility* is being liable for the consequences of one's actions or decisions. This can also include acts of omission, where by neglect or not taking any necessary action, a person was seen to suffer or resources damaged. *Professional responsibility* is the responsibility that each member of the health care team has for their own professional practice. Trained nurses are responsible to:

- their clients,
- their colleagues,
- their professional body, the UKCC,
- the organization in which they work.

In the United Kingdom, nurses are expected to conform to the Professional Code of Conduct issued by the UKCC. Nurse practitioners who fail to conform to the Code of Conduct or commit a serious offence may have disciplinary action taken against them by the UKCC, who can remove the right to practice.

The use and application of the concepts of accountability and responsibility to nursing practice reflects the growing confidence, identity and autonomy of professional psychiatric nursing practice. Being a primary nurse allocates responsibility in a very specific and visible way for the clients, their own practice and the actions of their team. It is a very demanding role development.

Advantages of Primary Nursing

1. It promotes nurse–client relationships and enhances the client's feeling of security.
2. The closer relationships increase nurses' job satisfaction.
3. Nurses feel a responsibility to the client and an involvement with him and his family through planning their care together.
4. Nurses appear more secure in their professional identity and recognize that they have a distinct role and skills.
5. Opportunities for learning are increased.
6. More economical use is made of time.
7. Communications are more effective.

Primary Nursing and Client Care: A Summary

1. The client and his family are introduced into the care network.
2. They are received by the primary nurse or team member, and introduced to the role of the nursing care team. Thus, the therapeutic relationship is initiated.
3. The nursing team and the client collaborate on identifying the client's needs and the planning of their care. If required, a key worker may be identified to work closely with the person.
4. An individualized care programme is implemented by the nursing care team and key worker through skilled nursing interventions.
5. The client's care is monitored daily by the nursing team and key worker, and the client's progress and needs are communicated to the nursing team and multidisciplinary team. On-going records are maintained of nursing interventions and the client's health care progress.
6. The individualized care programme is regularly evaluated by the nursing team and client, and it is modified and revised as necessary.

Suggested References

Altschul, A. (1980). The team approach to psychiatric care. *Nursing Times*, 1 May, Vol. 76, No. 18, pp. 797–798.

Armitage, P. (1985). Primary care: an individual concern. *Nursing Times*, 6 November, Vol. 81, No. 45, pp. 35–38.

Binnie, A. (1987). Structural Changes. *Nursing Times*, 30 September, Vol. 83, No. 39, pp. 36–37.

Bowers, L. (1987). Who's in charge: *Nursing Times*, 3 June, Vol. 83, No. 22, pp. 36–38.

Finch, J. (1983). Responsibility for others' mistakes. *Nursing Mirror*, 2 November, Vol. 157, No. 18, p. 40.

Godin, P., Pearce, I. and Wilson, I. (1987). Keeping the customer satisfied. *Nursing Times*, 30 September, Vol. 83, No. 38, pp. 35–37.

Green, B. (1983). Primary nursing in psychiatry. *Nursing Times*, 19 January, Vol. 79, No. 3, pp. 24–28.

Hyde, P. (1985). Accountability. *Nursing Mirror*, 17 April, Vol. 160, No. 16, pp. 24–25.

Matthews, A. (1982). *In Charge of the Ward*, Ch. 5, pp. 51–77. Blackwell Scientific, Oxford.

Narraidoo, A. (1985). Are we really accountable? *Nursing Times*, 16 January, Vol. 81, No. 3, p. 53.

Ritter, S. (1985). Primary nursing in mental illness. *Nursing Mirror*, 24 April, Vol. 160, No. 17, pp. 16–17.

Styles, M. (1985). Accountable to whom? *Nursing Mirror*, 30 January, Vol. 160, No. 5, pp. 36–37.

Sykes, M. (1985). *Licensed to Practice*. Baillière Tindall, London and San Diego.

UKCC (1984). *Code of Professional Conduct for the Nurse, Midwife and Health Visitor*, 2nd edition. UKCC, London.

Webb, C. (1987). Speaking up for advocacy. *Nursing Times*, 26 August, Vol. 83, No. 34, pp. 33–35.

Wright, S. (1987). Primary nursing: patient-centred practice. *Nursing Times*, 30 September, Vol. 83, No. 38, pp. 24–26.

If you are interested in particular aspects of management and team work then you may also find the following books useful:

Argyle, M. (1972). *The Social Psychology of Work*. Penguin, Harmondsworth.

Rees, W. D. (1984). *The Skills of Management*. Croom Helm, London.

Scott, J. and Rochester, A. (1984). *Effective Management Skills Series*: Sphere/BIM: Vol. 1: *What is a Manager*; Vol. 2: *Managing People*; Vol. 4: *Managing Work*. Sphere/BIM, London.
Walton, M. (1984). *Management and Managing: A Dynamic Approach*. Lippincott Nursing Series. Harper and Row, London.

Self-assessment Questions

SAQ 13. Define the term "primary nursing".
SAQ 14. Identify the three key roles of the primary nurse.
SAQ 15. Describe the ways in which psychiatric nurses are accountable for the care they give.
SAQ 16. List four advantages to clients of a primary nursing system.

Unit 1.4: Written Test

1. Describe the role of the primary nurse in relation to mental health care practice.
2. What are the advantages to both nurse and client of working in this way? What are the potential disadvantages of primary nursing in mental health practice and how can they be overcome?

TOPIC 2

Individualized Care in Mental Health Nursing Practice

At the end of this Topic the learner should aim to:

1. Describe the nursing skills required to assess a person's care needs.
2. Outline the stages involved in planning a nursing care programme.
3. Understand how nursing care programmes are implemented.
4. Describe methods of evaluation.

UNIT 2.1

Individualized Care and Assessment

Unit Objectives

At the end of this Unit the learner should be able to:

1. List the stages of the care planning process.
2. Describe the purposes of client assessment.
3. Outline the skills used to assess client needs.
4. Identify the range of information required for comprehensive assessment.

Individualized Care and the Nursing Process

Nursing care needs to be organized in a structured and systematic way if it is to meet the unique care needs of each individual. The nursing process provides such a framework for the delivery of comprehensive nursing care using a problem-solving approach.

The four stages of the nursing process are interrelated and several aspects of care may be involved in any nursing situation. The stages are:

1. *Assessment*: the collection and analysis of information to identify clients' care needs.
2. *Planning*: the formulation of a nursing care plan to meet clients' needs.
3. *Implementation*: putting the nursing care plan into action.
4. *Evaluation*: a continuous process of monitoring clients' progress and the effectiveness of nursing care interventions.

These stages are described in more detail in this and the following Units. As each mental health centre tends to use its own preferred terminology, commonly used words have been grouped together where appropriate.

The Characteristic Elements of the Nursing Process and Individualized Care

What specifically differentiates an approach to individualized nursing practice utilizing the nursing process is that:

1. The nursing care is designed to meet the unique care needs of each individual; it is a client-centred approach in which an attempt is made to identify the person's social, physical, psychological and spiritual needs. It is an "holistic" approach to care, in which practitioners work closely with their clients (see Unit 1.4: Primary Nursing).
2. Nursing care needs to be a collaborative process, i.e. clients and relatives have an equal and valid role to play in the caring process. It is seen as a "partnership in care".
3. Nursing interventions need to be based upon a sound knowledge and skills base – practitioners need continual professional development in order to make effective choices. Nurses need to develop a sound research base.
4. Nurses need to be accountable for their interventions, i.e. nursing care should be evaluated in order to maintain and develop the highest possible standards.
5. Nursing is an autonomous profession with a unique role and skills in the care of people.

Assessment

Assessment involves the collection of all the relevant information needed to give comprehensive, individual nursing care. It is the responsibility of the primary nurse/key worker to ensure the accuracy and thoroughness of this information as it forms the basis for the nursing care plan and nursing interventions. A poor database is likely to contribute to misunderstanding and misuse of human resources.

As a process, assessment does take time, but it should be viewed as an investment of effort that contributes significantly to the quality of care and practice. Assessment is an ongoing activity that can take place at each encounter between the client and care team. In many situations it is not always possible or desirable to collect all the relevant information required over a short period of time.

The Skills of Assessment

Assessment involves the application of a wide range of mental health nursing skills and professional experience. These include:

- observation,

- interviewing,
- teamwork,
- professional knowledge and experience,
- facilitating client self-assessment.

Observation

Observation is a key skill in mental health nursing practice. In residential settings, nurses are in client contact far more than any other members of the care team. In community practice, psychiatric nurses provide a major part of domiciliary based care and treatment programmes. Their observations, therefore, are important for:

1. *Skilled nursing practice* – the assessment, implementation and evaluation of care programmes.
2. *The client and their family*, who may find it difficult to communicate their needs. The quality of observation has implications for both care and treatment programmes. The nurse is also an advocate on the client's behalf for needs they cannot express.
3. *The multidisciplinary care team*, who are reliant upon the nurse's observations and feedback.

Observation is a continuous human activity from which we are constantly collecting and analysing visual information. Observation is both a personal and a selective process in which our perceptions are distorted and screened to meet our own needs. We all see things differently. Observation is influenced by the:

- level of concentration and attention given;
- attitudes and beliefs of the observer;
- presence of distractions in the environment;
- novelty of the situation and environment;
- emotional state and physical health of the observer;
- previous experience and knowledge of the observer;
- relationship with the person who is being observed;
- situation in which the observation takes place;
- expectations of the observer;
- individual differences in the way people perceive the environment.

The skill of observation

Because of these "observer variables", it is important that mental health nurses develop their skills of observation. This is to ensure that their observations are both accurate and objective. The skill of observation is enhanced by:

1. A knowledge of the psychology of perception.
2. A knowledge of human behaviour and non-verbal communication.
3. Insight and awareness of the nurse's own biases and emotional responses, i.e. not jumping to conclusions or making assumptions.
4. Systematic and structured observations that are goal-directed and purposeful.
5. The time committed towards observing, to ensure that what one sees is representative and in context.
6. Comparing the observations with other members of the care team.
7. Training in observational skills and strategies, preferably with video feedback or observed practice.
8. Recording the observations:

   - as soon as possible,
   - in descriptive not emotional terms,
   - legibly, clearly and concisely,
   - systematically,
   - what was actually seen.

The observations will contribute towards the development of a "baseline" of the person's current mental health status. It is important that the baseline is well-founded, because it will be used to determine and evaluate the person's care and treatment. In mental health practice dramatic changes are rarely seen. People often respond and change very slowly over a long period of time; hence the need for well-defined criteria in regard of the person's assessment.

Interviewing

Interviewing as an interpersonal skill is a structured situation in which the main objective is to collect information. It is an important mental health nursing skill that has particular implications for the nurse's ability to:

- identify and assess client's needs/problems;
- plan an individualized care programme;
- implement the care programme;
- evaluate the client's progress and the effectiveness of nursing interventions.

As a professional skill, interviewing is based upon the ability of the nurse to:

- establish a rapport and therapeutic relationship (see Unit 1.2);
- communicate effectively (see Unit 1.3);
- observe objectively and accurately (see "Observation", pp. 53);
- record information accurately and concisely.

Interviews may be organized in a variety of ways:

1. *Structured interview*: in which the areas of assessment and questioning are clearly identified and adhered to. In this setting the nurse may use pre-set questionnaires that may relate to the person's general background or specific needs. This approach is useful for special areas of practice and helps to promote accuracy.
2. *Open interview*: in which the nurse and the client are free to determine the type, style and format of the interview. This approach is useful where the nurse is a skilled interviewer.
3. *Semi-structured interview*: combining elements of the above two approaches. Typically, the nurse may start with a fixed agenda and move to a more open and discussive approach. This is probably the most commonly used approach.

Questioning technique

The ability to ask effective questions is a hallmark of skilled interviewing technique. Questions are used to:

- obtain information;
- ascertain the attitudes and expectations of the respondent;
- assess the extent of the respondent's knowledge and insight;
- identify the particular needs and problems of the respondent;
- focus attention on particular issues;
- promote self-appraisal;
- establish a rapport and express an interest.

The way in which questions are asked and phrased can also influence the reply that is given. To encourage good practice the following points should be borne in mind:

1. Questions should be seen to be valid, i.e. directly relevant and pertinent to the stated objectives and client's needs.
2. Questions should be non-threatening beyond the ability of the person to cope with them. Questioning about intimate and distressing matters may have to be delayed until trust has developed.
3. Questions should be unambiguous and kept brief.
4. Areas of questioning should be sequenced and flow into one another, not jump from topic to topic.
5. Closed questions – those that only require a short specific response – are useful for obtaining factual information. They can be prepared in advance and are useful where time is limited. They tend to be easier to answer and may help clients who are confused, withdrawn or over-talkative. Examples of closed questions are:

- "How old are you?"
- "Are you married?"
- "How long have you lived here?"

6. Open questions – which encourage a multiple word response – are useful for exploring a wider range of topics, thoughts and feelings. The client is given a freer choice on how they reply, which increases their feelings of control. They tend to encourage a higher degree of self-revelation and take longer to obtain the desired information. They also require the interviewer to be more attentive and skilful. Examples of open questions are:

   - "How would you describe your present relationship with your father?"
   - "In what ways has your drinking affected your family life?"
   - "When you first started to feel depressed how did you try to cope with your daily life?"

Conducting an interview
Pre-interview preparation

1. Collect and review necessary documentation, e.g. background information, referral agency, current difficulties leading to referral.
2. Prepare the environment to facilitate communication, e.g. seating, privacy, proximity.
3. Determine the recording method to be used, e.g. written, video, tape-recorder, checklist, questionnaire, forms.
4. Be clear about the objectives of the interview.
5. Be aware of how the interview setting might influence the person's behaviour and responses, e.g. home, clinic, ward, others present.
6. Keep an open mind and be objective – the aim is to collect information, not to make judgements.

Opening the interview

1. Use the interview to initiate and develop a therapeutic relationship.
2. Provide an opportunity for mutual introductions and use preferred names.
3. Explain own role in health care team.
4. State the purpose of the interview, i.e. stress that it is designed to benefit the person and improve the quality of their care.
5. Describe how the information will be used.
6. Define the time limit involved.
7. Reinforce the confidentiality of the material.

Developing the interview
1. Maintain a relaxed posture and movements.
2. Respect the person's personal space.

3. Speak clearly and concisely.
4. Use common words and simple language.
5. Modulate voice volume and tone to facilitate communication.
6. Give non-verbal signals to promote communication, e.g. eye contact, facial expression, nods.
7. Demonstrate active listening.
8. Skilful use of questioning technique.
9. Pace the interview to the person's responses, i.e. do not pressurize, be patient.
10. Seek clarification if information is not understood.
11. Help them to rephrase answers for a fuller response or where the reply is incomplete.
12. Keep focussed on the goals of the interview.
13. Demonstrate non-judgemental responses.
14. Reflect and re-state the person's statements carefully – do not over-use this technique.
15. Follow a systematic and logical sequence.

Ending the interview

1. Give the person an opportunity to provide further information and to ask any questions.
2. Draw to a close, do not end abruptly.
3. Keep to stated time limits.
4. Give clear verbal and non-verbal cues for ending: do not fidget, look bored or stare at the clock.
5. Thank them for their cooperation.
6. Emphasize the usefulness of the information
7. Be positive and impart hope.
8. Plan for the next meeting – enter it into your diary, give the client confirmation.
9. Make clear and accurate notes on appropriate documentation.

Teamwork

Depending upon the setting in which the assessment takes place it is quite likely to involve, at some stage, a number of other health care workers. This can include members of the nursing care team or other multidisciplinary team members. These groups of people, both from a personal perspective and with their differing professional backgrounds, can provide additional information that may be of value to the nursing assessment.

The specific skill of the nurse is to be able to:

- communicate effectively with co-workers;
- review existing written records for potentially useful information;
- identify and extract relevant information from these sources and members of the team.

Professional knowledge and experience

Assessment requires a sound knowledge and skills base. The standard of the assessment is directly related to the nurse's professional development. Practitioners who are motivated to update their knowledge and to enhance their skills are more likely to identify clients' needs accurately and to select appropriate interventions.

Self-assessment

Clients and relatives can contribute very meaningfully to the assessment process in a variety of ways. They can be asked to bring this information along with them, to complete it at the time of the interview, or to undertake it as a homework assignment. Both the information presented and the person's motivation in completing and complying with the self-assessment provide useful material. Self-assessment is also a very good way of promoting insight and understanding. People may be asked to:

1. Complete a questionnaire: ticking a response or writing an entry, e.g. anxiety assessment, orientation, social skills.
2. Keep a diary or log of their daily lives, specific difficulties, how they coped, their observations, thoughts and feelings, e.g. coping skills, relationship patterns, social activities.
3. Comment on video or cassette recordings of themselves or others in certain situations. They can be asked for their own perceptions or how they thought other people behaved.
4. Comment on the interviewer's transcript and summary. This can be useful in validating the nurse's perceptions and also to develop trust.

Nursing History

The information collected as part of the assessment is known as the "nursing history". This should contain a concise summary of the relevant information needed to:

1. Clearly identify the nature and extent of the difficulties and needs experienced by the individual, i.e. their understanding, expectations and perceptions of their health care difficulties.

2. Enable decisions to be made in regard of planning nursing interventions. It should be sufficiently detailed for appropriate interventions to be selected.

The format of the documentation used will vary between health care centres. However, it does need to be practical, easy to follow and relevant to the person's nursing care. It should not duplicate information readily available elsewhere.

The first step in using the collected information is to identify those areas of the person's life where they are experiencing difficulties or deficits and which are amenable to nursing intervention. Within a multidisciplinary care setting, other health care professionals may have the specific skills needed by the client for certain of their difficulties. The nurse can then refer the client as appropriate.

Depending upon the organization and the nurse's professional preferences, the person's difficulties or deficits may be described as either:

- *problems*: the specific difficulties being experienced by the person in relation to their mental health care problems; or
- *needs*: the specific deficits being experienced by the person in relation to their mental health care needs.

Whichever terminology is used by the nurse practitioner it is important that they can use it proficiently.

Needs/problems need to be described in sufficient detail to ensure that they are described accurately. This may require several sentences that detail the person's difficulties rather than one word, for example:

withdrawn/socialize	*vs*	avoids social contact with relatives, does not initiate conversation, speech unclear
anxious/freedom from psychological threat	*vs*	preoccupied with unpleasant anticipations, pacing and agitated movements, unable to leave house unaccompanied

Problems/needs which are described in such detail have several advantages:

1. They are unique to the individual and hence ensure real and valid difficulties have been identified.
2. Well-defined needs/problems suggest their own solution: most "general" problems/needs tend to be composed of several contributory difficulties. These are usually more manageable and amenable to nursing intervention.

Problems/needs may also be classified in terms of:

- actual, potential or possible,
- immediate/medium-term/long-term.

All needs and problems are attended to – classifying them further in this way can help to focus and emphasize certain aspects of nursing care. The definition of needs/problems will alter over time as they are resolved or reassessed.

The Range of Information

The information required may relate to the client's specific difficulties or include a more generalized assessment. This will be determined by the setting in which the nurse is working and organizational policies. Specialist clinical services may require a very detailed profile of the person's and relative's difficulties and needs that would be inappropriate in other settings. Elderly care, child and adolescent psychiatry and substance abuse are examples of services that may require very specific assessments to be completed. The information may include the following.

Behavioural assessment

What a person is seen to do. This is indicative of emotional and cognitive status. With all behaviour one needs to consider where, when, frequency, timing, duration, rate, speed, situation and context, preceding events, responses of others, potential reinforcers, and consequences.

General behaviour pattern

1. Organized and purposeful or disorganized and aimless.
2. Predictable and systematic or impulsive and unpredictable.
3. Conventional and accepted by others or leads to rejection.
4. Self-motivated and autonomous or needs prompting and guidance.
5. Level of energy – active, easily tired, retarded, persistent, easily gives up, goes from one thing to another, etc.

Verbal and non-verbal communication

1. Pattern of speech – slow, rapid, rhythm, pitch, tone, clarity, intonation, volume, emphasis, fluent, hesitant.
2. Content – comprehensible, relevant, dialect, slang, accent, topic.
3. Responsive, non-responsive, mute.
4. Non-verbal communication – eye contact maintained, avoided, overused; facial expression appropriate, fixed, blank; posture, gestures, hand movements, head movements.

Social interaction

1. Readily interacts with others, withdrawn, passive.
2. Assertive or aggressive. Social confidence and self-esteem.
3. Do they need prompting to join in with others?
4. Will they initiate conversations?
5. Do they seek or avoid social contacts?

Life skills

1. Autonomy and independence, i.e. ability to meet own care needs.
2. Able to use common domestic appliances.
3. Able to organize own activities of daily living.
4. Able to identify and use community resources.
5. Can organize and arrange own financial affairs.
6. Personal hygiene – self-maintained or dependent, specific problems, appear clean or neglected.
7. Personal appearance – self-maintained or dependent, groomed or untidy, shoes and clothing appropriate and fitted.

Cognitive assessment

1. Insight and understanding.
2. Concentration and attention.
3. Problem solving and decision making.
4. Creativity and imagination.
5. Memory – short-term and long-term, retentive or forgetful.
6. Orientation – date, time, place, person, situation.
7. Interest in the environment.
8. Level of consciousness and awareness – alert, drowsy, comatose, delirious.
9. Awareness of risks.
10. Thoughts, preoccupations, expectations, suspicions.
11. Evidence of delusions or hallucinations.
12. Perception of their health status and needs.
13. Coping skills used.
14. Perceived self-worth and self-esteem.

Emotional assessment

1. Normal pattern of emotional expression.
2. Current mood – depressed, tense, anxious, excited, elated, hostile, threatened, resentful.
3. Appropriateness of mood to situation.

4. Mood stable or liable to sudden changes.
5. Intensity of mood – lack of emotional response.
6. Emotional reaction to health care difficulties and interventions.

Social assessment

1. Married, single, divorced, widowed.
2. Sexual orientation and preferences.
3. Social support network – frequency of contact.
4. Close relationships – closeness, contact, problematic, conflict, stress.
5. Occupation – job satisfaction, stress, unemployed.
6. Financial status – debts, difficulties, coping.
7. Recreation – hobbies, interests, leisure activities.
8. Use of alcohol and drugs.
9. Education.
10. Social background and upbringing.
11. Housing conditions – comfortable, state of repair, heating, hygiene facilities, accessibility, isolated.

Physical assessment

1. General physical status

   - height, body build, colour of eyes and hair, any distinguishing features;
   - condition of skin – clear, rashes, bruises, swellings, pale, perspiring, scars, wounds;
   - weight – normal range, overweight, underweight, recent loss or gain;
   - eyes – clear, red, watery, dry, inflamed;
   - dentition – own teeth, dentures, oral hygiene;
   - menstruation – regular, irregular, amenorrhoea;
   - pregnancy – expected date of confinement, miscarriages, number of children;
   - blood pressure;
   - physical disability or existing medical condition;
   - medication – prescribed or self-administered.

2. Sleep pattern

   - normal rest and sleep patterns and preferences;
   - sleep disturbances – early waking, difficulty in falling asleep, restless, difficulty waking up in the morning;
   - dreams and nightmares;
   - night-time medication taken.

3. Appetite

   - normal dietary pattern – preferred foods, religious observances;
   - excessive appetite, loss of appetite;
   - eating habits;
   - problems or difficulties with eating;
   - nutritional knowledge.

4. Mobility

   - posture and gait, fully mobile and active;
   - dependency – need assistance, use of aids, confidence;
   - limitations or restrictions – contributory physical and sensory problems;
   - co-ordination of movement;
   - physical handicap.

5. Elimination

   - normal pattern – frequency, timing;
   - controlled or incontinent;
   - constipation, use of laxatives;
   - urinalysis;
   - nausea and vomiting.

6. Respiration

   - rate, depth, rhythm, symmetry;
   - breathless on exertion, recovery time;
   - respiratory difficulties – asthma, coughing, sputum;
   - smoke tobacco – how much, how long.

7. Senses

   - effectiveness of vision, hearing, taste, smell, touch;
   - use of aids for sight and hearing.

Unit Instructions

When you have researched the suggested references, have mastered the Unit Objectives and successfully answered the Self-assessment Questions, proceed with the Unit Written Test.

Suggested References

Altschul, A. and McGovern, M. (1985). *Psychiatric Nursing*, 6th edition. Baillière Tindall, London and San Diego.

Barker, P. J. (1985). *Patient Assessment in Psychiatric Nursing*. Croom Helm, London.

Barrowclough, C., Whitmore, B. and Tessier, I. (1984). The same, only different. *Nursing Mirror*, 24 October, Vol. 159, No. 15, pp. 28–30.

Bauer, B. and Hill, S. (1986). *Essentials of Mental Health Care Planning and Interventions*. W. B. Saunders, Philadelphia.

Campbell, C. (1978). *Nursing Diagnosis and Intervention in Nursing Practice*. John Wiley, New York.

Darcy, P. T. (1985). *Mental Health Nursing Source Book*. Baillière Tindall, London and San Diego.

Dexter, G. and Wash, M. (1986). *Psychiatric Nursing Skills: A Patient-centred Approach*. Croom Helm, London.

Doona, M. E. (1979). *Travelbee's Intervention in Psychiatric Nursing*, 2nd edition. F. A. Davis, Philadelphia.

Faulkner, A. (1981). Aye, there's the rub. *Nursing Times*, 19 February, Vol. 77, No. 7, pp. 332–336.

Hargie, O., Saunders, C. and Dickeon, D. (1987). *Social Skills in Interpersonal Communication*, 2nd edition. Croom Helm, London.

Hase, S. and Douglas, A. (1986). *Human Dynamics and Nursing*. Churchill Livingstone, Melbourne.

Hewitt, F. S. (1981a). Questions and listening. *Nursing Times*, 25 November, Vol. 77, No. 48, pp. 21–24. (Supplement "Communication Skills".)

Hewitt, F. S. (1981b). The interview. *Nursing Times*, 25 November, Vol. 77, No. 48, pp. 41–44. (Supplement "Communication skills".)

Hunt, G. and Eade, W. (1987). *Interviewing: A Communication Approach*. Holt, Rinehart and Winston, New York.

Irving, S. (1983). *Basic Psychiatric Nursing*, 3rd edition. W. B. Saunders, Philadelphia.

Lancaster, J. (1980). *Adult Psychiatric Nursing*. Henry Kimpton, London.

Lyttle, J. (1986). *Mental Disorder*. Baillière Tindall, London and San Diego.

McFarland, G. and Wasli, E. (1986). *Nursing Diagnoses and Process in Psychiatric Mental Health Nursing*. J. B. Lippincott, Philadelphia.

Martin, P. (Ed.) (1987a). *Psychiatric Nursing: A Therapeutic Approach*. Macmillan, London.

Martin, P. (1987b). *Care of the Mentally Ill*, 2nd edition. Macmillan, London.

Pelletier, L. (Ed.) (1987). *Psychiatric Nursing Case Studies, Nursing Diagnoses and Care Plans*. Springhouse Corporation, Springhouse, Pennsylvania.

Priestley, P. and McGuire, J. (1983). *Learning to Help: Basic Skills Exercises*. Tavistock, London.

Priestley, P. *et al.* (1978). *Social Skills and Personal Problem-solving*. Tavistock, London.

Robinson, J. (Ed.) (1978). *Documenting Patient Care Responsibly*. Springhouse Corporation, Springhouse, Pennsylvania.

Robinson, L. (1983). *Psychiatric Nursing as a Human Experience*, 3rd edition. W. B. Saunders, Philadelphia.

Roper, N., Logan, W. and Tierney, A. (1983a). Problems or needs? *Nursing Mirror*, 8 June, Vol. 79, No. 23, pp. 43–44.

Roper, N., Logan, W. and Tierney, A. (1983b). Identifying the goals. *Nursing Mirror*, 15 June, Vol. 79, No. 24, pp. 22–23.

Salisbury, D. (1985). Don't waste the process. *Nursing Times*, 6 March, Vol. 81, No. 10, p. 42.

Sencicle, L. (1982). A double-edged weapon. *Nursing Mirror*, 4 August, Vol. 155, No. 5, pp. 42–43.

Simmons, S. and Brooker, C. (1986). *Community Psychiatric Nursing: A Social Perspective*. Heinemann Nursing, London.

Stockwell, F. (1982). The nursing process in a psychiatric hospital. *Nursing Times*, 25 August, Vol. 78, No. 34, pp. 1441–1442.

Sundeen, S. *et al.* (1981). *Nurse–Client Interaction*, 2nd edition. C. V. Mosby, St. Louis.

Tierney, A. (1984). Defending the process. *Nursing Times*, 16 May, Vol. 80, No. 20, pp. 38–41.

Ward, M. (1984). Teaching the teachers. *Nursing Times*, 20 June, Vol. 80, No. 25, pp. 46–48.

Ward, M. F. (1985). *The Nursing Process in Psychiatry*. Churchill Livingstone, Edinburgh.

Whyte, L. and Youhill, G. (1984). The nursing process in the care of the mentally ill. *Nursing Times*, 1 February, Vol. 80, No. 5, pp. 49–51.

Self-assessment Questions

SAQ 1. Identify six ways of promoting accurate and objective observations.

SAQ 2. Outline the sequence of an interview with four specific factors relevant to each stage.

SAQ 3. Describe five factors that promote skilled questioning techniques.

SAQ 4. List four observations that can be made in each of the following areas: emotions, behaviour, thoughts, physical status and life-style.

Unit 2.1: Written Test

1. How can mental health nurses ensure that their observations are accurate and objective?

2. What skills and approaches can mental health nurses use to facilitate communication during an interview?

3. Describe the role of self-assessment in the identification of clients' health care needs.

The Planning of Nursing Care

Unit Objectives

At the end of this Unit the learner should be able to:

1. List the stages involved in the process of planning of care.
2. Outline the criteria used to select nursing interventions.
3. Describe how desired outcomes/nursing objectives are established.
4. State the purpose of identifying priorities.

The Planning Process

In designing an individualized care programme, the nurses are using their professional judgement to select specific nursing interventions, to identify desired outcomes and to assign priorities that will meet the client's needs.

The planning of care should be a collaborative partnership between the nursing team, the client and his relatives. If the person is involved in the planning process this helps to promote cooperation and to prevent misunderstanding. It also permits the planning process to be used for increasing the client's understanding of his own health care needs.

The Structure of a Nursing Care Plan

The specific layout and terminology used in nursing care plans will vary according to established practice and the documentation supplied. Generally, a nursing care plan will incorporate the following:

1. *Needs/problems, personal difficulties*: a detailed description of the person's needs/problems/difficulties that require nursing intervention (see Unit 2.1).
2. *Objectives/goals/desired outcomes*: a detailed description of the person's and nurse's intended target behaviour.
3. *Priorities*: identification of a hierarchy of needs in terms of their importance to the person's health care status.

4. *Nursing interventions/nursing orders*: a detailed description of the nursing interventions required for each need/problem.
5. *Nursing notes/progress notes*: a section for documenting the ongoing nursing interventions and the person's responses (see Unit 2.3).
6. *Evaluation/review*: a section for including information relating to the evaluation of the person's progress and nursing interventions (see Unit 2.4).

Objectives/goals/desired outcomes

The statement of objectives for each need/problem identified is an important step in the care planning process. The stated outcomes:

1. Provide goal direction and purpose for the nursing interventions.
2. Influence the choice of nursing interventions.
3. Assist in the evaluation of the person's progress.
4. Facilitate in the evaluation of the effectiveness of the nursing interventions.

Setting objectives/desired outcomes

The objectives/outcomes that are set need to be realistic and attainable in terms of:

- the person's aspirations and potential;
- the skills and resources of the care team.

The setting of unrealistic and unattainable objectives can be very demoralizing and demotivating. Equally, if the outcomes are too minimal, then they can create false expectations of progress and the effectiveness of interventions.

The outcomes/objectives should be expressed sequentially and in terms of graded progression. They may be written as:

- short-term objectives/outcomes,
- medium-term objectives/outcomes,
- long-term objectives/outcomes.

Providing an overview of the caring process in this way gives further structure to the planning process and expectation of outcomes. This is particularly significant in mental health nursing practice in relation to mental health problems which, by their very nature, tend to be long-term. Giving a time boundary focusses the efforts of the care team.

The objectives or desired outcomes should be stated in such a way that the required response and the conditions under which it should occur are clearly described. Written this way, in behavioural terms, there is a well-defined target behaviour (see Exhibit 2.2.1).

Exhibit 2.2.1 Objectives and desired outcomes

Need/problem	Possible desired outcomes/objectives
1. To develop a positive self-image/low self-esteem	To make positive self-statements without prompting within 6 weeks. To decrease by 50% the number of self-critical statements within 6 weeks.
2. To initiate social contacts/lacking in confidence	To maintain eye contact during a conversation. To approach others without prompting. To make multiple word responses
3. Promote orientation/disorientated and confused	To locate own room unaided. To state correctly the day in response to questioning. To identify and name their primary nurse.

Priorities

In the process of planning nursing interventions it may be necessary to identify specific needs/problems that should be given a higher priority by the nursing team. Priorities may be selected in terms of:

1. The safety of the person – if their behaviour or physical condition puts them at risk.
2. Minimizing distress – if the person and the staff identify specific needs/problems that cause particular stress to the individual.
3. Utilizing resources effectively – if limited resources are available, including staff time, then they should be focussed on needs/problems that are most amenable to intervention or are likely to contribute most to recovery.
4. The objectives that are set – the attainment of specific objectives may be linked sequentially. Resolution of certain problems may also facilitate meeting other related needs.

If priorities are identified then they need to be clearly indicated on the care plan and made known to the care team and the client. Priorities may be described as high, medium or low. As the person's needs are met and problems are resolved then the priorities will alter.

Nursing interventions/nursing orders

Specific nursing interventions are selected for each identified need/problem. The interventions are chosen by the primary nurse/key worker, either as an individual practitioner or in collaboration with the nursing care team. The interventions are selected in terms of:

1. Effectiveness in meeting the person's needs/resolving their problems.
2. The skills, knowledge and experience of the nurse practitioners.
3. The resources available and the policies of the organization.
4. The approval and acceptability of the client and family.

Once the nursing interventions have been selected and written down, they then become the nursing orders. The nursing orders should be written as precise instructions as to how the care is to be given. This is to ensure that the interventions are carried out consistently by the nursing staff (see Exhibit 2.2.2).

Exhibit 2.2.2 Nursing orders

Need/problem	Possible nursing orders
1. To develop communication skills/ poor communication skills	Ask open-ended questions. Positively reinforce unprompted contact. Give feedback and guidance on communication skills. Use video feedback of role plays of identified social situations
2. Provide a safe and secure environment/ avoid self-injurious behaviour	Observe at all times. Remove potential risks. Engage in diversional activities. Encourage to talk about self-harmful thoughts and feelings

The Nursing Care Plan

The nursing care plan when written is a tool that should provide for:

1. Individualized nursing care – tailored to meet the unique needs of each client.
2. Co-ordination and continuity of care – the document facilitates communication among the care team and promotes consistency of approach.
3. Evaluation of client progress and nursing care interventions – the quality of the nursing care plan is directly related to the quality of care that is given.

The nursing care plan needs to be:

- readily available and accessible,
- easy to follow,
- flexible and adaptable with space for additions and alterations.

When completed the written care plan should be signed and dated by the responsible nurse practitioner who is accountable for the client. Later additions and alterations should be clearly indicated and each entry signed and dated.

Unit Instructions

When you have researched the suggested references, have mastered the Unit Objectives and successfully answered the Self-assessment Questions, proceed with the Unit Written Test.

Suggested References

Altschul, A. and McGovern, M. (1985). *Psychiatric Nursing*, 6th edition. Baillière Tindall, London and San Diego.

Barnett, D. (1985). Making your plans work. *Nursing Times*, 9 January, Vol. 81, No. 2, pp. 24–27.

Bauer, B. and Hill, S. (1986). *Essentials of Mental Health Care Planning and Interventions*. W. B. Saunders, Philadelphia.

Campbell, C. (1978). *Nursing Diagnosis and Intervention in Nursing Practice*. John Wiley, New York.

Darcy, P. T. (1985). *Mental Health Nursing Source Book*. Baillière Tindall, London and San Diego.

Dexter, G. and Wash, M. (1986). *Psychiatric Nursing Skills: A Patient-centred Approach*. Croom Helm, London.

Hampshire, G. (1983). Defining goals. *Nursing Times*, 16 March, Vol. 79, No. 11, pp. 45–46.

Hase, S. and Douglas, A. (1986). *Human Dynamics and Nursing*. Churchill Livingstone, Melbourne.

Irving, S. (1983). *Basic Psychiatric Nursing*, 3rd edition. W. B. Saunders, Philadelphia.

Lancaster, J. (1980). *Adult Psychiatric Nursing*. Henry Kimpton, London.

Lyttle, J. (1986). *Mental Disorder*. Baillière Tindall, London and San Diego.

McFarland, G. and Wasli, E. (1986). *Nursing Diagnoses and Process in Psychiatric Mental Health Nursing*. J. B. Lippincott, Philadelphia.

Manchester, J. (1983). A framework for planning. *Nursing Mirror*, 13 April, Vol. 156, No. 15, pp. 34–36.

Marriner, A. (Ed.) (1979). *The Nursing Process*. C. V. Mosby, St. Louis.

Martin, P. (Ed.) (1987a). *Psychiatric Nursing: A Therapeutic Approach*. Macmillan, London.

Martin, P. (1987b). *Care of the Mentally Ill*, 2nd edition. Macmillan, London.

Pelletier, L. (Ed.) (1987). *Psychiatric Nursing Case Studies, Nursing Diagnoses and Care Plans*. Springhouse Corporation, Springhouse, Pennsylvania.

Robinson, L. (1983). *Psychiatric Nursing as a Human Experience*, 3rd edition. W. B. Saunders, Philadelphia.

Schröck, R. A. (1980). Planning nursing care for the mentally ill. *Nursing Times*, 17 April, Vol. 76, No. 16, pp. 704–706.

Somociuk, G. (1985). Concept meets reality. *Nursing Mirror*, 11 September, Vol. 161, No. 11, pp. 29–33.

Ward, M. F. (1985). *The Nursing Process in Psychiatry*. Churchill Livingstone, Edinburgh.

Yura, D. and Walsh, M. B. (1978). *The Nursing Process: Assessing, Planning, Implementing and Evaluating*. Appleton Century Crofts, New York.

Self-assessment Questions

SAQ 5. State each of the stages involved in completing a nursing care plan.

SAQ 6. List five criteria used to select nursing interventions for specific problems/needs.

SAQ 7. Identify four factors that the nurse needs to consider when establishing nursing objectives/desired outcomes.

SAQ 8. List four factors that need to be considered when determining priorities.

Unit 2.2: Written Test

1. Describe in detail the factors that influence the choice of nursing intervention for a specific client need/problem.
2. What purpose do desired outcomes/nursing objectives have in the care planning process? What factors need to be taken into account when trying to identify appropriate outcomes/objectives?
3. How does the setting of priorities within the care plan influence a person's nursing care?

UNIT 2.3

The Implementation of Nursing Care

Unit Objectives

At the end of this Unit the learner should be able to:

1. Outline the responsibilities of the primary nurse/key worker for the implementation of care.
2. State methods for ensuring continuity of care.
3. Describe the purposes of nursing team meetings.
4. List criteria for maintaining effective written records.

Implementation

Implementation involves the activation and initiation of the nursing care plan. Each intervention should be purposeful and goal-directed towards helping the person meet their health care needs. Through their skilled interventions, mental health nurses are trying to influence positively the person's:

1. Emotions – their expression and appropriateness.
2. Behaviour – their actions, skills, verbal and non-verbal behaviour.
3. Cognitions – their thoughts, perceptions, understanding and knowledge.
4. Physiological status – their physical health status, basic physical needs.

The interventions are based upon the clinical skills and knowledge of the psychiatric nurse. The most important skills that the psychiatric nurse uses are those involved with therapeutic relationships and communication.

The Primary Nurse/Key Worker

The designated primary nurse/key worker is responsible for ensuring the implementation of the nursing care plan. Either as a practitioner in their own right or as a leader of a team of nurses, they need to ensure that the nursing care plan is implemented consistently. They need to confirm that those involved in the caring process, themselves and their nursing team:

1. Develop an effective therapeutic relationship with the clients and relatives.
2. Understand the objectives and interventions required for each person in their care.
3. Have the skills and knowledge to implement the nursing care programme.
4. Recognize the need for consistency and continuity of care.
5. Work effectively as a team.
6. Comply with the stated nursing orders.
7. Give feedback and communicate effectively with members of the nursing and multidisciplinary care team on their interventions and the client's responses.
8. Maintain accurate written records.
9. Have a clear understanding of their role and responsibilities.
10. Have the opportunity for regular clinical supervision of their nursing practice.

Nursing Team Meetings

The nursing care team need to meet regularly to facilitate communication and to co-ordinate their activities. The timing, duration and frequency of meetings should be sufficient to ensure that there is adequate time for:

- information to be exchanged and discussed;
- priorities to be determined;
- client progress to be monitored;
- peer support and team development;
- promoting free discussion;
- professional development and education.

Nursing Written Records

The written records that are maintained have an important role in psychiatric nursing practice. They need to be written in a systematic way if they are to meet the needs of:

1. *Communication* among the nursing and multidisciplinary care teams.
2. *Continuity and consistency* of nursing care by those involved.
3. *Accountability* for nursing decisions and actions.
4. *Evaluation* of client progress and nursing practice.

The format of nursing records or progress notes will vary depending upon local practice and documentation. In order to meet the required criteria the written records need to be:

1. Written by the person's key worker or by a member of the same nursing team who has worked with the client.
2. Written by or under the supervision of a trained nurse.
3. Legible and comprehensible.
4. A detailed record of the nursing interventions.
5. A detailed record of the person's responses to the nursing interventions.
6. Purposeful statements of the person's current health status and significant events in their care.
7. Objective descriptions of what the nurse actually saw.
8. Written as soon as possible after significant events to avoid distortions or omissions due to memory loss.
9. Signed and dated after each entry.
10. Readily accessible to the nursing care team.

Unit Instructions

When you have researched the suggested references, have mastered the Unit Objectives and successfully answered the Self-assessment Questions, proceed with the Unit Written Test.

Suggested References

Altschul, A. and McGovern, M. (1985). *Psychiatric Nursing*, 6th edition. Baillière Tindall, London and San Diego.

Bauer, B. and Hill, S. (1986). *Essentials of Mental Health Care Planning and Interventions*. W. B. Saunders, Philadelphia.

Campbell, A. (1978). *Nursing Diagnosis and Intervention in Nursing Practice*. John Wiley, New York.

Darcy, P. T. (1984). *Theory and Practice of Psychiatric Care*. Hodder and Stoughton, London.

Darcy, P. T. (1985). *Mental Health Nursing Source Book*. Baillière Tindall, London and San Diego.

Dexter, G. and Wash, M. (1986). *Psychiatric Nursing Skills: A Patient-centred Approach*. Croom Helm, London.

Hase, S. and Douglas, A. (1986). *Human Dynamics and Nursing*. Churchill Livingstone, Melbourne.

Irving, S. (1983). *Basic Psychiatric Nursing*, 3rd edition. W. B. Saunders, Philadelphia.

Lancaster, J. (1980). *Adult Psychiatric Nursing*. Henry Kimpton, London.

Lyttle, J. (1986). *Mental Disorder*. Baillière Tindall, London and San Diego.

McFarland, G. and Wasli, E. (1986). *Nursing Diagnoses and Process in Psychiatric Mental Health Nursing*. J. B. Lippincott, Philadelphia.

Martin, P. (Ed.) (1987a). *Psychiatric Nursing: A Therapeutic Approach*. Macmillan, London.

Martin, P. (1987b). *Care of the Mentally Ill*, 2nd edition. Macmillan, London.

Pelletier, L. (Ed.) (1987). *Psychiatric Nursing Case Studies, Nursing Diagnoses and Care Plans*. Springhouse Corporation, Springhouse, Pennsylvania.
Robinson, L. (1983). *Psychiatric Nursing as a Human Experience*, 3rd edition. W. B. Saunders, Philadelphia.
Sundeen, S. *et al.* (1981). *Nurse–Client Interaction*, 2nd edition. C. V. Mosby, St. Louis.
Ward, M. F. (1985). *The Nursing Process in Psychiatry*. Churchill Livingstone, Edinburgh.

Self-assessment Questions

SAQ   9. What are the responsibilities of the primary nurse/key worker in ensuring continuity of care.
SAQ 10. List five characteristics of effective staff meetings.
SAQ 11. State four reasons for maintaining comprehensive written records.
SAQ 12. Identify five criteria of comprehensive written nursing records.

Unit 2.3: Written Test

1. How can the primary nurse as an individual practitioner and team leader ensure continuity and consistency of care?

UNIT 2.4

The Evaluation of Nursing Care

Unit Objectives

At the end of this Unit the learner should be able to:

1. Describe the uses of evaluation in mental health nursing practice.
2. Identify ways in which nursing care can be evaluated.
3. Demonstrate how evaluation can be used to revise a nursing care programme.
4. Outline the implications of evaluation for mental health nursing practice.

Evaluation

Evaluation is an ongoing process of review. Every interaction with the person and with other members of the care team provides the opportunity to evaluate critically:

1. The person's current health status.
2. Their progress towards stated health care goals/desired outcomes.
3. The validity of the nursing care programme.
4. The effectiveness of nursing care interventions.
5. The quality of nursing care practice.

Evaluation should be part of the person's daily care programme. It also needs to be augmented by regular care planning or review meetings when the person's nursing care programme can be reviewed and discussed in detail.

Evaluation of Nursing Care Programmes

The evaluation of nursing care programmes is a process that reviews:

1. *The assessment of the person's care needs/problems*

   • were the needs/problems identified valid?

- were they accurately described?
- were sources of information used constructively?
- were the skills of observation and interviewing demonstrated?
- is the nurse's knowledge and skills base up to date?
- were the records accurately completed?
- how much involvement did the person and their family have?

2. *The care planning process*

- were appropriate nursing care interventions selected for the identified needs/problems?
- were the goals and criteria set realistic in terms of the person's potential and the resources available?
- were the priorities valid in terms of the person's needs/problems?
- how much was the person and their family involved in the planning of their care?
- how accurately is the care plan documented?

3. *The implementation of care*

- were the nursing care team consistent in their approach?
- did they communicate effectively with one another?
- were they flexible in response to changing circumstances?
- were accurate ongoing records kept of nursing interventions and the person's responses?
- are the team able to demonstrate the skills and knowledge base of their interventions?

4. *The evaluation of care*

- were complete and accurate records kept?
- how was the information that was collected used to revise the nursing care programme?
- how frequently were the person's needs re-evaluated?
- what feedback was given to the person in regard of their progress?

Sources of Evaluation

Evaluation is a process of using feedback from:

1. *The client and their family*

- their comments and suggestions in relation to their health care needs;
- their perceptions of the nursing care they have received;
- their perceptions of care they have received from other health care workers;
- their perceptions of the progress they are making;
- completion of self-administered questionnaires and satisfaction surveys;

- monitoring of any formal complaints that are made.

2. *The key worker/primary nurse*

  - their observations on whether the person's needs have been met;
  - their observations on the person's current health status;
  - their evaluation of the progress made towards stated objectives;
  - reviewing the information collected to date;
  - critical self-evaluation of nursing interventions;
  - peer review and clinical audits.

3. *The clinical supervisor*

  - their comments on the key worker's relationship with the client;
  - their evaluation of the effectiveness of the key worker's interventions;
  - their suggestions for developing the key worker's skills and knowledge.

4. *The nursing care team*

  - their combined observations on the person's current health status;
  - their combined evaluation of the person's progress towards stated objectives;
  - their combined review of the information collected to date;
  - critical evaluation of the team's nursing interventions;
  - peer review, quality circles, clinical audit.

5. *Multidisciplinary care team*

  - individual observations and comments from specialist practitioners;
  - team review meetings.

6. *The organization*

  - re-referral and readmission rates;
  - length of waiting lists;
  - service priorities and resources available;
  - demands being made upon the service;
  - complaints made to the organization.

7. *The community*

  - opportunities for feedback and participation;
  - accessibility to care and treatment resources;
  - incidence of complaints;
  - relationship with the neighbourhood.

Evaluation Skills

The skills used in evaluation include:

1. *Observation* of the person in relation to:

- their initial assessment;
- their current health status;
- the objectives for care;
- the progress being made.

2. *Interviewing* the person and their family to elicit their perceptions of:

- their current health care status;
- their health care progress;
- the care they have received.

3. *Discussion* with members of the nursing and multidisciplinary health care team.

4. *Analysis* of sources of available information:

- written records;
- charts;
- verbal.

5. *Knowledge* – the nurse's professional knowledge base and experience in relation to client care.

Outcomes of Evaluation

As a consequence of evaluation the following actions may be necessary:

1. *Redefining the person's health care needs/problems.* The nature of the person's needs are likely to change over time. Some needs may have been met while others have since become evident.

2. *Redesignating the priority of health care needs/problems.* Both the person's and the nurse's priorities are likely to alter over time. This may be in relation to their current health status or in terms of having resolved previous high-priority needs.

3. *Selecting alternative nursing care interventions.* Current interventions may be proving to be ineffective or inappropriate. Other interventions may need to be selected that are more likely to achieve the desired outcomes.

4. *Setting revised nursing care objectives/desired outcomes.* As objectives/outcomes are attained, then further ones need to be set. It may also be necessary to set more realistic objectives if existing outcomes appear in retrospect to be unattainable.

5. *Stating appropriate review criteria and dates.* Revised objectives/outcomes will also have to have their own criteria set in terms of time boundaries and standards of performance.

6. *Selecting another key health worker.* The visiting key worker may be proving ineffective due to relationship problems or lack of skills. In such a case, it may be preferable to designate someone who is better equipped to work with the person.

7. *Discharging the person from nursing care.* If the person and their family

are now able to meet their own health care needs independently, then their need for care should be terminated. This should be presented positively to the person as a significant step in their health care progress and recovery.

Implications of Evaluation

Evaluation of nursing interventions and care programmes has implications for many areas of mental health nursing practice.

1. *Reviewing the quality of client care.* Feedback from clients and their relatives may be used together with self and peer review to monitor the quality of care that is provided. Services may need to be reappraised in order to promote consumer satisfaction and to ensure that each practitioner is aware of the need to strive continually to improve standards.
2. *Identifying the need for professional development.* Evaluation may identify the need for individuals or teams to update and develop their skills and knowledge. The information can also be used by managers to plan educational programmes in line with service developments.
3. *Reviewing the management and organization of the care team.* The evaluation process may indicate the need to review the way that the nursing care team co-ordinate, communicate and liaise among themselves and with their co-workers.
4. *Developing a research base for nursing practice.* Most areas of mental health nursing practice have yet to be fully researched. Much of existing practice relies on "experience" and "common sense" rather than on a sound rational basis. Some of the available research indicates that nurses do not fully use the therapeutic potential of their contacts with clients. There is also potentially available a vast range of effective nursing care interventions that remain undocumented and could be usefully shared. There is an urgent need for nurses to identify, develop and validate the skills and knowledge base of their practice.
5. *Developing a philosophy and models of mental health nursing practice.* The professional development of psychiatric nursing practice is identifying the need to formulate a sound philosophical and practice base. Mental health nurses need a clear understanding of their own role in the caring process and to develop models of care that are both valid and promote a sound professional identity.

Unit Instructions

When you have researched the suggested references, have mastered the Unit Objectives and successfully answered the Self-assessment Questions, proceed with the Unit Written Test.

Suggested References

Altschul, A. and McGovern, M. (1985). *Psychiatric Nursing*, 6th edition. Baillière Tindall, London and San Diego.

Bauer, B. and Hill, S. (1986). *Essentials of Mental Health Care Planning and Interventions*. W. B. Saunders, Philadelphia.

Campbell, C. (1978). *Nursing Diagnosis and Intervention in Nursing Practice*. John Wiley, New York.

Darcy, P. T. (1985). *Mental Health Nursing Source Book*. Baillière Tindall, London and San Diego.

Dexter, G. and Wash, M. (1986). *Psychiatric Nursing Skills: A Patient-centred Approach*. Croom Helm, London.

Hase, S. and Douglas, A. (1986). *Human Dynamics and Nursing*. Churchill Livingstone, Melbourne.

Hurst, K. (1983). The quiet revolution. *Nursing Mirror*, 26 October, Vol. 157, No. 17, pp. 36–40.

Irving, S. (1983). *Basic Psychiatric Nursing*, 3rd edition. W. B. Saunders, Philadelphia.

Jackson, M. (1986). On maps and models. *Senior Nurse*, October, Vol. 5, No. 4, pp. 24–26.

Johnson, M. (1986). Model of perfection? *Nursing Times*, 5 February, Vol. 82, No. 6, pp. 42–44.

Kershaw, B. and Salvage, J. (Eds) (1986). *Models for Nursing*. John Wiley, Chichester.

Kitson, A. (1986a). The methods of measuring quality. *Nursing Times*, 27 August, Vol. 82, No. 35, pp. 32–34.

Kitson, A. (1986b). Taking Action. *Nursing Times*, 3 September, Vol. 82, No. 36, pp. 52–54.

Kitson, A. and Kendall, H. (1986). Quality assurance. *Nursing Times*, 27 August, Vol. 82, No. 35, pp. 29–31.

Lancaster, J. (1980). *Adult Psychiatric Nursing*. Henry Kimpton, London.

Loughlin, M. (1988). Modelled, muddled and befuddled. *Nursing Times*, Vol. 84, No. 5, pp. 30–31.

Luker, K. (1988). Do models work? *Nursing Times*, Vol. 84, No. 5, pp. 26–29.

Lyttle, J. (1986). *Mental Disorder*. Baillière Tindall, London and San Diego.

McFarland, G. and Wasli, E. (1986). *Nursing Diagnoses and Process in Psychiatric Mental Health Nursing*. J. B. Lippincott, Philadelphia.

Marriner, A. (Ed.) (1979). *The Nursing Process*, 2nd edition. C. V. Mosby, St. Louis.

Martin, P. (Ed.) (1987a). *Psychiatric Nursing: A Therapeutic Approach*. Macmillan, London.

Martin, P. (1987b). *Care of the mentally ill*, 2nd edition. Macmillan, London.

Miller, A. (1985a). Are you using the nursing process? *Nursing Times*, 11 December, Vol. 81, No. 50, pp. 36–39.

Miller, A. (1985b). Does the process help the patient? *Nursing Times*, 26 June Vol. 81, No. 26, pp. 24–27.

Pearson, A. (Ed.) (1987). *Nursing Quality Measurement: Quality Assurance Methods for Peer Review*. John Wiley, Chichester.

Pearson, A. and Vaughan, B. (1986). *Nursing Models for Practice*. Heinemann Nursing, London.

Pelletier, L. (Ed.) (1987). *Psychiatric Nursing Case Studies, Nursing Diagnoses and Care Plans*. Springhouse Corporation, Springhouse, Pennsylvania.

RCN Society of Psychiatric Nursing (1986). *Standards of Care in Psychiatric Nursing Practice*. Royal College of Nursing, London.

Smith, L. (1986). Issues raised by the use of nursing models in psychiatry. *Nurse Education Today*, Vol. 6, No. 2, pp. 69–75.

Ward, M. F. (1986). *The Nursing Process in Psychiatry*. Churchill Livingstone, Edinburgh.

Waters, K. (1986). Cause and effect evaluating patient care. *Nursing Times*, Jan 29 Vol. 82, No. 5, pp 28–30.

Wright, S. (1985). Nursing process a rich experience. *Nursing Times*, Sept 4, Vol. 81, No. 36, 38–39.

Wright, S. (1986). *Building and Using a Model of Nursing*. Edward Arnold, London.

Yura, D. and Walsh, M. B. (1978). *The Nursing Process: Assessing, Planning, Implementing and Evaluating*. Appleton Century Crofts, New York.

Self-assessment Questions

SAQ 13. Identify five skills that are used in the evaluation process.

SAQ 14. List six sources of information that can be used to evaluate nursing care.

SAQ 15. Describe four possible outcomes that may be necessary as a result of evaluating a nursing care programme.

Unit 2.4: Written Test

1. Describe the methods that are used to evaluate nursing care programmes in mental health practice.
2. In what ways may the evaluation be used to revise a nursing care plan.
3. What implications does evaluation have for the practice of mental health nursing?

TOPIC 3

The Skills of the Mental Health Nurse

At the end of this Topic the learner should aim to:

1. Describe the use of counselling techniques in mental health practice.
2. Outline the potential uses of group work in mental health practice.
3. Identify the role of mental health education and promotion.
4. Describe how social skills training programmes are organized and conducted.

UNIT 3.1

Counselling Skills

Unit Objectives

At the end of this Unit the learner should be able to:

1. Describe the uses of counselling in mental health practice.
2. Identify the skills used in counselling.
3. Specify counselling interventions to facilitate client communication.
4. Outline strategies that are used in counselling.

Counselling

Counselling is potentially a very effective therapeutic approach in which a trained therapist or counsellor uses communication and relationship skills to enable clients to:

1. Review their life-style and relationships.
2. Explore, clarify and resolve personal difficulties.
3. Develop their strengths and resources.
4. Promote their well-being.
5. Express their thoughts and feelings.
6. Increase their insight and self-awareness.

In the client-centred approach, the counsellor acts as a sounding board against which clients can express their concerns in an atmosphere of acceptance, trust and confidentiality. Crucial to this process is the counsellor's ability to understand the client's internal frame of reference – the person's unique subjective perception of their situation and the personal meanings they attribute to their experiences.

The relationship between counsellor and client is carefully structured to promote personal growth and to enable clients to arrive at their own solutions. The counsellor is a resource in the therapeutic process with the primary aim of facilitating this process. Characteristically, counsellors work in a non-directive style, although there may be situations in which they need to impose a more structured approach.

Counselling may form the main therapeutic approach in working with a client or may be used in conjunction with other therapies. Clients may be referred by other practitioners or, increasingly, through self-referral to statutory or voluntary agencies. The counselling may be done face-to-face or, in some situations, over the telephone. In either case the general principles, objectives and strategies are similar.

Counselling in Mental Health Practice

There are many opportunities for using counselling in mental health practice. Counselling may form part of a preplanned and ongoing programme or may be used in a more informal and spontaneous way. Depending upon the setting in which the counsellor practises, a wide variety of approaches may be used to facilitate relatively enduring changes in clients' thoughts, feelings and behaviour. In mental health practice the objectives may include:

- promoting insight and self-awareness;
- increasing self-confidence and self-esteem;
- developing social understanding;
- enhancing decision-making, problem-solving and coping skills;
- increasing personal responsibility and autonomy;
- resolving emotional distress;
- facilitating and supporting change;
- developing healthier and more effective relationship-making skills;
- improving social and communication skills;
- maintaining hope and motivation.

The Skills of the Counsellor

Effective counselling requires a broad repertoire of interpersonal and specialist skills and a sound knowledge base. These need to be used sensitively, selectively and with flexibility. The skills include:

1. *The ability to form therapeutic relationships with clients.* To demonstrate empathy, acceptance, genuineness, warmth, understanding and non-judgemental responses. To be perceived as a caring and supportive person. To create a safe and trusting climate. To meet the person's needs for security, self-awareness and insight (see also Unit 1.2).
2. *The ability to communicate clearly.* To speak clearly, to utilize their own non-verbal communication. To maintain an open posture, to demonstrate active listening. Observing the verbal and non-verbal communication of the client. Questioning technique. Pacing to the clients' responses (see also Unit 1.3).
3. *Specific counselling skills.* Planning and preparation for counselling sessions, to clarify client concerns, provide reassurance for people in

distress, to facilitate problem solving, awareness of strategies and resources, monitoring client progress and giving feedback, supporting client change, challenging, self-disclosure, techniques to facilitate client communication and understanding, to promote personal responsibility and mastery, appropriate use of audio-visual aids and written information, instructional skills, role modelling.
4. *Specific knowledge and skills related to the area of practice.* Drug or alcohol problems, crisis intervention, bereavement, relationship or sexual problems, advocacy, occupational problems, victim support, personal growth, learning difficulties, anxiety management, carer support, rape or incest, welfare benefits, social skills' training, self-harm.

Some counsellors may also work within a specific theoretical model or use a more generalized approach. Models used include humanistic, gestalt, behaviourist, cognitive, transactional analysis, rational emotive therapy.

Frequency, Duration and Number of Sessions

The frequency, duration and number of sessions are influenced by a number of factors:

1. The nature and severity of the client's problems – longstanding, degree of distress, crisis situation.
2. The resources available – counsellor's time, availability of rooms, client support network.
3. The client's progress during counselling – this can be very variable.

In clinical practice, 45–50 minutes once or twice a week at a prearranged time is common. It is important to keep to stated time boundaries. The environment used for counselling needs to be conducive to promoting security and suitable for client work – space, freedom from interruptions, minimal external distractions, privacy, warm, light, appropriate furniture, available as required.

Preparation for Client Work

1. *Personal preparation*: reviewing own experience and knowledge base in relation to client work, awareness of own feelings and expectations about client, previewing available information on client.
2. *Arranging clinical supervision from an experienced practitioner*: to provide support, to validate interventions and perceptions, to cope with the emotional demands, to reflect on experiences, to facilitate problem solving and decision making, to monitor client work, to enhance professional development.

3. *Recording of counselling sessions*: determining the nature of the records to be kept and the methods to be used – during or after sessions, written notes, audio or visual recording, use of appropriate rating scales, questionnaire or diary.
4. *Confirmation*: written information to client of appointment times, confirmation to co-ordinator or administration.

Stages in Counselling

The process of counselling, like that of therapeutic relationships, can be viewed as a series of stages that need to be worked through. The key elements are the development of the counsellor–client relationship and the strategies used to resolve the client's problems. The progress made in counselling may be very uneven and the relationship may also experience cycles of development and regression (see also Units 1.2 and 1.3).

Assessment

The first meeting with the client is particularly significant as it influences their expectations and attitudes towards future contacts. A range of strong emotions are likely to be evoked that may include guilt, apprehension, anger, hope, relief and bewilderment. The counsellor needs to be aware of how the client is likely to feel and behave at this stage. With skill these reactions can be used to facilitate the development of their relationship and to promote the client's self-awareness and understanding.

Initially, anxiety and defensiveness are likely to limit self-disclosure by clients to safe and non-threatening topics. The counsellor will also be closely scrutinized and watched by the client in an attempt to appraise the counsellor's personality and attitudes. As the relationship develops, the client will feel more confident about disclosing more intimate details about themselves. The key elements of this stage are:

1. Interventions to facilitate the development of the counsellor–client relationship.
2. Attempting to explore and understand the issues that brought the client to counselling.
3. Developing a baseline assessment and definition of the client's needs and problems.

A broad range of relationship and communication skills may be used, including:

1. Arranging the environment to facilitate communication and comfort.
2. Putting the client at ease – introductions, welcoming, acknowledgement, preferred name.

3. Clarifying the objectives of the counselling relationship and the counsellor's role.
4. Reassuring the client about the boundaries of confidentiality.
5. Demonstrating motivation and hope.
6. Role modelling desirable social skills.
7. Demonstrating active listening and attending.
8. Specifying and maintaining time boundaries.
9. Giving information as requested and required.
10. Reassuring the client that their problems or needs are not unique.
11. Negotiating a contract.
12. Using interventions to facilitate and reinforce client communication and self-disclosure:

   - skilled questioning technique;
   - restating – repeating the main ideas expressed by the client using their own words;
   - reflecting – accurately identifying and directing back to the client the feelings they are expressing;
   - summarizing – bringing together, simply and clearly, the main details expressed by the client;
   - paraphrasing – using other words, to rephrase briefly the essential meaning expressed by the client;
   - using verbal and non-verbal prompts;
   - demonstrating non-judgemental responses;
   - encouraging the client to describe their perceptions and experiences;
   - focussing on specific issues as appropriate;
   - pacing the session to the client's responses and allocating time;
   - coping with resistance and silence.

Action

From the groundwork of an established relationship and a degree of understanding of the client's presenting concerns, progress can be made towards identifying potential courses of action and implementing agreed strategies. Working at this more meaningful level can be much more stressful to both counsellor and client alike, and both will require support. While the counsellor's role is to provide support to their client, they will need to ensure that they have access to effective supervision. The key elements of this stage are:

1. An established relationship characterized by trust, intimacy and openness, with the resilience to withstand stress and confrontation.
2. Focussing and working on the client's concerns, promoting problem resolution and personal growth.

A broad range of communication and relationship skills may be used in addition to those from the previous stage:

1. Promoting continuity between sessions.
2. Supporting and encouraging problem solving and decision making.
3. Negotiating an action plan.
4. Supporting implementation of chosen strategies.
5. Encouraging self-evaluation and appraisal.
6. Monitoring and reviewing client progress.
7. Giving positive feedback and encouraging self-reward.
8. Ensuring the client has access to sources of information and recourses that are available.
9. Developing the client's coping skills.
10. Identifying and exploring themes that the client raises.
11. Interpreting themes and verbalizing what the client is implying.
12. Providing an alternative frame of reference and interpretations of the client's experience and perceptions.
13. Responding with immediacy, where appropriate – recognizing what is going on at a particular moment and communicating this constructively to the client.
14. Making observations of their behaviour and reactions which the person may not be aware of.
15. Focussing and exploring areas of significant meaning for the client.
16. Seeking clarification where the client is unclear or confused.
17. Confronting or challenging the client when they are evasive, resistant, hostile or when there are discrepancies in their behaviour, thoughts and feelings.
18. Providing support when the client is vulnerable or under stress.
19. Using counsellor self-disclosure with discretion where it would be helpful.
20. Making transitional statements and moving the conversation on.
21. Setting boundaries on potentially disruptive or threatening behaviour.
22. Ensuring compliance with negotiated contract.
23. Consistently maintaining time boundaries.
24. Reviewing homework and progress between each session.
25. Setting homework and planning for next session.
26. Drawing each session to a close with clear verbal and non-verbal signals for termination.
27. Closing each session with a summary of the areas covered.
28. Ending on a positive note.

Resolution

The ending of the counselling relationship may be:

1. Planned and predetermined, possibly part of a fixed term contract; or
2. Abrupt and unexpected, due to the client's sudden withdrawal or circumstances beyond the counsellor's control.

In either case it has to be recognized and acknowledged by both the client and the counsellor that their relationship is inevitably time-limited. The main factors that influence its duration are the client's progress and development and the counselling resources available, i.e. time, place and workload.

In practice the client should be prepared for ending the counselling relation well in advance. Impending closure can evoke powerful feelings that need to be acknowledged, used productively and resolved. Some clients may regard this as indicative of growth and progress and feel excited and pleased; others may feel extremely anxious and interpret this process as rejection, which may lead to feelings of hurt and loss. Attempts may be made to prolong the counselling by requests for further help, regression or the appearance of sudden additional problems. The key elements of this stage are:

1. Preparation of the client for the ending of counselling support.
2. Reinforcing client autonomy and mastery.
3. Acknowledging the progress and personal development made by the client.

A broad range of relationship and communication skills may be used in addition to those from previous stages:

1. Specifying from the start the time-limited nature of counselling.
2. Periodically drawing the client's attention to impending end.
3. Reviewing and summarizing progress towards stated personal goals.
4. Reflecting on experiences during counselling.
5. Giving constructive feedback.
6. Encouraging personal evaluation.
7. Allocating time for the discussion and evaluation of issues related to termination of counselling.
8. Providing opportunities to work through and resolve feelings related to termination of counselling.
9. Providing emotional support and practical advice.
10. Assisting clients to plan for the future.
11. Giving details on how to seek counselling help in future, if necessary.
12. Acknowledging the value of having worked with the client.
13. Bringing the relationship to a close.

Counselling Strategies

A wide range of strategies and interventions are used by counsellors. These are related to the counsellor's skills and knowledge base, the client's needs and the immediate situation. Some of those that are commonly used include the following.

Use of contracts

Some counsellors, where appropriate, develop therapeutic contracts with clients. The contract may be verbal or written and the process of constructing the contract may be used as part of the therapeutic process to facilitate understanding, to reinforce commitment and to set clear expectations from the start. The contract may specify:

1. The rights of the client as a consumer of the service.
2. The rights of the counsellor as a practitioner.
3. The purpose and rationale of the counsellor's therapeutic approach.
4. What will be required of the client in terms of participation and homework.
5. The confidentiality of any information.
6. The need to keep appointments and who to contact if unable to do so.
7. Practical issues, e.g. time, place, frequency, duration of sessions, availability of support between sessions during a crisis.

Problem-solving and decision-making strategies

In many counselling situations clients seek help with problem solving and decision making. Their difficulties may arise from their perception of a situation, a lack of information, indecisiveness, feeling trapped and helpless, or great stress. The counsellor's role in these cases is to enable the client to take personal responsibility for their own lives and to arrive at the decisions and solutions that are best for them. The counsellor may utilize a problem-solving strategy to facilitate this process:

1. Assessment

Through skilled communication, empathy and clarification to identify and define the nature of the problems. To provide an environment and relationship that facilitates trust, openness and honesty. Using questionnaires, diary, video, role play, checklists or other techniques to facilitate expression. This stage may take some time and it may be beneficial to use this process to increase the client's understanding and self-awareness.

2. Planning

(a) To generate and explore potential options using the client's experience, the counsellor's skills and knowledge and the use of specific techniques, e.g. brainstorming, research, use of contacts, potential resources.
(b) To evaluate potential options and alternatives in terms of the client's value system, the resources available and their attainability.
(c) To enable the client to make realistic choices in relation to their unique situation and their personal preferences. Exploring feelings about the choices made to ensure the client's commitment.

(d) Identifying the resources required to implement these choices – information, new skills, changes in life-style or relationships, support from others, counsellor's time.

(e) Collaborating with the client to develop a planned programme with step-by-step goals that are clear, realistic and measurable.

(f) Reinforcing the client's commitment through formulating a verbal or written contract.

3. *Implementation*

(a) Supporting the carrying out of the action plan.
(b) Giving guidance as required.
(c) Giving positive reinforcement – counsellor approval is a very potent reinforcer to facilitate and promote change.
(d) Encouraging client self-reward and reinforcement.
(e) Giving ongoing constructive feedback.
(f) Acknowledging and working through any difficulties experienced by the client in relation to the planned programme.
(g) Reinforcing the fact that change is possible.
(h) Promoting personal responsibility for the client's own actions.

4. *Evaluation*

(a) Monitoring compliance with the action plan and any set homework.
(b) Affirming and validating attainment of goals and client progress.
(c) Utilizing appropriate methods to evaluate progress – questioning, checklists, diary, audio-visual recording.
(d) Reviewing goals and replanning for client growth, mastery and autonomy.

Working with client resistance

Clients are not always able or willing to communicate with a counsellor. The processes of seeking and needing help can evoke powerful feelings that may be directed towards the counsellor. Clients may also lack insight into themselves or the nature of their difficulties. In particular, distress and guilt can, consciously and unconsciously, reduce self-awareness. These feelings may be expressed in a variety of ways, e.g. resistance, resentment, silence, lateness or non-attendance, hostility, challenging the credibility and validity of the counsellor's interventions.

It is important for the counsellor to acknowledge the validity of these feelings for the client and to use constructively the process of working through these difficulties to promote the client's mental health. It takes considerable skill and experience to feel comfortable with these strong feelings and to feel confident about the interventions chosen.

The specific counselling interventions will depend upon the nature of the client's needs and the stage of the helping relationship. Interventions that may be useful include:

- acknowledging the client's feelings and accepting them as normal;
- demonstrating non-judgemental and empathic responses;
- working on the therapeutic relationship to develop trust;
- reassurance about confidentiality;
- facilitating client disclosure and expression of feelings;
- giving positive feedback;
- working on small goals;
- limiting client distress;
- reframing overwhelming difficulties into more realistic and manageable perspectives.

Challenging and confrontation

At times during the counselling relationship the counsellor may become aware that the client has difficulty acknowledging or focussing upon certain areas. They may be evasive, dismissive or defensive about these topics. There may be times when firmly entrenched self-defeating attitudes, expectations or a negative self-image are also maintaining or contributing towards personal difficulties. Discrepancies and incongruities may also be identified in the client's thought processes, behaviour and feelings. These client responses indicate that the counsellor is approaching very sensitive areas that are important to the client's integrity. However, if these areas are negatively influencing the client's mental health, then the counsellor may need to challenge or confront the person with these distortions in order to:

1. Promote self-awareness and understanding.
2. Facilitate the development of more reality-based and helpful expectations and attributions.
3. Promote the development of a more positive and realistic self-image.
4. Enhance the person's sense of control and mastery and thereby their sense of personal responsibility.
5. Facilitate problem solving and decision making.
6. Support desired behavioural and emotional changes.

Challenging and confrontation are powerful interventions that need to be used with sensitivity if the outcomes are not to be destructive or negative. Clients can respond in a number of ways that may include:

1. Acceptance of the challenge and a desire to work through the issues.
2. Rejection of the challenge – dismissiveness, complacency, procrastination, blaming others, superficially agreeing, refusing to accept the challenge.

3. Counter-attacking the counsellor – doubting the counsellor's credibility, hostility and abuse.

Effective confrontation requires:

1. A well-established therapeutic relationship, particularly empathy and trust.
2. An ability to identify situations when challenging is appropriate.
3. Care in the way that the challenge is made – specific, direct, honest, non-destructive, strengths rather than weaknesses.
4. Being prepared for self-challenge – able to validate and assert your interpretations and perceptions, acceptance and non-judgemental responses.
5. Allowing time to work through and resolve positively any feelings that are evoked, and to remain focussed on the issues.

Counselling strategies for thinking difficulties

Many people experience difficulties in everyday life due to the way that they perceive and interpret situations and their own personal value system and expectations. Common difficulties include:

1. *Negative and disabling self-talk*: attributing inevitable difficulties and failure to intended personal actions. This reinforces feelings of hopelessness and helplessness.
2. *Low self-esteem*: personal devaluation of own self-worth. This can adversely influence attainment of personal needs and relationships with others.
3. *Punitive expectations*: constant expectations of negative and stressful outcomes in all situations. Expriences are anticipated and interpreted in relation to this negative value system.
4. *Unrealistic and overdemanding personal standards*: personal actions are invariably perceived as falling short of very high and harsh self-imposed standards. This can create considerable stress as the person strives to attain these demanding standards.
5. *Irrational beliefs and values*: these may complicate patterns of everyday living and relating to others. Such beliefs may be illogical and ill-founded and yet have a profound influence.

A wide range of counselling interventions may be used that aim to help the person:

1. Formulate more realistic and helpful standards and expectations.
2. Develop a more positive self-image and raise their self-esteem.
3. Correct factual inaccuracies in their belief system.
4. Develop positive coping self-statements and expectations.

Techniques used to facilitate the exploration of alternative frames of reference and to re-frame new beliefs and value systems include:

- focussed exploration and specificity;
- mental health education and promotion to correct misinformation and to develop the person's self- and social understanding (see Unit 3.3);
- challenging irrational beliefs;
- providing alternative and more helpful interpretations of perceptions and experiences;
- use of feedback – using structured diaries and homework assignments;
- role play and social skills training;
- development of coping skills;
- cognitive rehearsal and visual imagery;
- anxiety management and relaxation training.

Counsellor self-disclosure

Counselling is a two-way relationship. As much as the counsellor is attempting to understand and appraise the client, the client likewise is attempting to understand and appraise their counsellor. Clients observe counsellors' verbal and non-verbal behaviour, their clothing and manner, the decor of the office or counselling room and make various assumptions about them as people. Generally, the emphasis in the counselling relationship is upon the client's perceptions and experiences. However, there may be situations when self-disclosure by the counsellor can be used to attain therapeutic objectives.

Self-disclosure by helpers needs to be used carefully within the counselling relationship to avoid burdening or threatening the client, losing credibility or shifting the emphasis away from the client. Skilfully used, self-disclosure can be used to:

- model a useful social skill;
- facilitate disclosure by the client;
- increase the client's social awareness and understanding;
- develop the counselling relationship;
- maintain hope and demonstrate that positive change is possible.

In using self-disclosure the counsellor needs to be aware of:

1. The timing and appropriateness of the examples given.
2. The relevance and accessibility of the experiences shared.
3. The need to be selective and to limit the number of times they use self-disclosure.
4. The need to present positive outcomes as a result of difficulties faced.

Evaluating client progress and counsellor effectiveness

The client's progress and counsellor effectiveness needs to be monitored carefully and evaluated. A wide range of methods and sources of feedback may be used:

1. Self-analysis – critical self-appraisal of own practice.
2. Post-counselling evaluation and discussion with colleagues.
3. Analysis and feedback from supervisor.
4. Analysis of written records, process recordings, checklists or charts that are completed either during or after counselling sessions.
5. Comments and feedback from clients – completion of assignments and homework, statements made during sessions, questionnaires and rating scales, diary, observation of non-verbal behaviour, development of trust, and compliance with agreed programmes.
6. Comments and feedback from carers and relatives where appropriate.
7. Statistical information – punctuality, lateness, non-attendance, drop-out rate, number of sessions per client, recurrence of client problems.

When feedback is given to the client it is more effective if:

- the client requests it,
- it focusses on positives,
- it is concrete and specific,
- it is used selectively,
- the counsellor checks out and verifies the client's understanding.

See also Unit 3.4 "Social Skills Training" on methods and presentation of feedback.

Referral of clients to other agencies

Clients may need to be referred to other agencies for a variety of reasons. These may include:

1. The need for specialist help for specific problems – occupational, marital, sexual, medical, spiritual, learning difficulties, financial.
2. Reaching the limits of the counsellor's experience and knowledge.
3. Difficulty in working with the client – lack of progress, personality clash, over-identification with the client's problems.

The need for referral may be apparent early on in the counselling relationship or may become increasingly evident over a period of time. Referral may be a difficult issue to raise and some clients may react strongly to what they might perceive as rejection or negative feedback. Some counsellors may also feel strongly about referral. Feelings on both sides need to be acknowledged and worked through. If referral is necessary, then:

1. A suitable agency needs to be identified in relation to the client's needs.
2. The reasons need to be explained and discussed with the client.
3. Arrangements need to be confirmed with the new agency and passed on to the client.
4. A summary needs to be prepared for the referral agency.

Unit Instructions

When you have researched the suggested references, have mastered the Unit Objectives and successfully answered the Self-assessment Questions, proceed with the Unit Written Test.

Suggested References

Brearley, G. and Birchley, P. (1986). *Introducing Counselling Skills and Techniques*. Faber and Faber, London.

Burnard, P. (1987). The right direction. *Senior Nurse*, Vol. 7, No. 1, pp. 30–32.

Buckroyd, J. (1987). The nurse as counsellor. *Nursing Times*, 15 July, Vol. 83, No. 28, pp. 42–44.

Dexter, G. and Wash, M. (1986). *Psychiatric Nursing Skills: A Patient-centred Approach*. Croom Helm, London.

Dobson, M. (1987). Hindrance or help? *Senior Nurse*, Vol. 6, No. 6, pp. 18–19.

Egan, G. (1986). *The Skilled Helper*, 3rd edition. Brooks/Cole, Monterey.

French, P. (1983). *Social Skills for Nursing Practice*. Croom Helm, London.

Inskipp, F. (1986). *A Manual for Trainers: A Resource Book for Setting Up and Running Basic Counselling Courses*. Alexia Publications.

Kagan, C., Evans, J. and Kay, B. (1986). *A Manual of Interpersonal Skills for Nurses: An Experiential Approach*. Harper and Row, London.

Munro, E. A., Mantrel, R. J. and Small, J. J. (1983). *Counselling: A Skills Approach*, revised edition. Methuen, New Zealand.

Murgatroyd, S. (1985). *Counselling and Helping*. British Psychological Society and Methuen, London.

Nelson-Jones, R. (1982). *The Theory and Practice of Counselling Psychology*. Holt, Rinehart and Winston, London.

Nelson-Jones, R. (1983). *Practical Counselling and Helping Skills*. 2nd edition. Cassell, London.

Nelson-Jones, R. (1986). *Human Relationship Skills*. Holt, Rinehart and Winston, London.

Priestley, P. and McGuire, J. (1983). *Learning to Help*. Tavistock, London.

Stewart, S. (1983). *Counselling in Nursing: A Problem-Solving Approach*. Harper and Row, London.

Stewart, W. (1987). Counselling is not discipline. *Nursing Times*, 13 May, Vol. 83, No. 19, pp. 30–31.

Tschudin, V. (1987). *Counselling Skills for Nurses*, 2nd edition. Baillière Tindall, London and San Diego.

Wilson, H. and Kneisl, C. (1988). *Psychosocial Nursing Concepts: An Activity Book*. Addison-Wesley, New York.

Self-assessment Questions

SAQ 1. List four potential uses of counselling in mental health practice.
SAQ 2. Identify four interventions that facilitate client self-disclosure.
SAQ 3. Outline four factors that need to be considered when using confrontation or challenging.
SAQ 4. Describe four ways of evaluating client progress in counselling.

Unit 3.1: Written Test

John Stewart, aged 20, is studying for a degree in computing at a local university. He has been referred for help from the University Welfare Service to the Community Mental Health Centre. They indicate that he is feeling unnecessarily depressed and anxious about his studies, perceiving himself to be behind everyone else. He is also experiencing difficulties forming relationships with female students and is worrying that he may be a homosexual.

During counselling he appears to be very mixed up and finds it difficult to talk and express himself.

1. What counselling strategies can be used to facilitate John's self-expression and communication?
2. How can John be helped to gain a more realistic self-appraisal of his academic progress.
3. What approaches may be helpful in enabling John to clarify his sexual identity and to facilitate his ability to form relationships with female students?

Group Work Skills

Unit Objectives

At the end of this Unit the learner should be able to:

1. Outline the uses of group approaches in mental health practice.
2. Describe the characteristics of effective group leadership.
3. Specify the stages of group development and interventions to facilitate this process.
4. Identify ways that the effectiveness of a group can be evaluated.

The Nature of Groups

Groups can exert a powerful influence over members' behaviour. People have a natural tendency to form into groups and strong forces and motivations draw people together. These processes are complex and individuals vary considerably in their understanding and awareness of such group dynamics. Through membership of various groups, people attempt to meet basic social needs for security, belonging, approval and esteem. These compelling needs for affiliation, recognition and social contact, together with the forces that try to maintain and perpetuate a group, give groups their great potential to influence members. Used carefully and with skill, group processes can be utilized to attain positive outcomes for group members and to enhance the potential of a number of therapeutic approaches. The characteristics of a group include:

1. *Defined membership*: a boundary that differentiates members from non-members, an awareness of membership, stability and continuity of membership, identification with the group, rewards and benefits of group membership, e.g. acceptance, inclusion, regard.
2. *Time spent together*: shared experience of membership, time to develop relationships and roles within the group, group history, planned or ongoing life-span, sense of continuity, progress on task attainments.
3. *Common goals and purpose*: focus on specific group tasks and objectives, presence of an organizing influence, suppression of individual needs to work together, creation of a shared hidden agenda.

4. *Interaction*: opportunity for face-to-face contact with other members, participation and communication with fellow members.
5. *Development of norms*: standards or ground rules that govern behaviour, communication and beliefs in the group, and upon which member's behaviour is judged; sanctions and controlling processes that are used to enforce compliance; facilitating or negative influence of norms; explicit, conscious or spoken nature of norms, or implicit, subconscious and non-spoken nature of norms.

Groups in Mental Health Practice

There are many opportunities for using group approaches in mental health practice. Many nursing activities in particular involve working with groups of people. The group may be a planned and structured experience or may be more informal and spontaneous. Although there are a number of approaches to group work they do have certain commonalities in terms of group processes and development. Within the group approach the primary focus may be:

1. To facilitate other activities – social events, domestic and household tasks, committee meetings, care conferences, health education, training sessions.
2. To support a specific therapeutic approach – reality orientation, social skills and assertiveness training, problem-solving group, anxiety management, music and drama therapy, self-help.
3. Upon the group dynamics and processes – encounter group, group psychotherapy, support group.

Group approaches can be used in mental health practice to facilitate relatively enduring changes in members' thoughts, feelings and behaviour. Depending upon the nature of the group and its objectives, the outcomes may include:

- increased insight and self-awareness;
- increased self-confidence and self-esteem;
- increased understanding and awareness of others;
- enhanced problem-solving and coping skills;
- healthier and more effective relationship-making skills;
- improved social and communication skills;
- raised hope and motivation;
- willingness to take and accept responsibility;
- improved knowledge and skills in relation to group tasks and objectives;
- more realistic attitudes and expectations.

There are a number of processes whereby groups facilitate personal change. Depending upon the nature of the group these may include:

1. *Observational learning*: imitation, role modelling, demonstration, identi-fication, internalization.
2. *Information*: instruction, advice, shared experience, discussion, sugges-tion, learning new concepts.
3. *Universality*: the awareness that others also have difficulties, sharing of problems and experiences with others, reduced feelings of isolation, understanding of personal limitations and development of realistic expectations.
4. *Altruism*: helping and supporting others, the chance to be valued, reassurance and aid, developing trust with others, cooperation.
5. *Catharsis*: emotional release, the opportunity to work through unresolved issues, discussion of feelings, the chance to talk.
6. *Opportunities for new and differing experiences*: chance to try out new patterns of relating and emotional expression, risk taking in a safe and supportive environment, behavioural rehearsal and practice, explore solutions and alternatives, reality testing.
7. *Instillation of hope*: awareness of the potential for positive change, maintaining motivation and commitment to the group.
8. *Feedback*: observations and comments from group leaders and fellow members on person's behaviour, perceptions and emotional reactions, guidance and suggestions, positive reinforcement, public esteem.
9. *Group cohesiveness*: common sense of purpose, support and closeness, acceptance, trust in the group, rewards of group membership, attractive-ness of the group, intimacy, inclusion. (There is a paradox that if the group becomes too cohesive then members will attend to the processes of group membership at the expense of task attainment.)

Effective Group Leadership

The effectiveness of a group is primarily related to the skills and sensitivity of the group leader. This requires systematic training and supervised experience in the area of group work in which the person intends to practise. Unfortunately, the skills of group work are often learnt through trial and error and the potential inherent in groups is often not realized.

Depending upon the nature of the group and his/her own personality, the leader may adopt a particular leadership style – democratic, informal and facilitative or formal and directive. The chosen style needs to be one that the leader feels comfortable with and is appropriate to the group's aims and objectives. Generally, group processes are facilitated if the leader is non-authoritarian and is able to delegate leadership functions to the group as it develops.

In practice, leadership styles are highly individualistic and there is little consensus from research on which is the most effective. None the less, there are certain responsibilities and obligations placed upon leaders which they need to consider. Additionally, members may have expectations about the role of the leader which can lead to a strong reaction if the leader does not behave as anticipated.

The specific leadership interventions that are appropriate at a given moment will relate to the situation and the stage of development of the group. Overall, to be an effective group leader, the nurse needs to be able to:

1. *Form therapeutic relationships with the group*: to demonstrate empathy, acceptance, genuineness, warmth, to be perceived as a caring and supportive person. To create a safe and trusting climate. To meet member's needs for security and belongingness. To relate equally to all members and not to focus on individuals or show preferences.
2. *Communicate clearly*: to speak clearly, attend to their own non-verbal communication. To demonstrate active listening and acknowledge contributions by members. To utilize exercises, audio-visual aids and other sources of information to facilitate understanding. To give practical advice and information, to refer members to available resources. To explain and clarify issues.
3. *Facilitate group development*: to orientate individuals to the group, to enhance relationships and trust within the group. To encourage communication and participation. To facilitate self-disclosure and openness. To demonstrate enthusiasm for the group. To interpret and analyse group dynamics. To challenge and stimulate.
4. *Demonstrate competence in the group activity*: planning and preparation, to demonstrate and give guidance on tasks. To clarify and suggest approaches to tasks. To monitor and give feedback. To facilitate transfer and generalization of learning, to act as a role model. To be knowledgeable and skilful in task activity.
5. *To implement executive functions of leadership*: to define and clarify their role as group leader. To imitate and specify tasks. To reinforce group rules and norms. To set limits on behaviour, to manage time and maintain time boundaries. To challenge group members and to cope with leadership challenges. To resist manipulation.

Co-leadership

In a number of group situations there may be advantages in working with a co-leader. These can include:

1. Mutual support, particularly in potentially stressful group settings.
2. An increased range of skills and experience to bring to the group.
3. Feedback on interventions from the other leader.
4. Learning opportunities for trainee group leaders.
5. Observations and interpretations from two perspectives.
6. Opportunities to work in sub-groups to increase participation and feedback.
7. Providing two role models to group members.
8. Demonstrating a cooperative relationship to the group.

9. Ensuring continuity of leadership in case one leader is absent or leaves.
10. Dividing leadership functions and tasks.

To work effectively, the two group leaders need to ensure that they:

- are familiar with each other's style of leadership and working;
- follow similar approaches and can complement each other;
- present a balanced team appropriate to the group, e.g. male and female, two therapists of same gender;
- are both committed to working together and can agree on an appropriate style of partnership, e.g. egalitarian, leader plus observer, trainer and trainee;
- have time to plan in advance and to develop their own relationship.

Planning and Preparation for Group Work

Careful planning and preparation are important to ensure the effectiveness of any group approach. There are a number of factors that need to be considered.

Type of group

1. *Open group*: where members may join or leave the group at any stage during the group's lifetime. An open group can often be run for an indefinite period and cater for a changing client group. However, the frequent changes of membership can inhibit the development of cohesion and trust, limiting its potential.
2. *Closed group*: where the membership is fixed throughout the lifetime of the group. Once begun, no new members can be accepted, and great emphasis is laid on continuity of membership. The advantages of this stability are the increased opportunities for cohesion and trust to develop between members.

Whether a group is open or closed will depend on the purposes and objectives of the group and on the nature of the client group.

Group size

Group processes and interaction are considerably influenced by the number of members. Generally, smaller groups with 6–10 members plus leader(s) are more effective in therapeutic and educational settings because:

1. Relationships, and hence trust and cohesion, develop more quickly. Large groups tend to be inhibiting.

2. Within a small group it is possible to maintain face-to-face communication with all the other members. With greater numbers there is a tendency for sub-groups to form which may have competing objectives with the overall purpose of the group.
3. Opportunities for participation and individual recognition are greater. This enhances personal satisfaction and commitment to the group.
4. Leaders are able to give more effective direction, to monitor group processes and task attainment and to give more valid feedback.
5. There is an optimum balance between the resources that members are able to contribute to the group and their utilization through discussion and decision making. In larger groups there is potentially a greater range of ideas, but consensus becomes more problematic.

Larger groups may also be used effectively for specific purposes. Leaders may also use methods within a large group setting to facilitate personal involvement and to develop relationships. Exercises and tasks may be set that require people to pair off or work in small numbers and then to feedback to the main group.

Selection of members

The membership of any group is a critical factor in determining how effectively it can operate. The opportunities for selection, though, may be limited by self-selection, referral or the presence of a resident population. This is not necessarily a disincentive for group work, as what may appear to be a random mix of personalities can work very effectively, whereas an apparently well-selected group may fail to develop.

In terms of selection the leader has to consider not only the individuals' past history and current needs but also their potential in terms of how they are likely to relate and interact with other possible members. The selection also needs to consider the overall objectives of the group activity and the person's potential to benefit from such an approach. In some settings it may be possible to have a pre-selection interview or meeting with candidates so that both have the opportunity to preview each other.

The leader should ensure that the composition of the group does not vary to the extent that one or more of the members would be readily identified as being significantly different from the rest. A degree of homogeneity is important in promoting relatedness and identification within the group. Members who are perceived as "deviant" may be isolated from the others and be a focus for hostile feelings in the group – "scapegoating".

Factors that may need to be considered are:

1. *The range of problems, needs and abilities*: specific behaviour and emotional problems or a wide range; similar or dissimilar needs; similar or mixed ability.

2. *Age range*: specific age group, e.g. children, teenagers, young adults, middle-aged or elderly, or people of various ages.
3. *Racial and cultural origins*: mixed race, ethnic group.
4. *Socio-economic status*: employed, unemployed, social class, education.
5. *Sex distribution and gender*: all male or female, mixed, heterosexual or other sexual preferences.
6. *Motivation*: high motivation, limited commitment, voluntary or forced attendance.

Group aims and objectives

The leaders need to be clear as to the overall purpose of the group activity and the structure of the programme. The particular goals of the group will be influenced by:

- the characteristics of the group members;
- the purposes and objectives of the group activity;
- the skills and experience of the group leaders.

These will influence the specific methodology used by the leaders to attain the group objectives and meet the members' needs. General objectives may include:

- the development of the members' knowledge, skills or self-awareness;
- the provision of a safe environment where members can develop relationships with one another. .

Group leaders may also need to consider whether additional personal support may be necessary for individuals outside of the group setting and the resource implications of this.

Frequency, duration and timing of meetings

The frequency, duration and timing will depend upon:

- the nature of the group;
- the aims and objectives of the group;
- the resources available – group leaders' skills and availability of time, space and rooms, equipment.

For effective group development the members will need to meet fairly regularly for a sufficient period of time. In practice, weekly or bi-weekly meetings for 1–2 hours over several months enable group processes to operate and to attain desired objectives.

Once planned, it is important that the agreed timing is strictly adhered to. Starting on time and finishing promptly are significant time boundaries that need to be maintained by the leader. This also helps to give structure to the group sessions and to enhance members' security.

Place

The setting and the environment need to be conducive to promoting security and group development. The factors to be considered are:

- suitability,
- space,
- freedom from interruptions,
- minimum external distractions,
- privacy,
- warm,
- light,
- furniture,
- wall coverings and posters,
- adaptability of environmemnt.

Where possible the furniture should be rearranged to facilitate group interaction and eye-to-eye contact. The room should be available at the specified time for the duration of the group activity and anticipated life-span.

Leadership preparation

The style of leadership selected needs to be appropriate to the group members, the objectives of the programme and the personal characteristics of the group leader, e.g. permissive, directive, facilitative. These will also influence the desirability and appropriateness of co-leadership. Other leadership issues may include:

1. *Personal preparation*: reviewing their own experience and knowledge in relation to the intended group work, being aware of their feelings and expectations.
2. *Supervision*: an experienced supervisor should be identified who is available for regular supervision. Group work in any context is a complex process and sensitive supervision is required to validate their interventions and perceptions, cope with the demands made, reflect on their experiences, help with decision making, monitor their work and facilitate professional development.
3. *Recording of group work*: what records will be kept, methods to be used – written, audio or video tape, diary, rating scales, questionnaires – and

the issues to be recorded – cohesion, interaction between members, levels of participation, attendance, group climate, decisions, themes, group development, changes, informal rules, plans made, roles adopted by members, specific problems.

Contracts with members

The function of a contract with group members is to ensure that they are clear about:

1. The purposes and rationale of the group activity.
2. What will be required of them in terms of participation and possible assignments between groups.
3. The need for regular attendance and commitment.
4. Specific issues related to the group objectives and processes, if appropriate, e.g. confidentiality, contact between members outside of group settings.
5. Practical issues, e.g. time, place, frequency, duration.

Group leaders may formulate a preliminary contract either to discuss with individuals at a pre-selection interview or for subsequent negotiation with the group. The use of a contract in this way:

- reinforces understanding of the function and role of the group;
- reduces anxiety and also any potential drop out rate;
- facilitates attainment of group objectives by setting clear expectations for members.

Confirmation

All details related to the group should be confirmed with colleagues and any other key individuals in the organization. Where appropriate, relatives should also be notified.

Stages in Group Development

Groups, characteristically, evolve and work through a series of stages of development. The rate at which a group progresses can vary considerably and at times there may be setbacks which will need to be resolved before the group can recover its momentum.

Group formation: introductory, early or beginning phase

The first meeting of any group is extremely important in influencing the expectations, attitudes and behaviour of the members towards future meetings. Hence, it is particularly important that the group leaders are aware of how members are likely to feel and behave at this stage and to be able to work with these reactions to facilitate group formation.

The group may consist of people who have never met before or who already have a working relationship with one another. In either case, meeting together in a new situation can create strong feelings. Depending upon the nature of the group and the individual members' expectations, the range of emotions could be anxiety, excitement, puzzlement, apprehension, anger or suspicion.

Anxiety is particularly high during the early stages of the group and people are likely to behave in a guarded and defensive manner. Attempts will be made to increase feelings of security by efforts to form relationships and to impose a sense of structure on the situation. Clues will be sought on how to behave and on what to say within the group setting. Other group members and, in particular, the leaders, will be closely observed, tested out and evaluated. From this appraisal the person will attempt to define for themselves an appropriate personal role and to negotiate a group consensus.

Self-disclosure is limited to social and non-threatening topics and members will try to ensure that they project a favourable image. While people have a strong need to affiliate with their fellow group members there is also the fear of rejection and embarrassment.

The role of the leaders at this stage are:

1. To create a non-threatening and trusting climate in which the members can give support and encouragement to one another. Various strategies may be used, e.g. "ice breakers", group activities or other specific techniques.
2. To facilitate interaction and to promote intimacy. Establishing a groundwork of working rules or a contract on how to achieve the group's aims and to promote group relationships, are likely to be a particular focus of activity during the early stages. Leadership interventions at this stage which can help group formation and may also be appropriate at other stages of the group include:

   - pre-planning practical and attainable group activities that can accommodate change and promote spontaneity;
   - arranging the environment to facilitate group interaction;
   - clarifying for group members the role and function of the group, the aims and objectives, the methods and activities that will be used;
   - specifying from the start the period when the group will end;
   - introducing and defining their own role in the group;
   - role modelling desirable group behaviour – acceptance, non-judgemental, enthusiasm;
   - participating themselves in group activities and sharing their feelings with the group;
   - encouraging members to participate and to develop relationships through activities, discussion and reflecting questions to the group, acknowledging contributions;

- promoting feelings of security, reducing feelings of anxiety and offering support by creating a climate of trust;
- giving recognition and positive reinforcement to members;
- observing participation and communication between members, verbal and non-verbal;
- actively listening to contributions and identifying themes in what is said;
- maintaining time boundaries for the commencement and ending of group sessions.

Group development: middle, working or active phase

With the development of a climate of trust and a basic structure of relationships and norms, the group becomes a more productive unit and members are able to work together more effectively. Paradoxically, some of the signs of this growing closeness, security and trust are demonstrated by the members' confidence in being able to confront, challenge and criticize other members and the group leaders. However, members are also much more open with others and feel able to offer emotional and practical support.

During this stage the leaders are increasingly able to delegate aspects of group leadership to the members to enable the group to become self-perpetuating. The leaders, though, still need to be alert to group feelings and progress and to provide sufficient direction, where required, to facilitate attainment of group objectives.

Leadership interventions at this stage which can help group development and may also be appropriate at other stages of the group include:

- Ensuring that the programme for each session is clear and sufficient for the time available.
- Utilizing a variety of techniques to increase stimulation.
- Maintaining time boundaries for the starting and finishing of group activities.
- Periodically reminding members of future group termination.
- Promoting continuity of group themes and activities by reviewing the previous session, recalling details from previous groups and linking current activities to the overall group programme.
- Promoting and facilitating participation by all members.
- Encouraging group members to share their observations, ventilate their feelings and express their opinions by supporting self-disclosure.
- Redirecting and reflecting enquiries back to the group, where appropriate.
- Providing positive reinforcement and opportunities to participate to increase member satisfaction.
- Protecting and supporting members when they appear to be vulnerable or under stress.
- Offering accurate feedback and tentative interpretation to group

members on their behaviour, relationships and communication within the group.

- Focussing on specific issues which need to be worked through and which others may wish to avoid.
- Confronting and challenging members, if required, pointing out what they are doing and its effects on others.
- Setting boundaries on potentially disruptive and threatening behaviour.
- Encouraging comparisons of group and personal experiences.
- Stressing that members' problems and difficulties are not unique.
- Testing members' understanding and group consensus; seeking and giving clarification.
- Listening for, identifying and exploring group themes.
- Supporting and encouraging problem solving and decision making; encouraging members to share strategies and personal solutions.
- Delegating leadership functions on to the group as it is able to cope with them.
- Encouraging evaluation by members of the group's progress.
- Periodically reviewing the group's progress towards stated goals.
- Drawing the group to a close at the end of each session, summarizing the group's activities and themes.
- Planning with group members for the next group session and any homework assignments.

Group termination: closure or final phase

The ending of the group may result from a planned and foreseen event due to reaching the end of the programme or as an unexpected closure due to, for example, falling membership, staff or organizational changes, or sickness of group leaders. If the group activity has been planned for a fixed period, or even if it is premature, then it is very important that members have the opportunity to prepare as far as possible in advance for the ending of the group.

Closure of the group can evoke powerful feelings that need to be acknowledged, used productively and resolved. If the group has been a positive experience, then members are likely to feel a sense of loss and insecurity. These may be expressed as sadness, grief, anger, regression, disruption of task activities, withdrawal and apathy. Attempts may be made to prolong the life of the group through requests to extend the programme or to plan reunions with members. Members may also feel excited or pleased at the progress they have made or at the opportunity to cease attending.

Leadership interventions which can help group members to prepare and cope with termination include:

- specifying from the start when the group will end;
- periodically drawing the group's attention to the impending end of the group;

- reviewing and summarizing the progress made by the group;
- giving feedback to members on their progress in the group;
- reflecting on group experiences;
- devoting time for the discussion and evaluation of specific issues related to termination of the group;
- offering opportunities to work through and resolve feelings related to the termination of the group;
- providing emotional support and practical advice to members;
- helping members to plan for the future;
- bringing the group to a close.

Problems in Groups

If a group works well it can be a very productive and rewarding experience. However, for a variety of reasons, a group can also be very frustrating and negative. Problems can arise from a number of sources:

1. *Poor planning and organization*: confused arrangements, unclear instructions, inappropriate or unrealistic tasks, lack of resources, environmental distractions, poor selection of members for group objectives.
2. *Lack of skilled leadership*: inability to direct the group, inappropriate interventions, inaccurate analysis and feedback, demonstrating favouritism, colluding with the group, over-controlling and inability to delegate.
3. *Membership difficulties*: practical external difficulties, conflict of personal and group goals and needs, hostile expectations, unrealistic preconceptions about group roles and functions, compulsory attendance, previous negative experiences of group situations, newcomers to the group, stresses experienced in joining and staying within the group, lack of trust in the group.

The problems can be expressed in a variety of ways:

1. *Attendance issues*: persistent absences and lateness, attempts to finish early, blaming the group, doubts about validity of group membership, threatening to leave. Non-attendance can exert a powerful influence even though the member is not present.
2. *Apathy and withdrawal*: low participation, lack of enthusiasm, lack of volunteers, yawning, gaps in conversation, inattention, poor recall of previous groups.
3. *Silence*: a very powerful form of expression that may indicate a wide range of emotions, e.g. resistance, disinterest, aggression, or positive feelings such as reflection, calmness or thought. It takes considerable experience to feel comfortable with silence and to identify its nature. Depending upon the type of group, the way that members cope with the silence and the way it is resolved can be particularly significant.
4. *Avoidance of tasks and issues*: distracting, challenging value of group,

not planning ahead, avoiding pressing issues, extreme caution and reluctance to take risks, misunderstandings, denial of tasks or problems, inhibitions.

5. *Over-dependency on the leader*: not taking responsibility, reliance on leader for decisions, lack of initiative, over-supportive leader, collusion.
6. *Scapegoating*: focussing of negative and unacceptable feelings on to a vulnerable member, constant blaming of certain individuals, rejecting or ostracizing an individual from full group membership.
7. *Conflict between members*: hostility, ridicule, impatience, not listening, misunderstandings, challenging, threatening, lack of trust, withdrawal and apathy, rejection of ideas and suggestions.
8. *Conflict with group leaders*: challenging, doubts on competence, lack of trust, hostility, withdrawal and apathy, silences, rejection of ideas and suggestions, attempts to divert group away from tasks, competition for leadership by dominant members, attacks on leadership style.

The presence of difficulties within the group does not necessarily indicate a failure or setback. The issues raised and the way that they are resolved can be a useful learning experience for members and leaders alike. The group's ability to cope constructively with problems can provide useful feedback on its progress and the levels of trust that exist between members. Paradoxically, the experience of conflict may also serve to increase cohesion within the group and to promote solidarity. Total resolution of problems may not always be desirable or possible and members may have to learn to tolerate or cope with the presence of unresolved issues.

Depending upon the type of group it is important for the leaders to accept that it is not always either their responsibility or possible to resolve all issues. In many situations it is far more productive for the group to be allowed or facilitated to work on the issues and to arrive at a group solution. Problems may be resolved through:

1. *Communication*: discussion, acknowledgement, negotiation, support, reassurance, compromise, validation, emotional release, sharing experiences and solutions, questioning, feedback, voting.
2. *Specific techniques*: sculpting, role reversal, psychodrama, positive reinforcement, reframing, problem solving, teaching new skills, developing awareness and insight.

Evaluating Group Work

The process and progress of a group needs to be carefully monitored and evaluated. This feedback should then enable the group leaders to ensure that the group is able to attain its maximum potential. The methods available to evaluate the leadership interventions and the group's progress include:

- self-analysis of observations of group members and personal interventions;

- post-group evaluation and discussion with their co-leader, peer review of each other's contributions;
- analysis of written records, checklists and charts that are completed after group sessions by the group leaders;
- analysis and feedback from their supervisor;
- feedback from video recordings, audio tapes or observations from behind two-way mirrors;
- comments and feedback from group members – completion of assignments and homework, statements made in the group, question-naires and rating scales filled in by participants.

Observations and recordings may be made of both the process and content of the group sessions. The specific information that is collected will depend upon the nature of the group and its objectives. Useful feedback for evaluation can be made from studying:

1. *Patterns of attendance and punctuality*: regularity, absences, notification given, times of arrival, enforcement or challenge to time boundaries.
2. *Communication patterns within the group*: who talks to whom, what they say, how they say it, frequency of communication, periods of silence.
3. *Participation within the group*: whether all members contribute equally, which people attempt to dominate others, who remains silent, influence of members upon each other.
4. *The feelings that are expressed*: whether they are expressed openly or indirectly, whether are shared by other members, negative or positive, and whether trust and openness are expressed.
5. *Atmosphere*: warm, friendly, supportive and sensitive or cold, threaten-ing and intimidating, and morals of the group.
6. *Content of discussions*: group- or task-orientated, practical and specific or vague and unhelpful.
7. *Interest level shown*: high or low, boredom and fatigue, drifting to unrelated and irrelevant material, concentration on group activities, enthusiasm and motivation.
8. *Decision-making process*: made by a dominant few or by all, whether decisions are avoided, decisions clear or confused and fudged, degree of influence of individual members.
9. *Rate of progress*: slow or hurried, stuck, intermittent, objectives attained.
10. *Leadership within the group*: shared, dominated, flexible.
11. *Attainment of tasks*: effective use of resources, cooperation shown.

The characteristics of an effective group which give feedback to the leaders and members alike include:

1. The members are able to identify and acknowledge the other group members.
2. Members are punctual and attendance levels are high.

3. The atmosphere is relaxed and comfortable.
4. Members settle quickly to task activities and maintain focus on group objectives during meetings.
5. High levels of participation and communication between group members.
6. Creativity and initiative are encouraged.
7. Members demonstrate active listening when other members speak.
8. An increased ability and willingness to share and test out all aspects of their concerns.
9. Efforts are made by group members to encourage fellow members to participate.
10. Members work together to solve problems and to make decisions.
11. Support, reassurance and assistance are offered to fellow group members when appropriate.
12. Conflict is tolerated, examined and resolved.
13. The group demonstrates more initiative and gradually takes over delegated leadership functions.
14. Members express satisfaction and make positive statements about group membership and task attainment.
15. Group objectives are attained and a desire expressed for further progress.
16. Members are able to evaluate their own behaviour and reactions and that of the group.

Unit Instructions

When you have researched the suggested references, have mastered the Unit Objectives and successfully answered the Self-assessment Questions, proceed with the Unit Written Test.

Suggested References

Adamson, K. (1978). Silence in psychotherapy groups. *Nursing Mirror*, 18 May, Vol. 146, No. 20, pp. 25–27.

Argyle, M. (1983). *The Psychology of Interpersonal Behaviour*, 4th edition. Penguin, Harmondsworth.

Bauer, B. and Hill, S. (1986). *Essentials of Mental Health Care Planning and Interventions*. W. B. Saunders, Philadelphia.

Bion, W. R. (1961). *Experience in Groups*. Tavistock, London.

Bond, M. (1988). Setting up NT Assertiveness Training Groups. *Nursing Times*, 3 February, Vol. 84, No. 5, pp. 57–60.

Burnard, P. (1985). *Learning Human Skills*. Heinemann Nursing, London.

Burrows, R. (1985). Group therapy. *Nursing Mirror*, 3 April, Vol. 160, No. 14, pp. 41–43.

Darcy, P. T. (1985). *Mental Health Nursing Source Book*. Baillière Tindall, London and San Diego.

Douglas, T. (1976). *Groupwork Practice*. Tavistock, London.

Douglas, T. (1983). *Groups: Understanding People Gathered Together*. Tavistock, London.

Grant, P. (1982). The art of working together. *Nursing Mirror*, 3 March, Vol. 154, No. 9, Education forum, (ii)–(v).

Houston, G. (1984). *The Red Book of Groups*. Rochester Foundation.

Howden, C. and Levinson, A. (1987). Coping with stress – sharing and learning. *Senior Nurse*, August, Vol. 7, No. 2, pp. 6–8.

Klein, J. (1963). *Working with Groups*. Hutchinson, London.

Llewelyn, S. and Fielding, G. (1982). Under the influence. *Nursing Mirror*, 28 July, Vol. 155, No. 4, pp. 37–39.

Marram, G. (1978). *The Group Approach in Nursing practice*, 2nd edition. C. V. Mosby, London.

McFarland, G. and Wasli, E. (1986). *Nursing Diagnosis and Process in Psychiatric Mental Health Nursing*. J. B. Lippincott, Philadelphia.

McMahon, B. (1985). Getting to grips with groups. *Nursing Mirror*, 21 August, Vol. 11, No. 8, pp. 38–39.

McManama, D. (1983). Working with groups. *In* Robinson, L. (Ed.), *Psychiatric Nursing as a Human Experience*, 3rd edition. W. B. Saunders, Philadelphia.

Milne, D., Walker, J. and Bentinck, V. (1985). The value of feedback. *Nursing Times*, 20 February, Vol. 81, No. 8, pp. 34–36.

Moores, A. (1987). Facing the fear. *Nursing Times*, 8 July, Vol. 83, No. 27, pp. 44–46.

Mottram, E. M. (1980). The sister's role in group therapy in a general practice. *Nursing Times*, 7 February, Vol. 76, No. 6, pp. 253–254.

Muir-Cochrane, E. (1987). Freezing and thawing behaviour. *Nursing Times*, 14 January, Vol. 83, No. 2, p. 55.

Murgatroyd, S. (1985). *Counselling and Helping*. British Psychological Society and Methuen, London.

Preston-Shoot, M. (1987). *Effective Groupwork*. Macmillan, London.

Priestley, P. and McGuire, J. (1983). *Learning to Help*. Tavistock, London.

Remocker, A. and Storch, E. (1982). *Action Speaks Louder*, 3rd edition. Churchill Livingstone, Edinburgh.

Sprott, W. (1958). *Human Groups*. Penguin, Harmondsworth.

Sugden, J., Besant, A., Eastland, and Field, R. (1987). *A Handbook for Psychiatric Nurses*. Harper and Row, London.

Thompson, R. (1980). A refined form of hell on earth. *Nursing Mirror*, 6 March, Vol. 150, No. 10, pp. 33–35.

Wilson, H. and Kneisl, C. (1988). *Psychosocial Nursing Concepts: An Activity Book*, 3rd edition. Addison-Wesley, New York.

Yalom, I. O. (1975). *The Theory and Practice of Group Psychotherapy*, 2nd edition. Basic Books, New York.

Self-assessment Questions

SAQ 5. Describe four ways in which group approaches can exert a beneficial influence.

SAQ 6. Identify four characteristics of an effective group leader.

SAQ 7. List three characteristics of each stage of group development.

SAQ 8. Outline four measures that can be used to evaluate the effectiveness of a group.

Unit 3.2: Written Test

You have been asked to facilitate a staff support group in a mental health hostel.

1. Describe what factors you will need to consider in terms of planning for this group.
2. The first meeting is particularly hostile and problematic. What is this likely to indicate and what can you do as group leader to resolve some of these feelings?
3. After 6 months you have to announce that you have to leave as you are taking up a promotion elsewhere. The group has to decide whether to terminate, find a new facilitator or to become self-maintaining. What are the likely reactions from following each of these courses of action?

Mental Health Promotion

Unit Objectives

At the end of this Unit the learner should be able to:

1. Identify factors associated with positive mental health.
2. Describe the uses of health education in mental health practice.
3. Identify potential resources for mental health promotion and education.
4. Outline the range of educational strategies used in mental health education.

Personal Health and Life Choices

A person's health is a significant resource in determining the quality of their life: it influences their sense of well-being, their ability to participate in daily activities and their physical comfort. In the longer term, it can facilitate or restrict their range of relationships, social experiences, occupation and self-perception. Despite the profound influence that their health has on all aspects of living, most people have only a limited understanding of the factors that contribute towards their health maintenance and fitness.

Although a high value is attributed towards being "healthy" and on avoiding illness, this is rarely reflected in the way that people actually conduct their life. Many aspects of their behaviour and beliefs can be readily identified as adversely influencing their health. Contradictory health values and a tendency to behave in irrational ways, likewise, may do little to promote personal health positively.

The outcomes of this can readily be identified from the disease patterns that exist in our culture. These indicate that many people are making ill-informed choices in relation to their behaviour and life-style that are adversely influencing their health. This may be due to a number of factors that limit their options, e.g. restricted access to information, faulty knowledge, limited social experience and a lack of education.

People rarely give much thought to their state of health unless they are currently experiencing problems with their fitness or feeling unwell. It is something that they tend to take for granted and to be attributed to external and random factors over which the person has little control or personal responsibility. Much faith is placed upon the medical profession's ability to find cures for diseases that in reality have their origins in our life-style, e.g. dietary patterns, use of alcohol, drugs and tobacco, stress, lack of exercise. Significant developments and improvements in these areas are going to come from changes in individual choices and behaviour, not from medical advances. In this respect, people can do more to influence their own state of health than any health care professional can do for them. In terms of health promotion, therefore, health care workers have two main areas of focus:

1. *Health education*: to supply accurate, comprehensible information in a way that will promote positive health choices.
2. *Developing a sense of responsibility and control over personal health*: to promote awareness and to challenge fatalistic and passive views of health, to demonstrate that individual behaviour can influence personal health positively.

Health Education and Health Promotion

Health education is concerned with the strategies and approaches used to:

1. Present up-to-date health-orientated information to people.
2. Facilitate healthy choices in relation to an individual's health needs.
3. Support health promotional changes in behaviour and attitudes.
4. Increase the range of health options open to people.
5. Promote the person's health awareness and control of their own health needs.
6. Maximize people's potential for health and fitness.
7. Enable people to take responsibility for their own health.

Implicit in a health promotional approach to care are the assumptions that:

1. People have a right to information about their health care.
2. People have the right to actively participate in their own health care.
3. A person's behaviour and attitudes and, thereby, their health status, can be purposefully influenced by skilful presentation of health promotional information in a supportive environment.

Changing a person's health attitudes and behaviour in relation to their life-style is, however, a very complex process. Established attitudes and behaviour patterns are very resistant to change and people need to be motivated in order to consider alternatives.

Evaluating Mental Health

A person may evaluate and monitor their mental health in a number of ways:

1. Their current sense of well-being in comparison with their past experiences of health or illness.
2. A comparison of their current emotional state and behaviour with the way that they think they should be.
3. Self-perception in comparison with significant others.
4. Self-appraisal in terms of their knowledge base and beliefs in relation to mental health.

From this "audit" a person may make a number of judgements about their current mental health status:

1. That they feel well and are unaware of any health difficulties.
2. That they feel reasonably well and are able to cope with any identified minor health problems.
3. That they are distressed but do not require any outside help.
4. That they have serious mental health problems and require help from others.

The outcomes of these judgements may influence their subsequent behaviour in terms of perceiving themselves as mentally healthy or as mentally unwell. However, for a number of reasons, both a person's self-appraisal and personal judgements may be faulty. Their own knowledge base may be inaccurate or based upon unsound beliefs, their social experience may be limited and based upon an unhealthy life-style and relationships, their insight and cognitive functions may be impaired. Additionally, the conclusions that an individual arrives at may not be validated externally. The person may actually feel very well indeed or be unaware of problems in relation to their own behaviour that may cause great concern to others. If their problems feel vague or have developed insidiously over a long period of time, this can cause delay in seeking help and an impaired level of functioning becomes incorporated into their criteria of "health".

Whatever the consensus of both individual and external appraisals, there does seem to be a high incidence of mental health problems that are not recognized or acknowledged by either party. Part of the difficulty in relation to mental health are the potential consequences of stigmatization and labelling of difficulties as mental health issues (see Units 4.2 and 4.4). None the less, even what may appear to be minor problems have the potential to cause extreme distress. A lack of overt symptoms does not mean that the individual may not experience severe dysfunction.

The shortfall between prevalence rates for mental health problems and the actual numbers seeking help also indicates that only about one in four people contact health and welfare agencies. Many of the rest are further distressed by a basic lack of information in relation to their difficulties and on what courses of action are open to them to help them cope. Even those that do seek help complain frequently about communication problems between themselves and health professionals that confuse and mystify them. That there is a need for mental health information can be gauged in part from the growing literature and resources on self-help approaches to mental health problems. Additionally, many people are beginning to identify in their own lives the need for mental health promotion – courses on anxiety management, coping with stress and assertiveness are now common. One street survey revealed that four out of five people wished to increase their self-esteem. All of the above indicate the need for mental health workers to become far more actively involved in mental health education and promotion.

Influences on Mental Health

Mental health is an integral part of a person's emotional, social and physical health. The interrelationship between these dimensions is such that adverse influences on any aspect of a person's existence can be detrimental to a person's entire state of health. Likewise, a positive sense of well-being in one of these areas will also positively influence other areas of their life.

A person's mental health is not static. It may fluctuate over time and can change profoundly. At times these changes may be related to significant life events the person is experiencing or as a response to time, place or situation. Some of the factors may appear to be related to the choices a person has made or to the operation of random external events. A number of the factors that can influence a person's mental health are given in the list below.

Exhibit 3.3.1 Influences on mental health

Factor	Positively associated with mental health	Negatively associated with mental health
1. Self-image	Realistic self-appraisal	Unrealistic self-evaluation
	Insight	Lack of insight
	Self-acceptance of own limitations	Not recognize own limitations, frustrated and blaming others for own shortcomings
	High self-esteem and positive self-concept	Low self-esteem and negative self-concept, devalues self

	Sense of attainment and self-worth	Sense of failure and worthlessness
	Feel valued by others	Feels inadequate, de-valued by others
	Consistent and stable personality, sense of own uniqueness	Changeable and inconsistent, lack of own individuality
	Respected by others	Lack of respect shown by others, feel stigmatized
2. Sense of security	Feel secure	Feeling insecure
	Confident and assertive	Lacking in confidence and assertiveness
	Able to trust others	Mistrustful of others
	Can take risks and let go	Rigid and clinging
	Can tolerate ambiguity and inconsistency	Requires everything to be clear-cut and ordered
	Can accept other's viewpoints	Dogmatic and prejudiced
3. Mastery and autonomy	Feels in control of own destiny	Feeling manipulated and helpless
	Able to adapt to changing circumstances	Difficulty in responding to changing circmstances
	Select own chosen goals	Controlled by others
	Cope effectively with demands	Inability to cope causing further stress
	Independence	High degree of dependence upon others
	Accept and take responsibility	Wants others to decide and control
	Potential for growth and development	Fixed and rigid
	Optimistic and hopeful	Pessimistic and self-defeating
	Can delay gratification of needs	Requires immediate gratification
	Realistic expectations	Unrealistic expectations
	Access to financial, social and physical resources	Limited resources and deprivation

4. Relation-ships	Ability to form close, lasting relationships	Unable to form relationships
	Supportive relationships	Isolated, lack of support
	Close, condifing partner or friendships	Critical and demanding relationships
	Experienced as positively rewarding	Damaging to self-esteem
	Trust and honesty	Mistrust and suspicion
	Open emotional expression	Shallow and manipulative, collusion
	Concern for other's welfare	Indifferent to other's distress
	Sense of security and stability	Insecurity and instability
	Marriage (for men)	Marriage (for women), family violence and sexual abuse, bereavement, separation and divorce
	Sense of belonging to family and peer groups	Feel alienated from others
	Member of socially valued group	Belong to minority, victimized group
5. Body image	Acceptance of own body physique	Prolonged distress with body physique
	Unselfconsciousness and uninhibited	Inhibited and selfconscious, shy
	Secure in own appearance	Insecure in appearance
	Realistic expectations about modifying body size and shape	Unrealistic expectations about modifying body, size and shape
	Body a source of pleasure	Body viewed with distaste
	Body conforms to social expectations of "normality"	Visible signs of deformity and deviation in body configuration
6. Expression of sexuality	Able to accept and express own sexual preferances	Sexual feelings a source of distress

	Lack of guilt and inhibition	Repressed and inhibited sexual feelings, feeling of guilt and shame
	Sexuality a source of pleasure	Sexual contact a source of distress
	Positive and rewarding sexual experiences	Victim of negative sexual experiences, i.e. incest, abuse, harassment, rape
	Acceptance of other's sexuality	Strong intolerance towards alternative expressions of sexuality
	Does not discriminate on basis of gender	Sexist and prejudiced attitudes
7. Emotional expression	Able to express feelings	Feelings over-controlled and repressed
	Feelings appropriate and proportionate to circumstances	Inappropriate emotional responses, lack of or exaggerated feelings
	Able to empathize with others	Not sensitive to others
8. Physical health	Sense of well-being and feeling "healthy"	Malaise and feeling "run-down"
	Can identify and meet own phsyical needs, e.g. balanced diet, sleep, warmth, hygiene	Unable to identify or meet own physical needs, e.g. malnourishment, insomnia, cold, unhygienic
	Healthy life patterns and values	Unhealthy life-style that damages physical health
	Promotes own health maintenance	Self-injurious behaviour
	Abstinant or controlled use of dependency forming substances	Excessive and uncontrolled use of dependency forming substances
	Cope with disabilities	Chronic disabling illness
	Sight and hearing effective	Severe sensory difficulties
9. Behaviour	Skilled verbal and non-verbal behaviour	Unskilled verbal and non-verbal behaviour

	Appropriate to situation, expectations, age and culture	Inappropriate behaviour patterns
	Adapt behaviour to changing circumstances	Fixed, rigid and inflexible
	Able to understand and identify own motivation for own behaviour	Responds in an automatic, non-thinking way
	Can use initiative	Lack of initiative
	Self-motivating and directing	Apathetic, requires repeated prompting and guidance
10. Early life experiences	Stable, caring parental figures	Maternal deprivation, separation anxiety, sexual abuse, family violence, rejection by parents, heavy drinking or drug taking by parents, fearful and anxious childhood
	Healthy role models	
	Expressions of love and affection between family members	
	Rewarding life experiences	Negative life experiences
	Absence of traumatic events	Traumatic events
	Friendships and identification with peer group	Isolated, lack of friendships, peer group promotes unhealthy or inappropriate
	Attainment of developmental milestones	Development blocked and inhibited
	Parental figures promote autonomy and independence	Parents reinforce dependency and will not "let go"
	Educational attainment	Lack of attainment and schooling experienced as negative
11. Perception and thought processes	Clear sensory perception	Experience of sensory distortions
	Acceptance of reality	Rejection of reality
	Conscious of experience	Diminished or clouded consciousness

	Sensory stimulation and novelty	Sensory deprivation and monotony
	Orientated to time and place	Disorientated and confused
	Rational and logical thought processes	Cognitive distortions – over-generalization, magnification, selective abstraction, arbitrary inference. Irrational and distorted thinking
	Effective problem solving and decision making	Unable to solve problems, poor judgement and decision making
	Positive and optimistic outlook	Negative and pessimistic outlook
	Learn from experience	Unable to learn from experience
	Effective recall from memory	Pathological loss of memory
12 Occupational and leisure	Work and leisure activities are rewarding and fulfilling, cope with occupational stresses	Occupation is stressful, demanding and unrewarding
	Good relationships with work colleagues	Conflict with people at work, poor relationships
	Opportunities for leisure activities	Limited opportunity for leisure
	Job is perceived by person and others as having value	Low value placed on occupation by self and others
	Being in employment	Unemployed
13 Living environment	Personalized environment and possessions	Barren environment, few or lack of possessions
	Feels secure in home and immediate vicinity	Feel insecure and threatened in home and external environment
	Opportunities for privacy	Lack of privacy
	Reasonable physical comfort	Cold, damp, unhealthy environment
	Space for the inhabitants	Overcrowded

Mental Health Nursing and Mental Health Promotion

Many aspects of mental health nursing practice are concerned with mental health promotion. Nurses continually advise clients, provide information, clarify beliefs and feelings and help people to modify their life-styles. Beyond the explicit message communicated in these ways nurses also give more subtle health promotional signals through their own behaviour, beliefs and values which they demonstrate. In order to be effective role models for mental health promotion, nurses need to be clear about their own values and commitment and to incorporate these into their own practice and life-styles.

The concept of individualized care also has implications for incorporating health promotional objectives into nursing practice. The partnership in care and promotion of client participation have the objectives of increasing their sense of mastery, facilitating informed choice and enabling positive changes in behaviour, beliefs and life-styles. As an advocate for their client's health care needs, the nurse also has an obligation to challenge other practitioners, organizations and political decisions if these stand in the way of health promotional objectives.

Recently, the health promotional aspects of nursing practice have been recognized legally and incorporated into the statutory framework that governs nurse education. Approved courses for nurses have to prepare them for a role in health promotion and maintenance and to be able to recognize situations that may be detrimental to an individual's well-being.

Health Promotion in Mental Health Practice

Health promotion is an implicit part of mental health nursing practice. The range of activities may include:

1. Teaching problem-solving and decision-making skills.
2. Improving self-awareness and self-understanding.
3. Developing the client's and carer's coping skills and mastery.
4. Promoting a healthy life-style.
5. Supporting changes in behaviour and life-style.
6. Developing realistic expectations.
7. Facilitating positive attitude changes.
8. Reviewing and developing personal relationships.
9. Promoting the client's and carer's health knowledge.
10. Developing awareness of health maintenance and potential health hazards.
11. Improving the client's ability to express their feelings.
12. Developing communication skills.
13. Facilitating the expression of sexuality.
14. Promoting their physical health.
15. Enabling the client to develop a realistic body image.

16. Regaining control of dependency forming habituations.
17. Developing anxiety and stress management skills.
18. Promoting the client's self-esteem, confidence and assertiveness.
19. Developing awareness of the health resources that are available.
20. Enhancing autonomy, independence and personal responsibility.
21. Facilitating active involvement in health care by clients and carers.
22. Developing the client's and carer's ability to cope with existing health problems.

Resources for Mental Health Promotion

A wide range of resources are available that may be used for mental health promotion. These may be specially prepared materials or packages compiled by health care workers for their clients. Potential resources include:

1. *Written material*: books, leaflets, pamphlets, newsletters, magazines, journals, newspapers, posters, charts. Available from public and medical libraries, bookshops, newsagents, HMSO, DHSS.
2. *Audio-visual material*: audiotapes, videotapes, tape–slide packages, films, television and radio programmes, telephone health lines.
3. *Advisory services*: self-help groups, voluntary services, community health councils, DHSS, health promotion departments, primary health care workers, hospital-based services, social services, pharmacists, Post Offices, Citizen's Advice Bureaux, College of Health, private practitioners, professional contacts, Well Women and Well Men Centres, librarians.
4. *Educational programmes*: courses on health promotion, courses for carers or sufferers, O.U. and other formal courses, field trips and visits.
5. *Support networks*: friends and relatives, self-help groups, voluntary agencies, social services, primary health care workers and other statutory agencies, private practitioners.

The Framework of Health Promotion

Primary

Primary health promotion is targeted at healthy people with the objectives of promoting the development of a healthy life-style and improving their quality of health. Particular attention is placed on developing awareness of health issues and on effective coping strategies for health maintenance. The intention is to reduce the probability of mental health problems occurring. Approaches used in mental health promotion may include advisory services, mental health promotional programmes and campaigns, counselling, self-help and support groups, educational programmes aimed at particular risk groups, and walk-in mental health facilities.

Secondary

Secondary health promotion is aimed at minimizing the effects, severity and duration of existing emotional and mental health problems. The mental health promotional interventions may form part of a comprehensive treatment programme to facilitate the early resolution of problems and to use the experience to enhance health awareness and coping skills. Clients at particular risk need to be identified and mechanisms established for early detection and intervention when required.

Tertiary

Tertiary health promotion is aimed at minimizing the residual effects of mental disorder and to prevent the development of avoidable complications or long-term disability. The objectivs are to ensure that the person is rehabilitated to their optimum level of functioning and to promote social reintegration and independence. Clients with potentially damaging mental health problems need to be identified and the resources available to provide long-term support and monitoring.

Facilitating Health Promotional Change

Any health promotional message has to be presented in such a way as to facilitate an internalization of desirable attitudes and to promote healthy changes in life-style and behaviour. While the basic health promotional material may be readily identified, the manner and style of presentation can do much to either enhance or negate its intended effects.

The skills of health promotion

To be an effective health educator the nurse needs a broad repertoire of skills that they can match to the client's needs and the health promotional objective. The skills' base includes:

1. *Relationship skills*: with groups or individuals. To promote trust in the clients, to be seen to be understanding, non-judgemental and accepting. To respect the audience's beliefs and to promote their self-esteem.
2. *Communication skills*: to speak clearly in a way that is readily understood by their clients. To demonstrate active listening and responsiveness and to observe closely their non-verbal behaviour. To utilize this feedback to modify their own presentation.
3. *Educational skills*: to identify accurately the client group's educational needs, to set realistic health promotional goals, to select appropriate educational resources and approaches, to plan and identify the most

appropriate setting, to monitor and evaluate the health promotional outcomes.
4. *Knowledge and resource base*: to maintain and develop their own knowledge base and to be able to identify the appropriate reasons for client's needs.

The techniques of presentation

The manner in which the message is presented can do much to influence its effectiveness. In health promotion the following factors are particularly important:

1. *The credibility of the presenter*: health promotional messages need to come from a source that is respected both for its integrity and prestige. This is enhanced if the nurse is also observed to role model the values and behaviour that they are trying to facilitate in others.
2. *The relevance of the material*: pre-assessment and planning is necessary to ensure that the information is perceived by the clients as relevant to their needs. The content needs to be given careful consideration as does the language used.
3. *Attainability and desirability*: the client group need to feel that the messages being communicated are both attainable and represent desirable changes in life-style. If the gap between their existing beliefs and those they are being presented with is felt to be too great or involve too much sacrifice then the message will be rejected out of hand. It requires careful assessment of the target group and an understanding of the health issue in question to present a realistic message.
4. *Balanced presentation*: the presentation needs to be perceived as even and balanced. If the message is too dogmatic then it will have the counter-effect of increasing resistance to change. People need to know they are making a choice between alternatives in which the health promotional option is the most preferable.
5. *Order of presentation*: the sequence is important in facilitating attitude change. Important issues need to be presented first, as do the most agreeable and favourable parts of the health promotional message. The drawbacks and less acceptable aspects should be presented afterwards.
6. *The medium*: personal contact and active participation through discussion, role play and demonstration are far more effective than passive approaches such as talks, reading, etc. Where audio-visual material is used it should be carefully utilized to reinforce the message and not as the sole means of presentation.
7. *The message*: the information needs to present specific advice about what is required in terms of promoting health. Details of the actual steps required, ways of changing existing habits and how progress can be evaluated. Clear programmes rather than vague exhortations of health improvement are required.

The Educational Process in Health Promotion

Assessment

1. *Identify*:

   - existing client skills, knowledge and attitudes in relation to health needs;
   - process and acquisition of skills, knowledge attitudes – where and when;
   - how their knowledge and beliefs influence their health;
   - how strongly their beliefs are held and habits maintained;
   - motivation and commitment to change;
   - self-perception and self-esteem as a client and learner.

2. *Clarify and define*:

   - the target group;
   - strengths and assets in existing life-style and beliefs in relation to health;
   - deficits and needs for health promotional change;
   - potential and motivation for change.

Planning

1. *Specify*:

   - the health promotional objectives, the desirable outcomes;
   - the criteria of attainment.

2. *Self-preparation*:

   - review own knowledge and skills, and update if necessary;
   - identify available resources, e.g. audio-visual aids, experts, etc.
   - prepare necessary resources, e.g. handouts, reading lists, activities.

3. *Select appropriate instructional methods*:

   - relevant to the health promotional goals, the needs of the client group, within available resources and the expertise of the health worker. In making a choice of method the nurse needs to consider that:

     (i) active methods are more effective in producing attitudinal and behavioural change. These include: role play, simulation, games, group exercises, discussion;
     (ii) activities need to be varied periodically to maintain attention and motivation;

(iii) informality and humour are perceived as less threatening.

4. *Decisions*:

- timing – will clients be available, does it conflict with other demands;
- who to include, numbers you can cope with;
- place – comfortable, quiet, free from interruptions, appropriate for clients and method, booking of room.

5. *Notification*:

- clients – where, when, why, what is expected of them;
- significant others – family members, other care workers, administrative staff.

6. *Written plan and notes*:

- specify the sequence and timing of activities, key points that you wish to make.

Basically, the more thought and attention that is given to preparation and planning:

- the less anxious you are likely to be;
- confidence and mastery are enhanced;
- the more likely are the objectives to be attained.

Implementation

- Communicate clearly – volume, clarity, pace, tone.
- Appear confident and sure of what you are doing.
- Put people at their ease, be non-threatening.
- Gain and hold their attention.
- Encourage participation and involvement.
- Ask questions, check understanding, clarify misunderstandings.
- Be alert to feedback.
- Keep a structure.
- Periodically summarize.
- Give clear, precise information where required.
- Use exercises to promote understanding and awareness – role plays, games, simulation.
- Use aids to facilitate and reinforce understanding.
- Opportunities to rehearse new skills.
- Identify situations in real life where new knowledge and skills are applicable and can be used to consolidate learning.
- Opportunities for further self-development.

Evaluation

1. *Tools of evaluation*:

   - observation of newly acquired skills and changes in life-style and relationships;
   - evidence of attitude change through statements and behaviour;
   - recall and utilization of knowledge and information;
   - questions to assess understanding;
   - interest shown by clients for further development;
   - utilization of health-promoting resources;
   - follow up questionnaires;
   - diaries or records kept by clients.

2. *Educational process*:

   - organization and preparation;
   - content, methods and activities in relation to the client group's health promotional needs;
   - relationship with the group and credibility of the instructor;
   - attainability and realism of the objectives;
   - suitability of the time and place;
   - teaching style and communication with the group.

Unit Instructions

When you have researched the suggested references, have mastered the Unit Objectives and successfully answered the Self-assessment Questions, proceed with the Unit Written Test.

Suggested References

Antrobus, M. (1987). The neglected sex. *Nursing Times*, 4 February, Vol. 83, No. 5, pp. 31–33.

Carson, J., Low, S. and Thompson, M. (1987). Workshops on distress. *Nursing Times*, 24 June, Vol. 83, No. 25, pp. 32–35.

Clark, J. (1986). Heading off a breakdown. *Nursing Times*, 6 August, Vol. 82, No. 32, pp. 33–34.

Coutts, L. C. and Hardy, L. K. (1985). *Teaching for Health. The Nurse as Nurse Educator*. Churchill Livingstone, Edinburgh.

Coxon, J. (1986). Health education: A learning dilemma. *Senior Nurse*, July, Vol. 5, No. 1, pp. 22–24.

Distance Learning Centre (1986). *Teaching Patients and Clients*. Distance Learning Centre, London.

Dryden, W. (1984). *Rational–Emotive Therapy*. Croom Helm, London.

Ewles, L. and Simnett, I. (1985). *Promoting Health. A Practical Guide to Health Education*. John Wiley, Chichester.

Fox, J. C. (1986). Participating in change. *Nursing Times*, 18 June, Vol. 82, No. 25, pp. 33–34.

Gann, R. and Knight, S. (1986). *Consumers' Guide to Health Information*. College of Health, London.

Girling, R. (1987). *The Sunday Times Life Plan*. Collins, London.

Hamachek, D. E. (1987). *Encounters with the Self*, 3rd edition. Holt, Rinehart and Winston, New York.

Hase, S. and Douglas, A. (1986). *Human Dynamics and Nursing*. Churchill Livingstone, Melbourne.

Holland, S. (1986). Teaching patients and clients – 1. Teaching, learning or both?' *Nursing Times*, 3 December, Vol. 82, No. 49, pp. 33–37.

Holland, S. (1987a). Teaching patients and clients – 2. Encouraging participation. *Nursing Times*, 21 January, Vol. 83, No. 3, pp. 59–62.

Holland, S. (1987b). Teaching patients and clients – 3. The benefits of communicating. *Nursing Times*, 4 March, Vol. 83, No. 9, pp. 56–58.

Hume, C. and Pullen, I. (1986). *Rehabilitation in Psychiatry*. Churchill Livingstone, Edinburgh.

Irving, S. (1983). *Basic Psychiatric Nursing*, 3rd edition. W. B. Saunders, Philadelphia.

Jahoda, M. (1956). *Current Concepts of Positive Mental Health: A Report to the Staff Director*. Basic Books, New York.

Kent, G. and Dalgleish, M. (1986). *Psychology and Medical Care*. Baillière Tindall, London and San Diego.

Lyttle, J. (1986). *Mental Disorder: Its Care and Treatment*. Baillière Tindall, London and San Diego.

Melvin, B. (1987). Promoting health by example. *Nursing Times*, Vol. 83, No. 17, pp. 42–43.

Nelson-Jones, R. (1982). *The Theory and Practice of Counselling Psychology*. Holt, Rinehart and Winston, New York.

Norman, A. (1987). Divided we fall. *Nursing Times*, 29 April, Vol. 83, No. 17, pp. 16–18.

Pothier, P. (1987). Preventive measures. *Nursing Times*, 28 January, Vol. 83, No. 4, pp. 42–43.

Pownall, M. (1986). The advertising myth. *Nursing Times*, 20 August, Vol. 82, No. 34, pp. 19–20.

Price, B. (1986). The sickness, health – and in between. *Nursing Times*, 16 April, Vol. 82, No. 16, pp. 32–34.

Robinson, L. (1983). *Psychiatric Nursing as a Human Experience*, 3rd edition. W. B. Saunders, Philadelphia.

Seedhouse, D. (1986). A universal concern. *Nursing Times*, 22 January, Vol. 82, No. 4, pp. 36–38.

Shillitoe, R. (1985). I think, therefore I'm ill. *Nursing Times*, 20 February, Vol. 81, No. 8, pp. 24–26.

Shives, L. R. (1986). *Basic Concepts of Psychiatric – Mental Health Nursing*. J. B. Lippincott, Philadelphia.

Smith, R. E. and Birrell, J. (1986). Encouraging compliance. *The Professional Nurse*, September, Vol. 1, Issue 12, pp. 335–336.

Stanfield, I. (1984). Weeding out the victims. *Nursing Times*, 11 July, Community Outlook, Vol. 80, No. 27, pp. 238–240.

Sugden, J., Bessant, A., Eastland, M. and Field, R. (1986). *A Handbook for Psychiatric Nurses*. Harper and Row, London.

Taylor, C. M. (1981). *Returning to Mental Health*. Stanley Thornes, Cheltenham.

Townsend, P. and Davidson, N. (1982). *The Black Report, Inequalities in Health*. Penguin, Harmondsworth.

Vousden, M. (1985). Wise counsel. *Nursing Mirror*, 26 June, Vol. 160, No. 26, pp. 46–48.

Whitehead, D. (1987). *The Health Divide: Inequalities in Health in the 1980's*. Health Education Council, London.

Wilson, H. and Kneisl, C. (1988). *Psychosocial Nursing Concepts: An Activity Book*, 3rd edition. Addison-Wesley, New York.

Self-assessment Questions

SAQ 9. Identify eight factors associated with positive mental health.

SAQ 10. State six potential objectives for mental health promotion in nursing practice.

SAQ 11. List six potential sources of information for health education.

SAQ 12. Identify four factors that influence the choice of educational strategies used in mental health promotion.

Unit 3.3: Written Test

You have been invited to give a talk to a relatives support group on "Mental Health Promotion". The primary objectives are to help the carers develop their understanding of the resources available to them and to be aware of factors that influence mental health.

1. What key factors would you wish to present as having a key role in mental health promotion.

2. Identify the potential resources and sources of information that they might find useful.

3. What particular educational approaches are useful in promoting understanding and awareness.

Social Skills Training

The Nature of Social Skills

Interaction with others is an integral part of everyday living. In a wide range of situations and settings people utilize very diverse and complex patterns of behaviour in order to communicate and relate to others. The ability to do this effectively is dependent upon the possession of a sophisticated repertoire of social skills and an understanding of human behaviours that enable the person to:

1. Observe, analyse and assess interpersonal and social situations.
2. Determine what their own needs and objectives are in specific situations.
3. Select from their appraisal and personal experience the responses that are situationally appropriate and are intended to achieve their desired response.
4. Initiate and carry through the chosen course of action through their verbal and non-verbal behaviour.
5. Monitor the situation and responses of others and to modify their own behaviour accordingly.
6. Evaluate the outcomes in terms of meeting their needs and complying with social expectations.

As can be inferred from the above list, social behaviour also involves a complex network of cognitive, personal belief and emotional processes:

1. *Cognitive aspects*: perception of social situations, the ability to discriminate between patterns of observed behaviour and speech content, the ability to generate possible alternative courses of action and outcomes, to select situationally appropriate courses of action, to synchronize with others' expectations about the outcomes of their behaviour in specific situations, self-monitoring of their own behaviour, perceiving situations and outcomes as personally rewarding or not, exercising of restraint and self-control, cognitive rehearsal.
2. *Personal value system*: beliefs about the appropriateness of specific behaviour patterns, value placed on compliance with social expectations, feelings of mastery and control *vs* helplessness, self-esteem and confidence.
3. *Emotional responses*: the range and strength of emotional expression displayed, appropriateness of emotional response to situation, degree of emotional restraint.

Verbal and Non-Verbal Communication

Observation and analysis of interpersonal behaviour reveals a complex pattern of verbal and non-verbal communication. While verbal communication is primarily used to convey information, the non-verbal elements that accompany verbal speech have a particularly important role in human interaction. Non-verbal communication includes:

1. *Gaze and eye contact*: used to initiate interaction, facilitate turn taking, show interest or disinterest, nature of the participant's relationship, dominance or submissiveness, to provide feedback and to co-ordinate the interaction.
2. *Gestures*: hand and arm movements in conjunction with other bodily movements are used to add emphasis, reinforce verbal statements, maintain attention, demonstrate intimacy. Can be very distracting if used inappropriately, excessively or if completely lacking.
3. *Posture*: the posture adopted helps to define the situation, i.e. standing, sitting or lying down. Whether the posture is open, closed, rigid, slouched or relaxed can demonstrate warmth, ease, congruence, mirroring, social status, emotional state, self-esteem.
4. *Facial expression*: very important in emotional expression and demonstrating attentiveness. Needs to correspond to verbal messages and to be appropriate to the situation.
5. *Physical proximity and orientation*: the distance and positioning between participants. The closer the distance the more intimate the relationship. The angle of body that is adopted can facilitate or hinder communication.
6. *Body contact and touch*: this can be a very potent means of communication that is used to convey intimacy, affection, consolation, social ritual, warmth, aggression.
7. *Head movements*: to prompt, encourage and acknowledge communi-

cation. To add emphasis to positive or negative statements or expressing doubt.

8. *Appearance*: physical appearance and clothing have considerable social influence. First impressions, based on appearances, have a particularly powerful influence. Attractiveness is an important social resource. Appearances can indicate group and personal identity, age, status, social values, emotional state, social class and occupation.

9. *Para-language*: these are non-verbal aspects of speech that are used to emphasize meaning, maintain attention and express emotions. They include pitch, tone, volume, rate, fluency, clarity, inflection and intonation.

A high value is attributed towards non-verbal communication in confirming verbal messages and in communicating the real attitudes and feelings of the participants. In terms of this it is generally anticipated that there will be a high degree of congruence between the verbal and non-verbal messages that are sent. However, while people can regulate to a high degree what they choose to say, they have less control over their non-verbal communication. Given the reflex and habitual nature of human interaction people may not even be particularly aware of the non-verbal messages they are in fact communicating. At times of stress, the person's ability to control their non-verbal behaviour becomes even more tenuous.

In situations where there is perceived to be a significant difference between the verbal and non-verbal message, people will focus upon the non-verbal element. They will regard it as communicating the emotional status and true intent of the communication. This non-verbal "leakage" will also be used to make judgements about the person's sincerity and confidence.

Other significant functions of non-verbal communications include:

- giving vocal and postural cues;
- providing feedback to the participants;
- regulating and controlling the flow of communication – pacing, turn taking, synchronizing, meshing;
- defining the nature of the relationship between the participants – gender, intimacy, dominance, submissiveness.

The Range of Interpersonal Skills

In order to communicate and relate effectively to others, people need a broad range of interpersonal skills. These consist of complex patterns of verbal and non-verbal behaviour that are situationally appropriate and comply with social expectations. Some of the principal skills include:

1. *Social introductory and parting skills*: these are particularly important as people are profoundly influenced by the first few moments of meeting

with others. The elements include sighting and recognition, determining their response, approach and positioning, posture, verbal and non-verbal cues given to open and close the interaction.

2. *Observational skills*: self-observation, observation of the other participants, recognition of emotions, identifying attitudes, patterns of gaze and eye contact.
3. *Conversational skills*: appropriateness of content, power of self-expression, length of sentences, generality, formality, turn taking, degree of self-disclosure, amount of information, vocabulary, asking questions.
4. *Social reinforcement*: the ability to make the interactions rewarding. Interest shown, eye contact, head nodding, leaning forward, praise, focussing on speaker, relaxed open posture, reflecting statements and feelings, emotional expression, smiling, facial expression, verbal and non-verbal prompting, proximity and orientation, acknowledgement, offering physical or social rewards, demonstrating active listening skills, expressing empathy.
5. *Assertiveness and confidence*: maintaining eye contact, balanced posture, making and refusing requests, use of word "I", maintaining personal values, exercising control, avoiding manipulation.
6. *Meshing and synchronizing skills*: giving clear verbal and non-verbal cues to facilitate turn taking, continuity of conversational themes and to avoid participants all talking at the same time.

The Acquisition and Development of Social Skills

Patterns of social behaviour are developed from early infancy and throughout adult life. The primary processes involved in the acquisition of social skills include:

1. *Guidance and instruction*: advice and information on how to behave in specific situations; social "rules" and expectations.
2. *Demonstration and modelling*: where a person observes another's behaviour and attempts to reproduce their actions. Passive modelling, whereby a person is unconsciously influenced by the behaviour of those around them, can also exert a significant influence.
3. *Reinforcement*: the experience of the consequences of specific actions also influences which patterns of behaviour are likely to become established:

   - Positive reinforcement from which a person experiences a favourable outcome is particularly effective in increasing the probability of a specific behaviour pattern recurring and becoming established.
   - Negative reinforcement which prompts a person to behave in a particular way in a specific situation in order to avoid an unpleasant outcome.

4. *Feedback*: information on the effectiveness and outcomes of specific behaviour. This may come from personal appraisal or evaluations supplied by others.

These are discussed in more detail later in this Unit in the section on "Social Skills Training", see p. 144.

The repertoire of social skills that an individual develops is very dependent upon their range of social experience and interaction with others. The primary influences are:

1. Parental and family figures who are particularly important as role models and for the guidance and instruction they give in early life.
2. Peer group: as a person grows up they are exposed to a broader range of social experiences and role models. Schoolmates and personal friends are particularly significant influences during adolescence.
3. Occupation socialization: the person may acquire a new vocabulary, social values and specific patterns of interpersonal behaviour as they assimilate the prevailing culture of their work-place.
4. Adult personal relationships: partners and close relationships can act as powerful influences on the social skills that a person develops.

From each of these sources the person acquires a range of social behaviour and interpersonal skills that also indicate their:

1. *Cultural and geographical origins*: patterns of verbal and non-verbal behaviour are very culture-specific, e.g. language, dialect, gestures that are used.
2. *Gender*: male and female behaviour patterns tend to be differentiated from an early age. There are strong social expectations and prohibitions applied to what is regarded as gender-appropriate behaviour.
3. *Self-esteem and confidence*: the self-worth and value that a person places upon themselves is a key factor in influencing their interpersonal behaviour, social ease and assertiveness. High self-esteem is associated with the experience of a more positively rewarding social life.
4. *Value system*: attitudes and prejudices are communicated both verbally and non-verbally.
5. *Social class and education*: these can influence the person's speech patterns, vocabulary, linguistic code and non-verbal behaviour.

Individuals vary considerably in the range and effectiveness of their social skills. People are highly motivated in a variety of ways to meet their social needs – affiliation, security, acceptance, esteem and status, sexual expression, recreation, relationships. The repertoire of social skills that they possess will considerably influence the quality of their life through the socially rewarding and satisfying relationships that they are able to experience.

Social Skills Problems

A wide range of difficulties may be caused or exacerbated by a lack of social competence and awareness. These may cause periodic stress for individuals when confronted with specific situations or more serious social difficulties that cause long-term problems. The consequences may be experienced as subjective dissatisfaction, anxiety, loneliness, rejection, frustration, low self-esteem, shyness, isolation, relationship difficulties. The origins of social skills difficulties may include:

1. *Limited social development*: inappropriate or poor role models, absence of role models, limited social experience and lack of opportunities, chronic ill-health during infancy and adolescence.
2. *Social skills deficits*: limited repertoire of skills, inappropriate responses, maladaptive behaviour, lack of rewardingness, failure to reciprocate, poor communication skills, incongruent verbal and non-verbal behaviour, poor non-verbal communicators and perceivers.
3. *Cognitive factors*: irrational beliefs, faulty interpretation of social situations, poor interpersonal perception, negative self-talk, external locus of control, low self-esteem, limited insight, memory impairment.
4. *Social role*: gender, membership of a minority group, stigmatization.
5. *Environmental factors*: institutionalization, social deprivation and isolation.
6. *Mental health difficulties*: anxiety, depression, confusion, lack of insight, perceptual distractions, thought disorders.
7. *Physical health problems*: chronic, disabling illness, sensory deficits, mobility problems.

Social Skills Training

Social skills training is a therapeutic approach towards teaching the skills of social interaction, communication and relationships in a systematic way. Depending upon the setting – education, management training, life enhancement or clinical practice – and the needs of the client group, programmes may be focussed upon very specific aspects of behaviour or may have a broader application. Examples can include assertiveness, interviewing, communication and relationship skills, public speaking and salesmanship. There are also a broad range of clinical applications. Whatever the setting, the broad objectives of social skills programmes are to increase the person's repertoire of interpersonal skills and social awareness by:

- increasing their perception, analysis and understanding of interpersonal situations and patterns of behaviour;
- developing new social skills;
- enhancing existing skills to increase their effectiveness;
- correcting behavioural deficits or specific behavioural problems.

The focus of social skills training may appear, primarily, to be directed towards the modification of observable behaviour and the learning of new adaptive skills. However, there are coincidentally internal cognitive and emotional changes that serve to support, consolidate and maintain the development of new social skills. These may form an explicit part of the programme or be part of the "hidden agenda". Some of the changes may include:

- a shift from irrational, disabling self-talk towards more realistic and enabling expectations;
- enhancing self-esteem, feelings of mastery and personal control;
- increasing the range of options open to them and the ability to generate alternative responses.

Preparing a Social Skills Programme

Each interaction between a client and a therapist has the potential to modify the client's behaviour. However, unless this process is consciously used with clear objectives, then it does not achieve its full therapeutic potential and may even prove counterproductive. Running a social skills programme requires careful preparation and planning to achieve maximum effectiveness and to facilitate systematic social skills development. There can also be further benefits if the social skills programme is used in conjunction with other therapeutic approaches. Some of the key stages involved in preparation include:

1. *Identifying an experienced trainer and co-therapist*: the trainers need to understand the principles involved in social skills training and to have had some experience participating in a social skills group. Supervision should be arranged with an experienced trainer (see Unit 1.3). Other decisions involve the respective roles of the trainers and whether they should both be of the same sex or not.
2. *Group size*: social skills programmes can be run individually. However, for a number of important therapeutic reasons group approaches tend to be preferred. A small group size (4–8) provides a range of role models, increased potential for reinforcement and feedback from peers, and support from fellow group members. Once started the group is more effective if membership is closed.
3. *Determining the objectives:* the potential client groups needs, attainability and appropriateness of intended outcomes, therapeutic approaches to be used.
4. *Environment for the training sessions*: privacy, space, physical comfort, freedom from noise, accessibility.
5. *Resources required*: teaching aids, e.g. blackboard, flip charts, overhead projector, video recorder and camera, props and materials for role plays, stopwatch, timer and counter.

6. *Planning the programme*: designing a specific programme or using/ modifying an existing programme. Frequency, duration and timing of sessions. In practice most social skills sessions are conducted on a weekly basis for between 1 and 2 hours. Each session may have a particular theme or may be run in terms of the clients' progress and needs. The length of the programme may vary from a few sessions to a longer term arrangement.

7. *Selection of clients*: to match the therapeutic objectives, the resources available and to meet their needs.

8. *Preparation of clients*: notifying them of the arrangements, i.e. time, place, duration, number of sessions. Details on the aims of the programme and what they will be expected to do.

9. *Informed consent*: this will be required if the sessions are to be videoed and shown to an external audience. It also provides a further opportunity to ensure the clients' understanding of the programme and to gain their cooperation. Establishing a therapeutic contract if appropriate.

10. *Notifying significant others*: staff, carers, relatives, others who may also use the resources, administration.

Assessment of Clients' Social Skills

A wide variety of assessment methods may be utilized to establish a clear description and baseline of a person's current social skills repertoire and difficulties (see also Unit 2.1). Common methods used, often in combination, include:

1. *Interviewing*: focussing particularly on the social skills aspects of their difficulties, their emotional responses and understanding of interpersonal situations.

2. *Observation*: by relatives or care staff as unobtrusively as possible in the person's natural environment. Time sampling or periodic observation may be used to provide an overall view of a person's behaviour when continuous assessment is not possible or suitable.

3. *Role play*: specific or general situations may be role played to facilitate a detailed assessment and analysis of the person's social skills and difficulties.

4. *Questionnaires, check lists and rating scales*: related to social behaviour, they may be used in conjunction with other assessment methods.

5. *Self-reporting and self-monitoring*: clients are instructed in how to record their behaviour, thoughts, feelings and situations in a diary, log book or checklists. An advantage of using this approach is that if the person is well motivated, then the act of recording tends to lead to an improvement in the behaviour under scrutiny.

Whichever methods are used the information collected may include:

1. A detailed analysis of the person's social behaviour and situations they find difficult:

   (a) *antecedents*: place, situation, time, who else is involved, what they were doing, thoughts and feelings, expectations.
   (b) *behaviour*: detailed description of person's verbal and non-verbal behaviour under real-life or simulated conditions, appropriate and inappropriate responses, facilitating and dysfunctional thoughts, effectiveness of person's behaviour and responses, physiological responses, emotions expressed.
   (c) *consequences*: self-appraisal of performance, thoughts and feelings afterwards, responses of others.

2. Details of social environment: relationships, home, workplace.
3. Nature of identified problems: social skills deficits, dysfunctional thoughts, emotional problems.
4. History of identified problems: when and where they first developed or the person became aware of their difficulties.
5. Previous or current strategies to cope with problems: success or otherwise in resolving or adding to difficulties.
6. Potential for behaviour change: cues or trigger situations in the environment amenable to modification, external and internal reinforcers that maintain current behaviour, person's motivation and commitment for change, resources available within the person's relationships and environment.

The collected information is used to develop a profile or baseline of the person's:

- existing social skills repertoire;
- identified deficits or problem behaviours within their social skills;
- needs and potential for social skills development.

Designing the Social Skills Programme

The design of the programme should, as far as possible, involve the client, as this helps to increase motivation and commitment. It can also serve as a useful mental health promotional exercise. The programme will need to be planned in terms of:

1. The client's social skills training needs.
2. Realistic and attainable objectives expressed in behavioural terms to facilitate implementation and evaluation.
3. Selecting the most appropriate social skills techniques for the client's needs and the identified objectives.

4. Structuring the programme to facilitate the gradual and systematic development of the client's social skills, usually from the simple to the more complex. This will require detailed analysis of the desired social skills into their constituent verbal, non-verbal, cognitive and affective elements. The smaller "sub-units" of the total skill can then be learnt individually and then gradually linked together to form the total skill, e.g. assertiveness = eye contact, posture, gestures, voice tone, proximity, facial expression, self-belief, calmness.

5. Providing opportunities to rehearse and consolidate the new skills. The programme should be paced to avoid overloading and thereby stressing the client. There needs to be time for the skills to become gradually incorporated within their behavioural repertoire and for them to become generalized to other real-life situations.

6. Determining the methods of feedback that will be used and how progress will be monitored and evaluated.

Conducting a Social Skills Training Session

Introduction

The initial sessions may prove highly anxiety-provoking to participants. They need time to work through these anxieties and to develop trust in the trainers and fellow group members. This can be facilitated by the use of warm-up and trust exercises that are intended to put people at their ease and to develop relationships. As social anxiety is a common problem, aspects of anxiety management may be incorporated in the programme.

The objectives of the programme and the methods to be used should be discussed with the participants and expectations clarified. Emphasis should be placed on the need for active involvement and commitment for behavioural changes to take place. A written hand-out and outline of the programme is useful.

Briefing and instruction

The participants should be briefed on the particular skills that are to be practised during that session. These should include:

1. Specific details on the verbal and non-verbal behaviour to be developed.
2. The role of the behaviour in human interaction.
3. Details of the scenes and situations to be rehearsed. The role play may be structured with brief outlines or a script provided. Unstructured role play allows the participants more room for self-expression. Specific objectives should be set that enable the clients to:

   • focus on one aspect of the behaviour at a time;
   • gradually build up and develop the skill in a systematic way;

- actively participate in a variety of roles – main participant, supportive role, observer.

Behavioural rehearsal or role play

The opportunity to rehearse and practise new behaviours is essential to the process of social skills development. Role play and simulated exercises can be used to:

1. Represent real-life situations and task demands as closely as possible.
2. Provide the opportunity for repeated practice utilizing the same or modified strategies.
3. Rehearse situations in a safe setting where stresses can be reduced and risks avoided, e.g. damage to relationships or career, before transferring them to real life.
4. Give clients the opportunity to make decisions in response to their assessment of situations.
5. Modify or manipulate situations to enhance their educational value.
6. Enable clients to experience the simulated consequences which relate to their decisions and actions.

Role plays require careful preparation in order to achieve the maximum learning potential:

1. The environment and equipment need to be prepared beforehand.
2. The trainers should be clear on the objectives of the exercise.
3. Participants should be briefed as clearly and as concisely as possible on the aims of the practice and their roles. This should focus their attention on the behaviour being studied.
4. Others not directly involved can be given subsidiary roles that enable them to assist, e.g. as bystanders or observers. Observers may need preparation on what to focus upon and how to record their observations.
5. Scenes need to be graded from the simple and structured to the more complex and spontaneous to match the client's progress and learning needs.
6. The scene should attempt to resemble as closely as possible situations people encounter and the problems they might experience in real life.
7. The performance should be as brief as possible in order to achieve the desired objectives and to provide material for feedback and analysis. A surprising amount of information can be gained from even brief role plays. Sufficient time, therefore, needs to be allowed for this.
8. After feedback and analysis the scene can be repeated with either the same or different participants until the objectives are attained. Role-reversal, in which the main participants exchange roles for a re-run of a particular scene, is especially useful in facilitating empathy and social sensitivity.

Some clients may express considerable reservations about participating in role play. They tend to believe that the anxiety they experience will make their behaviour unrepresentative. However, if the situation is well planned and managed there is a strong correlation between a client's behaviour in role play and in real life. An additional benefit of role play is that it also reveals the participant's degree of insight, ability to empathize and their interpersonal perception.

With careful preparation and increased familiarity people's resistance to role play can be worked through and overcome. An indication of this is the client group's willingness to volunteer for specific roles.

Modelling

One of the advantages of role play as an educational approach is that it gives the participants the opportunity to study closely the behaviour of others. This provides the opportunity for observational learning or modelling which is a potent method of learning social behaviours. It is based upon the ability of the trainee to observe, recall and to reproduce significant aspects of the role model's behaviour. The model may be:

1. *A person*: the trainers, potentially very potent models, or fellow group members.
2. *An audio-visual model*: audio- or video-taped models. Tapes may be prepared in advance, made during role play sessions or commercially obtained.
3. *Written or diagrammatic material*: photographs, diagrams, written material or transcripts of situations may be used to increase knowledge and awareness.
4. *Covert*: in which the person visualizes themself or someone else modelling the desired behaviour in specific scenes. This cognitive rehearsal facilitates the development of positive expectations.

In order to be fully effective there are certain characteristics of modelling that can enhance the potential for learning:

1. The model should be credible to the client and someone with whom they can identify, i.e. similar in terms of age, sex, race, socio-economic background.
2. The model should be perceived as someone who has similar problems to the trainee.
3. The model should demonstrate how to cope rather than demonstrating mastery and excellence – this can be very intimidating to potential trainees.
4. A variety of potential role models should be offered as this increases the potential range of behaviours that can be learned. This may be achieved by one role model repeating a scene several times or by having several

role models demonstrating how they would handle the situation.

5. The models should be seen to demonstrate positive and appropriate examples of how to deal with situations.
6. The models should be seen to be clearly and positively rewarded as promptly as possible.

Feedback and debriefing

Feedback and debriefing are the most important part of the role play cycle. Knowledge of results and detailed guidance are essential to develop and improve any skill. The feedback may be given concurrently during the role play in the form of prompts and guidance or immediately after the role play (terminal feedback).

The feedback that is given should be prompt, detailed, focussed and clear to the participants. It should focus on the significant features of the behaviour and task rather than on the person. There should be ample opportunity to discuss and analyse the events. Initially, the participants may need to be brought out of role (de-roled) and anxieties resolved.

The forms of feedback that are available and a common sequence include:

1. *Self-analysis by key role players*: on how they perceived their own behaviour and that of the other principal players. Details should be sought not only on their actions but also on their thoughts and feelings. Participants have the potential to be very perceptive and also extremely harsh self-critics.
2. *Observations by trainers and observers*: on their perceptions of both the content and process of the role play. Notes and social interaction chats or inventories may be used to enable detailed analysis.
3. *Audio-visual*: video is a particularly potent form of feedback that is increasingly being used. The visual replay facilitates in-depth analysis and gives trainees the opportunity for critical self-confrontation. It may need to be used with care and tact to avoid the trainees focussing on negative aspects or rejecting the feedback altogether.
4. General discussion by all involved.

The role of the feedback and debriefing is to:

1. Provide positive reinforcement through praise, encouragement and non-verbal signals. Initially, the reinforcement is primarily external from the other participants and trainers. As the person develops their social skills they should also be encouraged to develop methods of self- or intrinsic reinforcement.
2. Give guidance and information on how to improve and modify their behaviour to enhance their interpersonal functioning.
3. Generate potential alternative ways of behaving. Other responses can be discussed and compared with the person's original behaviour.

4. Link the new skill with previous learning to show the relationships that exist between patterns of behaviour.
5. Suggest opportunities in real life for trying out the skills.

After feedback the scene can be repeated with the same or different participants to provide the opportunity to rehearse and consolidate their skills. The cycle of "role play – feedback – repeated role play – further feedback" is followed until the objectives are achieved by the participants.

Facilitating Transfer and Generalization of Learning

The ultimate test of the effectiveness of a social skills training programme lies in the ability of the clients to:

1. Transfer the skills learnt in the training sessions to the real world and to a variety of different situations where the behaviour is appropriate.
2. Consolidate and maintain the skills after the programme is completed. This requires the new skills and facilitating cognitions to become integrated into the person's everyday living patterns and to be reinforced in the natural environment.

The processes of transfer and generalization are facilitated by:

1. Ensuring that the clients understand the principles involved in the programme.
2. A supportive group climate and good relationships with fellow group members and trainers.
3. Utilizing a wide range of practical exercises that closely resemble real-life situations.
4. Working with a variety of role models during training sessions.
5. Providing adequate opportunity to rehearse the skills during training sessions.
6. Gradually reducing external feedback and developing the person's ability to reinforce themself.
7. Using a wide variety of methods of feedback.
8. Discussion and sharing with group members to prompt attitude change and cognitive restructuring.
9. Accompanying residents on practice sessions in real life situations.
10. Availability of practice opportunities for homework between sessions.
11. Periodic follow-up training sessions.

Homework

Homework is an integral part of any social skills training programme. It provides the opportunity to try out in real-life settings the skills and approaches that have until now been practised in role play. To be effective, homework has to be carefully structured:

1. Specific instructions need to be given in relation to the times, places, situations and frequency of practise of skills. These may need to be written down.
2. The tasks need to be graded in difficulty to have a high probability of reinforcement and to develop progressively the person's skills.
3. Relatives and significant others need to be informed of the homework requirements and the ways in which they can support and maintain the development of the person's skills.
4. The person should understand the relevance of the homework to their social skills programme and should be involved in identifying and selecting potential learning opportunities.

Homework facilitates the transfer and generalization of skills. In this process there is also a transition from explicit feedback and reinforcement towards self- and social reinforcement in the natural environment.

Opportunity should be provided at each therapy session for the individual or group to report on their homework and to share any difficulties.

Evaluation

The client's progress should be monitored throughout the programme. This is facilitated by:

- observation of clients during role plays;
- attending to the feedback from participants;
- reviewing the client's homework;
- consultation with co-therapist and supervisor.

Many of the techniques of assessment – interview, diary, rating scales, self-appraisal – can be used to make a summative evaluation of the client's overall progress. Clearly defined profiles of the client's baseline social skills and behavioural objectives for desired outcomes give a standard to measure progress against. Judgements can be made about:

- the accuracy of the assessment;
- the attainability of the objectives;
- the effectiveness of the training programme;
- the client's overall progress and need for further social skills training, if indicated.

Unit Instructions

When you have researched the suggested references, have mastered the
Unit Objectives and successfully answered the Self-assessment Questions,
proceed with the Unit Written Test.

Suggested References

Argyle, M. (1983). *The Psychology of Interpersonal Behaviour*, 4th edition. Penguin,
Harmondsworth.

Bandura, A. (1977). *Social Learning Theory*. Prentice Hall, Englewood Cliffs, N.J.

Barker, P. J. (1982). *Behaviour Therapy Nursing*. Croom Helm, London.

Barker, P. J. (1985). *Patient Assessment in Psychiatric Nursing*. Croom Helm,
London.

Barker, P. and Wilson, L. (1985). New wine in old bottles. *Nursing Times*, 25
September, Vol. 81, No. 39, pp. 31–34.

Bolton, R. (1979). *People Skills*. Prentice-Hall, Englewood Cliffs, N.J.

Briggs, K. (1986). Speak your mind. *Nursing Times*, 25 June, Vol. 82, No. 26, pp.
24–26.

Dainow, S. (1986). Believe in yourself. *Nursing Times*, 2 July, Vol. 82, No. 27, pp.
49–51.

Darcy, P. T. (1985). *Mental Health Nursing Source Book*. Baillière Tindall, London
and San Diego.

Davis, B. D. and Ternulf-Nyhlin, K. (1982). Social skills training. *Nursing Times*,
20 October, Vol. 78, No. 42, pp. 1765–1768.

Dickson, A. (1982). *A Woman in Your Own Right*. Quartet Books, London.

Ellis, R. and Whittington, D. (1981). *A Guide to Social Skill Training*. Croom Helm,
London.

Fensterheim, H. and Baer, J. (1975). *Don't Say 'Yes' When You Want to Say 'No'*.
Futura, London.

Hargie, O., Saunders, C. and Dickson, O. (1987). *Social Skills in Interpersonal
Communication*, 2nd edition. Croom Helm, London.

Kagan, C., Evans, J. and Kay, B. (1986). *A Manual of Interpersonal Skills for
Nurses: An Experiential Approach*. Harper and Row, London.

Kingston, B. (1987). *Psychological Approaches in Psychiatric Nursing*. Croom Helm,
London.

Knibbs, J. and Hardiman, F. (1983). A sense of security. *Nursing Mirror*, 21
September, No. 157, Vol. 12, Mental Health Forum, pp. vii–viii.

Le Lievre, J., Gilbert, M. T. and Reavley, W. (1983). Social skills training. *Nursing
Times*, 18 May, Vol. 79, No. 20, pp. 46–48.

Liberman, R., King, L., Derisi, W. and McCann, M. (1975). *Personal Effectiveness*.
Research Press.

Lyttle, J. (1986). *Mental Disorder – Its Care and Treatment*. Baillière Tindall, London
and San Diego.

Mercer, I. (1985). Striking the right balance. *Nursing Times*, 20 November, Vol.
81, No. 47, pp. 58–59.

Murgatroyd, S. (1985). *Counselling and Helping*. British Psychological Society and
Methuen, London.

Nelson-Jones, R. (1986). *Human Relationship Skills*. Holt, Rinehart and Winston, London.

Paul, N. (1985). *The Right to Be You*. Chartwell-Bratt, Bromley.

Pope, B. (1986). *Social Skills Training for Psychiatric Nurses*. Harper and Row, London.

Priestley, P., McGuire, J., Flegg, D., Hemsley, V. and Welham, D. (1978). *Social Skills and Personal Problem Solving*. Tavistock, London.

Rawat R. (1983). Social skills training. *Nursing Mirror*, 21 September, Vol. 157, No. 12, Mental Health Forum 9, pp. i–iii.

Rose-Neil, S. (1986). Just how assertive are you? *Nursing Times*, 25 June, Vol. 82, No. 26, pp. 28–30.

Smith, M. J. (1975). *When I Say 'No', I Feel Guilty*. Bantam, New York.

Trower, P., Bryant, B. and Argyle, M. (1978). *Social Skills and Mental Health*. Methuen, London.

Vousden, M. and Fisher, P. (1983). Actions speak louder than words. *Nursing Mirror*, 21 September, Vol. 157, No. 12, Mental Health Forum 9, pp. iii–vii.

Wilkinson, J. and Canter, S. (1982). *Social Skills Training Manual*. John Wiley, Chichester.

Self-assessment Questions

SAQ 13. List six non-verbal behaviours that have a role in human communication.

SAQ 14. Describe briefly six stages involved in the planning of a social skills programme.

SAQ 15. Outline six factors that need to be considered when utilizing role play.

SAQ 16. State four ways in which transfer and generalization of newly acquired skills can be facilitated.

Unit 3.4: Written Test

You are working with a small group of residents who are being prepared for a move from a ward in an isolated hospital to a hostel in the nearby town. As part of the process of preparation for this move the residents would appear to need to develop their social skills.

1. Describe in detail how you can evaluate the residents' level of social functioning.
2. What planning and preparation are necessary before beginning the programme?
3. Taking one common social skill as an example, describe how you would teach this skill to the resident.
4. How can you ensure that the newly acquired skills are transferred from role play to real-life situations?

TOPIC 4

The Nature of Mental Health Problems

At the end of this Topic the learner should aim to:

1. Recognize the importance of effective coping strategies in dealing with stress.
2. Describe the processes whereby individuals come into contact with health care agencies.
3. Outline how differing perspectives of mental health problems influence treatment and care.
4. Identify the basis upon which mental illnesses are classified.

UNIT 4.1

Stress and Coping

Unit Objectives

At the end of this Unit the learner should be able to:

1. Describe the relationship between coping and mental health.
2. Differentiate between effective and ineffective coping strategies.
3. Outline factors that influence a person's perception and response to stressful situations.
4. List the stages of development of a crisis.

Coping and Mental Health

Relationships and the activities of daily living pose continual demands and problems for the individual: situations have to be responded to; relationships have to be negotiated; physical, social and psychological needs have to be met. Certain situations may be anticipated by individuals and form part of a process of social maturity and development. Other situations may be completely unexpected and experienced as ill-timed accidents or personal tragedy.

A person's ability to cope with these demands and with specific life events would appear to be directly related to the quality of their life and to the maintenance of their mental health. Surveys tend to reveal that the experience of difficulty in coping with certain aspects of living are quite common in the "normal" population. There is also growing evidence that many people with mental health problems, for a variety of reasons, have significant deficits in their ability to cope effectively with both expected and unexpected life events.

Coping Strategies

Responding to situations and life events in order to avoid stress and to meet basic needs involves a complex process. The person has to initiate a problem-solving process in order to master the demands being made. Each individual develops unique ways of coping with the demands that they experience and in the strategies that they use to meet their needs. Behaviour, emotions and cognitions have to be organized into appropriate patterns to facilitate coping and to minimize the potential for emotional distress. The required responses may or may not be part of a person's existing repertoire of coping strategies. These may include:

1. *Cognitive responses*: thinking through potential courses of action, possible outcomes, identifying priorities and risks, decision making.
2. *Emotional responses*: coming to terms with loss, expressing feelings appropriately, re-evaluating the emotional significance of relationships.
3. *Behavioural responses*: taking action to implement a chosen strategy within a person's capabilities, using specific skills.

Effective coping strategies

Responding effectively to demands should ensure that:

1. The experience of stress is resolved or reduced through either problem solving, reducing the influence of adverse conditions, redefining the problem to a more manageable perspective or accepting situations that cannot be altered.
2. A sense of mastery is experienced, i.e. that the person feels in control of their own life and their self-esteem is enhanced.
3. Learning takes place, i.e. the person's ability to deal with future similar situations is enhanced. This increases their ability to cope with stress and to resolve potential crises. They feel less vulnerable and are able to be more objective about situations and to be more open with others.

Ineffective coping strategies

Responding ineffectively may have the following consequences:

1. Further increasing the experience of stress and thereby further reducing the person's ability to cope.
2. Creating feelings of loss of control and of being trapped and helpless.
3. Increasing the likelihood of making inappropriate compromises or decisions; repressing or denying unresolved conflict. This further increases the potential for subsequent crises.

If a person's existing coping strategies and skills are ineffective then they need to be helped to develop new resources. This is inherent in many therapeutic approaches including counselling, group work, social skills training, cognitive therapy and health education.

Coping and Mental Illness

People will tend to use a variety of coping methods for a given situation. However, it would appear that those with mental health problems frequently have difficulty coping because their:

- appraisal of situations is inaccurate and distorted;
- range of potential responses is limited and often maladaptive;
- ability to select appropriate coping responses is restricted.

Many of the symptoms of "mental illness" may be viewed as ineffective or inappropriate coping methods. The symptoms for the individual may represent a way of coping but they can also severely impair their interpersonal functioning and activities of living. For example, it would appear that those with mental health problems tend to make excessive use and be reliant upon short-term coping methods at the expense of long-term problem solving (see Exhibit 4.1.1).

Exhibit 4.1.1 Coping strategies

Short-term coping strategies	Long-term coping strategies
Crying	Seeking information
Sleeping	Talking to others
Withdrawing	Exploring alternatives
Rationalizing, denial projection	Making plans, setting goals
Displacement, diversional activity	Re-evaluation
Anger, aggression	Learning new skills
Alcohol, cigarettes, drugs	Anticipatory rehearsal
Eating more or eating less	Taking direct action
Spending money	Going for help
Humour	Attempting to change situation

Coping with Stress and Life Events

Assessment

In order to respond appropriately to situations the individual has initially to assess and analyse what significance an event has for them. From this appraisal the person can then select what seems to them an appropriate coping response. Each person formulates a unique assessment that is influenced by a number of factors that can interfere with their perception:

1. *Past experience*: new situations may be inaccurately attributed with similarities to previous experiences. Traumatic past events and early experiences may also distort the person's perception of the present.
2. *Subjective involvement*: being actively involved in situations limits the amount of objectivity that the person can have.
3. *Relationship with the person or events being appraised*: people or events that have a particularly high emotional relevance to the person will not be viewed clearly.
4. *Value and belief system*: strongly held beliefs may influence the person's perspective, e.g. personal moral codes, religious beliefs, prejudices, gender and occupational roles.
5. *Cognitive framework*: a person's cognitive framework may be such that it distorts their perception. Frequently this gives a negative bias and limits the individual's belief in the possibility of taking effective action. Cognitive distortions may include helplessness, over-generalization, selective abstraction, arbitrary inference, magnification, minimization, dichotomous thinking, personalization, delusional thinking, confusion.
6. *Sensory and perceptual distractions*: the experience of illusions and hallucinations seriously interferes with the ability of a person to make an accurate assessment.
7. *Mental defence mechanisms*: these are unconsciously activated psychological mechanisms that attempt to preserve the integrity of the individual. They endeavour to protect the individual from threat by distorting an individual's perception of events or by psychologically redirecting the stress. Mechanisms may include:

    - *repression*: unacceptable and anxiety-producing impulses are completely blocked from awareness;
    - *denial*: threatening events are warded off by denying that they happened or by not acknowledging other people's perception of their behaviour;
    - *displacement*: feelings that cannot be expressed towards the intended person are diverted towards more readily accessible and vulnerable people or objects;
    - *rationalization*: seeking socially acceptable reasons as to why unattainable goals are no longer desired or why certain courses of action were followed;
    - *projection*: unacceptable personal impulses are externalized and other people incorrectly attributed with them;
    - *conversion*: psychological stress is converted and expressed as physical symptoms;
    - *sublimation*: redirecting personally unacceptable drives into more socially acceptable channels.

Responding to stress and life events

From their appraisal the person's chosen response is influenced by a number of factors.

Past experiences

The person may be able to reproduce strategies that they found successful before or to use their experience to generate alternative solutions. However, learning from experience is not always very effective because:

1. A person's experience may be limited.
2. The outcomes of stressful situations may have been distressing and unpleasant rather than a positive learning experience.
3. People tend to lack full insight into situations in which they are subjectively involved.
4. Learning tends to take place slowly and a little at a time.
5. People rarely review life experiences in order to identify how they could have improved their response; the more distressing the situation the more likely is the person to try and "put it all behind them".

Repertoire of coping strategies

The greater the range and effectiveness of potential responses available to the person, the more likely are they able to select an appropriate response. A limited choice of responses seriously handicaps a person's ability to cope effectively.

Resources available

The availability of personal and practical resources are significant factors in determining a person's ability to cope with difficulties. Resources include:

1. *Self-esteem and sense of mastery*: a high degree of self-belief and confidence are especially important. In particular, a person needs to perceive themself as being able to influence positively their own life events and to have a degree of mastery over their destiny.
2. *Network of supportive social relationships*: close, confiding relationships where the person is valued and given emotional support; where practical help and assistance is available.
3. *Financial resources*: which remove a source of worry to many people and increase the options available – access to private care, buying in practical services, taking a holiday, moving house, improving their environment, treating themself.
4. *Accessibility to support services*: the availability of treatment and social

support agencies, the identification and acknowledgement of the individual's difficulties.

5. *Occupational status*: more highly skilled professionals are more likely to be tolerantly supported during periods of stress. They are also more likely to be able to redesign aspects of their work role to reduce stress, particularly if they are of value to the organization or are self-employed.

Personal and social value of finding a solution

Each person has their own value system that determines what is classified as stressful and how important it is for them to resolve their difficulties. What may seem trivial to outsiders may be a source of major stress for the individual. Alternatively, what others may regard as intolerable circumstances may be viewed with equanimity by the person. There may also be occasions when the person's individual value system may be in conflict with those of other agencies and workers who believe they are trying to help.

Situation in which the problem occurs

Specific situations may be the cause of great stress to the person. However, the perceived consequences may impose severe constraints upon the way that the individual can respond. For example, work conflict with a superior, family violence or sexual abuse in which the person fears further violence or unwarranted guilt and shame.

The demands being made

Each person has a limit as to how much stress they can tolerate and cope with effectively. Some people and families may at great cost be able to cope with quite severe levels of stress. Frequently, in such a situation, the addition of even a seemingly minor difficulty may precipitate a crisis. Changes in the person's self-perception, support network, environment or physical health are significant additional stressors. People are particularly affected by:

1. *The severity of the life event*: Some situations are generally acknowledged to be particularly stressful. These include bereavement, divorce, imprisonment, personal injury or illness, redundancy, retirement, pregnancy, moving house, changing jobs.
2. *The number of stressful life events and their closeness in time*: A succession of stressful life events occurring closely together can overwhelm a person, whereas in isolation they could possible have coped with the individual events.
3. *The time available for a response.* The more time available for a person to respond, the less stressful the experience and the more time to seek an effective solution. However, when people are under great stress their perception of time becomes distorted and they generally want to resolve

the situation as soon as possible. However, this may not always be the best course of action.

State of physical health

An optimum state of physical health is important in coping with stressful life events. A person's health tends to suffer when under stress, causing fatigue, malaise, lethargy and insomnia.

Taking action

From their appraisal and the coping strategies available to them people will initiate a response. Initially they will resort to their habitual coping methods and, where possible, replicate past responses to similar situations. If these are not successful, then the individual may need to consider alternative ways of coping. The outcomes may be that:

1. *The situation is successfully resolved*. The person perceives the outcomes as desirable and favourable. They may experience a sense of mastery and enhanced self-esteem. It may have been a situation from which the person has been able to learn and add to their repertoire of coping strategies – "nothing succeeds like success".
2. *The situation is contained*. The person is able to limit the extent of disruption by redefining or accepting the situation. This may mean coming to terms with and tolerating a long-term demand upon their resources. Depending upon their nature, the problems may gradually resolve over time or be a source of mounting stress.
3. *The situation is not coped with*. Increasing stress causes further disruption to the person's social, psychological and physical well-being. Mounting stress may then precipitate a crisis which the person is not able to cope with on their own or with the resources available to them.

Phases of a Crisis

A crisis can be an overwhelming experience for a person that may leave them psychologically and socially damaged. It can also be an opportunity for personal growth and greater maturity. Crises can be viewed as a series of phases of mounting distress with characteristic patterns of behaviour and response. The crisis may be resolved at any of the stages or may proceed unabated.

A. Impact

Habitual coping strategies are used to try and restore equilibrium and to resolve the stress experienced. These are found to be ineffective and the individual experiences stress and strain. The individual may or may not be aware of the cause of their stress and may exhibit a wide range of psychological and physical signs. These can include:

1. *Psychological*: anger, irritability, impatience, temper, moodiness, indecision, restlessness, inability to concentrate, forgetfulness, sensitivity to criticisms, jealousy, grief, shame, excitability, impulsiveness, worrying, feeling tense, depression, loss of libido, drinking and smoking more.
2. *Physical*: headaches, loss of appetite or overeating, loss of sleep or sleeping more, fatigue, tiredness, aches and pains, indigestion, palpitations, nausea, breathlessness, dizziness, diarrhoea, stomach upsets.

B. Recoil

Continued failure to cope with the crisis causes increasing disorganization and mounting anxiety. These further inhibit the ability of the person to respond effectively. Increasing desperation may force the person to try novel ways of coping.

C. Disorganization

Severe stress causes high levels of tension and impairment of functioning. The person's behaviour becomes increasingly disorganized and purposeless.

D. Inertia and exhaustion

Continued failure to resolve the crisis causes progressive deterioration and exhaustion. Physical signs and symptoms of exhaustion are evident. Psychologically the person feels helpless, trapped and ready to give up.

Unit Instructions

When you have researched the suggested references, have mastered the Unit Objectives and successfully answered the Self-assessment Questions, proceed with the Unit Written Test.

Suggested References

Adams, G. A. & Macione, A. (Eds) (1983). *Handbook of Psychiatric Mental Health Nursing*. John Wiley/Fleschner, New York.

Aguilera, D. C. and Messick, J. S. (1982). *Crisis Intervention Therapy for Psychological Emergencies*. New American Library/Mosby, St. Louis.

Argyle, M. (Ed.) (1981). *Social Skills and Health*. Methuen, London.

Atkinson, R. L., Atkinson, R. C. and Hilcard, E. R. (1983). *Introduction to Psychology*, 8th edition. Harcourt Brace Jovanovich, London and San Diego.

Bond, M. (1986). *Stress and Self-Awareness: A Guide for Nurses*. Heinemann Nursing, London.

Booth, A. L. (1985). *Stressmanship*. Seven House, London.

Bowron, B. (1980). Recognising the presence of stress. *Nursing*, Vol. 1, No. 10, pp. 428–430.

Burnard, P. (1985). How to reduce stress. *Nursing Mirror*, 6 November, Vol. 161, No. 19, pp. 47–48.

Caplan, G. (1968). *An Approach to Community Mental Health*. Tavistock, London.

Castledine, G. (1985). Taking a rest from stress. *Nursing Times*, 20 March, Vol. 81, No. 12, p. 22.

Clarke, M. (1980). Psychological aspects of stress. *Nursing*, Vol. 1, No. 10, pp. 426–27.

Coleman, V. (1982). Stress can kill. *Nursing Mirror*, 6 October, Vol. 155, No. 14, p. 41.

Consumer's Association (1982). *Living with Stress*. Consumer's Association/Hodder and Stoughton, London.

Cooper, C., Cooper, R. and Eaker, L. (1988). *Living with Stress*. Penguin, Harmondsworth.

Cox, T. (1978). *Stress*. Macmillan, London.

Cranwell-Ward, T. (1987). *Managing Stress*. Pan, London.

Ekberg, T. Y. (1986). Spouse burnout syndrome. *Journal of Advanced Nursing*, Vol. 11, pp. 161–165.

Evison, R. (1985). Self-help in preventing stress build up. *The Professional Nurse*, March, Vol. 1, No. 6, pp. 157–159.

Gillespie, C. (1987). Stress reducing strategies. *Nursing Times*, 30 September, Vol. 83, No. 39, pp. 30–32.

Hase, S. and Douglas, A. (1986). *Human Dynamics and Nursing*. Churchill Livingstone, Edinburgh.

Hingley, P. and Cooper, C. (1986). *Stress and the Nurse Manager*. John Wiley, New York.

Hingley, P. and Harris, P. (1986). Lowering the tension. *Nursing Times*, 6 August, Vol. 82, No. 32, p. 52.

Hobbs, T. (1985). Stress among the staff – who looks after the nurse? *Nurse Education Today*, Vol. 5, No. 5, pp. 201–209.

Hughes, B. and Boothroyd, R. (1985). *Fight or Flight? Mastering Problems of Everyday Life*. Faber and Faber, London.

Kowalski, R. (1987). *Over the Top*. Avalon Press/Winslow Press. Bristol/Bicester.

Lombardi, T. (1987). Under control. *Senior Nurse*, May, Vol. 6, No. 5, pp. 8–9.

Lyttle, J. (1986). *Mental Disorder*. Baillière Tindall, London and San Diego.

Mapanga, M. (1985). Caring for Learners. *Nursing Mirror*, 26 June, Vol. 160, No. 26, pp. 44–46.

Milne, D., Burdett, C. and Beckett, J. (1986). Assessing and reducing the stress and strain of psychiatric nursing. *Nursing Times*, 7 May, Vol. 82, No. 19, pp. 59–62.

Montague, S. (1980a). The physiological basis of the stress reaction. *Nursing*, Vol. 1, No. 10, pp. 422–425.

Montague, S. (1980b). Measuring stress. *Nursing*, Vol. 1, No. 10, p. 430.

Morrice, J. K. W. (1976). *Crisis Intervention Studies in Community Care*. Pergamon Press, Oxford.

Murgatroyd, S. (1985). *Counselling and Helping*. British Psychological Society and Methuen, London.

Murgatroyd, S. and Woolfe, R. (1982). *Coping with Crisis – Understanding and Helping Persons in Need*. Harper and Row, London.

Murgatroyd, S. and Woolfe, R. (1985). *Helping Families in Distress: An Introduction to Family Focused Helping*. Harper and Row, London.

Nicklin, P. (1987). Violence to the spirit. *Senior Nurse*, May, Vol. 6, No. 5, pp. 10–12.

Nursing Skill Book Series (1983). *Using Crisis Intervention Wisely*. Nursing 83 Books, Springhouse, Pennsylvania.

Orme, J. E. (1984). *Abnormal and Clinical Psychology: An Introductory Text*. Croom Helm, London.

Porritt, L. (1984). *Communication: Choices for Nurses*. Churchill Livingstone, Edinburgh.

Priestley, P., McGuire, J., Flegg, D., Hemsley, V. and Welham, D. (1978). *Social Skills and Personal Problem Solving*. Tavistock, London.

Rowan, F. P. (1980). *The Chronically Distressed Client*. C. V. Mosby, St. Louis.

Sheehy, G. (1974). *Passages – Predictable Crises of Adult Life*. Bantam, New York.

Shepherd, G. (1984). *Institutional Care and Rehabilitation*. Longman, London.

Taylor, A., Sluckin, W., Davies, D. R., Reason, J. T., Thomson, R. and Colman, A. M. (1982). *Introducing Psychology*, 2nd edition. Penguin, Harmondsworth.

Thomas, M. (1980). Stress and mental illness. *Nursing*, February, Vol. 1, No. 10, pp. 438–440.

Trower, P., Bryant, B. and Argyle, M. (1978). *Social Skills and Mental Health*. Methuen, London.

Tschudin, V. (1985a). Too much pressure. *Nursing Times*, 11 September, Vol. 81, No. 37, pp. 30–31.

Tschudin, V. (1985b). Warding off a crisis. *Nursing Times*, 18 September, Vol. 81, No. 38, pp. 45–46.

Vousden, M. (1985). Taking the strain. *Nursing Mirror*, 14 August, Vol. 161, No. 7, pp. 25–28.

Watson, J. (1986). A step in the right direction. *Senior Nurse*, Vol. 5, No. 4, pp. 12–14.

Wilson-Barnett, J. (1979). *Stress in Hospital: Patients' Psychological Reactions to Illness and Health Care*. Churchill Livingstone, Edinburgh.

Wilson-Barnett, J. (1980). Prevention and alleviation of stress. *Nursing*, Vol. 1, No. 10, pp. 432–436.

Self-assessment Questions

SAQ 1. Identify four characteristics of ineffective coping skills.

SAQ 2. List and describe four mental defence mechanisms.

SAQ 3. Describe four factors that may influence how an individual responds to a stressful situation.

SAQ 4. List in order and describe the stages of a crisis.

Unit 4.1: Written Test

1. In what ways can a person's repertoire of coping skills influence their mental health?

2. Describe the factors that determine how an individual appraises a situation and identifies an appropriate response.

Pathway to Care

Unit Objectives

At the end of this Unit the learner should be able to:

1. Describe the factors involved with the self-assessment of mental health problems.
2. Identify the courses of action open to people with mental health difficulties.
3. Outline influences which determine whether help is sought.
4. State the steps required for intervention in a crisis.

Self-assessment and Mental Health

The experience of stress or long-term difficulties may alert an individual or family to the need to make adjustments in their life-style or to seek help. Social surveys repeatedly reveal high levels of mental ill-health morbidity in the population for which outside assistance is not sought. This would indicate that the majority of these people are attempting to deal with their difficulties themselves or are unable or unwilling to seek help. As most problems are short-lived and not too severe, most people are probably able to contain or resolve their difficulties. However, this still leaves a significant degree of personal suffering and distress for which potential resources are not utilized.

Initially, in order to seek help or even to tackle their own problems, the person and their family have to be in a position to recognize the nature of their difficulties. However, this process of recognition is complicated by a number of factors:

1. *The difficulty of objective personal appraisal.* Insight and self-awareness are often limited or restricted when experiencing mental health problems (see unit 4.1).
2. *The ability of the family and person to cope with stresses.* There is a lot of stress even in "ordinary families" who develop their own ways of maintaining equilibrium: most can tolerate minor difficulties, some can tolerate and cope with quite severe problems. A number of families cope

with a considerable burden for a prolonged period, often at considerable personal expense and detriment to the quality of their lives and relationships.

3. *The insidious nature of many mental health problems.* The problems that develop are often gradual and evolve over a long period of time. This gives time for the family to adjust to changed demands and to accommodate and tolerate changes in behaviour, emotions, performance and rhythms. The nature of these difficulties may not be recognized and have adverse effects on family life and relationships. Gradually, mounting emotional, social, sexual and economic problems may cause severe stress and tend to make others withdraw.

4. *The perceived short-term nature of difficulties.* Most mental health problems are short-term and not necessarily severe. In the majority of cases most people attempt to deal with their problems unaided or hope that they will soon pass. However, the experience of repeated "short-term" difficulties may disguise the presence of more fundamental long-term problems.

5. *Family defence mechanisms.* As with individual mental defence mechanisms, close groups of people can, consciously and unconsciously, collusively respond to defend their integrity. Reactions may be attempts to misperceive or "ignore" the problems:

   - *normalize* – other people behave like this;
   - *attenuate* – the problems are not that bad or serious;
   - *balancing* – balancing out a person's "bad" or "difficult" behaviour with aspects of their behaviour that are "good" or approved of;
   - *denial* – not accepting that anything is actually wrong.

6. *Personal and family value systems and expectations.* Against this criteria the person and their family may compare themselves against:

   (a) Their previous level of functioning and assess their past performance in relation to their current difficulties. They may or may not be able to identify significant changes in their behaviour, emotions, thoughts and physical health, which could indicate the presence of severe difficulties.

   (b) Significant others and compare how others seem to be coping with life events in relation to assessments of their own performance. Friends and relatives may be approached for advice, help and opinions.

   (c) Their knowledge, experience and attitudes towards mental health problems. General levels of knowledge about mental health problems tend to be inaccurate and distorted. This, together with the stereotype of mental illness as gross "insanity", rarely provides a suitable criteria for evaluating their own difficulties. Previous experiences with mental health services may have been limited or negative. Most clients and families complain of difficulty in gaining access to services and of not being kept informed. These experiences colour future responses to difficulties and on seeking help.

7 *The high personal and social costs of labelling their difficulties as mental health problems.* The stigma attached to mental illness is such that it acts as a powerful disincentive.

Seeking Help

A decision may be made that the person or family is experiencing severe difficulty in coping. Several courses of action are then open.

Not to seek help

As a consequence of this they may find that:

1. The problems resolve themselves.
2. They find ways of coping unaided that reduce the demands being made.
3. The problems continue and create chronic misery and distress.
4. The problems increase in severity and eventually create a crisis such that the family is ultimately forced to seek help.

To seek help

Depending upon the nature of the stress, access may be sought to available sources of help. However, this does not necessarily ensure that the problems will be resolved. Seeking help may cause strong feelings among those concerned, e.g. guilt, shame, disbelief, embarrassment, loss of face, sense of failure, anger, confusion. Approaches may be made to the following:

1. A support network of close friends and relatives who may not have been previously involved. These may be able to offer practical advice and support through the period of crisis. This is probably the most commonly used resource.
2. Voluntary agencies may be approached depending on the presenting problems or their local accessibility, e.g. Samaritans, A.A., Help the Aged, Marriage Guidance. They may be seen as more approachable, appropriate and less stigmatizing than statutory services.
3. Emergency services, e.g. police, casualty departments or ambulance services, may be approached if the situation is perceived as a crisis with possible life-threatening consequences.
4. The person's General Practitioner is probably the most readily known and accessible health care professional.
5. Statutory services, for example:

- psychiatric hospitals;
- community mental health centres, possibly with self-referral facilities;
- Local Authority Social Services departments, most of which offer an emergency service out of office hours.

The General Practitioner

The person's GP has a key role in determining whether the person's difficulties will be identified and on their access to other services. In these respects the GP has an important "gate-keeper" role. The person's visit to their GP may be self-initiated or, if they are unwilling or unable, may be organized by their relatives. Actually seeing a doctor or other health care worker requires a lot of skill on the part of the client for a successful consultation. The average contact time is limited and in that time the person has to communicate difficulties of which they may have only limited awareness and a limited vocabulary. Yet the recognition of mental health problems takes a lot of time and skill. The person's previous relationship with their GP is an important factor in this consultation.

Visits tend to be precipitated by social and interpersonal problems and the person may present a wide range of difficulties. A person's perception of their difficulties may be in contrast to the views held by others (see Exhibit 4.2.1).

Exhibit 4.2.1 Contrasting perceptions of mental health problems

Experienced by person	*Perceived by others*
Feel unwell, tired insomnia, fatigue, fed up, run down, poor concentration, strain in relationships, loss of appetite and interest, sexual problems, difficulty in coping, feeling changed or different, excessive smoking and drinking, hearing and seeing things	Miserable, lazy, poor hygiene and appearance, off their food, changed for the worse, withdrawn, forgetful, up all night, loss of affection, irritable, seem different or changed in some way that they cannot easily describe, irresponsible

Initially, people tend to present with physical signs and symptoms as this is how they conceptualize their difficulties and experience them. Such perceptions also strongly influence their expectations on treatment. Many want tablets to make them feel better and GPs are under a lot of pressure to prescribe. Any suggestions by the GP that the person's difficulties may be mental health problems are likely to come as a shock to the person. The GP's response may be to:

1. Focus on the presenting physical symptoms and to prescribe a variety of tonics, vitamins, laxatives or placebos. Large numbers of people repeatedly attend the GP's surgery with vague and non-specific symptoms. Often, the underlying mental health problems are not recognized or acknowledged.
2. Attempt to treat the underlying difficulties. The limited time available and the nature of the presenting problems are such that over-reliance on minor tranquillizers and antidepressants is common. Vast numbers of prescriptions for psycho-active medications are given annually. There is some evidence of poorly supervised and inappropriate medication given to people for many years. Many of these tablets are subsequently used when people overdose and attempt suicide.
3. Reject the presenting symptoms and not to validate the person's perceptions, especially if they are seen as non-medical in origin, e.g. financial, occupational, housing, relationship.
4. Refer to the Community Mental Health team for assessment and intervention.
5. Refer to a psychiatrist. The pattern of referral by GPs is not consistent, with some referring too readily and others hardly referring at all. The person is likely to have to wait some time for an appointment. Many keep their appointment secret and do not in the end attend. Most are unaware of the role of the psychiatrist or what treatments are available.
   The purpose of this diagnostic process by both the GP and the psychiatrist is to validate the person's difficulties and to legitimize the person's "sickness role". This confirms that the person is not responsible for their behaviour and is in need of treatment. From his/her assessment the psychiatrist will identify an appropriate medical course of action.

Social Intervention

The individual and their family may have varying degrees of success in their attempts to resolve and contain their difficulties. Their ability to do this may eventually determine whether outside intervention is necessary. Minor deviations in behaviour may be tolerated by the local community. If the person's behaviour is perceived as threatening or self-injurious then outside agencies may intervene. This recognition factor is important because most classifications of mental health problems are made in the community by lay people and not by professionals. Factors related to this include:

1. *Visibility*: how much of their behaviour is seen by others and is perceived as threatening or damaging to the community or individual.
2. *Not fulfilling social obligations*: if the person is perceived as being unable,

reluctant or unwilling to make expected social responses or to meet social expectations. A perceived failure by the person to recognize that they are not fulfilling these obligations is also significant.

3. *Social distance*: the frequency and intensity of social contacts and relationships. A relative degree of isolation or social anonymity may mean that the individual's behaviour can remain "hidden" in certain environments.

Psychiatric emergencies

Many people referred to mental health services are in a state of crisis. Common presenting emergencies include:

- attempted suicide,
- extreme personal distress,
- family conflicts,
- interpersonal difficulties,
- danger to self or others,
- psychotic episode,
- aggressive behaviour,
- work problems.

Crisis Intervention

Individuals experiencing a crisis require help. It is important that crisis intervention services are accessible and are able to offer a prompt response to people in need to re-establish equilibrium. By this stage of crisis, people's behaviour is frequently disorganized and they are in an unstable state. Their situation can rapidly improve or deteriorate.

The primary role of the helping agency is to guide the person constructively through this experience. The objectives of crisis intervention are to:

1. Resolve the immediate crisis and restore normal functioning as quickly as possible.
2. Facilitate the development of the person's and family's coping skills.

The purpose of crisis intervention is primarily to deal with that specific situation. The client and family may have other related problems, but unless they are contributing directly to their current crisis they are best dealt with afterwards. Long-term therapy may subsequently be required, but this is not part of crisis intervention.

If the crisis is viewed as a temporary difficulty, it is more likely to be resolved quickly and without after-effects; hence the need to provide intensive short-term interventions for the crisis. In this way recovery tends to be quicker and more complete than if the individual is treated as "ill" and forced into a sick role.

The majority of crises are self-limiting; most are resolved with or without intervention within 6 weeks. The participants may be able to work out their own solution unaided. However, there is also the risk that inappropriate solutions and compromises may be made that can increase their psychological and social vulnerability. This increases the likelihood of further and major crises.

Crisis intervention is an active process that is based upon the principles that people have the capacity for growth and the ability to regain control of their lives. In the short-term, assistance is required to clarify and to seek solutions to immediate problems. Any solution may ultimately require changes in the participant's behaviour, emotions, relationships, perception or environment.

Assessment

1. *Identify precipitating factors*: what exactly happened in the preceding 48 hours, and what demands are being made that they cannot cope with?
2. *Identify who is involved*: who are the participants, are they helping or hindering, and what is their relationship with the person and the crisis?
3. *Identify the consequences*: how is the person being affected, what is the extent of their distress and disorganization, and what are the reactions of their family and friends?
4. *Identify any risks to the person or family*: are there any life-threatening risks, self-injurious intent, confusion, psychologically damaging situations, extreme distress, what is their state of physical health and do they have the ability to meet their needs?
5. *Ascertain the individual's perception of events*: is it realistic, are their thoughts, feelings and actions congruent, have they experienced similar situations in the past?
6. *What coping skills are being used by the person*: what are their personal strengths and weaknesses, are they able to carry out any practical steps immediately?
7. *Identify the resources and support available*: who do they live with, who is trusted, are there any close confiding relationships, what resources do they think they need?

Intervention

1. *Establish rapport*: initiate a therapeutic relationship with the participants. Demonstrate acceptance and non-judgemental responses (see Unit 1.2). Be aware of own reactions. Communicate clearly and listen actively (see Unit 1.3).
2. *Explain the role of the agency in the situation*: the time limits and the

resources available. Be realistic about the potential of the agency to alter circumstances. Emphasize the objectives of helping the clients to work out their own solutions. Advise that seeking help is a positive step. Explain in advance all actions that are to be taken.

3. *Calm the participants*: relieve their anxiety and stress, limit the extent of their disorganization. Role model calmness. Demonstrate confidence in yourself and in the credibility of the helping agency. Reaffirm hope in the potential for a positive outcome.

4. *Clarify the situation*: encourage the participants to speak freely and to ventilate their feelings. Stay with the crisis and focus on the actual events and issues of the current situation as closely as possible. Do not deal with irrelevant material or spend too much time analysing why the person has failed. Assist the participants to arrive at an objective assessment of their difficulties. Help them to clarify and define their stresses. Try to turn vague worries into specific problems that can be dealt with.

5. *Seeking solutions*: identify and explore possible solutions. Explore means of achieving solutions. Identify key priorities. Assess availability of required resources. Maintain positive self-esteem. Help the participants to regain and develop sense of mastery and autonomy. Emphasize the educational aspects of dealing with the crisis and the steps required to resolve it. Offer constructive advice, if required. Decide whether it is necessary in the short-term for mutual relief to remove the person from a stressful situation.

6. *Implementing solutions*: set realistic and attainable goals. Set a specific timetable. Make written or verbal communications with the participants. Facilitate the development of coping strategies and decision-making skills. Teach appropriate practical skills to the participants. Enlist aid from friends and relatives not already involved. Refer to appropriate agencies for practical assistance or specialist resources. Make necessary practical arrangements. Modify environmental conditions where possible to reduce stress. Isolate from individuals or environments that are exacerbating the stress. Support implementation of chosen strategies and newly developed skills. Encourage to work through the crisis. Resist attempts to withdraw too early. Challenge attempts at denial, scapegoating or endless attribution of blame. Evaluate the outcomes of the participants' attempts to resolve the crisis. Provide ongoing feedback to the participants. Encourage self-evaluation.

Resolution

1. Compare the initial objectives with the actual outcome of the situation. Evaluate whether:

   - the crisis has resolved;
   - the client is now able to cope unaided with their current situation;
   - longer-term support is required by an appropriate agency.

2. Review with the client the changes and mechanisms that have been useful.
3. Initiate anticipatory planning with the client to promote learning and to enhance their coping strategies.
4. Promote the client's recognition and understanding of stresses in their life-style.
5. Advise the client on ways of gaining access to support services in the event of future crises.

Unit Instructions

When you have researched the suggested references, have mastered the Unit Objectives and successfully answered the Self-assessment Questions, proceed with the Unit Written Test.

Suggested References

Aguilera, D. C. and Messick, J. M. (1982). *Crisis Intervention Therapy for Psychological Emergencies*. New American Library, C. V. Mosby, St. Louis.

Caplan, G. (1974). *An Approach to Community Mental Health*. Tavistock, London.

Carr, P. J., Butterworth, C. A. and Hodges, B. E. (1980). *Community Psychiatric Nursing*. Churchill Livingstone, Edinburgh.

Consumer's Association (1982). *Living with Stress*. Consumer's Association/Hodder and Stoughton, London.

Gibbs, A. (1986). *Understanding Mental Health*. Consumer's Association/Hodder and Stoughton, London.

Goldberg, D. and Huxley, P. (1980). *Mental Illness in the Community*. Tavistock, London.

Hughes, B. and Boothroyd, R. (1985). *Fight or Flight? Mastering Problems of Everyday Life*. Faber and Faber, London.

Hume, C. and Pullen, I. (1986). *Rehabilitation in Psychiatry*. Churchill Livingstone, Edinburgh.

Lyttle, J. (1986). *Mental Disorder*. Baillière Tindall, London and San Diego.

Mangen, S. (1982). *Sociology and Mental Health*. Churchill Livingstone, Edinburgh.

Miles, A. (1981). *The Mentally Ill in Contemporary Society*. Martin Robertson, Oxford.

Morrice, J. K. W. (1976). *Crisis Intervention – Studies in Community Care*. Pergamon, Oxford.

Murgatroyd, S. and Woolfe, R. (1982). *Coping with Crisis – Understanding and Helping Persons in Need*. Harper and Row, London.

Peterson, L. C. (1983). *Clients in situational/developmental crisis*. In Adams, C. G. and Macione, A. (Eds), *Handbook of Psychiatric Mental Health Nursing*. John Wiley/Fleschner, New York.

Rowan, F. P. (1980). *The Chronically Distressed Client*. C. V. Mosby, St. Louis.

Scheff, T. J. (Ed.) (1967). *Mental Illness and Social Processes*. Harper and Row, New York.

Simmons, S. and Brooker, C. (1986). *Community Psychiatric Nursing: A Social Perspective*. Heinemann Nursing, London.

Sugden, J. (1986). Psychiatric emergencies. *In* Sugden, J., Bessant, A., Eastland, M. and Field, R. (Eds), *A Handbook for Psychiatric Nurses*. Harper and Row, London.

Tuckett, D. (Ed.) (1976). *An Introduction to Medical Sociology*. Tavistock, London.

Wright, B. (1986). *Caring in Crisis: A Handbook of Intervention Skills for Nurses*. Churchill Livingstone, Edinburgh.

Self-assessment Questions

SAQ 5. List and describe four factors that influence the recognition of mental health problems.

SAQ 6. Outline three possible outcomes of not seeking help for mental health problems.

SAQ 7. Identify five support resources available to the family and person experiencing distress.

SAQ 8. Describe briefly the stages and processes of crisis intervention.

Unit 4.2: Written Test

1. What factors influence a person's self-assessment of their mental health problem and in deciding whether to seek help?

2. GPs receive a lot of visits from clients with mental health problems. What difficulties are there for the GP and client in recognizing and identifying the nature of the person's difficulties?

3. Describe in detail the skills used by health care workers in attempting to resolve a crisis situation.

Models of Mental Illness

Models of Mental Illness

There are a wide range of views as to the nature, causes and treatment of mental illnesses. In theoretical terms, they can be considered as "models" in which an attempt is made to consider the implications and validity of the contrasting viewpoints. The most common models can be considered under the following headings:

- medical model,
- social model,
- psychological models,
- anti-pyschiatry movement.

Medical model

The medical model views mental illnesses as conditions in which the primary cause is essentially physical and arises from a fault in the structure or function of a specific tissue or organ. This physical pathology is then regarded as contributing to the changes in behaviour, mood, perception and thoughts that are characteristic of mental illness. Sufferers are regarded as being "ill" and requiring medical treatment and intervention.

Medical concept of mental illness

1. Underlying physical pathology – where the cause is already known or remains to be discovered:

- biochemical,
- endocrine,
- genetic,
- trauma,
- infection,
- diet,
- toxins.

2. People's behaviour, emotions, thoughts and perceptions are interpreted as "signs and symptoms". These are then classified into a specific "diagnosis".
3. Mental illness is then regarded as a medical speciality which should be treated in a medical setting by doctors, nurses, etc. The doctor is perceived as the expert and uses physical methods of treatment, e.g. chemotherapy, ECT, psychosurgery.
4. The sufferer is defined as a "patient" who is expected to cooperate, be grateful and is relieved of responsibility for their behaviour.
5. The anticipation is that the person will be "cured" or "relieved of symptoms" following the medical intervention.

The medical model is the one that currently predominates in the organization of the National Health Service and allocation of resources. The hospital sector still attracts most of the resources and most of the research has been orientated towards identifying undiscovered phsyical causes or consequences of mental illness.

Social model

The social model of mental illness is one in which our relationships and the environment are seen as crucial to our mental well-being. Disruptions in either of these causes stress, which results in an impaired ability to relate to others and to function independently. The primary focus is on family and group relationships. Critical factors include:

1. *Early life experiences*:

- upbringing,
- the values and attitudes imparted,
- presence of a caring parent,
- relationships between the parents.

2. *Adolescence*:

- peer group influences,
- education,
- self-esteem and self-image,
- sexual experiences.

3. *Adulthood*:
    - relationships – supportive, conflict, over-demanding,
    - marriage – unstable, divorced, separated,
    - bereavement – grief reactions to loss,
    - occupational stress,
    - unemployment,
    - financial problems,
    - helplessness and lack of control over life situation,
    - unexpected crises that overwhelm the person.

4. *Environment*:
    - individual's perception – pleasant, unpleasant,
    - safe or insecure
    - state of housing – well maintained, deteriorated, cold, clean
    - overcrowding

5. *Social class*: certain social classes seem to be at more risk than others of developing certain mental illnesses. Reasons for this seem to be uncertain and tend to be viewed as certain classes and minority groups being disadvantaged in some way.
6. *Gender differences*: there is a clear gender bias in the incidence of certain types of mental illness. Women in particular appear to be particularly vulnerable. In social terms, this is explained in terms of the excess stress and lack of support available to women. Women are viewed in a stereotyped way as "neurotic", are expected to be passive and have conflicting sexual pressures on them. Social institutions treat women as inferior to men, and women are educationally and legally disadvantaged.

Social intervention

The objectives of social intervention are to facilitate the development of the individual's coping skills and social awareness to enable them to remain autonomous. This is achieved through:

1. *Community care and support* in the person's own home from the community mental health and primary health care teams.
2. *Group therapy* in which the objectives are to increase the person's insight into their own behaviour and its effects upon others.
3. *Social skills training* in which individuals are taught the skills of relating to others.
4. *Life skills*: people are taught the necessary life skills and activities of daily living to maintain their independence and ability to cope.
5. *Health education*: the individual's life-style and coping strategies are reviewed. Education is aimed towards promoting the healthy aspects of the person's life-style and teaching them ways of identifying and coping with potential stress.

6. *Family therapy, couple's therapy*: families and couples are helped to work through and resolve their stresses and to develop more effective ways of coping and relating. People are enabled to communicate more effectively and to provide effective support to other family members.
7. *Therapeutic community*: if people do require residential care then it should be in an environment in which their ability to communicate and relate to others is given priority. In a therapeutic community people are given considerable autonomy in creating their own rules and are expected to work together to solve problems. Role barriers between staff and residents are minimal and the staff primarily try and create the conditions conducive for therapeutic change.
8. *Voluntary work*: the community is seen as a resource in which there is a lot of mutual support and goodwill. In particular, the development of self-help groups is encouraged.

The social model has had a considerable influence on broadening the perspective of hospital-based care. With the move towards community-based care it is likely that the resources and ranges of services available in the community will increase considerably.

Psychological models

As with each of the other "models" the label "psychological model" encompasses a wide range of opinions that are not necessarily in agreement with each other. Under the loose heading "psychological models" there are a number of divergent views:

Behavioural theories

Behaviour is learned from the individual's upbringing, role models and life experiences. Mental health requires the individual to have been exposed to a variety of adaptive models which facilitate the development of the person's social and coping skills. "Mental illness" is regarded as being characterized by inappropriate behaviour learned from negative life experiences. Behavioural therapies, therefore, focus on the need to re-learn more adaptive and appropriate patterns of behaviour. Approaches include:

- social skills training,
- communications skills,
- assertiveness,
- life skills,
- anxiety management,
- role play,
- operant conditioning,
- classical conditioning.

Cognitive theories

The focus is upon the way that an individual perceives and interprets the world. The thought processes are then seen as instrumental in determining how an individual behaves and their emotional reactions. Mental stress is seen as the result of dysfunctional cognitions in which perceptions are interpreted in an inappropriate and disabling way. Interventions are designed to examine and alter a person's internal cognitive framework. Therapeutic strategies include:

- cognitive therapy,
- rational emotive therapy,
- personal construct therapy,
- transactional analysis,
- neurolinguistic programming (NLP).

Psychoanalytic theories

These originate from the work of Sigmund Freud and have been a powerful influence on the development of psychology and psychiatry. This theory stresses the early stages of psychosexual development that an individual passes through in order to reach maturity. "Fixation" at one of the stages can cause problems in later life. Early childhood is regarded as a particularly vulnerable period in which certain traumatic experiences can become repressed and emerge later in adult life. These unresolved conflicts can cause anxiety and other emotional problems in adult life.

Individuals are seen as having an unconscious mental life in which mental defence mechanisms operate to protect the individual from stress and to maintain their integrity. Problems arise if the defence mechanisms are used excessively or seriously distort an individual's perception or ability to cope.

Therapy is directed towards helping the person gain insight into their mental life and towards identifying unresolved conflicts. The therapeutic approach of "psychoanalysis" is usually a long-term method. Therapeutic methods include free association, dream analysis and transference. Although rarely available to NHS patients it has had a considerable influence on other psychotherapeutic approaches. Therapeutic methods influenced by these perspectives include:

- art therapy,
- music therapy,
- individual psychotherapy,
- group analytic psychotherapy,
- psychodrama,
- hypnosis.

Anti-psychiatry movement

This small but vocal group question both the existence of mental illness and the way that in their view psychiatry is used as a means of social control. Psychiatry is perceived as being eager to justify its own existence and power base by incorporating all sorts of social and personal problems within its area of practice. All types of deviant behaviour are then classified as "mental illness".

Mental illness is viewed as an understandable reaction to pathological relationships or social repression. Intervention is required in terms of altering the fabric of social relationships, personal expectations and limiting the power of mental health professionals.

Although generally regarded as "fringe" viewpoints, they have served a useful purpose in challenging existing perspectives. Mental health care workers need to be able to validate their interventions and to justify the resources allocated to psychiatric services.

Unit Instructions

When you have researched the suggested references, have mastered the Unit Objectives and successfully answered the Self-assessment Questions, proceed with the Unit Written Test.

Suggested References

Altshul, A. (1980). The care of the mentally disordered: three approaches. *Nursing Times*, 13 March, Vol. 76, No. 11, pp. 452–454.

Argyle, M. (1981) (Ed.). *Social Skills and Health*. Methuen, London.

Bloch, S. (Ed.) (1986). *An Introduction to the Psychotherapies* 2nd Edition. Oxford University Press, Oxford.

Clarke, A. (1980). *Psychiatry in Dissent*, 2nd edition. Tavistock, London.

Cochrane, R. (1983). *The Social Creation of Mental Illness*. Longman, London.

Davis, R. (1984). *An Introduction to Psychopathology*, 4th edition. Oxford.

Jones, R. K. and Jones, P. (1975). *Sociology in Medicine*. English University Press, London.

Kingston, B. (1987). *Psychological Approaches in Psychiatric Nursing*. Croom Helm, London.

Lang, R. D. (1964). *Sanity, Madness and the Family*. Penguin, Harmondsworth.

Margen, S. P. (1982). *Sociology and Mental Health*. Churchill Livingstone, Edinburgh.

Miles, A. (1981). *The Mentally Ill in Contemporary Society*. Martin Robertson, Oxford.

Szasz, T. (1970). *Ideology and Insanity*. Pelican, Harmondsworth.

Trower, P., Bryant, B. and Argyle, M. (1978). *Social Skills and Mental Health*. Tavistock, London.

Tuckett, D. A. (Ed.) (1976). *An Introduction to Medical Sociology*. Tavistock, London.

Wing, J. K. (1978). *Reasoning about Madness*. Oxford.

Self-assessment Questions

SAQ 9. List four characteristics of the medical model of mental illness.

SAQ 10. Identify four therapeutic approaches used to facilitate social functioning.

SAQ 11. Differentiate three main differences between behavioural and psychoanalytic theories of mental illness.

SAQ 12. State two criticisms that the anti-psychiatry movement makes against the practice of psychiatry.

Unit 4.3: Written Test

1. What are the main differences between the medical and social models of mental illness?

2. Describe in detail the approaches used in the social model of psychiatry.

The Classification of Mental Illness

Unit Objectives

At the end of this Unit the learner should be able to:

1. Differentiate between neurotic and psychotic illnesses.
2. Define the terms "organic" and "functional".
3. Describe the effects of labelling a person as "mentally ill".
4. List the diagnostic labels used in psychiatry.

Diagnosis in Mental Illness

Mental illnesses are classified and identified in terms of their effects upon a person's:

- behaviour,
- thought (cognitive) processes,
- emotions (affect),
- physical health.

Specific disturbances in each of the above areas are then compared with standard classifications of mental illnesses in order to arrive at the medical diagnosis. The two main systems of classification currently in use are the:

1. *International Classification of Diseases*, 9th revision, World Health Organization – known as the ICD 9.
2. *Diagnostic and Statistical Manual of Mental Disorders*, 3rd edition, American Psychiatric Association – known as the DSM III.

Both manuals give extensive and definitive details in regard to the classification and diagnosis of mental illnesses.

The limitations of diagnosis

The use of diagnostic labels in classifying mental health problems is not without its limitations:

1. *The validity and reliability of diagnosis*. The situation is improving but there is evidence that diagnostic labels are used inaccurately and inconsistently. Different professionals have been shown to give different diagnostic labels when presented with the same data.
2. *Social influences*. There is a tendency for women to be labelled as neurotic irrespective of the nature or validity of their symptoms. Other variables such as social class, education and occupation can also influence the diagnosis made.
3. *Labelling*. Once a person has a diagnosis or label attached to them there are a number of consequences. The person's self-perception and that of others towards them undergoes a significant change. Behaviour, emotions and thoughts, past and present, are reinterpreted in terms of illness. The stigma of mental illness also tends to isolate the person and their family from other people. These reactions serve to reinforce the person's image and role as an "ill person" and tend to inhibit their return to "normal life".
4. *Perjorative*. Some diagnoses are used in a negative way to imply value judgements, such as "psychopath" and "hysterical".
5. *Individuality*. The diagnosis is a medical judgement that indicates the appropriate medical treatment. However, each person's experience and needs are unique. People present with a range of problems that extends far beyond the boundaries of their diagnosis. In terms of planning a person's nursing care, the diagnosis is only an indicator that may or may not be useful.

The uses of diagnosis

The use of diagnostic labels can serve certain useful functions:

1. *Communication*: between members of the health care teams is facilitated.
2. *Predictive*: it will give some indication of the course of the illness and the treatment required.
3. *Validation*: a person and their family may be relieved that they have a problem which is recognized and confirmed by outsiders.
4. *Research and planning*: medical and epidemiological studies can be made of people with similar conditions.

The classification of mental illness

The primary diagnostic labels used relate to the degree of insight present, common presenting symptoms and in terms of the known pathology.

Neurosis

Neurosis is used to describe those mental illnesses where:

1. The person retains insight into their condition. They are aware that they have mental health problems, though their actual perception and understanding may be limited.
2. The person remains in contact with reality and may be able to continue functioning normally, albeit in a restricted way.
3. Anxiety is a common feature. The emotional experience is regarded as one which differs from normal reactions in terms of the degree of emotion experienced rather than on its nature.
4. The symptoms tend to be less severe than with psychotic illnesses. This should not be taken to mean that the person suffers any less. Some people with neurotic illnesses can be extremely distressed and socially unable to function.
5. Cognitive functions, such as memory, intelligence and judgement, are minimally affected.
6. There is little change in personality. However, the long-term effects of neurosis can considerably alter a person's self-image, their relationships with others and their life-style. The effects of these can be to affect adversely a person's self-esteem, motivation, interests and ability to cope.
7. The symptoms are viewed as arising from internal psychological stress. They may be due to early life experiences, current stress in a person's life or relationships, or with maladaptive patterns of behaviour.
8. The conditions may be amenable to treatment, such as psychotherapy, behaviour therapy or medication. Many people do not seek help for neurotic illnesses and either suffer with chronic difficulties or find that the symptoms clear up spontaneously.

Diagnostic categories

- anxiety states or anxiety neurosis or anxiety reaction,
- reactive or psychoneurotic depression,
- phobia, phobia anxiety or phobic reaction,
- obsessional neurosis or obsessional-compulsive reaction,
- hysteria or hysterical reaction.

Psychosis

Psychosis is used to describe those mental illnesses where:

1. The person loses or only has limited insight into their condition. They may not be aware that they are ill and require help.
2. The person progressively loses contact with reality as others perceive it. This seriously inhibits their ability to communicate and relate with others. They may experience sensory hallucinations.
3. There may be extreme disturbance of the person's behaviour and emotions. These may be regarded by others as inappropriate and bizarre.
4. Thought processes can be seriously affected and disturbed in a variety

of ways. Concentration, judgement and memory can be grossly impaired.
5. Their personality as perceived by others can undergo profound changes, such that they seem a fundamentally different person.
6. The condition is viewed as progressive with treatment primarily aimed at preventing further deterioration and stabilizing the person's current condition, if possible.

Psychoses are further sub-divided into two main categories in terms of their psychopathology:

(a) *Organic psychoses*: where there is an identifiable physical cause:

- chronic confusional states (dementia),
- acute confusional states (delerium).

(b) *Functional psychoses*: where the cause remains unknown:

- affective – endogenous depression,
        manic-depressive psychosis,
        mania,
        hypomania.
- schizophrenia – simple
        hebephrenic,
        catatonic,
        paranoid.

Other diagnostic categories

Other diagnostic categories commonly used in psychiatry include:

1. *Psychopathy*: in which the person is viewed as behaving in an irresponsible and antisocial way. They have difficulty in forming relationships and are frequently in conflict with others. They are viewed as having a low tolerance to stress and in needing to satisfy their needs immediately.
2. *Dependency on alcohol or drugs*: which can cause physical and social damage to the user and others. The person experiences withdrawal effects if they do not continue taking the substance and are thereby driven to take more.
3. *Anorexia nervosa and anorexia bulimia*: both of these are associated with extreme disturbances in the person's eating behaviour. Serious physical consequences, even death, can arise from nutritional deficiencies.
4. *Sexual disorders*: changing attitudes towards sexual behaviour usually mean that someone is more likely to require help for the anxiety, depression or other consequences of their sexual preferences rather than the preference itself. People may require specialised help for paedophilia or trans-sexualism.

Unit Instructions

When you have researched the suggested references, have mastered the Unit Objectives and successfully answered the Self-assessment Questions, proceed with the Unit Written Test.

Suggested References

Alker, A. (1988). What will happen to Jane? *Nursing Times*, 3 February, Vol. 84, No. 5, pp. 63–65.

Altschul, A. and McGovern, M. (1985). *Psychiatric Nursing*, 6th edition. Baillière Tindall, London and San Diego.

Cochrane, R. (1984). *The Social Creation of Mental Illness*. Longman, London.

Fernando, L. (1986). What is normal? *Nursing Times*, 8 January, Vol. 82, No. 2. pp. 58–59.

Goffman, E. (1963). *Stigma*. Penguin, Harmondsworth.

Hume, C. and Pullen, I. (1986). *Rehabilitation in Psychiatry*. Churchill Livingstone, Edinburgh.

Manchester, J. (1985). The nature of psychiatric disorders. *Nursing*, February, Vol. 2, No. 34, pp. 991–992.

Mangen, S. (1982). *Sociology and Mental Health*. Churchill Livingstone, Edinburgh.

Miles. A. (1981). *The Mentally Ill in Contemporary Society*. Martin Robertson, Oxford.

Sugden, J. (1985). Labelling theory. *Nursing*, March, Vol. 2, No. 35, p. 1021.

Szasz, T. (1970). *The Myth of Mental Illness*. Paladin, London.

Trethowan, W. and Sims, A. (1983). *Psychiatry*, 5th edition. Baillière Tindall, London and San Diego.

Tuckett, D. (Ed.) (1976). *An Introduction to Medical Sociology*. Tavistock, London.

Voudsen, M. (1987). *Is there racism on the wards? Nursing Times*, Oct 21, Vol. 83, No. 42, p. 18.

Willis, J. (1976). *Clinical Psychiatry*. Blackwell Scientific, Oxford.

Self-assessment Questions

SAQ 13. List four characteristics of a psychotic illness.

SAQ 14. Identify four neurotic illnesses.

SAQ 15. Define the terms "organic" and "functional" mental illness.

SAQ 16. What are the potential hazards involved in diagnosing someone as mentally ill?

Unit 4.4: Written Test

1. What are the characteristic features of a neurotic illness?
2. What are the limitations of medical diagnosis for nursing practice?
3. How can labelling a person as mentally ill influence their relationships and self-image?

TOPIC 5

The Care of People with Mental Health Problems

At the end of this Topic the learner should aim to:

1. Describe the range and functions of primary health care services.
2. Identify the resources available for community mental health care.
3. Appreciate the developments in community-based care and their effects on public attitudes.
4. Outline the features of a therapeutic care environment.

Primary Health Care

Unit Objectives

At the end of this Unit the learner should be able to:

1. Define the term "primary health care"
2. Identify the members of the primary health care team.
3. Describe the roles of the members of the primary health care team.
4. List the range of voluntary organizations and their services.

Definition

Primary health care refers to the range of health care services available in the community which:

1. Provide a first point of contact for those with health care needs.
2. Offer a range of home- and health centre-based support and treatment services.
3. Monitor the health status of specific client groups.
4. Offer a referral service to more specialist treatment and care services.
5. Liaise and co-ordinate care and treatment programmes with hospital-based services.

Community-based primary health care provides a complementary service with both local authority and hospital services to provide a comprehensive health service to the local community. The care given covers preventive, therapeutic and rehabilitation services. The services cater for a wide range of potential health care needs that also includes mental health problems. Specialist community services for the mentally ill are gradually being expanded to cater for this client group.

Primary Health Care Team

The team may be based within a health centre, surgery, clinic or have separate premises. The services are provided by both the Local Health

District and the Social Services who have specific responsibilities for certain aspects of care provision. Increasingly, Social Services and health authorities are collaborating in joint ventures throughout the field of health care provision.

Members

The primary health care team consists of the following members:

- general practitioners,
- health visitors,
- district nurses,
- midwives,
- practice nurses,
- specialist nurses.

Some health centres also have facilities for preventive health services, such as occupational therapy, family planning and cytology, speech therapy, pharmaceutical services, physiotherapy, chiropody, ophthalmic services, dental services, ante- and post-natal care facilities, child health care services, laundry services for incontinent people, health education classes, physical fitness classes, and voluntary and support groups.

1. *General practitioners* are responsible for:

- diagnosis, management and treatment of illness in patient's home;
- referral to hospital if necessary for specialist opinions or treatment;
- supervision of convalescence and return to work;
- health education.

2. *Health visitors* are responsible for:

- domiciliary visiting following childbirth, regular visiting to families with small children, casework with actual and suspected cases of non-accidental injury or sexual abuse of children, visits to pregnant mothers, nurseries, play groups, etc.
- children's health and development until school age. Advising and supporting mothers and families with children who have health problems;
- identification of potential risk factors to child health;
- support and care of the whole family;
- health assessments of the elderly;
- health education, e.g. ante-natal classes, clubs for the elderly, etc.;
- school health service;
- liaison with hospitals and participation in training of students (medical, nursing, social work, etc.);
- involvement in research projects.

3. *District nurses* are responsible for:
   - assessing and meeting the needs of people at home with physical health problems;
   - providing home-based nursing care;
   - monitoring and promoting the health of the chronically sick, elderly, terminally ill and bereaved;
   - referral to other agencies and liaison with residential services;
   - health education and promotion participating in professional training;

4. *Midwives* are responsible for:
   - care of mothers and newborn babies;
   - ante-natal education;
   - working closely with health visitors;
   - family planning.

5. *Specialist nurses*
   - community psychiatric nurses (see Unit 5.2);
   - community mental handicap nurses;
   - school nurses;
   - nurses with specialist clinical skills – terminal care, pain control, continence advisors, diabetes, sexually transmitted diseases, stoma-therapist.

6. *Social workers* are responsible for a wide range of activities including:
   - family case work, family therapy
   - individual case work, counselling;
   - applications for home helps, meals on wheels, support facilities;
   - housing and financial problems;
   - health education;
   - specialist services, e.g. child abuse, mental health problems, clients with visual, auditory or physical handicaps.

Statutory bodies

The services are provided through various departments to meet the needs of certain care groups:

1. *Central government*
   - Department of Health and Social Security; benefits and allowances as currently available:
       Income Support, Family Credit, Housing Benefit, Maternity Grant, Statutory Maternity Pay, Funeral Grant, Widows Benefit. Social Fund–Community Care Grants, Crisis Loans, Budgeting Loans.

- Department of Employment: Job Centres, Training Commission, unemployment benefit offices;
- Home Office: probation and after-care services.

2. *Local health authorities*

- hospital accommodation;
- medical, nursing and other services;
- specialist services at health centres, day hospitals, out-patients' departments and community care;
- ambulance services;
- occupational health services for staff
- after-care services.

3. *Local authorities*

- *environmental health*: housing, food control, water supplies, pollution, refuse and sewage disposal, prevention and control of infectious diseases, health education;
- *social services*: children and families; the elderly; the physically disabled; mentally disordered and handicapped; social workers; adult training workshops; day centres; hostels; residential care; domiciliary occupational therapy, home helps and other assistance (meals on wheels, home adaptations, etc.), applicance centres (aids and devices), recreational and travelling facilities, books, radio, television, telephone and special equipment for home use, and holidays, social clubs, outings, social centres, etc.

Voluntary organizations

The voluntary and non-statutory bodies act as pressure groups for social reform and actively campaign for improved welfare provision for their client groups. They provide many care and supportive services for client groups in need that are not catered for by statutory services.

Although statutory and voluntary services occasionally overlap, the main contribution of the voluntary organizations is aimed at improving the quality of life for individuals and their families.

The services provided

1. *Relationship and stress problems*

- Samaritans,
- Marriage Guidance Council: Relate
- National Association of Young People's Counselling and Advisory Services,
- victim support schemes,
- Catholic Marriage Advisory Council,
- Family Planning Association,
- National Council for the Divorced and Separated.

2. *Women*

- Women's Refuges,
- Rape Crisis Line,
- Mastectomy Association of Great Britain,
- Miscarriage Association,
- National Association for Pre-menstrual Syndrome,
- National Childbirth Trust,
- Women's Health Concern.

3. *Mental health problems*

- MIND (National Association for Mental Health),
- Psychiatric Rehabilitation Association,
- Richmond Fellowship,
- Mental After-care Association,
- Depressive Anonymous,
- Open Door (agoraphobia),
- National Schizophrenic Fellowship,
- Alcohol Concern,
- Alcoholics Anonymous, Al-Anon, Al-Teen,
- Councils on Alcoholism,
- Cyrenians,
- Anorexic Aid and Anorectic Family Aid,
- National Autistic Society,
- Ex-services Mental Welfare Society,
- Gamblers Anonymous.

4. *Elderly*

- Age Concern,
- Help the Aged,
- carer's support groups,
- Alzheimer's Disease Society.

5. *Children*

- National Society for the Prevention of Cruelty to Children,
- Save the Children Fund,
- Church of England Children's Society,
- Dr Barnardo's Homes,
- Child Poverty Action Group,
- School Playgroup's Association,
- Invalid Children's Aid Association,
- Hyperactive Children's Support Group.

6. *Social and welfare services*

- British Red Cross Society,
- Women's Royal Voluntary Service,
- Salvation Army,
- St John's Ambulance.

7. *Physical health problems*

- Disablement Income Group,
- Spastics' Society,
- Muscular Dystrophy,
- Physically Handicapped and Able-bodied (PHAB),
- British Epilepsy Association,
- Marie Curie Memorial Foundation,
- Parkinson's Disease Society.

8. *Visual handicap*

- The Royal National Institute for the Blind,
- The Partially Sighted Society.

9. *Hearing loss*

- The Royal National Institute for the Deaf,
- The British Deaf Association,
- National Deaf Children's Society,
- The National Deaf–Blind Helper's League.

10. *Advice and information services*

- Association of Carers
- Citizen's Advice Bureau,
- Shelter,
- Royal Society for the Prevention of Accidents,
- Association of Self-help and Community Groups,
- Charities Aid Foundation.

Unit Instructions

When you have researched the suggested references, have mastered the Unit Objectives and successfully answered the Self-assessment Questions, proceed with the Unit Written Test.

Suggested References

Barefoot, P. and Cunningham, P. J. (1977). *Community Services*. Faber and Faber, London.

Blaxter, M. (1976). *The Meaning of Disability*. Heineman Educational, London.

Boswell, D. M. and Wingrove, J. M. (Eds) (1974). *The Handicapped Person in the Community*. Tavistock/Open University Press, London/Milton Keynes.

Briggs, A. and Oliver, J. (1985). *Caring*. Routledge and Kegan Paul, London.

Brown, M. (1982). *Introduction to Social Administration in Britain*, 5th edition. Hutchinson, London.

Butler, J. R. and Vaile, M. S. (1984). *Health and Health Services*. Routledge and Kegan Paul, London.

Consumer's Association/Patients Association (1983). *A Patient's Guide to the National Health Service*. Consumer's Association/Hodder and Stoughton, London.

Davies, B. M. (1977). *Community Health and Social Services*, 3rd edition. Hodder and Stoughton, London.

Gibbs, A. (1986). *Understanding Mental Health*. Consumer's Association/Hodder and Stoughton, London.

Marsh, D. (Ed.) (1979). *Introducing Social Policy*. Routledge and Kegan Paul, London.

Mellor, H. W. (1985). *The Role of Voluntary Organisations in Social Welfare*. Croom Helm, London.

Room, G. (1979). *The Sociology of Welfare*. Basil Blackwell/Martin Robertson, Oxford.

Townsend, P. and Davidson, N. (Eds) (1982). *Inequalities in Health: The Black Report*. Penguin, Harmondsworth.

Wilmott, P. (1978). *Consumer's Guide to the British Social Services*. Penguin, Harmondsworth.

Young, P. (1985). *Mastering Social Welfare*. Macmillan, London.

Self-assessment Questions

SAQ 1. Describe four functions of the primary health care services.

SAQ 2. Identify four members of the primary health care team and briefly describe their roles.

SAQ 3. List three main statutory bodies and identify the services they provide to the community.

SAQ 4. List the range of services provided by six voluntary organizations.

Unit 5.1: Written Test

1. Describe the function of the primary health care team in preventive medicine.
2. Discuss the roles of:
   - the health visitor,
   - the social worker,
   - district nurses in the primary health care team.
3. Identify four specific problems which may be experienced by a physically disabled man, aged 36, who is married with two young children. Describe briefly the services available in the community for help with the problems you have identified.

Community Mental Health Care

Unit Objectives

At the end of this Unit the learner should be able to:

1. Describe the advantages of community care.
2. List the community resources available for the care and treatment of people with mental health problems.
3. Outline the working of a community mental health centre.
4. Identify the skills of the community mental health nurse.

Community Care

Community care refers to the full range of support and treatment services provided for people with mental health problems in their own homes and within the community. Community and hospital services are complementary elements of a comprehensive mental health service to the local population. Community care resources are provided by both statutory and voluntary agencies.

Aims of community care

1. To provide a comprehensive domiciliary and community-based care, support and treatment service.
2. To enable the sufferer and their family to function at an optimum level in their own home and in the community.
3. To provide support during periods of crisis to people and their family in their own home environment.
4. To give advice and information on mental health problems. To promote positive mental health in the community.
5. To liaise with hospital-based services to provide continuity and aftercare for former residents.

Advantages of community care

1. Increased accessibility to mental health /health care services for potential consumers.
2. Problems are dealt with in the environment in which they have caused difficulties for the person and their family and in which the person will continue to live.
3. Social and family networks are maintained.
4. Independence and autonomy are promoted.
5. Reduces the stigma associated with mental health problems.
6. Research shows community-based care to be an effective, acceptable and safe alternative to hospital-based treatment, regardless of diagnosis.

Statutory Health Care Services

Social Services Departments (Local Authority)

1. *Social workers*. Advisory and supportive service to patients and family. Statutory duties under the Mental Health Act 1983 (as mental welfare officers, approved social worker).
2. *Day centres*. Rehabilitation programmes for those able to return to work (e.g. occupational therapy). Sheltered employment or occupation for those suffering from chronic mental health problems.
3. *Adult training centres*. Provision of training and sheltered employment or occupation for those unable to cope with open employment.
4. *Social clubs*. Recreational and social activities are provided by both statutory and voluntary organizations.
5. *Residential accommodation*. Both statutory and voluntary organizations provide residential accommodation, e.g. hostels, half-way houses, group homes, sheltered accommodation. The private sector also has a significant role in providing accommodation for people with mental health problems. The range of accommodation includes licensed nursing homes, hostels, bedsits, reitrement homes, sheltered accommodation.
6. *Practical help*. Home help service, home library, incontinent laundry service, meals on wheels. Voluntary services may be able to offer various practical services such as shopping, gardening, visiting and befriending, trips out, and "sitting" for dependent people while the relatives go out for the day or evening.

District health authorities

1. *Out-patient clinics*. These may be held at the general hospitals in the health district or at the psychiatric hospital itself. New clients are referred

by their General Practitioner for assessment, diagnosis and treatment. People recently discharged from hospital are followed up. Many people are able to continue with their employment until fully recovered.

2. *Day hospitals.* As the name implies, people attend during the day and return home in the evening. The service may be based within a general or psychiatric hospital site or may be attached to other health care facilities such as health centres, homes for the elderly confused, or hostels. Day hospital services may offer a broad range of services related to the specific client group. They provide:

- long-term support and care;
- assessment and monitoring of psychological and physical health;
- programmes of treatment and rehabilitation;
- recreational and social activities;
- physical care;
- relief for the family and relatives.

3. *Specialized centres.* Services may be available for a wide range of specific problems. They are based within existing mental health facilities or have separate accommodation. Clients may be seen individually or as groups on an appointment or sessional basis. Facilities may be available for:

- alcohol-related problems,
- drug abuse,
- counselling,
- psychotherapy,
- family therapy,
- couples' therapy,
- sex therapy,
- anxiety management,
- social skills training,
- group work.

4. *Community psychiatric nurses.* The community psychiatric nurse (CPN) is a member of a multidisciplinary team providing mental health care to the population of a health district. CPNs are probably the single most important profession involved in community mental health care. Their numbers have increased considerably with the growing trend towards community-based care. They are all qualified psychiatric nurses, some of whom have undertaken post-basic ENB courses in community psychiatric nursing.

Settings for community care

The community mental health service may be based within a variety of settings. The siting of the base tends to influence the role of the team and also the client group that are referred to them. They may work from the following.

1. Community mental health centre

This is a centre away from the main hospital and sited within the locality that it serves. A full range of mental health professionals provide an easily accessible and comprehensive service. Members of the multidisciplinary team may include CPNs, psychologists, occupational therapists, social workers and centre support staff.

Staff from the centre may visit clients in their own homes or provide a treatment service based within the centre. Members of the team may also have a sessional input to local health centres to see people with mental health problems. Some centres offer a self-referral or "walk-in" service, whereby people are able to come to the centre on their own initiative for help with mental health problems.

The community mental health centre can also act as a local focus on issues and services related to mental health. It can be used as a resource for education and also to co-ordinate and liaise with voluntary agencies.

2. Community health centre

CPNs may be based in the centre alongside other members of the primary health care team or provide a sessional input.

3. Psychiatric hospital, unit or day hospital

Community services based within hospital settings have the advantage of easier communication and liaison with hospital services. However, they are not as easily accessible to the public and retain an identification with existing hospital services.

4. Specialist treatment centre/client group

Many CPNs working from health centres and hospitals have a generic case load and deal with a wide range of clients. An increasing number are based within specialist centres or work primarily with a specific client group. Areas of speciality include:

- elderly care,
- rehabilitation,
- drinking problems,
- drug abuse,
- child and adolescent services,
- behavioural psychotherapy,
- forensic psychiatry,
- family therapy,
- anxiety management.

Referral

Sources of referral

1. Primary health care teams, particulary GPs.
2. Consultant psychiatrist.
3. Social Services departments.
4. Other community agencies, e.g. schools, probation, occupational health.
5. Self-referral.
6. Other professional sources.

In a community mental health centre the potential client may be referred to the multidisciplinary team. From an initial assessment of the person's needs by the team they may then be taken on by the person within the team who has the requisite therapeutic skills to help the client. In this approach members may work in a very specialized way with clients that transcends traditional role boundaries.

Reasons for referral

1. Personal stress and decreased ability to manage daily living.
2. Life crises, e.g. family violence, bereavements, self-injurious behaviour, redundancy, relationship problems.
3. Support network unable to cope or near exhaustion.
4. Concern by relatives and family at person's behaviour, thoughts or mood.
5. Assessment and background information.
6. Advice and information on coping and available community resources.
7. To ensure compliance with treatment and medication programmes.
8. To monitor mental and physical health.
9. Recurrence of previous mental health problems.

Community Psychiatric Nursing

The practice of psychiatric nursing in the community requires an extended skills and knowledge base. In particular, CPNs need to be aware of family dynamics, community resources and to be able to work autonomously. They need a broad base range of clinical skills and to be able to apply these to a home and community setting. In order to work effectively, they need to be familiar with the social and physical geography of the health district in which they are based.

The Skills of the Community Psychiatric Nurse

Mental health nursing skills

1. Assessment in a home and community setting.
2. Planning care programmes for home- and community-based clients.
3. Implementing care programmes for home- and community-based clients.
4. Evaluating care programmes for home and community based clients.

Clinical skills

1. Support to individuals and their families.
2. Counselling and psychotherapy.
3. Group work and family therapy.
4. Behavioural approaches

   - anxiety management
   - social skills training
   - individual programmes

5. Supervision of medication.
6. Pre-admission and pre-discharge work.
7. After-care and follow-up.
8. Rehabilitation.

Educational skills

1. Health education and promotion of mental health.
2. Preventive interventions:
   - *primary prevention*: to reduce the chances of mental health problems developing and identifying potential risk groups;
   - *secondary prevention*: to minimize the effects of established problems.
   - *tertiary prevention*: to reduce the residual effects of mental health problems through rehabilitation and therapy.

3. Knowledge of the resources available in the community and in hospital.
4. Consultant and resource to other members of the care team.
5. Professional self-development of skills and knowledge.

Managerial skills

1. Time management.
2. Identification of priorities.
3. Record keeping.

4. Liaising with members of the community team.
5. Co-ordinating with hospital-based team.
6. Case work management.
7. Supervision of case load.
8. Peer and team support.

Research skills

1. Utilising existing research findings.
2. Researching own clinical practice and client group.
3. Critically evaluating existing community mental health services.

Voluntary Organizations

Voluntary organizations make an important contribution to the provision of services to people with mental health problems. Some health districts have appointed a co-ordinator of voluntary services to co-ordinate the services offered by the different organizations. Some organizations involved specifically with mental health problems include:

1. *MIND (The National Association for Mental Health)*. This offers an advisory service, promotion of mental health, practical help, group homes, publications, conferences and pressure groups.
2. *Richmond Fellowship*. This offers residential accommodation (hostels), therapeutic care, an advisory service and courses in mental health and group work.
3. *Samaritans*. Trained volunteers offer a 24-hour telephone and personal listening service to the suicidal and despairing.
4. *Schizophrenia Association*. This offers support for families, promotion of a better understanding of schizophrenia and publications.
5. *Alcoholics Anonymous, Al-Anon, Al-Teen*. These offer support for people and their families affected by dependency on alcohol.
6. *Alzheimer's Disease Society*. This offers support groups for relatives, literature and information, and financial assistance.
7. *Anorexic aid and anorexic family aid*. These offer support groups for anorexics and their families, an information service and a telephone help line.

There are voluntary organizations, support groups and charities for most types of mental health problems. Many are set up on a local, county or regional basis. Citizen's Advice Bureaux should be able to advise you of the voluntary services available locally.

Unit Instructions

When you have researched the suggested references, have mastered the
Unit Objectives and successfully answered the Self-Assessment Questions,
proceed with the Unit Written Test.

Suggested References

Altschul, A. and McGovern, M. (1985). *Psychiatric Nursing*, 6th edition. Baillière
    Tindall, London and San Diego.
Bouras, N. and Kember, S. (1985). A suitable case for day care. *Nursing Times*, 17
    July, Vol. 81, No. 29, pp. 43–44.
Brewer, C. (1983). Social workers v CPNs. *Nursing Times*, 15 June, Vol. 79, No.
    24, p. 76.
Brooker, C. (1984a). Bloomsbury's set of problems. *Nursing Times*, 24 October,
    Vol. 80, No. 43, pp. 24–26.
Brooker, C. G. (1984b). Some problems associated with the measurement of
    community psychiatric nurse intervention. *Journal of Advanced Nursing*, Vol. 9,
    No. 2, pp. 165–174.
Brooker, C. G. and Simmons, C. M. (1985). A study to compare two models of
    community psychiatric nursing care delivery. *Journal of Advanced Nursing*, Vol.
    10, No. 3, pp. 217–223.
Brough, R. (1982). The community psychiatric nursing service at Prestwich hospital.
    Nursing Times, 12 May, Vol. 78, No. 19, pp. 784–788.
Caplan, G. (1969). *An Approach to Community Mental Health*, 2nd edition.
    Tavistock, London.
Carr, P. J., Butterworth, C. A. and Hodges, B. E. (1980). *Community Psychiatric
    Nursing*. Churchill Livingstone, Edinburgh.
Cohen, D. (1978). Psychiatry at home. *New Society*, 2 March, Vol. 43, No. 804,
    pp. 486–487.
Corrigan, J. and Soni, S. D. (1977). Community psychiatric nursing: an appraisal
    of its impact on community psychiatry in Manchester, England. *Journal of
    Advanced Nursing*, Vol. 2, No. 4, pp. 347–354.
Coverdale, P. R. (1980). New patterns of contact. *Nursing Times*, 12 June, Vol. 76,
    No. 24, pp. 1061–1062.
Dexter, G. and Wash, M. (1986). *Psychiatric Nursing Skills: A Patient-centred
    Approach*. Croom Helm, London.
Dyke, B. (1984). CPNs and primary health care teach attachment. *Nursing Times*,
    7 March, Vol. 80, No. 10, pp. 55–57.
Fenton, F. R. *et al*. (1982). *Home and Hospital Psychiatric Treatment*. Croom Helm,
    London.
Gibbs, A. (1986). *Understanding Mental Health*. Consumer's Association/Hodder
    and Stoughton, London.
Godin, P., Pearce, I. and Wilson, I. (1987). Keeping the customer satisfied. *Nursing
    Times*, 23 September, Vol. 83, No. 38, pp. 35–37.
Gunstone, S. (1983). The scope for prevention. *Nursing Times*, 14 September, Vol.
    79, No. 37, pp. 42–43.

Hall, V. and Russell, O. (1982). The community mental health nurse: a new professional role. *Journal of Advanced Nursing*, Vol. 7, No. 1, pp. 3–10.

Hendon, J. (1984). Liaising with the community. *Nursing Mirror*, 30 May, Vol. 158, No. 22. Psychiatry forum (pull-out supplement), pp. vii–viii.

Leopoldt, H. (1979a). Community psychiatric nursing – 1. *Nursing Times*, Vol. 75, No. 13. Occasional Papers.

Leopoldt, H. (1979b). Community psychiatric nursing – 2. *Nursing Times*, Vol. 75, No. 14. Occasional Papers.

Lim, D. (1985). Imprisoned by fear. *Nursing Mirror*, 24 July, Vol. 161, No. 4, pp. 18–19.

Lyttle, J. (1986). *Mental Disorder*. Baillière Tindall, London and San Diego.

Manchester, J. (1985). But what do CPNs actually do? *Nursing Mirror*, 29 May, Vol. 160, No. 22, pp. 37–38.

McKendrick, D. (1981). Statistical returns in community psychiatric nursing – 1. *Nursing Times*, 16 September, Vol. 77, No. 26, pp. 101–104.

Sharpe, D. (1982). GP's view of community psychiatric nursing. *Nursing Times*, 6 October, Vol. 78, No. 40, pp. 1664–1666.

Sharpe, G. (1985). Effective and efficient. *Nursing Mirror*, 10 July, Vol. 161, No. 2, pp. 39–41.

Simmons, S. and Brooker, C. (1986). *Community Psychiatric Nursing: A Social Perspective*, Heinemann Nursing, London.

Simmons, S. and Brooker, C. (1987). Making CPNs part of the team. *Nursing Times*, 13 May, Vol. 83, No. 19, pp. 49–51.

Skidmore, D. (1984). Muddling through. *Nursing Times*, 9 May, Vol. 80, No. 19, pp. 179–181. Community Outlook.

Thomas, W. (1984). Depot drugs in community psychiatry. *Nursing Times*, 18 January, Vol. 80, No. 3, pp. 43–46.

Whitehead, A. (1984). A personal view of CPNs. *Nursing Times*, 18 January, Vol. 80, No. 3, p. 64.

Williamson, F., Little, M. and Lindsay, W. (1981). Two community psychiatric nursing services compared. *Nursing Times*, 23 September, Vol. 77, No. 27, pp. 105–107.

Self-assessment Questions

SAQ 5. List four services provided by the following bodies in community care for people with mental health problems:

- social services,
- local health district,
- voluntary organizations.

SAQ 6. Identify five reasons why people may be referred to the community psychiatric team.

SAQ 7. Describe briefly four services provided by the community mental health centre.

SAQ 8. Identify the skills of the community psychiatric nurse in relation to:

- nursing care,
- clinical work,
- education,
- management,
- research.

Unit 5.2: Written Test

Thomas Brown, aged 45, has been referred to the community mental health centre for assessment. He has been unemployed for 3 years and has made numerous unsuccessful attempts to find work. He has become increasingly despondent and complains of feeling anxious in social situations. His relationship with his wife, Jenny, is under stress, and she is threatening to leave him if he does not "pull himself together".

1. What community resources may be useful in this situation?
2. What skills will the community psychiatric nurse require to use in order to help the couple cope with their situation?

UNIT 5.3

Issues in Community Care

Unit Objectives

At the end of this Unit the learner should be able to:

1. Describe the problems experienced by families and individuals in coping with mental health problems.
2. Identify the reactions of staff to developments in community care.
3. Outline public attitudes towards mental illness.
4. Define the term "stigma".

Family and Self-care

The concept of community care may seem a recent development to health care professionals and planners but it is something that individuals and families have always had to cope with. The majority of families and individuals with mental health problems do not make use of the limited community resources available. Frequently lacking in skill or information they are, none the less, expected to cope with the problems they are experiencing. Some families may manage quite effectively and develop appropriate coping strategies. For most, though, they find themselves progressively burdened with long-term and seemingly intractable problems. These can cause considerable stress and seriously interfere with their own mental health and the quality of their lives.

Common difficulties experienced by individuals and families include:

1. Feelings of distress and anxiety.
2. Feelings of helplessness and not knowing what to do.
3. Stress and disruption in close relationships and family life.
4. Physical exhaustion and a lack of support.
5. Social isolation – from the need to be in constant attendance, loss of friends and visitors, secondary stigma.
6. Guilt and ambivalence towards the sufferer.
7. Occupational difficulties and restrictions.
8. Financial problems.

Prolonged stress, desperation and a decreasing ability to cope may eventually cause the family to seek help. However, the resources presently allocated to community care are insufficient to meet the current level of need that exists. People may find themselves receiving limited support from an overstretched community care team.

The Transfer of Care

The number of patients resident in psychiatric hospitals has fallen considerably over the past 30 years, from 154 000 in 1954 to 70 000 in 1983. These numbers are still decreasing. Many of these people are now either:

- living independently;
- living in other health care residential accommodation with full-time care;
- supported by community care services in a range of residential settings.

The transfer of care on this scale forms part of a policy by successive governments to promote the development of community care services for the mentally ill as a preferential alternative to hospital-based care. Such a development has been facilitated by:

1. The recognition of the potentially harmful effects of long-term residential care.
2. The advantages of caring for people in their own home environment, maintaining family and social links.
3. The improvement of methods of rehabilitation and treatment.
4. Changes in attitudes and expectations by health care staff and people at large.
5. Legislation that encouraged community alternatives for care.

A common misconception held by both staff and the public is that the move towards community care is being made in order to save money. The economic realities of a comprehensive community care system are that the provision of a fully resourced community programme costs some 10% more than hospital-based treatment. The actual transfer of resources on its own would, therefore, be insufficient to provide the level of care required. It will require a greater investment in resources.

Another issue that relates to the level of resources required includes an increase in the demand for psychiatric services from:

1. Greater accessibility of services so that more people are inclined to use them.
2. Increased recognition and identification of mental health problems by health care professionals and the public.
3. The increasing numbers of elderly people with mental health problems.

Staff Reactions to Developments in Community Care

The developments in community care have considerable implications for health care staff who work in established services. Most have been trained to work in a hospital setting and have years of institutionally-based experience. The prospect of a radical change in role can seem quite threatening. Reactions can include:

1. *Insecurity*: a fear of the unknown.
2. *Stress*: from the strain of adjustment.
3. *Feeling de-skilled*: their existing skills and knowledge are of limited use in a community-based residential or domiciliary service.
4. *Feelings of loss*: grieving for the institution, loss of institutional-based status, role, relationships.
5. *Isolation*: having to take on greater responsibility with a lack of immediate support.
6. *Apathy and disillusionment*: not being in harmony with these developments, which causes bitterness and resentment.

The staff involved in such developments need to be adequately prepared for their new roles. Other staff have found the change of role and pattern of care a great stimulus and have used the opportunity to revise radically their skills and expectations. Learners who train in such an environment are also at an advantage in adapting to community-based roles.

Public Attitudes Towards Mental Illness

Social attitudes towards those with mental illness are not favourable. The mentally ill are regarded as a dangerous and disturbed group of people who pose a potential threat to others. The mentally ill are to be feared, avoided and treated with suspicion or derision.

The existence of such hostile attitudes or "negative stereotypes" towards the mentally ill are essentially a product of ignorance, folklore and sensationalism by the media. People are brought up to fear mental illness and to associate it with unpleasant, dangerous and frightening behaviour: murder, rape, violent assault, arson and sex offences are frequently associated with "madmen", "lunatics" and "psychopaths". Selective reporting in newspapers, fictional books, horror movies and television plays also serve to further confirm for people the dangerous nature of "insanity". Psychiatrists and psychologists are involved in sensational court cases. Convicted people are sent for "treatment" to special hospitals. It is little wonder then that the public's perception of mental health problems is so distorted.

It will take much social and health education to ensure that attitudes towards the mentally ill are more humane and based upon accurate information and understanding rather than prejudice and fear.

Public Reactions to Community Care Development

With such widespread negative attitudes being held by many people towards the mentally ill, it is hardly surprising that the move towards community care can evoke very strong reactions. People are mystified and frightened by the planner's desire to encourage community care for a group of people that they basically think should be kept locked up. Local reactions to planning applications for new hostels, units and other developments are usually extremely hostile. People fear for the safety of their families and for their property values. Inevitably any location chosen is "inappropriate" and "too near" to local schools, nurseries, residential estates, etc. They refer to the increasing number of homeless psychotics and others with mental health problems that they see in town centres, shopping precincts and libraries.

Staff involved with the development of community services find, therefore, that one of their first tasks in any programme is to promote public awareness and understanding of the client group and the service to be offered. It can take a lot of effort, perseverence and courage for the staff to initiate and set up a hostel or services in an unwelcome environment.

Stigma

The very strong and negative images held of mental illness ensure that sufferers are identified as being different from other "normal" people. They are seen as having a "spoiled" social identity and are disqualified from full social acceptance. On the basis of this difference or "stigma", they are also treated as if they are intellectually subnormal, untrustworthy and morally suspect. Other people try to avoid them and interactions frequently reinforce the concept of the sufferer as a person of little social worth.

The existence of these attitudes causes great distress to both the sufferers and their families. At the same time that they are trying to cope with their own mental health problems they have the added burden of shame and guilt. In order to cope with this "stigma", they adopt defensive strategies in order to try and hide their problems from others. They feel that they have to avoid "normal" people in case they are found out and exposed to ridicule or shame. This withdrawal can lead to social isolation. Contact may be limited to others with similar problems who will accept them non-judgementally. Relatives of the affected person may also find that their own lives and relationships are adversely influenced by their association with the sufferer.

Unit Instructions

When you have researched the suggested references, have mastered the Unit Objectives and successfully answered the Self-assessment Questions, proceed with the Unit Written Test.

Suggested References

Anderson, G. (1984). Changing attitudes, taking risks. *Nursing Times*, 29 August, Vol. 80, No. 35, pp. 19–21.

Barnett, C. (1987). What will the neighbours say? *Nursing Times*, 24 June, Vol. 83, No. 25, pp. 31–32.

Broadley, K. (1985). Shelter or suffering. *Nursing Mirror*, October, Vol. 161, No. 18, pp. 40–43.

Brown, P. (1985). *The Transfer of Care*. Routledge and Kegan Paul, London.

Gaze, H. (1985). Countdown to Closure. *Nursing Times*, 22 May, Vol. 81, No. 21, pp. 18–19.

Gaze, H. (1987). Community care-less. *Nursing Times*, 7 January, Vol. 83, No. 1, pp. 20–21.

Gibbs, A. (1986). *Understanding Mental Health*. Consumer's Association/Hodder and Stoughton, London.

Goffman, E. (1963). *Stigma*. Penguin, Harmondsworth.

Goldberg, D. and Huxley, P. (1980). *Mental Illness in the Community*. Tavistock, London.

Heywood-Jones, I. (1987). Prisoners of care. *Nursing Times*, 22 April, Vol. 83, No. 16, pp. 44–45.

Laurance, J. (1986). The 'scandal' of Lincoln's suicides. *New Society*, 20 June, Vol. 76, No. 1225, pp. 15–16.

Mangen, S. P. (1982). *Sociology and Mental Health*. Churchill Livingstone, Edinburgh.

Miles, A. (1981). *The Mentally Ill in Contemporary Society*. Martin Robertson, Oxford.

Morris, P. (1984). Mentally ill and homeless. *Nursing Times*, 29 August, Vol. 80, No. 35, pp. 16–17.

Naughtie, J. (1985). For once, a unified front. *Nursing Times*, 27 March, Vol. 81, No. 13, pp. 22–23.

New Society (1987). The crisis in community care. *New Society*, 18 September, Vol. 81, No. 1290. Special Supplement.

Psychiatric Nurses' Association (1985). Boarded out or shunted on? *The British Journal of Psychiatric Nursing*, April, Vol. 2, No. 12, pp. 1–2.

Shepherd, G. (1984). *Institutional Care and Rehabilitation*. Longman, London.

Sines, D. (1984). Change for the better? *Nursing Times*, 15 August, Vol. 80, No. 33, pp. 42–44.

Social Services Select Committee Report on Community Care (1985). House of Commons Paper 13–1, HMSO, London.

Vousden, M. (1984). Community care is not a cheap option. *Nursing Mirror*, 13 March, Vol. 160, No. 11.

Vousden, M. (1987a). Out of MIND. *Nursing Times*, 26 August, Vol. 83, No. 34, pp. 18–19.

Vousden, M. (1987b). Haven of care. . .or sick joke? *Nursing Times*, 24 June, Vol. 83, No. 25, pp. 28–30.

Self-assessment Questions

SAQ 9. List five problems experienced by families caring for someone with mental health problems.

SAQ 10. Identify four reactions that hospital-based staff might experience in the move towards community care.

SAQ 11. State four reasons why public views of mental health problems are so hostile.

SAQ 12. Define the term "stigma" and the effects that it can have on a person's self-perception and behaviour.

Unit 5.3: Written Test

You are working on a hospital ward for long-stay residents that is shortly to move to a hostel in a local town.

1. What are the possible reactions of the local community? Why do people have this set of attitudes?
2. What actions can be taken to ensure that relationships with the local community are positive?
3. How might the hospital staff affected by this move react to working in a community-based hospital? How can the staff be prepared for this transition?

Residential Care

Residential Care

People with mental health problems may require residential care for a variety of reasons:

1. Lack or exhaustion of available support network.
2. An inability to cope any longer with the stress of mental health problems.
3. Acutely disturbed, self-injurious or confused behaviour, where the person is a risk to themselves or to others.
4. Access to specialist assessment and treatment facilities.

The changing pattern of care provision in mental health services means that admission to a psychiatric hospital may not be necessary or desirable for many people. Their needs for residential care may be met within the increasing diversity of alternative residential facilities. For most people, anyway, residential care will form just a short interlude in the care and treatment of much longer-term mental health problems. Staff in residential care and treatment settings need to keep in perspective the fact that they are only dealing with a small percentage of the total number of people wth mental health problems. The residential client group is also not necessarily formed of the most disturbed or dependent people.

The range of residential care facilities can include:

1. Psychiatric hospital or DGH psychiatric units where the person may be admitted formally or informally.
2. Specialist treatment units either attached to or independent of other hospital facilities, e.g. alcohol treatment unit, detoxification centre, regional secure unit, drug dependency unit, family therapy unit, therapeutic community child and adolescent psychiatry units.
3. Health and Social Service community-based residential facilities, e.g. purpose-built or adapted homes for the elderly confused (HEC), halfway home, group home, hostel or other supervised or non-supervised accommodation. These exist for people with a wide range of problems, differing needs and abilities. In these settings the residents may still be under the care of a psychiatrist or be discharged and paying rent to the health authority or housing association. In these situations the hostel is their home until they are ready to move on to more independent facilities.
4. Many voluntary organizations run hostels for people with specific problems or for those who are experiencing mental health difficulties. Examples are hostels organized by the Richmond Fellowship, MIND and county-based councils on alcoholism.

Influence of the Care Environment

The environment of a care area can exert a powerful influence upon the behaviour, thoughts and feelings of both the staff and residents. Used constructively, the environment of any care area can be carefully utilized to exert a powerful therapeutic effect.

Conversely, the environment can also exert very damaging and debilitating effects on both residents and staff. Prolonged exposure to an insular and rigid care regime can create additional problems of "institutionalization" or "institutional neurosis". This is a pattern of behaviour characterized by a loss of independence, initiative, individuality, motivation, self-esteem, social and life skills, interest in personal appearance and hygiene, and an interest in the future.

Environmental factors which create institutionalization have been identified as loss of contact with the outside world, social isolation, enforced dependency, rigid, unvarying routines, strict conformity, environmental poverty, strong barriers between staff and residents, no involvement or choice in the organization of the care area, depersonalization with little personal recognition, few possessions and hospital clothes. The longer residents remain in such an environment the more dependent they become and the less likely they are to leave.

Massive efforts to rehabilitate this group of long-stay institutionalized residents have reduced bed numbers considerably in mental hospitals. Many residents are now living in supervised hostel accommodation or are now independent of care services. Hopefully, the mistakes of the past will not be repeated and there are now a number of identified sound principles upon which to base therapeutic residential care.

The charge nurse/manager/team leader

All of the research available indicates that the person in charge of care exerts a considerable influence on the clinical, work and learning environments. Their personality, management style, clinical skills and commitment to education are crucial contributing factors.

1. *Personality*

   - Need to be motivated, enjoy and be interested in their work.
   - Need to be kind, patient, firm, consistent, calm and sensitive, able to form effective working relationships, approachable, sense of humour, open, flexible, receptive, able to express concern for the welfare of others.

2. *Management style*

   - To give personal recognition to staff, provide support and encouragement, to use people's time and skills to the best effect, to plan ahead.
   - Organize, co-ordinate and lead the staff team.
   - Delegate and give responsibility to staff.
   - Initiate change and to follow it through.
   - Ensure good communications with all staff.
   - Promote the identity of the staff team.
   - Monitor staff performance and to give feedback.
   - Resolve conflicts between staff and to promote harmony.
   - Make decisions, to manage and not administrate.

3. *Clinical skills*

   - To promote good relationships and a high quality of care.
   - Give a high orientation and contact time with residents.
   - Demonstrate good nursing skills and high standards.
   - Need to be clinically experienced and skilful.
   - Ensure that residents are treated as people and individuals.
   - Reinforce the staff's recognition that nursing care is important and is effective in helping people.

4. *Education*

   - To maintain their own professional development.
   - Instruct other staff and learners.
   - Explain how and why things are done.
   - Help and encourage other people to learn.

Reception and orientation of residents

For many people the experience of coming into care represents a real life crisis and can be a traumatic time. Most people are anxious about being admitted and the stigma of being associated with psychiatric services. People need to be received in a reassuring and calming way. The staff need to be positive about their role and to use their first contacts to initiate a therapeutic relationship. Newcomers should be introduced to the other residents and staff, shown around the care area and given an explanation of the daily routine. They should, if possible, be admitted by the primary nurse or someone from the nursing team who will subsequently be working with them. The information should be backed up by written information that lists all the key points. They should also be given an explanation of the nursing care programme and treatment regime. The whole experience should be approached in a humane, kind and understanding way.

Maximum opportunity for staff–resident contact

Barriers between staff and residents should be minimized to promote contact. Titles, uniforms, keys and separate "territories" all keep staff and residents apart. Interaction is facilitated if staff are confident enough to work with people without these professional props and to share space and time with the residents. The staff should use each contact constructively to develop therapeutic relationships and to work towards the attainment of the residents' needs. Positive reinforcement should be given to adaptive and healthy behaviour. Non-adaptive and dependent behaviour should not be reinforced.

Residents should be kept fully informed through daily meetings and notice boards of all relevant issues and given the opportunity to discuss them. The community meeting should also be a forum for decision making, planning and resolving conflicts.

Planned individual care programmes

Each person should have a specific nurse as a primary nurse or key worker with whom they can identify. They should have the opportunity to meet with them on a regular and planned basis for support, guidance, feedback, problem solving and to monitor their progress. Staff duty times and shifts should be organized to ensure that someone from each team is on duty at all times if possible. The staff and residents of a particular care team should also meet regularly as a group to facilitate peer support and relationships. Each resident's care programme should be orientated towards meeting the person's social, psychological and physical needs and towards maximizing their potential.

Individual recognition and identity

Residents should be treated with respect and dignity. Their individuality should be reinforced through their contacts with staff, through the use of their own clothes and possessions and from being able to personalize some part of the environment as their own. Individual choice and preferences in relation to food and use of recreation should be supported. The need for privacy should be respected. Significant personal events and dates, such as birthdays and anniversaries, should be identified and celebrated.

Maximum degree of choice and responsibility

Any rules, routine or restrictions should only exist in terms of safety or by the consent of the whole resident and staff community. Such rules that do exist should be stated clearly in a statement of policy that is consistently applied. In terms of care activities, the nurses should not do anything for the residents that they are capable of doing for themselves. Residents should be encouraged to participate in the activities of the care area and should be given specific re-training and education to promote their independence.

Residents should be encouraged to do their own laundry, make their own beds, do basic household chores, buy and cook their own food, decide meal-times, buy their own clothes, have access to money and a bank account, decide how to spend their leisure time, determine when they want to go to bed, participate in decision and policy making, participate in their own care and treatment programmes, and comply with self-medication programmes. These activities should represent positive care and practice choices by the staff who are committed to promoting autonomy and independence. Both staff and residents should also take responsibility for their choices and to experience the consequences of their actions. A degree of risk is a very real part of life and of therapy. In many ways, the range and degree of choice available to residents is a good indicator of the quality of care.

Home-like atmosphere

Most care areas are stuck with their existing layout and decor and many do not facilitate modern care practices. However, even given this restriction, it is how the available environment is used that is important. Efforts should be made to create a non-institutional environment through the layout of available furniture, the use of ornaments, pictures and flowers, and the siting of televisions and radios. There should be a choice of daytime areas and places for specific activities or privacy. Large areas should be divided into smaller sitting areas with the furniture positioned to facilitate communication. Meal-times should be used as a social and therapeutic occasion in which tablecloths and cruets are used, and eating skills reinforced in an unhurried atmosphere.

Friendship and recreational activities between residents should be facilitated for them to meet their social needs. In longer-term care facilities the residents' need for physical affection and sex should be respected in a sensitive and non-judgemental manner. Sex education and contraceptive advice should be given if needed.

Contact with the outside world

Family and friends should be encouraged to visit with minimal restrictions. Where possible the residents should likewise be encouraged to visit their home and family for the day, weekend or longer. Relatives should be kept fully informed about the resident's progress. A relatives' support group should be formed or the relatives put in touch with other self-help or voluntary organizations. Volunteers should be welcomed and given a part to play in the care area. Residents should have access to a telephone and to writing materials. A choice of books, newspapers and TV should be available.

Use of local community facilities should be encouraged, e.g. libraries, swimming pools, cinemas and clubs. Where access is difficult, transport should be organized to take residents on outside visits. Staff should make themselves fully aware of the range of voluntary and statutory resources that are available locally and to draw the resident's attention to them or to organize their use.

Contacts with local community groups should be encouraged through inviting visits, open days and organizing joint events.

Unit Instructions

When you have researched the suggested references, have mastered the Unit Objectives and successfully answered the Self-assessment Questions, proceed with the Unit Written Test.

Suggested References

Altschul, A. and McGovern, M. (1985). *Psychiatric Nursing*, 6th edition. Baillière Tindall, London and San Diego.

Baker, P. J. (1985). *Patient Assessment in Psychiatric Nursing*. Croom Helm, London.

Barker, P. J. and Fraser D. (Eds) (1985). *The Nurse as Therapist: A Behavioural Model*. Croom Helm, London.

Barton, R. (1959). *Institutional Neurosis*. John Wright, Bristol.

Beardshaw, V. (1981). *Conscientious Objectors at Work*. Social Audit, London.

Bloor, M. (1986). Who'll make the tea? *New Society*, 31 January, Vol. 75, No. 1205, pp. 185–186.

Butler, R. J. and Rosenthal, G. (1985). *Behaviour and Rehabilitation*, 2nd edition. John Wright, Bristol.

Burrows, R. (1985). Reflective image. *Nursing Times*, 15 May, Vol. 81, No. 20, pp. 61–62.

Clark, D. H. (1981). *Social Therapy in Psychiatry*. Churchill Livingstone, Edinburgh.

Dexter, G. and Wash, M. (1986). *Psychiatric Nursing Skills: A Patient-centred Approach*. Croom Helm, London.

Dietrich, G. (1976). Nurses in the therapeutic community. *Journal of Advanced Nursing*, 1976, Vol. 1, No. 2, pp. 139–154.

Durham, R. C. (1985). Creating Therapeutic Environments. *In* Barker, P. J. and Fraser, D. (Eds), *The Nurse as Therapist: A Behavioural Model*. Croom Helm, London.

Fenton, F. R. *et al.* (1982). *Home and Hospital Psychiatric Treatment*. Croom Helm, London.

Fretwell, J. (1982). *Ward Teaching and Learning*. Royal College of Nursing, London.

Frois, M., Kole, B., Jack, H. and Harries, C. (1983). A hospital-hostel. *Nursing Times*, 14 September, Vol. 79, No. 37, pp. 44–45.

Goffman, E. (1961). *Asylums*. Penguin, Harmondsworth.

Jansen, E. (Ed.) (1980). *The Therapeutic Community*. Croom Helm, London.

Kennard, D. (1983). *An Introduction to Therapeutic Communities*. Routledge and Kegan Paul, London.

Krzyszkowski, S. and Carnell, R. (1985). Long-stay break. *Nursing Mirror*, 8 May, Vol. 160, No. 19, pp. 40–42.

Leopoldt, H. and McStay, P. (1980). The psychiatric group home – 1. *Nursing Times*, 8 May, Vol. 76, No. 19, pp. 829–832.

Lindsay, M. (1982). A critical view of the validity of the therapeutic community. *Nursing Times*, 22 September, Vol. 78, No. 38, pp. 105–107. Occasional Paper.

Mercer, I. (1985). Striking the right balance. *Nursing Times*, 20 November, Vol. 81, No. 47, pp. 58–59.

Orford, J. (1982). Institutional Climates. *In* Hall, J. (Ed.), *Psychology for Nurses and Health Visitors*. Methuen/The British Psychological Society, London.

Orton, H. D. (1981). *Ward Teaching Climate*. Royal College of Nursing, London.

Thornicroft, G. (1979). Group homes – a success? *Nursing Times*, 11 January, Vol. 75, No. 2, pp. 84–85.

Towell, D. and Harries, C. (1979). *Innovations in Patient Care*. Croom Helm, London.

Wilkinson, D. (1987). Busy doing nothing. *Nursing Times*, 10 June, Vol. 83, No. 23, pp. 30–31.

Wolkowski, A. (1986). A life of rejection. *Nursing Times*, 16 April, Vol. 82, No. 16, pp. 35–38.

Self-assessment Questions

SAQ 13. List five factors involved in creating a therapeutic environment.

SAQ 14. How does the manager of a care area influence its therapeutic potential?

SAQ 15. Identify ten areas in which residents can be given choice.

SAQ 16. Describe four ways that residents can be involved in the management of a residential care facility.

Unit 5.4: Written Test

You have been invited to give a talk on a study day devoted to creating a therapeutic environment.

1. Identify the key areas involved in creating a therapeutic environment.
2. Describe in detail how four of the key areas you have identified contribute to promoting resident welfare.

TOPIC 6

Anxiety-related Problems

At the end of this Topic the learner should aim to:

1. Describe the physical, psychological and behavioural effects of anxiety.
2. Be aware of factors that can precipitate anxiety.
3. Outline the range of therapeutic interventions available for helping people to resolve their anxiety.
4. Identify the nursing care needs and interventions required for the person suffering from anxiety.

The Nature of Anxiety

Unit Objectives

At the end of this Unit the learner should be able to:

1. Differentiate between the facilitating and distressing effects of anxiety.
2. Describe the effects of anxiety upon a person's behaviour, emotions and physiology.
3. Outline the factors that can contribute towards the experience of anxiety.
4. Describe the classification of anxiety in mental health practice.

Anxiety

Anxiety is a normal emotional and physical response to situations that are perceived as potentially threatening. The function of anxiety is to mobilize the person's resources to cope with threats which may be of a social, physical or psychological nature.

Perception of a threat stimulates the autonomic nervous system and the release of adrenaline and noradrenaline from the adrenal glands. The effect of this is to initiate a wide range of physiological responses. These increase a person's alertness and ability to respond to identified threats. This is sometimes described as the "fight or flight" reaction.

However, the same physical and psychological responses that in most situations facilitate coping can also, under certain conditions, pose problems for the individual. Primarily intended to deal with immediate or short-term situations, the responses can also become distressing and counterproductive if:

1. The duration of the threat is prolonged or continuous, creating a long-term anxiety response that becomes exhausting and distressing.
2. The intensity of the reaction is disproportionate in terms of the potential threat posed, so that the person becomes overwhelmed by their anxiety.
3. The person is unable to identify the nature of the threat that is making them feel anxious – the feelings disappear to arise spontaneously and cause generalized distress.

4. The person is aware of the nature of the threat posed but is unable to control purposefully their anxiety-specific situations, which may trigger off an anxiety response that the person may recognize as inappropriate.
5. Anxiety is not an appropriate response to the situation, i.e. other responses and behaviour may be more effective in that situation.

The boundary at which the anxiety ceases to facilitate a response and that at which it becomes subjectively unpleasant is a fine one. This will be influenced by the individual's perception and interpretation of their personal experiences.

Exhibit 6.1.1 The effects of anxiety

Facilitating effects of anxiety	*Distressing effects of anxiety*
1. *Physical*	
Increased pulse rate	Palpitations
Raised blood pressure	Headache
Raised muscle tone	Tension and rigidity
Blood flow increased to large muscle groups	Tremor
	Dizziness and fainting
Blood flow decreased to non-essential organs	Weakness and loss of energy
	Difficulty in breathing
Increased respiratory rate	Hyperventilation
Diminished awareness of pain	Cold clammy skin, perspiration
	Pale skin
Pupils dilated to increase perceptual field	Frequency of micturation
	Diarrhoea or constipation
Sensory alertness	Dry mouth, difficulty in chewing and swallowing
Faster reaction time	Difficulty in speaking
Short-term increase in physical endurance and stamina	Churning stomach, gastro-intestinal upsets
	Nausea
	Loss of appetite
	Blurred vision
	Sleep disturbances, insomnia, tiredness and fatigue
	"Freezing" – rigid with fear
	Sexual and orgasmic dysfunction
2. *Psychological*	
Focusses attention on threat	Thought blocking – "mind going blank"
	Totally preoccupied with anxiety
Rapid decision making	Poor concentration
Enhanced problem solving	Poor memory
Increased motivation	Indecisiveness

Facilitating effects of anxiety	Distressing effects of anxiety
Increased learning	Hopelessness and helplessness
Prepared to take risks	Fearful and frightened
Accept challenges	Panic stricken
Aspire to high achievement	

Recognizing Anxiety

The effects of anxiety may be evident in a number of ways. Some clients may be able to describe fully the influence of anxiety upon their thoughts, feelings and behaviour. Others may be severely distressed but not recognize the nature of their anxiety. However, with skilful observation, interviewing technique and other assessment tools, the nurse can identify the extent to which a client is experiencing anxiety.

1. *Physical effects*: verbal complaints of the distressing effects of anxiety, muscular tension, headaches, non-specific physical symptoms, aches and pains. Hypochondriacal concerns. Psycho-somatic reactions. Exacerbation of pain and discomfort from any pre-existing physical disease.
2. *Emotional effects*: fear, panic, distress, unease, apprehension, easily upset, low tolerance for stress, on edge, impatient, irritable, shame, embarrassment, unsettled, agitated, depression, guilt.
3. *Cognitive effects*: dread of the future, foreboding, anticipating the worst, guilt, constant preoccupation with anxious thoughts, fears of going "mad", loss of self-esteem, negative and self-defeating perceptions, feeling trapped and helpless, wanting to escape, inattentive, poor concentration, forgetful, reduced powers of reasoning and problem solving, loss of usual interests.
4. *Behavioural effects*: facial expression tense, biting lips, constant eye movements, eye lids twitching, crying, tearfulness, posture rigid, tremor, awkward movements, clumsiness, poor co-ordination, tapping fingers, wringing hands, sweating palms.

    Speech–increased rate, raised pitch, frequent speech errors, erratic rhythm, increased rate of breathing, sighing, hyperventilating.

    Fidgeting, rocking backwards and forwards, pacing up and down, restlessness, aimless movement, agitation, loss of control.

    Clinging and demanding, seeking constant reassurance, overtalkative, withdrawal, avoidance of potentially threatening situations.

Sources of Anxiety

There are many potential factors that can contribute towards the experience of anxiety.

Early upbringing

1. Experience of parental conflict, material deprivation or separation anxiety as an infant. This predisposes to insecurity, low self-esteem as an adult and relationship difficulties in adult life.
2. Parental role models that continually demonstrate and reinforce anxious behaviour.
3. Traumatic incidents in early life that interfere with the individual's social developments and self-esteem – situations of failure, serious accidents, child abuse, incest and sexual abuse, prolonged physical illness.
4. Limited range of social experience – overprotected, limiting learning opportunities.

Threats to security needs

1. Stressful life events and difficulty in coping.
2. Relationship conflict and marital stress.
3. Occupational stress, fear of redundancy, unemployment.
4. Perception of the environment as threatening – feeling at risk, new and unknown environments.
5. Situations of loss.
6. Threats to self-esteem.
7. Financial problems.
8. Frustration and inability to meet basic needs.
9. Victim of crime – burglary, rape, assault.
10. Prolonged debilitating physical illness.

Learned fear

1. Anxiety learned as a maladaptive, inappropriate response to situations where other reactions would be more appropriate.
2. Traumatic life events that sensitize the person to react anxiously upon repeated exposure to similar situations. This may also lead to more generalized feelings of anxiety and insecurity.

Perception of self- and life events

1. Lack of self-esteem and confidence.
2. Unrealistically high personal expectations that person is unable to attain – perception of self as a "failure".
3. Negative, irrational thought patterns.
4. Limited range of coping strategies.
5. Perceiving life events as being randomly and externally controlled with themselves having little influence over the outcome.
6. Suspicion and lack of trust.

Sense of helplessness and lack of control

1. Inability to exert control or alter the outcome of stressful situations.
2. Feelings of impotence and helplessness.
3. Feeling overwhelmed by stress and life events.
4. Situations outside the person's experience.
5. Confusion and disorientation.
6. Inability to meet habituation needs – dependency on alcohol, cigarettes, drugs.

Personality

1. "Trait" anxiety – personality type characterized by persistent and enduring anxiety responses to many situations.
2. Type "A" personality – high drive and motivation to achieve, inability to relax, "workaholic", lives under continual stress and self-imposed demands.

Repressed conflict

1. Threats to the person's integrity that are moderated by mental defence mechanisms and expressed as more generalized anxiety.
2. Repressed desires and drives that cause frustration and tension.

Physical causes

1. Pre-menstrual tension, menopause.
2. Disease of the limbic structures of the brain.
3. Endocrine – thyrotoxicosis, tumours of the adrenal glands.
4. Side-effects of stimulants – excessive tea or coffee, amphetamines.
5. Withdrawal from dependency-inducing substances – tranquillizers, alcohol, drugs.

The Classification of Anxiety

In mental health practice anxiety may be classified as follows.

Anxiety state/anxiety reaction/anxiety neurosis

This is an emotional and behavioural state of continued and prolonged apprehension and fear. The individual's anxiety is out of all proportion to any precipitating stress that can be identified. In many instances there may be no apparent or recognizable threat. The individual's anxiety is free-floating and the person tends to be constantly preoccupied with worries about the future. The bodily discomforts associated with prolonged anxiety are present and may cause considerable distress. This degree of anxiety seriously interferes with a person's ability to meet their needs and can exert a crippling influence on the individual's life.

Phobic anxiety/phobic reaction/phobia

Most aspects of phobic anxiety are essentially the same as those of an anxiety state. However, whereas in an anxiety state the person's fears are generalized, in phobic anxiety they are focussed upon a very specific triggering event. Confrontation with this object or situation initiates a severe anxiety and panic attack. The object of fear may be almost anything in the person's environment, e.g. people, animals, insects, bacteria, dirt, open spaces, enclosed spaces, aspects of the weather. This list is almost infinite. However, irrespective of the stimulus that initiates this distressing reaction, a phobia is characterized by:

1. The subjective experience of a degree of panic, terror and fear that are out of all proportion to the potential threat posed.
2. Difficulty in being able to explain why they have this specific fear. Quite often at an intellectual level, the sufferer can appreciate that the fear must seem illogical and absurd.
3. An inability to limit or control the extent of the fear and panic when confronted with the triggering stimulus.
4. The strategies adopted to avoid the feared situation as far as possible. These strategies may involve elaborate precautions being taken by the sufferer and those that live with them. These may seriously disrupt and interfere with normal life and activities.

Incidence

In the field of health care practice, anxiety may be seen as a prominent feature of both mental and physical health problems. As a mental health problem it is estimated that about 2–5% of the total population suffer from severe anxiety. Only about 1% of these require treatment in a residential setting.

The diagnosis of anxiety, in clinical practice, is most frequently applied to women. Biologically, there are some physiological explanations (pre-menstrual tension, the experience of childbirth and motherhood, the menopause) that are specific gender stresses. However, sociologically, there appear to be a number of other explanations for the male–female differences:

1. Upbringing patterns and role modelling that:

- Reinforce open emotional expression in females and suppress it in males. Men are brought up to have other outlets for their feelings.
- Reinforce more positive self-esteem and social confidence in males than females.

2. Marriage and close relationships tend to be at the expense of the mental health of the female rather than the male partner. The woman is expected to provide emotional support for her male partner but frequently is not provided with support in return. Even in an age of increasing joint involvement in child-rearing activities, the demands made upon "mothers" still far exceed those of the father.
3. The tendency for female mental health problems to be prejudged and labelled as "neurotic", irrespective of their actual nature, by many health care workers.

Unit Instructions

When you have researched the suggested references, have mastered the Unit Objectives and successfully answered the Self-assessment Questions, proceed with the Unit Written Test.

Suggested References

Blenkinsop, J. (1986). There came a big spider. . .. *Nursing Times*, 8 January, Vol. 82, No. 2, pp. 28–30.

Campbell, C. (1978). *Nursing Diagnosis and Intervention in Nursing Practice*. John Wiley, New York.

Consumers' Association (1982). *Living with Stress*. Consumers Association/Hodder and Stoughton, London.

Cox, T. (1978). *Stress*. Macmillan, London.

Gibbs, A. (1986). *Understanding Mental Health*. Consumers Association/Hodder and Stoughton, London.

Goodwin, D. W. (1983). *Phobias the Facts*. Oxford Publications, Oxford.

Hughes, B. and Boothroyd, R. (1985). *Fight or Flight?* Faber and Faber, London.

Hughes, J. (1986). *An Outline of Modern Psychiatry*, 2nd edition. John Wiley, New York.

Hunter, C. (1985). Easing the tension. *Nursing Times*, 16 January, Vol. 81, No. 3, pp. 40–43.

Irving, S. (1983). *Basic Psychiatric Nursing*, 3rd edition. W. B. Saunders, Philadelphia.

Kowalski, R. (1987). *Over the Top*. Avalon Press/Winslow Press, Bristol/Bicester.

Lancaster, J. (1980). *Adult Psychiatric Nursing*. Henry Kimpton, London.

Lim, D. (1985). Imprisoned by fear. *Nursing Mirror*, 24 July, Vol. 161, No. 4, p. 18–19.

Lyttle, J. (1986). *Mental Disorder*. Baillière Tindall, London and San Diego.

Macphail, D. and McMillan, I. (1983). Fighting phobias. *Nursing Mirror*, Mental Health Forum 8, 17 August, Vol. 157, No. 7, Supplement (i)–(ii).

Martin, P. (Ed.) (1987). *Psychiatric Nursing: A Therapeutic Approach*. Macmillan, London.

Melville, J. (1977). *Phobias and Obsessions*. George Allen and Unwin, London.

Mitchell, R. (1982). *Phobias*. Penguin, Harmondsworth.

Murdoch, W. and Newton, A. (1985). High anxiety. *Nursing Times*, 30 January, Vol. 81, No. 5, pp. 26–28.

North, N. (1985). Phobias – the misunderstood fear. *Nursing Times*, 2 January, Vol. 81, No. 1, pp. 24–25.

Robinson, L. (1983). *Psychiatric Nursing as a Human Experience*, 3rd edition. W. B. Saunders, Philadelphia.

Seligman, M. (1975). *Helplessness*. W. H. Freeman, San Francisco.

Smail, D. (1984). *Illusion and Reality: The Meaning of Anxiety*. J. M. Dent, London.

Snaith, P. (1981). *Clinical Neurosis*. Oxford University Press, Oxford.

Trethowan, W. and Sims, A. (1983). *Psychiatry*, 5th edition. Baillière Tindall, London and San Diego.

Willis, J. (1976). *Clinical Psychiatry*. Blackwell Scientific, Oxford.

Note: Many of the references in Unit 4.1 may also be useful in gaining a greater understanding and awareness of anxiety.

Self-assessment Questions

SAQ 1. Identify eight distressing physical symptoms of prolonged anxiety.

SAQ 2. List ten aspects of a person's behaviour and emotions that would indicate anxiety.

SAQ 3. Outline six factors that can contribute towards anxiety.

SAQ 4. State four characteristics of a phobia that differentiate it from an anxiety reaction.

Unit 6.1: Written Test

Janice Marks has been referred to a community mental health centre. She complains that she has been suffering from severe anxiety for a number of years.

1. How is she likely to describe the effects of anxiety upon herself?
2. What observations could you make of her behaviour that would confirm her complaints?
3. What factors in her recent background may have contributed to her present experience of anxiety?

Care and Treatment of the Person with Anxiety-related problems

Care and Treatment

A wide range of therapeutic interventions may be used to help the person with anxiety or phobias. These may focus on both the presenting symptoms and the person's life-style and coping skills. The specific interventions will depend upon the assessment undertaken by the therapist and the skills and resources available to them. The general approach should be towards an integrated and readily accessible service that is able to support the person and their family in the community or in residential care, as required.

Therapeutic aims

1. To minimize the experience of distress.
2. To enable the person to regain control of their emotional, cognitive behavioural and physical reactions to stressors.
3. To facilitate the development of the person's and their family's coping skills.

Family and self-care

Minor anxieties in relation to many aspects of everyday life are common. A wide range of situations and activities may have the potential to evoke anxiety – social situations, relationships, decision making, work and irrational fears. Generally, they tend to make the person feel uncomfortable or awkward rather than distressed, and are often associated with a sense of embarrassment.

The experience of more severe anxiety is also quite common, particularly as a reaction to specific stressful life events. In these situations the symptoms may be extremely distressing, possibly even disabling for a limited period. However, for most people, the experience is short term and within a comparatively limited period of time a degree of equilibrium is regained.

There are a number of people, though, who for a variety of reasons, experience prolonged and intense feelings of anxiety that they cannot escape. This may be because of difficulties in coping, extreme fears of specific objects or of overwhelming feelings of anxiety from within. For such people the continual experience of anxiety is extremely distressing and draining.

Family life and activities of everyday living may be severely disrupted by the sufferer's agitation, intense dread and physical complaints. Very heavy demands may be placed upon the support network as those around the sufferer try to cope with the person. In particular the person's demands for continuous, yet ineffectual, reassurance and their clinging and demanding behaviour may prove exhausting.

Within the immediate network of the sufferer and their family the anxiety may be vaguely conceptualized as "nerves" or as to the person being "highly strung". Depending upon their resolve and perception the anxious behaviour may be accommodated to quite extreme degrees. In some ways, the allowances made, the practical help given and changes in expectations may even, unwittingly, reinforce the anxious person's behaviour. Over time, fairly significant changes may evolve within the pattern of relationships that reaffirm the person's anxious "identity" and minimize the risk of exposure to feared situations. However, some of those in close relationships with the sufferer may become increasingly intolerant and make demands that the person "snap out of" or "pull themselves together". To them the high levels of anxiety and phobic fears seem exaggerated and incomprehensible. Over time these difficulties can generate further problems and a deterioration in close personal relationships.

The person's anxieties may fluctuate over time or remain relatively unchanged. For some people there is a slow improvement and even spontaneous recovery.

Approaches may be made to the person's GP for symptomatic relief from the distressing physical effects of prolonged anxiety, e.g. malaise, insomnia, gastrointestinal upsets, headaches and other pains. Often, the sufferer repeatedly attends the surgery with a succession of ever-changing anxiety-related physical problems. The GP may attempt to treat these presenting symptoms or may recognize the underlying distress.

It is significant that there has been a rapid growth in the number of publications, audio-visual resource materials and support groups available for people with anxiety-related problems.

Initially, the person and their family can be helped considerably in coping with anxiety by:

1. Accurate information about anxiety and its effects.
2. Involvement in the care and treatment process.
3. Reassurance that effective intervention is possible.
4. The opportunity to talk freely about their problems.
5. The address of a local contact support group.
6. Developing the person's and family's coping skills.
7. Reviewing their life-style and expectations to promote their mental health.

Community care

Most people with anxiety do not approach community mental health services. They attempt in their own way to deal with the problems they experience. In clinical practice the majority of those with anxiety can be treated successfully and cared for at home. This will depend upon the support of the family, the severity of the symptoms and the skills and resources available within the community mental health team. The aims of community care are:

1. To support the person and their family.
2. To minimize the distress experienced.
3. To implement community-based treatment and care programmes.

The services available include:

1. The community mental health centre – with community psychiatric nurses, social workers, psychologists, occupational therapists and consultant psychiatrists working as a team to offer skills-based therapeutic interventions.
2. General practitioners.
3. Voluntary agencies – MIND, Open Door, Citizens' Advice Bureaux, Phobics Society, Tranx Release, Tranquillizer Withdrawal Support, contact and support groups for sufferers and relatives.
4. DHSS – benefits, allowances and grants as currently available to individuals and their families.
5. Out-patient clinics and day hospitals.

Residential care

The reasons for admission to a residential facility for care and treatment include:

1. Lack of support in the community.
2. Personal and family exhaustion.
3. The need to remove the person from an environment that is actively reinforcing the anxiety and making excessive demands.
4. Detailed assessment and the need for specific types of therapy. In relation to anxiety, it may also be necessary to undertake specific physiological investigations to exclude possible physical causes.

Treatment Interventions

Psychotherapeutic methods

1. *Skilled nursing care*: one of the most important therapeutic factors.
2. *Individual counselling and psychotherapy*: to increase insight, promote self-esteem and to release repressed emotion. To develop coping skills.
3. *Group therapy*: to increase insight and self-awareness, to share personal experiences and provide opportunities for social learning.
4. *Family or couples therapy*: to enable couples or families to be more supportive and to communicate more effectively. To help the family find ways of coping with stress and to adopt a more healthy life-style.

Behavioural approaches

A wide range of potential interventions may be used that aim to enable the client to:

- control their anxiety and phobic reactions;
- develop their social and physical skills;
- increase their self-awareness, self-esteem and self-confidence.

In combination with other approaches, they are probably the most effective therapeutic interventions for anxiety-related problems. The specific therapeutic programme will depend upon the history and nature of the client's problems and the therapist's skills.

Progressive relaxation

To learn to control anxiety and tension. Initially, the client is given an explanation of the relationship between their perception of stress-inducing situations and their physiological reactions. The client is introduced to the therapeutic approach and is given positive hope that they can re-learn non-anxious responses and the skills of relaxation.

In a quiet and distraction-free environment the client is made comfortable, either lying or sitting, and is given detailed instruction on specific relaxation skills and techniques. These may be focussed upon their body musculature, breathing cycle or thought processes.

Deep muscle relaxation

The client is asked to clear their mind of worries and to focus on the exercises. There is no rush and the person is asked to keep as calm as possible. Starting with one part of the body the person is asked to gently tense their muscles and to hold for a number of seconds. During this time they are asked to focus on the physical feelings of tension associated with that part of the body. From this awareness the person is then asked to slowly relax this part of the body and this time to focus upon the contrasting feelings of relaxation. They are then asked to compare the two feelings of tension and relaxation. With repeated practice and focussing the person is taught to discriminate between these two muscle states.

This process is repeated for each muscle group of the body until the client is able to consciously relax themselves. This will require the client to practice these exercises daily until these new skills become habitual. A complete relaxation cycle may require some 20–30 minutes.

During relaxation, the therapist may give a commentary to the client themselves or may use a specially prepared audio-tape. Such tapes are now widely available commercially. The tone of voice used is soft and contains detailed instructions on a relaxation programme. Clients can take these tapes home for use. Alternatively, detailed written guidelines may be given to clients.

The presence of a therapist is useful in both providing feedback to the client and in answering specific questions.

The use of "biofeedback" is also helpful in relaxation programmes. Electronic monitoring devices are available that are able to give visual or auditory feedback to the client on an aspect of their physical response to stress. The device may monitor the client's pulse rate, blood pressure, muscle tension, palmar sweat, skin conductance and resistance. Following explanation of the role of the machine in therapy the client is given a demonstration on themselves of the differing visual or auditory signal associated with both tension and relaxation. Using the device to give external feedback on their relative state of relaxation, in association with internal feedback from their nervous system, the client is encouraged to practice and discriminate between tension and relaxation. "Biofeedback" used in this way may be used as part of a relaxation programme or form an integral aspect of the therapy.

Breathing exercises

As with muscular relaxation, the client is instructed on the relationship between respiration and tension. Typically, anxiety is associated with rapid and shallow breathing patterns and relaxation with deep and slow, rhythmic breaths. The breathing exercises may be integrated within an overall programme of relaxation or may be taught as specific techniques to the client. There is a wide range of potential breathing exercises developed from clinical practice or adapted from yoga and other long-established practices.

The client needs to be comfortable in a quiet and interruption-free environment. The role of the therapist is to instruct the client in the specific technique, their uses and to give feedback to the client. Audio-tapes and written material may be used to supplement therapy and for the client to use at home. The exercises are practised until the client is proficient and is able to induce a relaxed state as required. Some exercises used are:

1. *Abdominal breathing*. Lying on their back, the client is instructed to rest their hands over their abdomen. They are asked to take a deep inhalation with the abdomen expanding outwards. This fully inflates the lungs and the hands will be pushed upwards. Steady exhalation reverses this process and the person is aware of their hands returning to their previous position. This cycle is repeated a number of times. The aim of this exercise is to increase the client's awareness of the physical feelings associated with deep and relaxed breathing.
2. *Breath holding*. From a comfortable posture the client is instructed to inhale deeply and to hold their breath for a number of seconds. They are then instructed to exhale and to focus on the physical sensations of tension release associated with this.
3. *Rhythmic breathing*. The client is asked to regulate their breathing in a steady and rhythmic way. As they do this they are asked to clear their mind and focus on the sensations associated with respiration. Specific words or numbers may be associated with both inhalation and expiration in order to regulate the breathing. Slow and rhythmic deep breathing has a calming effect and begins to demonstrate to the client, like other exercises, that they can begin to take control of their responses.

Whichever approach is used to teach relaxation, it is important that the client actively uses the skills and is able to integrate them into their everyday life.

Systematic desensitization

Interviewing techniques, rating scales and other assessment methods are used to help the person identify anxiety-provoking situations. They may also be asked to keep a detailed diary of their everyday experience of anxiety – situation, time, place, intensity of reaction, physical feelings, thoughts and behaviour. From this information a hierarchy of anxiety-provoking situations is identified, both imagined and real, as they affect that person.

Parallel to this the person is instructed in, and encouraged to develop, the skills of relaxation. When they are competent at this the therapy can then move on to deal with their specific anxieties.

The person is then presented with the least anxiety-provoking situation that they have identified. This may be a real-life situation or one in which they have to create a vivid and realistic image in their mind. Initially, they may find themselves tensing upon this exposure to an anxiety-inducing stimulus. However, at the same time they are encouraged to practice incompatible relaxation responses. This sequence is repeated until the person is able to confront the situation without reacting anxiously and to actively relax.

When the person has successfully mastered the least anxiety-provoking situation, they then progress to the next most anxiety-inducing situation. A similar sequence of exposure to stressor and practising relaxation is repeated until the person is comfortable with that situation. The full hierarchy of anxiety-provoking situations is worked through until the person has mastered their fears. This method of approach is successful in about 50% of clients.

Social skills and assertiveness training

Many anxious people find social situations stressful or have specific social fears. The objectives of social skills and assertiveness training are to:

- develop the person's social competence;
- enhance the person's self-esteem and confidence;
- raise the person's sense of control and mastery.
  (See also Unit 5.4.)

Modelling

The client watches the therapist model the desired behaviour and not react anxiously to objects or situations that the client finds frightening. The client is then encouraged to carry out the same behaviour and imitate the therapist – "participant modelling".

Flooding

The client agrees to prolonged exposure to situations that they find anxiety-provoking. After a short period of time the overwhelming feeling of anxiety subsides and the person also realizes that the previously feared consequences have not happened. It may require several repeated exposures for the person to overcome their fears and to regain control of their behaviour in this way.

Self-regulation and self-reinforcement procedures

All forms of therapy require the active participation of the client. If the person is given clear instructions they will be able to actively complete various homework assignments in relation to their therapeutic programme. It is possible to teach clients specific techniques that they can use as self-administered therapy and to complement therapist-initiated interventions.

Self-monitoring is one approach in which the person keeps a detailed record of the frequency, intensity and duration of their anxiety. Date, time, duration, situation, intensity, physical feelings, thoughts and behaviour may all be recorded.

Focussing on the anxiety helps to increase the client's awareness and, paradoxically, to reduce the effects of anxiety. Participation also helps to raise self-esteem and to promote cooperation. The data collected also provide useful information for the therapist.

Cue cards can be prepared and used as a self-instructional aid to reinforce positive behaviour and cognitions. Other applicable techniques can be taught to clients and their families.

Other therapeutic approaches

Problem-solving techniques

Many anxious people experience stress and anxiety due to difficulties in decision making and problem solving. These deficits further add to the experience of stress and create feelings of helplessness, low self-esteem and of being overwhelmed. Some people can be helped considerably from training in improved decision-making and problem-solving skills. Briefly, some of the stages include:

1. Assessing current worries – intensity, frequency, validity.
2. Defining specific problems – to turn vague worries into manageable problems.
3. Identifying which problems are or are not amenable to alteration or solution.
4. Determining the priority of the problems.
5. Generating as many solutions as possible to each problem, i.e. "brainstorming".
6. Evaluating the potential solutions in terms of the likely outcomes – consequences, practicality, likelihood of success, personal acceptability.
7. Selecting the most suitable solutions and compiling an action plan with desired outcomes and a timetable.
8. Initiating the action plan.
9. Evaluating the outcomes – modifying existing solutions, adopting new approaches if solutions are not successful.

Cognitive therapy

Many anxious people develop a perceptual set and belief system that actively generates and maintains their anxiety. Negative expectations – "this is going to be awful" – and disabling self-talk – "I can't do it" – undermine confidence and create unnecessary stress.

The objectives of cognitive therapy are to change these dysfunctional and automatic negative thoughts and to help the client develop more positive thought processes and expectations. This can then help to raise self-esteem and to increase a person's sense of mastery and control.

Cognitive approaches may be used in association with relaxation techniques to help the client overcome specific anxieties and fears. Relaxation skills may be taught that are associated with a specific cue word or to a calming scene. With practice, recall of the cue word or imagining the calm scene can promote relaxation. This may also be used as an approach to systematic desensitization when cognitive rehearsal of feared situations is used with a relaxing cue word or image. Ultimately, the person is able to visualize themself-coping competently with previously stressful situations.

Rational emotive therapy (RET)

Rational emotive therapy is another approach that is used to modify a person's perceptual set and belief system. In this approach, many people are viewed as having irrational thoughts and beliefs that create difficulties for them. Frequently, the irrational thoughts are reinforced by the negative outcomes that the person predicted for themself – "I just know this is going to be awful." This generates feelings of stress and anxiety before the situation occurs, yet the person associates the event rather than their thoughts as creating the tension.

The therapist helps the client to identify their irrational thoughts and to re-evaluate the validity of such assumptions. Clients are assisted to discriminate between rational and irrational thinking and to base their assumptions on a more sound basis.

Occupational therapy, art therapy and psycho drama

These are used to help develop emotional expression, to release feelings as diversional activities, and to promote insight.

Recreational and social activities

These are used to provide diversional activities, meet social needs, to provide positively reinforcing situations and opportunities to practice social skills.

Herbal remedies

To reduce anxiety and to help overcome withdrawal symptoms.

Voluntary organizations

MIND, Open Door, Tranx Release, selfhelp and support groups.

Reviewing life-style

1. Diet – to promote healthy nutrition and reduce caffeine intake.
2. Promoting physical health – exercise, regulating weight.
3. Reducing excessive cigarette smoking and intake of alcohol.
4. Reviewing self-imposed demands.
5. Increasing opportunities for relaxation in daily life.
6. Developing new interests for stress-reducing potential – new hobbies, meditation, yoga, shiatsu, t'ai chi ch'uan, massage, reflexology.

Physical Treatment Methods for Anxiety

Chemotherapy

1. Anxiolytics/minor tranquillizers — for short-term use only:

- Chlordiazepoxide (Librium),
- Diazepam (Valium),
- Lorazepam (Ativan).

2. Night sedation if insomnia is present:

- Nitrazepam (Mogodon).

Tranquillizer dependency (Benzodiazepine dependency)

Minor tranquillizers and night sedation are useful in providing short-term relief from the immediate effects of anxiety. Clinically, anxiolytics are only effective for the first few months and the use of night sedation becomes counterproductive after 3–12 days. However, there is growing concern about their use in clinical practice.

Statistics indicate a pattern of prescription and usage that far exceeds known safety levels. In the UK, 250 000 people have been taking tranquillizers for more than 1 year. A total of 23% of the adult population have taken tranquillizers at some time, i.e. approximately 10 million people, and 1 in 40 adults are taking tranquillizers every day of the year. Twice as many women are taking tranquillizers than men – 1 in 5 women and 1 in 10 men take tranquillizers each year. One-third of those taking tranquillizers have been taking them for more than the recommended limit of 4 months, i.e. about 3.5 million people.

Concern has grown due to:

1. The sheer number of prescriptions written each year for tranquillizers. They form one of the largest groups of drugs used in the NHS and many millions of prescriptions are written for them annually.
2. The inappropriate use of tranquillizers for people with chronic social and life problems.
3. Evidence of physical pathology from their long-term use for the user and of foetal damage in pregnancy.
4. The development of dependency upon tranquillizers by clients who experience psychological and physical withdrawal symptoms when they attempt to stop taking them.

The warning signs of an increased risk of dependency include:

1. Taking minor tranquillizers for more than 4 months.
2. An increased dosage due to loss of initial effect.
3. A change of brand due to reduced effectiveness of original medication.

Currently, the large numbers of people taking minor tranquillizers would indicate that it is potentially one of the world's major drug problems. Rather than repeated prescriptions being given for chronic anxiety, the initial therapeutic effect of tranquillizers needs to be used to facilitate longer-term psychotherapeutic interventions. Ultimately, the person needs to learn to live without their pills, learn to relax and to develop more appropriate stress management strategies.

Unit Instructions

When you have researched the suggested references, have mastered the Unit Objectives and successfully answered the Self-assessment Questions, proceed with the Unit Written Test.

Suggested References

Armstrong, P. (1987). Off the hook. *Nursing Times*, 11 November, Vol. 83, No. 45, pp. 34–35.

Bailey, R. D. (1985). *Coping with Stress in Caring*. Blackwell Scientific, Oxford.

Beech, H. R., Burns, L. E. and Sheffield, B. F. (1982). *A Behavioural Approach to the Management of Stress*. John Wiley, Chichester.

Blenkinsop, J. (1986). There came a big spider. . . *Nursing Times*, 8 January, Vol. 82, No. 2, pp. 28–30.

Bloch, S. (Ed.) (1986). *An Introduction to the Psychotherapies*, 2nd edition. Oxford Publications, Oxford.

Bolton, R. (1979). *People Skills*. Prentice-Hall, New York.

Bond, M. (1982). *The Art of Relaxation. Nursing Mirror*, October, Vol. 155, No. 14, pp. 29–31.

Bond, M. (1986). *Stress and Self-Awareness: A Guide for Nurses*. Heinemann Nursing, London.

Coleman, V. (1985). *Life Without Tranquillizers*. Piatkus, London.

Dickson, A. (1982). *A Woman in Your Own Right*. Quartet, London.

Dryden, W. (1984). *Rational-Emotive Therapy: Fundamentals and Innovations*. Croom Helm, London.

Dryden, W. and Golden, W. L. (1986). *Cognitive Behavioural Approaches to Psychotherapy*. Harper and Row, London.

Gillies, D. and Lader, M. (1986). *Guide to the Use of Psychotropic Drugs*. Churchill Livingstone, Edinburgh.

Goodwin, D. W. (1983). *Phobias: The Facts*. Oxford University Publications, Oxford.

Haddon, D. (1984). *Women and Tranquillizers*. Sheldon Press, London.

Harrison, A. (1986). Therapeutic Touch. Getting the massage. *Nursing Times*, November, 26, Vol. 82, No. 48, pp. 34–35.

Hughes, B. and Boothroyd, R. (1985). *Fight or Flight?* Faber and Faber, London.

Hughes, J. (1986). *An Outline of Modern Psychiatry*, 2nd edition. John Wiley, New York.

Irving, S. (1983). *Basic Psychiatric Nursing*, 3rd edition. W. B. Saunders, Philadelphia.

Jupp, H. and Dudley, M. (1984). Group cognitive/anxiety management. *Journal of Advanced Nursing*, Vol. 9, pp. 573–580.

Kowalski, R. (1987). *Over the top*. Avalon Press/Winslow Press, Bristol/Bicester.

Lacey, R. and Woodward, S. (1985). *That's Life!: Survey on Tranquillisers*. BBC Publications/MIND, London.

Liberman, R. P., King, L. W., Derisi, W. J. and McCann, M. (1975). *Personal Effectiveness*. Research Press, Champaign, Illinois.

Lim, D. (1985). Imprisoned by fear. *Nursing Mirror*, 24 July, Vol. 161, No. 4, pp. 18–19.

Lyttle, J. (1986). *Mental Disorder*. Baillière Tindall, London and San Diego.

Meichenbaum, D. (1979). *Cognitive Behaviour Modification*. Plenum, New York.

Mitchell, R. (1982). *Phobias*. Penguin, Harmondsworth.

Moores, A. (1987). Frightened of fear. *Nursing Times*, 2 April, Vol. 83, No. 13, pp. 34–38.

Murdoch, W. and Newton, A. (1985). High anxiety. *Nursing Times*, 30 January, Vol. 81, No. 5, pp. 26–28.

North, N. (1985). Phobias – the misunderstood fear. *Nursing Times*, 2 January, Vol. 81, No. 1, pp. 24–25.

Orr, R. (1984). The cost of blessed tranquillity. *Nursing Times*, 5 September, Vol. 80, No. 36, pp. 48–50.

Paul, N. (1985). *The Right To Be You*. Chartwell-Bratt, Bromley.

Priestley, P., McGuire, J., Flegg, D., Hemsley, V. and Welham, D. (1978). *Social Skills and Personal Problem Solving*. Tavistock, London.

Robinson, L. (1983). *Psychiatric Nursing as a Human Experience*, 3rd edition. W. B. Saunders, Philadelphia.

Silverstone, T. and Turner, P. (1982). *Drug Treatment in Psychiatry*. Routledge and Kegan Paul, London.

Snaith, P. (1981). *Clinical Neurosis,* Oxford University Press, Oxford.

Trethowan, W. and Sims, A. (1983). *Psychiatry*, 5th edition. Baillière Tindall, London and San Diego.

Self-assessment Questions

SAQ 5. List five ways in which severe anxiety can adversely affect the quality of personal and family life.

SAQ 6. Describe the sequence of a session designed to help a person learn deep muscle relaxation.

SAQ 7. Outline how systematic desensitization could be used to help a client overcome a fear of dogs.

SAQ 8. Identify three factors that may indicate a risk of "tranquillizer dependency".

Unit 6.2: Written Test

Jennifer Robinson, aged 25, has been taking anxiolytic medication for 6 months for moderate anxiety. She appears nervous and to be generally lacking in confidence. She has requested to see you as she has recently seen a television documentary about "benzodiazepine dependency", and wishes to discuss other therapeutic options for helping her resolve her anxiety. She has asked for an outline of alternative therapeutic approaches to anxiety, other than medication, in order to make an informed choice.

Describe briefly the range of therapeutic interventions that can be discussed with Jennifer and their role in the treatment of anxiety.

Nursing Care of the Anxious Person

Unit Objectives

At the end of this Unit the learner should be able to:

1. Identify the nursing care needs of the person with anxiety-related problems.
2. Plan an individualized care programme.
3. Select appropriate nursing care interventions for the person's needs.
4. Describe possible evaluation criteria for specific needs.

Mental Health Nursing Care

Each person's care needs are unique and have to be assessed individually. A range of potential care needs have been selected to illustrate the problems that the anxious person may experience and the potential nursing interventions that may help them. For the person with anxiety-related problems these may include the needs to:

A. Feel secure and free from threat.
B. Experience relief from physical stress and tension.
C. Freedom from persistent anxious thoughts.
D. Overcome their fear of specific situations.
E. Facilitate the development of the person's and family's coping skills.

A. Feel Secure and Free From Threat

Associated problems/personal difficulties

Person may feel insecure and threatened as a result of:

1. Continual apprehension and sense of dread about their future.
2. An inability to resist intrusive anxious thoughts and feelings.
3. Feelings of guilt and loss of self-esteem.

4. Anticipation of specific fear-inducing situations or objects.
5. Continual feelings of tension and physical discomfort.
6. Inadequate knowledge of their care and treatment programme.

Assessment

1. Person's description of their anxieties and worries.
2. Comments made by relatives and friends.
3. Nurse's observations of the person's:

   (a) Response to questions about their anxieties.
   (b) Understanding: questions asked and statements made in relation to their health care needs and treatment programme.
   (c) Emotions expressed: edginess, irritability, anxiety, tearfulness, dread.
   (d) Concerns expressed: apprehension, dread of the future, negative self-statements, specific fears.
   (e) Response to specific fear-inducing situations or objects.
   (f) Non-verbal behaviour indicating anxiety: posture, gestures, bodily movements, tremor, rigidity, eye movements, restlessness, pacing, fidgeting, fiddling, picking, excessive smoking.
   (g) Verbal pattern: rate, tone of voice, pitch, speech errors, hesitation, thought blocking, overtalkativeness.
   (h) Physiological responses: rate of respiration, perspiration, frequency of micturation, thirst, gastrointestinal upsets, palpitations.

4. Scores and responses to anxiety-related questionnaires and rating scales.
5. Support network available to the person – relationships with key people.
6. Identification of potential stressors in the person's current life experiences and life-style.

Desired outcomes

1. Person is more relaxed and feels free from threat.
2. Person and family's understanding of their health care needs are increased.

Nursing intervention	Rationale
1. Initiate a therapeutic relationship. Spend time with them. Be available and approachable.	Interventions more likely to be successful in an atmosphere of trust and cooperation. Also shows sense of worth and acceptance which helps to increase feelings of security and

Nursing intervention   *Rationale*

Demonstrate active listening. Involve person in the care planning process. Ensure non-judgemental and non-critical approach

safety. Being non-judgemental helps a person to deal with their guilt. Reduces feelings of anxiety and threat

2. Provide clear and understandable information about their treatment, health care and the roles of different health care workers. Encourage questions. Ask for feedback on their understanding. Clarify any misunderstandings

A lot of anxiety is associated with fear of the unknown. People have a right to information about their health care. The nurse is in an ideal position to use this process to facilitate the development of the person's understanding about their health care needs

3. Enlist the person's cooperation in the planning of their health care. Promote their autonomy and self-esteem

People are more likely to cooperate if they are well-informed and involved in the decision-making process. It also increases feelings of personal control

4. Explain all actions in advance

Interventions do not then come as an anxiety-provoking surprise. Promotes feelings of trust in carer.

5. Refrain from unnecessary procedures and interventions if person is extremely agitated

Unnecessary interventions would add to feelings of agitation. Wait till person is calmer and more receptive

6. Ensure that significant personal items are available

Familiar objects help to increase feelings of security

7. Provide support and reassurance to relatives and carers

Anxiety in relatives will communicate itself to person. Reassurance in carers also communicates positively to person

8. Encourage the person to talk about their stressful feelings. Encourage them to express their feelings in a more appropriate way. Provide feedback

Ventilating their feelings in this way may reduce some of the necessity for communicating through their anxiety. Provides an opportunity for health education in the appropriate expression of emotional stress. Promotes insight

Nursing intervention	*Rationale*
to the person on their behaviour and use it as a learning situation	
9. Role model calm behaviour. Adopt a non-threatening, open posture and tone of voice	Can have a powerful calming effect as people tend to be subconsciously influenced by the behaviour of those they are with and to "reflect" their behaviour. Behaving calmly then helps to facilitate less anxious thoughts
10. Use touch where appropriate	Therapeutic touch can have a very powerful calming influence and promote feelings of security and reassurance. Needs to be used with discretion because people have very different touch thresholds
11. Approach unhurriedly. Demonstrate calmness. Do not rush the person. Be aware of your own reactions and experience of stress. Be patient and aware of your own feelings of frustration in dealing with the person. Take periodic breaks if possible	Anxiety in the carer communicates itself to the person. Caring can be a stressful experience at times. This may unconsciously influence your interactions with others. The person may be very demanding and resistant. Find ways of coping with your own stress
12. Arrange for own clinical supervision	Supervision is an effective way of providing support and of personal development
13. Facilitate the development of the person's ability to communicate and relate to others	Helps the person to express and thereby release feelings of anxiety and tension
14. Encourage appropriate diversional, recreational and social activities	Helps to avoid boredom and to divert the person's thoughts away from stressful topics. Physical activity is also a beneficial channel for stress

Evaluation

1. Person demonstrates relaxed verbal and non-verbal behaviour.
2. Person demonstrates trust in their care and treatment.
3. Person makes positive statements about their future.

B. Experience Relief from Physical Stress and Tension

Associated problems/personal difficulties

Person may be experiencing continual stress and tension that:

1. Causes extreme physical discomfort and malaise.
2. May precipitate distressing physical responses to anxiety.
3. Interferes with the person's ability to meet their physical needs.
4. Reinforces their sense of apprehension and dread.
5. Interferes with their ability to participate in activities of daily life.

Assessment

1. Person's description of their physical stress and tension.
2. Comments made by relatives and friends.
3. Nurse's observations of the person's:

   (a) Response to questioning about their physical discomfort.
   (b) Physiological responses: rate of respiration, perspiration, frequency of micturation, thirst, gastrointestinal upsets, palpitations, headaches and other anxiety-related physical symptoms.
   (c) Physical need deficits: dietary, sleep, rest, comfort, hygiene.
   (d) Non-verbal behaviour: restlessness, agitation, pacing, hand movements, tremor, rigidity, clumsiness, co-ordination.

4. Responses to anxiety related questionnaires and rating scales.

Desired outcomes

1. Person experiences relief from physical stress and tension.
2. Person able to meet their physical needs.

Nursing intervention	Rationale
1. Initiate a therapeutic relationship. Spend time with them. Be	Interventions more likely to be successful in an atmosphere of trust and cooperation

Nursing intervention	*Rationale*
available and approachable. Ensure a non-judgemental and non-critical approach	
2. Advise the person on the importance of meeting physical needs and their role in mental health. Specify basic physical requirements with person and family. Negotiate a programme to meet physical needs	Person may not be aware of these needs or their role in health promotion. Prolonged anxiety may have disrupted normal patterns of meeting physical needs. Reintroducing a pattern helps to structure the person's day and to regain a sense of control
3. Advise on the importance of a regular healthy diet – fresh food, high fibre. Monitor nutritional intake. Monitor elimination. Monitor weight	Irregular food intake is stressful and may contribute to gastrointestinal problems, nausea, constipation, diarrhoea. Fresh and wholesome food is less likely to have artificial additives, which have been associated with behavioural disturbances and food allergies affecting mental health.
4. Advise on the need to reduce intake of coffee and of reducing cigarette smoking	Potential stressors. Caffeine and nicotine are both stimulants and can lead to dependency
5. Ensure that hygiene needs are met. Encourage use of warm baths for relaxation	Apart from cleanliness, hygiene also promotes self-esteem and sense of well-being. Makes person feel calmer
6. Reinforce compliance with programme to promote physical needs	Programme compliance is necessary to reach desired health care objectives
7. Encourage the person to rest or relax if they appear to be under stress. Provide feedback on their behaviour	Person may not be aware of the effect of anxiety on their behaviour
8. Assess person's need for sleep and rest. Identify person's preferred rest and sleep patterns. Advise person on physiological	Many people with insomnia under-report the actual amount of sleep that they actually have. Many people have unrealistic expectations of the total amount of sleep that they need and define themselves as "insomniacs"

Nursing intervention	*Rationale*
needs and differences for sleep. Explore with person options for meeting needs for rest	
9. Advise person on approaches to improve sleeping: • Ensure bed is comfortable, e.g. firm mattress, warm, quiet • Choose activities before bedtime that facilitate sleep, e.g. mild exercise, warm bath • Avoid stimulants at bedtime, e.g. tea, coffee • Do not go to bed too soon or too long after a meal because digestion and hunger both disrupt sleep	There may be simple environmental and behavioural changes that can enhance sleep
• Only use bed for sleeping, not for reading, watching TV or eating	Need to associate bed only with sleep, not other wakeful activities.
• Get up if person has not fallen asleep within 10 minutes, leave bedroom and do something in another room for a short while, return to bed and repeat this cycle, as necessary, until asleep	Need to learn to associate bed with falling asleep quickly
• Practice relaxation exercises while in bed and unable to sleep • Avoid worrying about not being able to sleep	Reinforces relaxation techniques. Likely also to foster sleep
• Set the alarm and get up at same time each day irrespective of actual sleep	Helps to re-establish a rhythm

Nursing intervention	Rationale
• Do not nap during the day	Reduces the need for sleep at night-time. Contibutes to insomnia
10. Role model calm behaviour. Approach unhurriedly. Do not rush or make sudden movements	Can have a powerful calming effect as people tend to be subconsciously influenced by the behaviour of those around them and to "mirror" this behaviour
11. Use touch where appropriate. Massage person's neck and shoulders. Teach the skills of facial and temple massage to the person and family	Touch can have a very potent effect in reducing tension. Touch and massage need to be used in a context where both the nurse and person are comfortable with this approach. Basic massage skills can be taught to the person and family, both as an aid to reducing stress and a mutually enjoyable activity
12. Recommend methods for reducing sensory stimulation. Recommend periods of quiet	Person's environment may be a source of stress. May have adapted to quite stressful stimuli, e.g. TV, records on all the time, etc.
13. Explain the relationship between stress and the physiological responses of anxiety. Provide appropriate resource material, e.g. diagrams, books, pamphlets, video. Check on person's understanding. Clarify any misunderstandings or misconceptions	Many people are unaware or have a confused idea on anxiety and body physiology. This forms the basis of providing a programme of health education that offers a longer-term strategy for dealing with anxiety in the person's life
14. Reassure the person that they can regain control of their physiological reactions to stress	Person may feel trapped into a cycle of chronic anxiety and feel helpless about their ability to take action
15. Explain the principles of deep muscular relaxation, breathing exercises, cognitive visualization, and their role in relaxation. Plan a relaxation programme with the	Method chosen will depend upon the client's needs and the skills of the nurse. All approaches may ultimately be used in order to provide the person with a comprehensive range of relaxation strategies. Person will need support and guidance in order to develop effective relaxation skills

Nursing intervention	*Rationale*
person using appropriate approach. Give clear instructions and guidance. Arrange and advise on suitable environmental conitions. Demonstrate and give clear instructions on the chosen approach to relaxation	
16. Provide guidance on implementation of programme. Give positive reinforcement for compliance with programme	Promotes compliance and rewards progress
17. Emphasize the importance of recognizing internal tension and external stressors. Encourage the discrimination between feelings of tension and relaxation	Helps the person to increase their insight and to identify potential stressors in their environment
18. Advise on the need to practice relaxation exercises regularly in order to develop and maintain these skills. Assist the person to identify opportunities for relaxation in their everyday life	To be effective and lasting the relaxation has to be integrated into everyday life and generalized to a number of situations
19. Inform person of side-effects of anxiolytic medication	Person may confuse side-effects with physical effects of stress
20. Observe for side-effects of anxiolytic medication	Certain side-effects may add to physical discomfort and personal stress
21. Encourage participation in appropriate diversional, recreational and social activities	Diverts thoughts away from anxious preoccupations. Also relaxing and physical activity is a beneficial channel for stress
22. Explore with the person the potential of	There may be a wide range of stress-reducing activities that the person has

Nursing intervention	Rationale
other activities to reduce stress and tension	never considered. These may have physical benefits in reducing tension and also in creating new interests, e.g. yoga, massage, reflexology

Evaluation

1. Person confirms and demonstrates reduced influence from the physical effects of anxiety.
2. Person is able to demonstrate and utilize relaxation skills.
3. Posture and non-verbal communication indicate personal calmness.

C. Freedom from Persistent Anxious Thoughts

Associated problems/personal difficulties

A person with anxiety-related problems may experience difficulties in relation to:

1. Constant preoccupation with anxious thoughts.
2. Emotional distress.
3. A continual sense of dread and foreboding.
4. Loss of self-esteem and self-confidence.
5. Difficulty in concentrating on other activities.
6. A cognitive framework that reinforces anxiety biased perceptions.

Assessment

1. Person's description of their anxious thoughts.
2. Information from relatives and friends.
3. Nurse's observations of the effects of anxiety upon the person's:

(a) Communication pattern:

- verbal expression: tone, volume, pitch, rate, errors;
- non-verbal communication: posture, facial expression, eye contact, gestures, hand movements, restlessness, fidgeting.

(b) Thought processes: content of anxious thoughts and preoccupations, interpretation of life and daily events, anxious predictions and anticipations, frequency of anxious thoughts and pattern throughout the day, association of anxious thoughts with external events.

(c) Emotional reaction to anxious thoughts: intensity and duration of emotional distress experienced as a result of anxious thoughts. Effectiveness of coping strategies for anxious thoughts.

4. Psychosocial environment: presence of identifiable eliciting stimuli or triggering cues. Reactions of others to person's anxiety. Potential reinforcers of anxious behaviour and thoughts. Presence of potential stresses in the person's environment and life-style.

Desired outcomes

1. To facilitate opportunities for emotionally positive experiences.
2. To reduce the influence of anxious cognitions on their emotions and behaviour.
3. To experience relief from anxious preoccupations.

Nursing interventions	Rationale
1. Initiate therapeutic relationship. Demonstrate active listening	Interventions more likely to succeed in an atmosphere of trust and cooperation
2. Spend time with them. Be available and approachable. Ensure non-judgemental and non-critical approach	To minimize distress and to create the potential for emotional change
3. Promote self-esteem	Improving self-esteem helps to raise their personal confidence and to influence their perceptions positively
4. Promote feelings of security and personal safety (see **A**). Promote relaxation and relief from physical tension (see **B**)	Person is unable to focus on psychological relief from anxiety until they are physically relaxed and feel secure
5. Provide opportunities for the person to express themselves openly and honestly	Helps to relieve tension and to demonstrate acceptance

Nursing interventions	*Rationale*
6. Provide reassurance about potential for positive change and for regaining control of their anxious thoughts and behaviour	Person may feel that their situation is hopeless after their own long-term inability to resist anxiety
7. Do not reinforce anxious behaviour	Person will be alert to cues from carers and sensitive to any negative messages
8. Encourage appropriate diversional activities. Identify activities that the person finds relaxing and provide relief	Diverts attention from anxious preoccupations
9. Utilize drama, art and music to encourage expression of anxious feelings	May provide outlets for the expression of anxious feelings and provide useful therapeutic material
10. Explore person's expectations and self-imposed standards	Many anxious people have very high and unattainable expectations
11. Assist the person to acknowledge the influence of their expectations and personal standards on their emotions. Explore alternative expectations and standards. Help person to develop more attainable expectations and standards. Encourage acceptance of self-limitations	This can create a great pressure on them. The person needs to be helped to reshape their beliefs about themself and to develop more valid and realistic expectations
12. Demonstrate how thoughts about situations influence the person's emotional reactions. Offer alternative non-anxiety-provoking interpretations of their perceptions. Assist the person to identify some positive anticipations	Many anxious people perceive things in a stress-inducing way. They focus selectively on negative aspects, exaggerate and over-generalize. They need to re-frame their perceptions and expectations

Nursing interventions	Rationale
13. Encourage awareness of positive responses from others. Offer hope	These can be used to raise their mood and reduce anxiety. Anxious people tend to focus on negative responses from others
14. Provide appropriate written cue cards that reinforce positive cognitions and non-anxious behaviour. Explain how to use cue cards	Cue cards provide a self-administered therapy that the person can use to regain control of their thoughts and behaviour
15. Teach the person how to keep a log or diary of their anxious thoughts throughout the day	Self-recording promotes insight and helps to reduce the frequency of anxious thoughts. Helps to promote a sense of mastery and self-control. Also provides useful data for the therapist
16. Assist the person to identify specific factors associated with their anxiety	Person may not be aware of the way that environmental factors are influencing their anxiety
17. Encourage the person to modify environmental factors, where possible, that are contributing to anxious thoughts and behaviour	Modification of contributing environmental factors may help to reduce stimuli that elicit anxious thoughts

Evaluation

1. Person appears more relaxed and less distressed.
2. Person able to interpret events in a non-anxious way.
3. Reduction in the frequency of anxiety-related statements.
4. Posture and non-verbal communication indicate personal calmness.

D. Overcome Their Fear of Specific Situations

Associated problems/personal difficulties

Person with anxiety-related problems may have specific difficulties in relation to:

1. Preoccupation with feared situations or objects.
2. Avoidance behaviour in relation to feared situations or objects.
3. Overwhelming fear and panic when confronted with feared situations.
4. Disruption to normal activities of living and relationships.
5. High levels of stress and tension.

Assessment

1. Person's description of specific anxiety-provoking situations.
2. Comments made by relatives and friends.
3. Nurse's observations of the person's:

   (a) Response to questioning about their specific fears.
   (b) Behavioural response to feared situations.
   (c) Emotional response to feared situations, i.e. intensity, duration.
   (d) Cognitions associated with feared situations.
   (e) Scores or responses to rating scales.

4. Detailed description of triggering stimulus:

   (a) What precisely the person fears.
   (b) Frequency of exposure to feared situations.
   (c) Situations in which it occurs.
   (d) Reactions of significant others, i.e. do they reinforce the reaction in any way.
   (e) Outcomes of exposure to feared objects/situations.
   (f) Potential for environmental modification.

Nursing intervention	Rationale
1. Initiate therapeutic relationship. Be available and approachable. Demonstrate active listening	Interventions more likely to be successful in an atmosphere of trust and cooperation
2. Reassurance, acceptance, ensure non-judgemental and non-critical approach. Promote feelings of security (see **A**)	To minimize anxiety and create the conditions for behavioural change. Effective learning can only take place if the person feels secure
3. Role model calm behaviour and communication	Modelling can be a powerful influence for positive behaviour change

Nursing intervention	*Rationale*
4. Negatively reinforce anxious behaviour and cognitions. Positively reinforce confident behaviour	Helps to decrease frequency of anxious behaviour
5. Teach family members the skills of giving reinforcement to non-anxious behaviour	Family members may be inadvertently contributing to the maintenance of anxious behaviour
6. Teach person the skills of progressive relaxation (see **B**)	Person will need to relearn the skills of relaxation in order to cope effectively with anxiety-provoking situations
7. Explain to the person the principles of systematic desensitization	Promotes cooperation and understanding
8. Identify with person significant fear-provoking situations	Person is likely to have a range of situations that cause differing degrees of anxiety and fear
9. Assist person to rank these situations from least to most anxiety provoking	These may be in terms of real or imagined situations. An anxiety ranking schedule or questionnaire may be helpful to achieve this
10. Expose person to least anxiety-provoking situation and at the same time encourage them to commence relaxation. Continue and practice until the person feels able to relax when exposed to least anxiety-provoking situation. Provide positive feedback on person's progress. Progressively work through hierarchy of anxiety-provoking situations. Ensure satisfactory coping at each stage	Systematic desensitization works as a process of gradual re-learning. The principle is for the person to gradually regain control and mastery over previously anxiety-provoking situations. Learning in small stages facilitates success and minimizes opportunities for failure. The physiological responses of relaxation are incompatible with being stressed by anxiety-eliciting stimuli. This also helps the person to develop more positive cognitions towards previously anxiety-provoking situations
11. Provide support when the person is attempting to confront feared situations	Confronting the feared situation is a very stressful experience. The person benefits from recognition and acceptance of this difficulty

Nursing intervention	Rationale
12. Reassure about the non-harmful consequence of confronting feared situations	Person may fear harmful consequences when confronted with feared situations
13. Facilitate the transfer of coping skills to real-life situations	Overcoming phobic anxieties needs to be generalized to the real world if the behaviour is to be maintained
14. Identify situations with the person in which they experience social anxiety or difficulty in relating to others	Social anxieties are a common source of stress or difficulty. They may relate to many aspects of both domestic and work life. Many people with mental health problems are either lacking in social skills or have problems relating to others
15. Explain the principles of assertiveness and social skills training	Social skills and assertiveness training help to develop communication and emotional expression skills (see Unit 3.4)
16. Role play with feedback these situations with the person. Give demonstration and guidance as required. Provide information on the nature of human interaction and the expression of feeling. Provide information on the principles and application of assertiveness skills	Role play provides safe learning opportunities and the ability to develop progressively social skills. In assertiveness and social skills training specific social skills are: • identified and defined; • divided into their constituent elements; • the elements are practised with feedback in role-play until competence is achieved; • the entire skill is practised with feedback until competence is achieved; • the skill is transferred to real life situations
17. Provide feedback on the development of social skills. Give positive reinforcement. Encourage the transfer of newly learned skills to real-life situations	Practice in this way can be a useful stage in regaining behavioural control. Promotes insight and shows that others are concerned for their welfare. Improved social skills also improve self-esteem, confidence and the ability to communicate. Enhances feelings of personal control
18. Reinforce person's self-esteem	Improving self-esteem helps to improve the person's self-image in relationships with others. More likely to relate to others in a confident way
19. Provide opportunities for the person to	Helps to relieve tension and to demonstrate acceptance

Nursing intervention	*Rationale*
express themselves openly and honestly	
20. Encourage the use of appropriate coping mechanisms in relation to anxiety-provoking situations (see **E**). Facilitate the development of emotional and behavioural coping skills/strategies	Need to develop and use effective ways of coping with stress. May be possible to make life-style changes that promote mental health. Limited coping skills increase their potential to react anxiously
21. Encourage acceptance of self-limitations. Encourage honesty in presenting self. Support a realistic assessment of their life circumstances	Person needs to develop a realistic image of themselves
22. Offer feedback on the person's behaviour	Person may not be aware of how others perceive them
23. Explore with the person the effects of their behaviour on their own and their family's life	Person may not be fully aware of how their behaviour is disrupting their life and relationships
24. Offer feedback on the person's behaviour and use it as a learning situation	Person may not be fully aware of how much their anxiety-related behaviour is dominating their life
25. Explore with the person the effects of their behaviour and emotions upon others	Person may not be aware of how their behaviour and emotional reactions affect others
26. Organize experiential exercises (drama, role-play, games) in which the person relates to others in an unstructured way and can express themselves freely	Structured and spontaneous experiential exercises can provide powerful feedback and personal learning opportunities. Specific exercises can be used to promote insight and social skills
27. Encourage social interaction with others. Organize group activities	Social activities can be very rewarding and also provide group dynamics that the person may find therapeutic

Evaluation

1. Person able to confront feared situations without panic.
2. Person able to demonstrate assertive behaviour.
3. Person able to interact with others with confidence.
4. Person demonstrates raised self-esteem and confidence in their verbal and non-verbal communication.

E. Facilitate the Development of the Person's and Family's Coping Skills

Associated problems/personal difficulties

The experience of anxiety-related problems may show that:

1. Existing methods of coping may be counter-productive and maladaptive.
2. Current life-style, expectations and relationships may be potential sources of stress.
3. The family may find it difficult to provide emotional support to the anxious person.
4. The person and their family may lack information about the resources available to help them.
5. There may be feelings of guilt in relation to their problems and asking for help.

Assessment

1. Person and family's perceptions of their current situation.
2. Existing coping methods used and their effectiveness.
3. Support available to the person and family.
4. Accuracy of the knowledge and information given by the person and their family.
5. Statements of guilt and stigma.
6. Awareness of resources available to them.
7. Previous experience, if any, of dealing with similar problems.

Desired outcomes

1. Person and family able to make an informed choice about the resources they require.
2. Person and family able to cope better with life and personal problems.

Nursing intervention	Rationale
1. Initiate therapeutic relationship. Involve person and family in the care and planning process	Interventions more likely to be successful in an atmosphere of trust and cooperation
2. Advise that seeking help and recognition of problems are a positive step towards finding solutions	Many people feel that seeking help is a sign of weakness and failure. Also helps to reduce guilt
3. Encourage questions. Provide accurate information. Identify appropriate health care resources	May have inaccurate knowledge and expectations. Fear of the unknown. Need to know what resources are available to them
4. Advise against early correction of problems	Under stress it is sometimes easier to make short-term adaptations that only store up future problems. It takes time to help the family to work out what is best for them
5. Reassure that there are ways of improving the situation	Family may feel that the situation is hopeless
6. Advise against recrimination and focussing on past problems	Need to focus on the present and future and to deal with anger and guilt in a more productive way
7. Advise on the need for acceptance and mutual support within their relationships	Family needs to come to terms with their situation. They are each other's primary source of support, which will need to be utilized to cope effectively
8. Explain the need to identify and recognize potentially stressful situations. Recommend methods for coping with stress	Mental health problems tend to be long-term in nature. In order to cope effectively, the family needs to be taught ways of making the necessary long-term adjustments
9. Teach methods for achieving relaxation. Teach how to use problem-solving methods for coping with difficulties. Assist	Most of the education needs to be directed towards coping methods. These include the way that the members of the family communicate, their expectations and the way that emotional support is given. Life-style

Nursing intervention	Rationale
the family to learn new coping and communications skills. Encourage the setting of realistic goals and expectations	and relationship changes may be necessary
10. Review occupational/ unemployment stresses. Encourage the development of appropriate work-related coping strategies	Work and unemployment can be major sources of stress. As these encompass such a wide range of life events, it is important that the person learns how to cope with these stresses constructively
11. Encourage the setting of progressive goals in small stages. Advise the family on how to give feedback and support to one another	The re-learning needs to be done in a gradual way in which the family provides the main support and reinforcement
12. Teach the family and person to recognize the limits of their ability to cope and when it is advisable to seek help.	The family should not overburden itself as this can damage relationships and its longer-term ability to cope.
13. Put family in contact with self-help and voluntary groups	Self-help groups are able to offer effective and understanding help.

Evaluation

1. Person and family able to identify their health care needs.
2. Person and family identify and select resources they require.
3. Person and family demonstrate use of improved coping methods.

Unit Instructions

When you have researched the suggested references, have mastered the Unit Objectives and successfully answered the Self-assessment Questions, proceed with the Unit Written Test.

Suggested References

Altschul, A. and McGovern, M. (1985). *Psychiatric Nursing*, 6th edition. Baillière Tindall, London and San Diego.

Barker, P. J. (1982). *Behaviour Therapy Nursing*. Croom Helm, London.

Barker, P. J. (1985). *Patient Assessment in Psychiatric Nursing*. Croom Helm, London.

Bauer, B. and Hill, S. (1986). *Essentials of Mental Health Care Planning and Interventions*. W. B. Saunders, Philadelphia.

Blenkinsop, J. (1986). There came a big spider. . . *Nursing Times*, 8 January, Vol. 82, No. 2, pp. 28–30.

Bond, M. (1986). *Stress and Self-awareness: A Guide for Nurses*. Heinemann Nursing, London.

Campbell, C. (1978). *Nursing Diagnosis and Intervention in Nursing Practice*. John Wiley, New York.

Darcy, P. T. (1985). *Mental Health Nursing Source Book*. Baillière Tindall, London and San Diego.

Dexter, G. and Wash, M. (1986). *Psychiatric Nursing Skills: A Patient-centred Approach*. Croom Helm, London.

French, H. P. (1979). Reassurance: a nursing skill? *Journal of Advanced Nursing*, Vol. 4, No. 6 pp. 627–634.

Harrison, A. (1986). Therapeutic Touch. Getting the massage. *Nursing Times*, 26 November, Vol. 82, No. 48, pp. 34–35.

Hase, S. and Douglas, A. (1986). *Human Dynamics and Nursing*. Churchill Livingstone, Melbourne.

Irving, S. (1983). *Basic Psychiatric Nursing*, 3rd edition. W. B. Saunders, Philadelphia.

Lancaster, J. (1980). *Adult Psychiatric Nursing*. Henry Kimpton, London.

LeMay, A. (1986). The human connection. *Nursing Times*, 19 November, Vol. 82, No. 47, pp. 28–30.

Lim, D. (1985). Imprisoned by fear. *Nursing Mirror*, 24 July, Vol. 161, No. 4, pp. 18–19.

Lyttle, J. (1986). *Mental Disorder*. Baillière Tindall, London and San Diego.

McFarland, G. and Wasli, E. (1986). *Nursing Diagnoses and Process in Psychiatric Mental Health Nursing*. J. P. Lippincott, Philadelphia.

Macphail, D. and McMillan, I. (1983). Fighting phobias. *Nursing Mirror*, Mental Health Forum 8, 17 August, Vol. 157, No. 7, (i)–(ii).

Martin, P. (1987a). *Care of the Mentally Ill*, 2nd edition. Macmillan, London.

Martin, P. (Ed.) (1987b). *Psychiatric Nursing: A Therapeutic Approach*. Macmillan, London.

North, N. (1985). Phobias – the misunderstood fear. *Nursing Times*, 2 January, Vol. 81, No. 1, pp. 24–25.

Pelletier, L. (Ed.) (1987). *Psychiatric Nursing Case Studies, Nursing Diagnoses and Care Plans*. Springhouse Corporation, Springhouse, Pennsylvania.

Robinson, L. (1983). *Psychiatric Nursing as a Human Experience*, 3rd edition. W. B. Saunders, Philadelphia.

Teasdale, K. (1987). Giving reassurance to anxious patients. *The Professional Nurse*, January, Vol. 2, No. 4, pp. 112–113.

Self-assessment Questions

SAQ 9. Describe six nursing interventions that can promote a sense of security in an anxious person.

SAQ 10. Outline six ways in which anxiety can disturb a person's physical comfort.

SAQ 11. List five observations that you would need to make if an anxious person had a specific situational fear.

SAQ 12. Identify four ways in which an anxious person and their family can be helped to improve their coping skills.

Unit 6.3: Written Test

John Anderson, aged 37, has been referred for help for long-term anxiety. He exhibits high levels of distress and agitation while he is being interviewed. He complains of constant worry and of a range of anxiety-related physical problems. His wife has threatened to leave him if he does not seek help, because she is fed up with his clinging behaviour and need for constant reassurance. His work has been suffering and he is not coping well with the increased responsibilities that he has recently been given. From your assessment, you identify that he needs:

- to experience relief from physical stress and tension;
- freedom from persistent anxious thoughts;
- to develop his coping skills;
- to increase his assertiveness.

Describe in detail potential interventions to enable him to meet each of the above needs.

TOPIC 7

Depression

At the end of this Topic the learner should aim to:

1. Describe factors associated with the development of depression.
2. Recognize the effects of depression upon a person.
3. Outline the range of therapeutic interventions available for people who are depressed.
4. Identify the nursing care needs and interventions required for the person who is depressed.

The Nature and Origins of Depression

Unit Objectives

At the end of this Unit the learner should be able to:

1. Identify factors associated with the onset of depression.
2. Outline the categories of depression in clinical practice.
3. Describe the relationship between depression and self-harm.

Depression as a Mental Health Problem

Depression and sadness are common emotional experiences in everyday life. These moods may arise from within, without apparent cause, or be seen as a reaction to disappointment, stress or loss. Despite these unpleasant feelings people are usually able to continue and cope with their daily lives.

Depression as an illness is characterized by a profound mood disturbance in which there is extreme distress, misery and despair. These overwhelming feelings negatively influence a person's thoughts, perceptions, feelings, behaviour and physiology. At its most extreme, the sufferer can believe that life is unbearable and may attempt to injure themselves or to take their own lives.

Depression may be regarded as pathological in terms of:

1. The intensity of the mood disturbance: it is an overwhelming and extreme experience of sadness, grief, hopelessness, despair and misery.
2. The duration of the mood disturbance: if it is long-term and interferes with a person's ability to meet their needs.
3. Onset: when it develops without apparent cause, or it can be seen to follow from a distressing or traumatic life event.
4. Risk: if the person's thoughts, feelings and behaviour indicate a life-threatening potential.

Incidence

Depression is one of the most common mental health problems. In any one year, 3–5% of the population receive treatment for depression. Social surveys indicate that 8–15% of the population experience a period of depression each year.

Aetiological Factors

There appear to be a number of factors which may contribute to the experience of depression. In many people it would appear that an interaction of personal and external events is involved.

Social factors

1. *Relationship problems*: conflict, disharmony, separation, divorce, affairs, loneliness, lack of support, sexual difficulties, insecurity, physical violence, psychological cruelty.
2. *Occupational problems*: work stress, frustration, conflict, insecurity, low occupational status, unemployment.
3. *Home problems*: overcrowding, poor living conditions, stress of child-rearing, isolation from relatives, child physical and sexual abuse, money problems.
4. *Experience of loss*: bereavement, divorce, redundancy, loss of health, loss of social status, grief reactions.
5. *Experience of stress*: frustration, difficulty in meeting demands, inability to cope, unexpected traumatic life events such as assault, rape, burglary, accidents.
6. *Helplessness*: inability to alter or escape adverse life conditions and relationships which leads to feelings of being "trapped" and hopelessness.
7. *Social class*: the evidence is conflicting. Clinically, people from the upper social classes have the highest incidence rates for referral to a psychiatrist. However, community surveys tend to show that people in the lower social classes have the highest incidence of depression. For a variety of reasons they do not seek or are not referred for treatment.

Gender

Women suffer from depression twice as commonly as men. The most vulnerable period for women is from puberty to 45. After the age of 55 the discrepancy narrows. Significant factors in depression in women include:

1. *Marriage*: tends to be detrimental to women's mental health. Married women suffer far more mental ill-health and stress than women who live alone. Conversely, married men have less mental ill-health than single men.
2. *Female role conflicts*: legal, educational and social discrimination against women, lower social and occupational status, sexual double standards and conflicts. Expectations and stress of mothering and working roles.

3. *Emotional expression*: women are brought up to express their feelings and hence their mood states are much more visible.
4. *Medical perceptions*: Tendency by doctors to regard female problems as emotional and neurotic.

Age

The incidence of depression overall increases with age. Reactive depression is more common in younger adults. The incidence of psychotic depression is higher in the middle-aged and elderly.

Biological factors

1. *Genetic*: some evidence for an hereditary association in severe psychotic or endogenous depression and in manic depressive psychoses. None identified for reactive depression.
2. *Side-effects*: certain drugs can cause a depressive-like reaction.
3. *Association of depressive symptoms with certain physical illnesses*: viral infections, Parkinson's disease, Cushing's syndrome.
4. *Hormonal*: post-natal depression, premenstrual tension, menopause, myxoedema (hypothyroidism).
5. *Chronic physical ill-health*: any long-term debilitating illness such as arthritis, heart disease, renal failure, chronic bronchitis, multiple sclerosis, cancer, disability.

Early life experiences

1. *Parental role models*: tendency to react depressively to life events, pessimistic, defeatist viewpoint.
2. *Separation anxiety*: main caring figure periodically absent with damaging emotional consequences for the child.
3. *Maternal deprivation*: lack of a caring parent in early life is associated with later problems of insecurity, low self-esteem and difficulty in forming relationships.
4. *Negative life events*: prolonged childhood illness, educational difficulties, conflict in the home, child physical and sexual abuse.

Cognition and thought processes

Some people appear to develop a predominantly negative perceptual set about themselves, the world and the future. Automatic negative thoughts and other dysfunctional thought processes render them prone to guilt, low self-esteem and self-defeating attitudes. Perceiving and interpreting life events in this way engenders depressive emotional reactions of despair, hopelessness and helplessness.

Loss of personal and social reinforcement

The behavioural viewpoint of depression is based upon the principle that in order to maintain our mental health we require positive reinforcement from our life experiences and relationships. People become depressed when there is:

1. *A reduction or reduced frequency of reinforcement*: as in bereavement, redundancy, relationship conflict, separation.
2. *A loss of effectiveness of the reinforcers*: occupational stress or "burn out", loss of interest in partner.
3. *Aversive control*: the person behaves in the same way but other's reactions change and are no longer reinforcing.
4. *A loss of reinforcible behaviour*: the person stops behaving in a way that others feel able to reinforce.
5. *Learned helplessness*: where the person expects that an aversive outcome of a situation is likely or that a desired outcome is unlikely. They also believe that they are unable to influence the outcome in any way.

Classification of Depression

In clinical terms, depressive signs and symptoms may be diagnosed in:

1. Reactive depression or neurotic depression.
2. Endogenous depression or psychotic depression.
3. Manic-depressive psychosis – in the depressive phase.
4. Involutional melancholia – depression associated with mid-life changes.
5. Post-natal depression – following childbirth (see also Unit 12.1.)

Within this classification system reactive and endogenous depression are the most commonly used diagnoses. In clinical terms, the following distinctions tend to be made:

1. *Reactive depression* is associated with:

    • reaction to adverse life events – a potential cause may be identified;
    • retention of insight – the person realizes they are ill;
    • milder mood disturbance;
    • less physiological function disturbances to appetite, energy, libido;
    • no diurnal variation;
    • frequent presence of other neurotic symptoms, e.g. anxiety, phobias, obsessions.

2. *Endogenous depression* is associated with:

    • spontaneous onset – no identifiable cause;
    • loss of insight – psychotic symptoms may be present, such as

hallucinations and delusions, particularly delusions of guilt, unworthiness, poverty, bodily changes;
- severe mood changes;
- presence of evident physiological disturbances, e.g. psychomotor retardation, constipation;
- diurnal variation.

Although this distinction is made between reactive and endogenous depression, in reality the diagnosis can be very difficult to make. In 40% of people with reactive depression there is no recognizable cause or event. In 37% of people with endogenous depression there is a clear precipitant.

A large number of people with reactive depression are often depressed before the "identified" life event. In these cases it is unclear whether the event caused the depression or vice versa. For many people with reactive depression there do not appear to be any precipitating events. Similarly, with psychotic depression, the person has often had a long period of neurotic depressive symptoms before being diagnosed.

Clinically, there are a number of divergent views regarding the classification and nature of depression that further complicate the distinction between reactive and endogenous depression. Briefly:

1. That reactive depression is similar to and a less severe form than endogenous depression.
2. That reactive and endogenous depression are totally separate clinical entities.
3. That there are a large number of undifferentiated types of depression that need to be more accurately classified.
4. That depression is an understandable reaction to life events (psychosocial viewpoint) that requires social and psychological intervention, contrasted by views that regard depression as a disease with biological pathology which requires physical intervention (medical model).

Differential Diagnosis

The wide ranging effects of depression are such that, particularly in the early stages, it may be difficult to differentiate it from certain other psychiatric illnesses. There is also the possibility too, that a person may be suffering from depressive symptoms in addition to their existing problems. In particular, depression may be confused with:

1. *Dementia*: in the early stages in an elderly person the presenting symptoms of self-neglect, loss of interest, poor concentration and loss of energy can seem very similar.
2. *Schizophrenia*: flattening of affect, apathy, self-neglect, loss of interests and withdrawal may be misinterpreted initially with depression.

Physical illnesses which may give rise to depressive-like symptoms include Addison's disease, myxoedema, Parkinson's disease.

Depression and Self-harm

In the depths of their despair, guilt and hopelessness, the depressed person may feel that the only way out of their misery is to kill or harm themselves. Frequently, though, their attempts at self-harm appear to be ineffectual and counterproductive. Most depressed people are too stressed and confused to undertake logically an act of self-destruction. The psychodynamics of self-harm are such that the person both wants to live and die at the same time. Uncertainty of outcome in such cases is common. Acts of self-harm would appear to be done:

1. Under extreme distress and desperation.
2. Impulsively, with a short time span between thought and action.
3. As a way of coping and resolving their situation in the short term.
4. As an act of communication, i.e. a call for help, seeking of attention.

A warning is invariably given – take all threats seriously.

Unit Instructions

When you have researched the suggested references, have mastered the Unit Objectives and successfully answered the Self-assessment Questions, proceed with the Unit Written Test.

Suggested References

Brown, G. W. and Harris, T. (1978). *Social Origins of Depression*. Tavistock, London.

Davis, D. R. (1984). *An Introduction to Psychopathology*, 4th Edition, Oxford University Press, Oxford.

Dominian, J. (1976). *Depression*. Fontana/Collins, London.

Farmer, R. and Hirsch, S. (Eds) (1980). *The Suicide Syndrome*. Croom Helm, London.

Fraser, M. (1982). *ECT, A Clinical Guide*. John Wiley, Chichester.

Gibbs, A. (1986). *Understanding Mental Health*. Consumers Association/Hodder and Stoughton, London.

Gillett, R. (1987). *Overcoming Depression*. Dorling Kindersley, London.

Goddard, A. (1982). Cognitive behaviour therapy and depression. *British Journal of Hospital Medicine*, March, Vol. 27, No. 3, pp. 248–253.

Goldberg, D. and Huxley, P. (1980). *Mental Illness in the Community*. Tavistock, London.

Goodwin, D. W. and Guze, S. B. (1979). *Psychiatric Diagnosis*. Oxford University Press, Oxford.

Hauck, P. (1973). *Depression, Why it Happens and How to Overcome It*. Sheldon Press.

Hawton, K. and Catalan, J. (1982). *Attempted Suicide*. Oxford University Press, Oxford.

Hayes, J. and Nutman, P. (1981). *Understanding the Unemployed*. Tavistock, London.

Hughes, J. (1986). *An Outline of Modern Psychiatry*, 2nd edition. John Wiley, Chichester.

Irving, S. (1983). *Basic Psychiatric Nursing*, 3rd edition. W. B. Saunders, Philadelphia.

Jacoby, R. J. (1981). Depression in the elderly. *British Journal of Hospital Medicine*, January, Vol. 25, No. 1, pp. 40–47.

Lancaster, J. (1980). *Adult Psychiatric Nursing*. Henry Kimpton, London.

Lyttle, J. (1986). *Mental Disorder*. Baillière Tindall, London and San Diego.

Mangen, S. (1982). *Sociology and Mental Health*. Churchill Livingstone, Edinburgh.

McCulloch, J. W. and Phillip, A. E. (1972). *Suicidal Behaviour*. Pergamon, Oxford.

McRae, M. (1986). *A State of Depression*. Macmillan, London.

Mitchell, R. (1975). *Depression*. Penguin, Harmondsworth.

Nairne, K. and Smith, G. (1984). *Dealing with Depression*. The Women's Press, London.

Parkes, C. M. (1986). *Bereavement, Studies of Grief in Adult Life*, 2nd edition. Penguin, Harmondsworth.

Pollit, J. (1982). Sadness. *British Journal of Hospital Medicine*, February, Vol. 27, No. 2, pp. 117–120.

Rees, L. (1982). *A Short Textbook of Psychiatry*. Hodder and Stoughton, London.

Robinson, L. (1983). *Psychiatric Nursing as a Human Experience*, 3rd edition, W. B. Saunders, Philadelphia.

Rowe, D. (1983). *Depression, the Way Out of Your Prison*. Routledge and Kegan Paul, London.

Rush, J. (1983). *Beating Depression*. Century Publishing, London.

Seligman, M. (1975). *Helplessness*. W. H. Freeman, San Francisco.

Snaith, P. (1981). *Clinical Neurosis*. Oxford University Press, Oxford.

Trethowan, W. and Sims, A. (1983). *Psychiatry*, 5th edition. Baillière Tindall, London and San Diego.

Williams, J. (1984). *The Psychological Treatment of Depression*. Croom Helm, London.

Willis, J. (1976). *Clinical Psychiatry*. Blackwell Scientific, Oxford.

Self-assessment Questions

SAQ 1. Define the term "depression".

SAQ 2. List ten factors which may contribute to depression.

SAQ 3. Why is depression diagnosed twice as commonly in women?

SAQ 4. How do a person's cognitions contribute to the experience of depression?

SAQ 5. Identify three factors as to why acts of self-harm are frequently ineffectual.

Unit 7.1: Written Test

1. What do you understand by the term "depression"?
2. Describe briefly factors which may contribute to depression.
3. What underlying reasons may be involved in acts of self-harm?

Recognizing Depression

Unit Objectives

At the end of this Unit the learner should be able to:

1. Describe the social effects of depression upon a person.
2. Outline the psychological effects of depression.
3. List the physical effects of depression.
4. Identify the influence of depression upon a person's behaviour.

Clinical Features

There is a wide range of potential symptoms that a person suffering from depression may complain of. These indicate both the severity of the depression and the individual's life situation and experience. Frequently, the symptoms develop insidiously and are only recognized in retrospect.

At times a person may be severely depressed in respect of their thoughts and intent for self-harm but may outwardly not show evidence of this. It requires considerable skill to identify the person's potential for self-harm in such cases.

Emotional

1. Indifference.
2. Fed up, browned off.
3. Sadness, despair, misery, dejection.
4. Grief, gloom and pessimism.
5. Hopelessness and helplessness.
6. Crying and tearful.
7. Flatness and unresponsive.
8. Little joy and pleasure in life.
9. Irritable, angry and aggressive.
10. Anxious, tense and irritable.
11. Agitation, particularly in the older person, with wringing of hands, moaning, rocking body and aimless activity, restlessness and pacing.

12. Diurnal variation, i.e. the mood may vary throughout the day. Characteristically the mood patterns may be:

- worse in the mornings and improve as the day goes on, or
- responsive to external events and deteriorate as the day progresses.

Social

1. Withdrawn and uncommunicative, avoid contact with others.
2. Loss of interest in family, friends and relationships.
3. Deterioration and conflict in relationships.
4. Loss of enjoyment in activities that previously gave pleasure.
5. Loss of interest in appearance and personal hygiene.
6. Loss of interest in hobbies and the outside world.
7. Difficulty in coping with demands at work.

Behavioural

1. Loss of energy and vitality, apathy.
2. Feel fatigued and weak, everything too much effort and burden.
3. Reduced levels of activity. At its most extreme the person may be inactive and unresponsive. This may be evidence of psychomotor retardation or depressive stupor in which a person remains aware of what is happening around them but is unresponsive.
4. Stooped posture, facial expression is dull, sad and non-responsive.
5. Slower, softer speech, monotonous tone, monosyllabic replies. In a depressive stupor the person may remain mute.
6. Potential self-injurious behaviour (viewed as either a way of communicating distress or internalized aggression).

Psychological

1. Slower thought processes, poverty of thought – difficulty in concentration.
2. Poor at problem solving and planning ahead.
3. Intellect and memory unaffected.
4. Interpret everything negatively.
5. Expect rejection and failure.
6. Self-doubt and indecision.
7. Perceive self as totally inadequate.
8. Profound loss of self-esteem and self-worth.
9. Self-deprecatory and self-reproachful.
10. Morbid thoughts and preoccupation with unpleasant events.
11. Suicidal preoccupation and intent.

Delusional ideas

These are more commonly associated with severe depression.

1. *Guilt*: deserves to be punished, sinful, wicked person. A burden to others. Confesses to "crimes".
2. *Hopelessness*: absolutely nothing can be done to improve their situation. Life not worth living for self.
3. *Worthlessness*: everyone else would be much better off if the person killed themself.
4. *Poverty*: bankrupt and unable to pay for their food and treatment.
5. *Hypochondriasis*: insides going "rotten". Believe they are suffering from cancer, venereal disease, contagious illness.

Perceptual

1. World seems grey, dull, dark, bleak, cold, cheerless.
2. Time: day too long, time drags, clock hands never move, seems as if the depression is never going to end.
3. Feel changed and cut off from others, depersonalized.
4. In extreme states of depression the person may, rarely, experience auditory hallucinations. The voices may condemn the person, accuse them of crimes and wickedness, prophesy doom. As a consequence, the person feels even more wretched.

Sexual

1. Loss of libido and interest in sexual activity.
2. Impotence in males, physiological non-arousal in women.

Physical

1. *Sleep disturbance*: Most depressed people complain of disturbed sleep. A pattern of either insomnia or early morning waking may predominate. The range of problems may include:
   - difficulty in falling asleep;
   - disturbed sleep throughout the night;
   - early morning waking and lying awake for several hours until it is time to get up;
   - feeling excessively tired and unrefreshed in the morning;
   - extreme difficulty in getting up in the morning;
   - feeling tired and worn out all day.

2. *Appetite*. In the early stages of depression a person may indulge in comfort eating which may cause further feelings of guilt and low self-esteem. As the depression becomes more pronounced there is a loss of appetite. Perceptually, food appears unappetizing and is tasteless to the person. Prolonged anorexia can lead to considerable weight loss and possible malnourishment and dehydration. Food may be actively refused. If there are delusions of poverty the person will refuse to eat as they believe that they cannot afford to pay for the food. The person may have delusions of guilt in which they believe that they do not deserve to eat and hence reject food. The person may believe that they have a terminal illness or that their "insides are blocked up". These may be evidence of either hypochondriacal delusions or of severe constipation. In both cases the person may refuse food or be unwilling to eat.

3. *Bowel activity*. Constipation is a common problem in depression. This can cause great discomfort and distress. There may be a gross preoccupation with bowel function which may reach delusional levels. Constipation arises from the reduced intake of food and reduction of physical activity and movement from retardation and stupor.

4. *Other physical complaints*:

   - general malaise and feeling unwell much of the time,
   - aches and pains in the body and joints,
   - headaches,
   - chest pains,
   - coldness,
   - dry skin,
   - stomach complaints,
   - dry mouth.

Identifying Potential for Self-harm

1. *Attempted suicide/self-injurious behaviour*: peak age group 20–35, females having a higher rate than males.
2. *Suicide*: incidence increases with age, males having a higher rate than females.
3. *Males tend to use more "violent" methods than women*: hanging, cutting, jumping from high places, firearms, drowning.
4. *Personal factors*: marital disharmony, financial difficulties, long-term unemployment, experience of loss, isolation, chronic ill-health, poor housing conditions. Family member attempted or committed suicide.
5. *Occupation*: certain occupations associated with higher suicide risk, e.g. psychiatrists, dentists, doctors, nurses, pilots and high stress jobs.
6. *Cultural factors*: higher rates in more affluent societies. Culture and availability of implements determines methods most frequently employed. Lower rates in those who are devoutly religious.
7. *Psychiatric factors*: depression, especially when recovering energy and motivation but thoughts still morbid and depressive. Where there are

ideas and delusions of guilt, hopelessness and worthlessness are present. Also low self-esteem, history of previous attempts, severe insomnia, severe hypochondriacal preoccupations, sociopathic personality disorders, alcohol and drug abuse (associated with high suicide rates) and chronic psychiatric illness.

Unit Instructions

When you have researched the suggested references, have mastered the Unit Objectives and successfully answered the Self-assessment Questions, proceed with the Unit Written Test.

Suggested References

Aguilera, D. C. and Messick, J. M. (1982). *Crisis Intervention, Therapy for Psychological Emergencies Methodology*. C. V. Mosby, New American Library, London, St. Louis.

Campbell, C. (1978). *Nursing Diagnosis and Intervention in Nursing Practice*. John Wiley, New York.

Consumer's Association (1982). *Living with Stress*. Consumer's Association/Hodder and Stoughton, London.

Davis, D. R. (1984). *An Introduction to Psychopathology*, 4th Edition. Oxford University Press, Oxford.

Farmer, R. and Hirsch, S. (Eds) (1980). *The Suicide Syndrome*, Croom Helm, London.

Gibbs, A. (1986). *Understanding Mental Health*. Consumer's Association/Hodder and Stoughton, London.

Gillett, R. (1987). *Overcoming Depression*. Dorling Kindersley, London.

Goodwin, D. W. and Guze, S. B. (1979). *Psychiatric Diagnosis*. Oxford University Press, New York.

Hauck, P. (1973). *Depression, Why it Happens and How to Overcome It*. Sheldon Press.

Hawton, K. and Catalan, J. (1982). *Attempted Suicide*. Oxford.

Hughes, J. (1986). *An Outline of Modern Psychiatry*, 2nd edition. John Wiley, Chichester.

Kreitman, N. and Dyer, J. (1981). Suicide and parasuicide. *Nursing*, October, Vol. 1, No. 30, pp. 1310–1312.

Mitchell, R. (1975). *Depression*. Penguin, Harmondsworth.

Nairne, K. and Smith, G. (1984). *Dealing with Depression*. The Women's Press, London.

Rees, L. (1982). *A Short Textbook of Psychiatry*. Hodder and Stoughton, London.

Robinson, L. (1983). *Psychiatric Nursing as a Human Experience*, 3rd edition. W. B. Saunders, Philadelphia.

Ross, T. (1982). Death wish. *Nursing Mirror*, 3 November, Vol. 155, No. 18, pp. 19–21.

Rowe, D. (1983). *Depression, The Way Out of Your Prison*. Routledge and Kegan Paul, London.

Rush, J. (1983). *Beating Depression*. Century Publishing, London,

Rushforth, D. (1985). Deliberate self-harm. *Nursing Times*, 18 September, Vol. 81, No. 38, pp. 51–53.

Snaith, P. (1981). *Clinical Neurosis*. Oxford University Press, Oxford.

Trethowan, W. and Sims, A. (1983). *Psychiatry*, 5th edition. Baillière Tindall, London and San Diego.

Walsh, M. H. (1981). Frequency of drug overdose. *Nursing Times*, 29 January, Vol. 77, No. 5, p. 202.

Walsh, M. H. (1982). Patterns of drug overdose. *Nursing Times*, 17 February, Vol. 78, No. 7, pp. 275–278.

Williams, J. (1984). *The Psychological Treatment of Depression*. Croom Helm, London.

Willis, J. (1976). *Clinical Psychiatry*. Blackwell Scientific, Oxford.

Wright, R. I. (1979). Self-poisoning trends and management. *Nursing Times*, 15 November, Vol. 75, No. 46, pp. 1966–1968.

Self-assessment Questions

SAQ 6. List five possible effects of depression on a person's behaviour.
SAQ 7. What delusions may be seen in severe depression?
SAQ 8. State five physical symptoms found in depression.
SAQ 9. Describe six factors associated with self-injurious behaviour.
SAQ 10. What are the emotional effects of depression?

Unit 7.2: Written Test

Janet Sprue, aged 26, and married with two young children, has been repeatedly attending her GP's surgery with a broad range of vague physical complaints. The GP thinks that these are an expression of underlying depression and has referred her to the community psychiatric nurse (CPN), who has a sessional input to the group practice.

1. What statements might Janet make that indicate that she is suffering from depression?
2. What observations might the CPN make while they are interviewing Janet that could confirm she is depressed?
3. What factors would the CPN have to consider in determining Janet's potential for self-harm?

Care and Treatment of the Person Who is Depressed

Unit Objectives

At the end of this Unit the learner should be able to:

1. Describe the range of therapeutic interventions available for the person who is depressed.
2. Identify the support required for the person and their family in the community.
3. List factors associated with the prognosis of depression.

Care and Treatment

There are a range of therapeutic interventions that are effective in depression. The general approach should be an integrated and readily accessible service to support the person and their family in the community or in residential care as required.

Therapeutic aims

1. To relieve the depressive symptoms as soon as possible.
2. To avoid acts of self-harm.
3. To facilitate the development of the person and their family's coping skills.

Family and Self-care

Social surveys indicate a high incidence of depression in the community (8–15%). However, only a small percentage (2–3%) are actually treated. This would indicate that most people who are depressed are not in contact with any health care agency. In reality, most people with depression are either trying to cope alone or are being looked after by their family under stressful conditions. For some of these depression can become a life of chronic misery.

The individual may experience insomnia, loss of energy and interests, sadness, problems at work and difficulty in coping. The family see someone who is possibly irritable, tearful, difficult to live with, neglectful and emotionally detached. Over time this can generate further problems and a deterioration in close personal relationships. Other people feel rejected, hurt and frustrated.

It is significant that there has been a rapid growth of publications on self-care in depression and in the number of support groups available (e.g. Depressives Anonymous).

People can be helped considerably in coping with depression by:

1. Accurate information about depression and its effects.
2. Involvement in the care and treatment process.
3. The opportunity to talk freely about problems.
4. Enabling the person and family to come to terms with their guilt and letting them talk openly about their experiences.
5. The address of a local contact support group.
6. Developing the person's and family's coping skills.
7. Reviewing their life-style and expectations to promote their mental health.

Community Care

Most people with depression are cared for in the community. Community care involves a wide range of statutory and voluntary services that aim to provide comprehensive treatment and support. Provided an accurate assessment is made of the person's potential for self-harm, it is possible for quite depressed people to be cared for at home. The aims of community care are:

1. To support the person and their family.
2. To enable the person to remain in their own home.
3. To monitor the person's mental and physical health.
4. To implement community-based treatment and care programmes.

The services available include:

1. The community mental health centre with community psychiatric nurses, social workers, psychologists, occupational therapists and consultant psychiatrists, working as a team to offer skills-based therapeutic interventions.
2. General practitioners
3. Voluntary agencies: MIND, Depressives Anonymous, DASS, Samaritans, Citizen's Advice Bureaux.
4. Out-patient clinics and day hospitals.

Residential Care

The reasons for admission to residential facilities for treatment include:

1. Lack of support in the community.
2. The need for intensive care when the person is severely depressed and is potentially suicidal.
3. History of previous suicidal and self-injurious behaviour.

Treatment Interventions

Physical treatment methods for depression

1. *Chemotherapy*

   (a) *Antidepressants*:

   (i) Tricyclics and tetracylics

   - imipramine (Tofranil),
   - amitriptyline (Tryptizol),
   - mianserin (Bolvidon),
   - dothiepin (Prothiaden).

These are the most widely used type of drugs for depression. They can take up to 2 weeks to have an effect. They are fairly safe in clinical use and generally have only mild and transient side-effects.

   (ii) Monoamine oxidase inhibitors (MAOI):

   - phenelzine (Nardil),
   - tranylcypromine (Parnate).

MAOIs are less frequently used now except in very specific cases. Their use is limited by the dietary prohibitions that people on MAOIs must follow. People must avoid cheese, marmite, bovril, aspirin and alcohol.

   (b) *Anxiolytics*: if anxiety is a prominent feature. For short period only.
   (c) *Night sedation*: if sleep disturbance is present. Only effective for short period after which use becomes counterproductive.

2. *Electroconvulsive therapy* (ECT). Informed consent required. Psychological and physical preparation of person. Treatment involves passing a

high-voltage electrical current across the forehead to induce a fit. The person is given a general anaesthetic and muscle relaxant to control muscular reaction, which is seen as slight twitch and contraction. Short recovery period in which person is confused and unsteady. Person may require 8–12 treatments, two or three times a week, for several weeks until the depression lifts. May be given either "unilaterally" or "bilaterally". Unilateral ECT tends to produce less confusion and memory loss afterwards. Some controversy surrounds the use of ECT.

Psychotherapeutic interventions for depression

1. *Skilled nursing care*: one of the most important factors.
2. *Individual psychotherapy*: to work through unresolved grief and other issues, to release repressed emotions, and to increase insight.
3. *Behavioural therapy*: to increase the incidence of positive reinforcement in the person's life-style. Avoidance of negatively reinforcing experiences.
4. *Cognitive therapy*: to develop more positive thought processes and expectations, and to change dysfunctional and automatic negative thoughts.
5. *Assertiveness training*: to help the person express their feelings and to raise their self-esteem.
6. *Family or couple's therapy*: to enable the couple to be more supportive and communicate more effectively.
7. *Development of coping and stress management skills.*
8. *Group work*: to help people share their experiences and work together to seek solutions.
9. *Occupational therapy*: to develop life skills and as diversional activity.
10. *Art therapy and psychodrama*: to help express and release their feelings.
11. *Recreational and social activities*: to provide positively reinforcing experiences.
12. *Voluntary organizations*: MIND, Samaritans, Depressives Anonymous.

Outcomes

In the majority of situations people find that their depression gradually lifts and their mood recovers. Those who seek treatment likewise find that the therapeutic interventions should enable them to recover in a shorter period of time. For a small number of people the depression may become a way of life of chronic misery and repeated prescriptions for antidepressants. Clinically, therefore, there is no doubt that intervention can be effective. However, given the broad range of social, relationship and personal factors implicated in the pathology of depression, the recovery may be short-lived if the person is returned to an environment that contributed significantly to the onset of depression. Significant changes may be needed in a person's

environment, relationships and life-style to avoid some of the causative factors. The potential for such real change may, however, be limited. This is one of the main dilemmas in attempting to treat people with depression.
Factors associated with a positive outcome include:

1. Mode of onset: an acute onset favours a speedy recovery.
2. Clinical features: the more definite the affective nature of the illness the better the prognosis.
3. History of previous similar illness from which they recovered.
4. Absence of complicating factors such as chronic debilitating physical illness, alcoholism or drug abuse.

Unit Instructions

When you have researched the suggested references, have mastered the Unit Objectives and successfully answered the Self-assessment Questions, proceed with the Unit Written Test.

Suggested References

Ashton, J. (1986). Preventing suicide in hospital. *Nursing Times*, 31 December, Vol. 82, No. 52, pp. 36–37.

Bailey, J. (1983). ECT or not ECT – that is the question. *Nursing Times*, 2 March, Vol. 79, No. 9, pp. 12–14.

Ballinger, B. R. (1985). Depression – effective alternatives to drug therapy. *Geriatric Medicine*, October, Vol. 16, No. 10, pp. 14–20.

Barker, P., Hume, A. and Robertson, W. (1985). Psychological therapy in affective disorders. *Nursing Mirror*, 29 May, Vol. 160, No. 22, pp. 34–36.

Beck, A. T. *et al.* (1979). Cognitive Therapy of Depression. John Wiley, New York.

Biley, F. (1985). Learn to believe in yourself. *Nursing Times*, 29 May, Vol. 81, No. 22, pp. 40–41.

Brooking, J. and Minghella, E. (1987). Parasuicide. *Nursing Times*, 27 May, Vol. 83, No. 21, pp. 40–43.

Carr, P. J., Butterworth, C. A. and Hodges, B. E. (1980). *Community Psychiatric Nursing*. Churchill Livingstone, Edinburgh.

Clare, A. (1980). *Psychiatry in Dissent*, 2nd edition. Tavistock, London.

Coupar, A. and Conway, C. (1986). Hospital admission for depression. *Journal of Advanced Nursing*, Vol. 11, No. 6, pp. 697–704.

Crossfield, T. (1988). Curse or cure? *Nursing Times*, 3 February, Vol. 84, No. 5, pp. 66–67.

Dryden, W. (1984). Rational-emotive Therapy. Croom Helm, London.

Dryden, W. and Golden, W. (Eds) (1986). *Cognitive-behavioural Approaches to Psychotherapy*. Harper and Row, London.

Fraser, M. (1982). ECT, A Clinical Guide. John Wiley, Chichester.

Gibbs, A. (1986). *Understanding Mental Health*. Consumer's Association/Hodder and Stoughton, London.

Gillies, D. and Lader, M. (1986). *Guide to the Use of Psychotropic Drugs*. Churchill Livingstone, Edinburgh.

Goddard, A. (1982). Cognitive behaviour therapy and depression. *British Journal of Hospital Medicine*, March, Vol. 27, No. 3, pp. 248–253.

Goldberg, D. and Huxley, P. (1980). *Mental Illness in the Community*. Tavistock, London.

Hauck, P. (1973). *Depression, Why it Happens and How to Overcome it*. Sheldon Press, London.

Hawton, K. and Catalan, J. (1982). *Attempted Suicide*. Oxford University Press, Oxford.

Hughes, J. (1986). *An Outline of Modern Psychiatry*, 2nd edition. John Wiley, Chichester.

Juniper, D. (1978). *How to Lift Your Depression*. Open Books, Wells, Somerset.

Lyttle, J. (1986). *Mental Disorder*. Baillière Tindall, London and San Diego.

MacKay, D. (1982). Cognitive behaviour therapy. *British Journal of Hospital Medicine*, March, Vol. 27, No. 3, pp. 242–247.

Mangen, S. (1982). *Sociology and Mental Health*. Churchill Livingstone, Edinburgh.

Mawson, D. (1985). Shock waves. *Nursing Times*, 13 November, Vol. 81, No. 46, pp. 42–44.

Mitchell, R. (1975). *Depression*. Penguin, Harmondsworth.

Moores, A. (1987). Walking back to happiness. *Nursing Times*, 21 October, Vol. 83, No. 42, pp. 55–57.

Nairne, K. and Smith, G. (1984). *Dealing with Depression*. The Women's Press, London.

Rees, L. (1982). *A Short Textbook of Psychiatry*. Hodder and Stoughton, London.

Rowe, D. (1983). *Depression, The Way Out of Your Prison*. Routledge and Kegan Paul, London.

Royal College of Nursing Society of Psychiatric Nursing (1982). *Nursing Guidelines for ECT*. Royal College of Nursing, London.

Rush, J. (1983). *Beating Depression*. Century Publishing, London.

Silverstone, T. and Turner, P. (1982). *Drug Treatment in Psychiatry*. Routledge and Kegan Paul, London.

Simmons, S. and Brooker, C. (1986). *Community Psychiatric Nursing – A Social Perspective*. Heinemann Nursing, London.

Snaith, P. (1981). *Clinical Neurosis*. Oxford University Press, Oxford.

Trethowan, W. and Sims, A. (1983). *Psychiatry*, 5th edition. Baillière Tindall, London and San Diego.

Vaughan, P. J. (1985). *Suicide Prevention*. PEPAR Publications, Birmingham.

Vissenga, C. and Whitfield, W. (1983). ECT: a balanced perspective? *Nursing Times*, 20 July, Vol. 79, No. 29, pp. 43–44.

Williams, J. (1984). *The Psychological Treatment of Depression*. Croom Helm, London.

Willis, J. (1976). *Clinical Psychiatry*. Blackwell Scientific, Oxford.

Self-assessment Questions

SAQ 11. What factors influence whether a person is treated at home or is advised to accept hospital treatment?

SAQ 12. What community support may be necessary for someone with depression?

SAQ 13. Identify two antidepressants and describe their usage, doses and side-effects.
SAQ 14. What psychotherapeutic interventions are helpful in depression?

Unit 7.3: Written Test

Peter Brown, aged 56, has been suffering from depression for 6 months following his redundancy. Despite numerous attempts he has been unable to find other work and now feels dejected and useless. His wife is concerned because he keeps saying that he "cannot go on much longer". He has lost weight and is sleeping badly. He has lost all his previous interests and is neglectful of his appearance. The GP has requested that the CPN visits and makes a psychiatric assessment.

1. What home-based interventions are possible in the community to help this couple?
2. Following an overdose, Peter is admitted to an acute psychiatric ward. He is prescribed antidepressants and ECT. How are these physical methods of treatment used to relieve depression?

Nursing Care of the Person Who is Depressed

Mental Health Nursing Care

Each person's care needs are unique and have to be assessed individually. A range of potential care needs have been selected to illustrate the problems that the depressed person may experience and the possible nursing interventions that may help them. For the person who is depressed these may include the needs to:

A. Promote their self-esteem.
B. Feel protected in a safe and secure environment.
C. Experience an uplift in mood.
D. Meet their basic physical needs.
E. Communicate and relate to others.
F. Facilitate the development of the person's and family's coping skills.

A. Promote Their Self-esteem

Associated problems/personal difficulties

Person may be experiencing a severe loss of self-esteem that can:

1. Cause him severe emotional distress, e.g. feelings of worthlessness, failure and guilt.

2. Distort his perceptions, i.e. interpret everything in a negative and self-defeating way.
3. Interfere with his ability to communicate.
4. Increase the risk of self-harmful or suicidal behaviour.
5. Interfere with his motivation to meet his basic needs independently.

Assessment

1. Person's description of their perceived self-worth at present.
2. Person's description of their earlier life experiences in relation to their self-esteem at the time.
3. Personal experiences of success, coping and failure.
4. Identify the criteria that the person uses to evaluate their self-esteem in relation to others.
5. Nurse's observation of the effects of low self-esteem upon the person's:

   (a) Communication: negative self-statements, self-criticism, inferiority and inadequacy. Statements of guilt, worthlessness and hopelessness. Volume, tone, clarity and rate of speech.
   (b) Behaviour: passive, non-assertive, social anxiety, withdrawn, submissive posture, avoiding eye contact.
   (c) Emotions: sadness, failure, rejection, hopelessness.
   (d) Reaction to situations that challenge their self-esteem.
   (e) Specific activities that influence the person's self-esteem.

6. Social reinforcement available to the person: partner, friends, personal possessions, personal events, activities, interests, financial, occupational.
7. Potential stressors in the person's life and their ability to cope with them.

Desired outcomes

1. To assist the person to formulate a more positive self-image.
2. For the person to make positive personal statements that indicate self-worth.
3. For the person to make positive future-orientated statements.
4. To avert the potential for self-injurious behaviour.

Nursing intervention	Rationale
1. Initiate therapeutic relationship. Involve the person in the care planning process	Interventions more likely to be successful in an atmosphere of trust and cooperation. Reinforces sense of self-worth and individuality

Nursing intervention	*Rationale*
2. Use the person's preferred name. Facilitate the use of personal belongings. Personalize the person's intimate environment. Show recognition of person's attainments. Emphasize the person's value as an individual. Spend time with them	Personal recognition of individuality reinforces sense of identity and promotes self-esteem. This also promotes the person's feelings of security and potential for change. Helps to promote self-esteem and show concern
3. Identify and help to celebrate significant personal dates, e.g. birthdays, anniversaries. Encourage personal interests. Promote contact with relatives and personal friends. Increase opportunities for group interaction. Increase environmental stimulation	Potential situations for personal reinforcement that may also help to raise mood. Helps to overcome feelings of isolation and rejection. Still valued by others. Avoids boredom and increases potential distractions
4. Gradually increase personal responsibility in small stages. Set graded task assignments	Need to avoid situations of potential failure and to increase the opportunity for experience of success. This can be very reinforcing
5. Explore self-criticism. Identify criteria used to evaluate self. Assist the person to acknowledge the influence of these criteria on their self-esteem. Explore alternative ways of evaluating their self-worth. Help person to develop internal sources of self-esteem. Encourage acceptance of self-limitations	Many depressed people have very harsh and unattainable expectations of themselves. Inevitably, this leads to feelings of failure, guilt, self-blame and worthlessness. The person needs to be helped to re-shape their beliefs about themself and to develop more valid and realistic expectations
6. Identify and work with their strengths and resources.	Depressed people often regard themself as totally worthless and need to be presented with personal attainments

Nursing intervention	*Rationale*
7. Offer alternative interpretations of life experiences that person uses to devalue themselves. Encourage awareness of positive responses from others. Promote a realistic assessment of situations. Explore previous achievements and successes	Depressed people tend to see everything negatively and to misperceive events in a way that is personally devaluing. They tend to devalue all past attainments
8. Increase personal responsibility in small stages. Reinforce initiatives taken by the person. Encourage gradual mastery of situations	Dependency and the restrictions imposed to avoid self-harm may also be damaging to person's self-esteem. Gradually need to reintroduce personal control over life circumstances. A degree of risk may be necessary to regain personal initiative
9. Teach the skills and principles of assertiveness (see Unit 3.4)	Increases personal control that can be expressed in a more effective way. Increases confidence, self-esteem and the ability to communicate more effectively
10. Identify options for work and leisure activities	Relieves boredom and helps to raise self-esteem if meaningfully employed
11. Enable person to meet their spiritual needs	May feel that their past behaviour is sinful and that they have been rejected by their faith. Contact with appropriate minister can help to promote spiritual welfare
12. Provide factual information about the incidence of depression in the community	Person may feel guilty and stigmatized about receiving psychiatric treatment. This can be damaging to their self-esteem
13. Encourage them to pay attention to their hygiene and appearance	Appearance and hygiene are two important factors in self-esteem. Feeling clean and looking presentable help to improve the person's self-image and the way they appear to others.

Evaluation

1. Increase in the frequency of positive personal statements.
2. Decrease in the incidence of negative self-statements.
3. Demonstrates more assertive verbal and non-verbal communications.
4. Makes future-orientated statements and plans.

B. Feel Protected in a Safe and Secure Environment

Associated problems/personal difficulties

Person may be feeling insecure and at risk as a consequence of:

1. Inadequate knowledge of their illness and treatment.
2. Thoughts of self-harm and suicide.
3. Feelings of guilt and worthlessness.
4. Extreme stress and frustration.
5. Inability to control their own emotions and behaviour.

Assessment

1. Person's descriptions of their anxieties and fear of threat.
2. Reactions of the person's relatives and friends.
3. Identify their potential for self-harm:

    (a) History of previous attempts at self-harm: methods used, planning, precautions taken, outcomes.
    (b) Delusions of guilt and worthlessness.
    (c) Severe stress in the person's life: recent crises including bereavement, redundancy, debts, miscarriage, etc.
    (d) Social and relationship isolation: lack of support.
    (e) Associated problems of alcohol abuse, drug abuse, chronic physical ill-health.
    (f) Stage of depressive illness: near recovery when motivation returns but still have morbid thoughts.

4. Nurse's observations of the person's:

    (a) Communications: statements of suicidal intent, guilt, hopelessness, helplessness, feeling trapped, rejection.
    (b) Behaviour: increasingly active, regaining energy, looking much better when recently very depressed, acting suspiciously, denial of any problems, attempts at self-injury, hoarding of tablets.

Desired outcomes

1. To reduce the potential for self-injurious behaviour.
2. To avoid self-injury.
3. To enable the person to communicate his thoughts and feelings in regard of self-harm.
4. To promote feelings of safety and security.

Nursing intervention	Rationale
1. Evaluate person's potential for self-harm. Ensure that all care workers are aware of any risk of self-harm. Co-ordinate all nursing care activities	The risk of self-harm needs to be clearly established to ensure appropriate care is given. Nursing team must be consistent and aware of any risk of self-harm
2. Initiate therapeutic relationship with key worker. Spend time with them. Be available and approachable. Use touch	Interventions are more likely to be successful in an atmosphere of trust and cooperation. This is especially true when trying to win the confidence of someone who is potentially suicidal. Reinforces sense of self-worth and individuality. Reduces feelings of anxiety. Promotes feelings of security
3. Demonstrate acceptance and non-judgemental responses. Be aware of own feelings and beliefs about self-injurious behaviour.	Being non-judgemental helps a person to deal with feelings of guilt. To promote own insight and effectiveness.
4. Ensure that all potentially harmful substances and implements are removed. Ensure that all medication is taken immediately. Ensure that the person is under observation at all times. Involve in group activities	Reduces the opportunity for self-harm. Prevents hoarding of drugs for possible overdose. The observation needs to be done in such a way that it is non-obtrusive and does not increase stress. Being involved in group activities helps to achieve this.
5. Provide clear and understandable	A lot of insecurity is associated with fear of the unknown and misconceptions.

Nursing intervention	*Rationale*
information about their care and treatment. Encourage questions. Ask for feedback on their understanding. Clarify any misunderstandings. Involve the person in the care planning process. Explain the need for any precautions	People have a right to information about their health care. The nurse is in an ideal position to use this process to facilitate the development of the person's understanding about their health care needs
6. Encourage the person to retain and use personal belongings	Familiar objects help to increase feelings of security
7. Provide support and reassurance to family and friends. Advise them not to bring in any medication or potentially harmful implements to the person without consulting the staff	Possible feelings of guilt, shock and ambivalence towards person who has expressed suicidal intent. Important that any existing social support network is maintained. Need for their cooperation
8. Ask the person if they are still contemplating suicide or self-injury. Identify the intensity and frequency of suicidal thoughts. Identify factors which appear to trigger suicidal thoughts. Identify potential factors that help to reduce suicidal preoccupation	All depressed people consider self-harm. It can be helpful to bring the topic out into the open. Many depressed people feel relieved about discussing the topic. Identifying factors that reinforce suicidal preoccupations helps to pinpoint risk situations. Person may suggest interventions that help to reduce suicidal thoughts. Self-harm is a form of communication. Talking about it is cathartic and may help to decrease the possibility
9. Make a verbal contract with the person not to harm themselves	Encouraging personal responsibility helps to raise self-esteem. This needs to be done with caution and with regard to the person's clinical condition. A professional judgement has to be made at some stage in the caring process to balance risk with potential therapeutic gain

Nursing intervention	Rationale
10. Set limits on potentially self-injurious behaviour	Person needs to be aware and acknowledge that you will intervene if their behaviour causes concern. This helps also to increase feelings of security if the person is shown that they will not be allowed to harm themselves
11. Approach unhurriedly. Demonstrate calmness. Do not rush the person. Be aware of your own reactions and experiences of stress. Take periodic breaks if possible	Anxiety in the carer communicates itself to the person. Caring for a depressed and suicidal person is a very stressful experience. This may unconsciously influence your interactions with them. Find ways of coping with your own stress
12. Encourage diversional recreational and social activities	Helps to avoid boredom and to divert the person's thoughts away from stressful topics. Physical activity is also a beneficial channel for stress
13. Encourage the person to rest or relax if they appear to be under stress. Provide feedback on their behaviour	Person may not be aware of the effect of anxiety on their behaviour

Evaluation

1. Person does not attempt acts of self-harm.
2. Person can safely be left unobserved.
3. Decrease in statements of suicidal intent.
4. Increase in future-orientated statements and plans.

C. Experience an Uplift in Mood

Associated problems/personal difficulties

Person may be experiencing profound feelings of sadness, misery and despair that:

1. Cause great emotional distress.
2. Increase their potential for self-harm.
3. Negatively influence the way they perceive their environment.
4. Reinforce feelings of hopelessness and helplessness.

5. Reduce their motivation to attend to their physical needs.
6. Interfere with their ability to communicate.

Assessment

1. Person's description of their depressive emotional experiences and thoughts.
2. Information from relatives and friends.
3. Nurse's observation of the effects of their mood upon the person's:

   (a) Communication pattern:
   - verbal expression: tone, volume, rate, rhythm, clarity;
   - non-verbal communication: posture, facial expression, eye contact, gestures, proximity, hand movements.

   (b) Thought processes: content of depressive thoughts and preoccupations, interpretation of life and daily events, depressive predictions and anticipations, frequency and pattern of depressive thoughts throughout the day, association of depressive thoughts with external events.
   (c) Emotional reaction to depressive thoughts: intensity and duration of emotional distress experienced as a result of depressive cognitions. Effectiveness of coping strategies for depressive cognitions.

4. Psychosocial environment: presence of identifiable eliciting stimuli or triggering clues. Reactions of others to person's depressive behaviour and statements. Potential reinforcers of depressive behaviour and thoughts. Presence of potential stresses in person's environment or lifestyle.

Desired outcomes

1. To facilitate opportunities for emotionally positive experiences.
2. To reduce the influence of depressive cognitions on their behaviour, emotions and communication.
3. To promote the person's control over their own cognitions and behaviour.

Nursing intervention	Rationale
1. Initiate therapeutic relationship	Interventions more likely to be successful in an atmosphere of trust and cooperation

Nursing intervention	Rationale
2. Offer reassurance. Demonstrate acceptance. Ensure non-judgemental responses. Avoid cliches, do not criticize. Be patient, tolerant and use touch, where appropriate	To minimize distress and to create the potential for emotional change
3. Empathize with their emotional experience. Take time out to review own emotional reactions. Review own coping strategies	Depression communicates to influence the carers. It can be a very demanding and draining experience. Important to be aware of the emotional demands being made. Easy to become tired, drained and irritable. Own reactions can distance you and reinforce a depressive mood. May engender feelings of frustration and impotence in the carer
4. Promote their self-esteem (see **A.**)	Self-esteem directly related to a person's emotional responses and perception of situations
5. Enhance feelings of security and safety (see **B.**). Ensure that basic physical needs are being met (see **D.**). Promote physical comfort	Important to ensure that basic psychosocial and physical needs are being met. This ensures the optimum conditions for promoting a positive emotional experience. If a person feels physically uncomfortable this will only add to their overall misery
6. Encourage appropriate diversional activities	Boredom and lack of social stimulation tend to reinforce sense of isolation and depressive mood
7. Do not reinforce depressive mood and behaviour. Model own behaviour and communications to demonstrate calmness and sense of proportion	Person will be alert to reactions and statements by carers. May unconsciously communicate verbally and non-verbally in a way that reinforces their feelings of depression
8. Provide opportunities for the person to express themselves openly	Helps to relieve tension and to demonstrate acceptance
9. Chart their mood throughout the day	Most depressed people have mood variations throughout the day

Nursing intervention	*Rationale*
10. Encourage person to keep an emotional diary/log throughout the day	Self-recording is both therapeutic and instructional. Provides useful feedback on progress
11. Identify with the person situations that lead to a depressive emotional reaction	Person may not be aware of these situations that add to their depression
12. Assist the person to avoid potentially depressing situations. Facilitate their emotional coping skills and behavioural strategies. Demonstrate how thoughts about situations influence the person's emotional reactions. Offer alternative non-depressive interpretation of their perceptions	May be possible to make life-style changes that promote mental health. Limited coping skills increase their potential to react depressively. Many depressed people perceive everything in a negative way. They selectively focus on negative aspects, exaggerate and over-generalize. They need to re-frame their perceptions and expectations
13. Encourage awareness of positive responses from others	These can be used to raise their mood
14. Identify activities and thoughts that raise their mood. Identify specific periods of the day when mood lifts	They can be even more effective if used during upswings in mood
15. Assist the person to identify some positive anticipations. Focus on the future. Offer hope	When depressed people focus on a very unpleasant present and guilt-ridden past. They need to have pleasant events to look forward to. This is positively reinforcing and diverts their depressive focus
16. Instruct in the skills of thought-blocking for depressive cognitions	Some people are able to use this for persistent morbid thoughts (see p. 332)
17. Give medication as prescribed. Observe for side-effects.	Antidepressant medication and other prescribed treatment helps to reduce the severity of depressive symptoms

Evaluation

1. Makes emotionally positive statements.
2. Posture and non-verbal communication indicate a raised mood.
3. Appears more relaxed and less distressed.
4. Able to interpret events in a non-depressive way.
5. Marked reduction in the frequency of depressive statements.

D. Meet Their Basic Physical Needs

Associated problems/personal difficulties

A person may be experiencing difficulty in meeting their physical needs due to:

1. Loss of appetite.
2. Sleep disturbances.
3. Loss of interest in personal hygiene.
4. Profound loss of energy and motivation.
5. Feelings of unworthiness and intent for self-harm.

Assessment

1. Person's statements in regard of meeting their needs for nutrition, fluids, hygiene, rest and sleep.
2. Information available from relatives and friends.
3. Nurse's observations of:

   (a) Person's self-initiated activities in relation to meeting their physical needs.
   (b) Level of prompting required to motivate the person.
   (c) Resistance demonstrated by person.
   (d) Behaviour of others in the environment in relation to the person's non-attainment of basic physical needs.
   (e) Possession and use of personalized hygiene facilities.
   (f) Dietary intake and elimination.
   (g) Sleep pattern and level of activity throughout the day.
   (h) Identified physical health deficits.

Nursing intervention	Rationale
1. Initiate therapeutic relationship	Interventions are more likely to be successful in an atmosphere of trust and cooperation

Nursing intervention	*Rationale*
2. Promote their autonomy and self-esteem (see **A.**)	Raising self-esteem increases the person's interest in their appearance and hygiene
3. Encourage their interest in how they appear to others. Make unprompted positive comments about their appearance and their behaviour	External social feedback in the form of recognition and comment is a powerful reinforcer in an environment that is perceived as non-rewarding. Even very depressed people can benefit from this feedback
4. Ensure that they are wearing clean and well-fitting clothes.	Helps to raise self-esteem.
5. Encourage the person to use personalized soap, flannel, towel, toothbrush, etc.	Person more likely to use items that belong to them
6. Ensure that dignity and privacy are respected and maintained	Intrusions into privacy can cause personal distress. If you treat people in a less than respectful way they will also feel devalued. This can be a very difficult situation when trying to promote self-esteem and yet, at the same time, be alert for potential risks. Only your detailed knowledge of the person and your relationship can help you determine which actions you take
7. Encourage choice and option over washing and bathing. Give positive feedback on personal initiatives	Facilitating control over their life increases motivation
8. Identify food preferences and previous eating patterns. Facilitate personal choice in regard of diet and meal-times. Provide opportunities for the person to take responsibility and book their own meals	More likely to eat preferred food and follow personal dietary pattern. Person will take more interest in food that they have selected and prepared

Nursing intervention	*Rationale*
9. Present food in an attractive manner and in a conducive environment. Small portions. Do not rush at meal-times. Positively reinforce all attempts at feeding. Be firm	Helps to create a conducive environment and person not put off by presentation of food. May be more prepared to eat at certain times of the day in relation to possible upswings in mood or previous dietary patterns
10. Monitor dietary and fluid intake. Weigh periodically	Avoid malnutrition, dehydration and further weight loss
11. Ensure adequate fibre is taken. Encourage regular activity	Helps to prevent constipation which can be very discomforting
12. Identify normal sleep pattern. Encourage participation in activities during the day and evening. Encourage them to stay up until a reasonable time. Avoid daytime sleeping or "retreating" to bed	Each person's pattern is unique. Daytime sleeping makes night-time sleep difficult. If they go to bed too early, bound to give the impression of "insomnia" if not really tired (see also p. 257)
13. Identify which factors promote sleep for that person. Identify factors that disturb their sleep. Promote physical comfort of their bedspace. Avoid noise at night. Switch off unnecessary lights	May be simple actions that can be taken to facilitate a good night's sleep. Noises can be very disruptive (see also p. 257)
14. Observe sleep pattern at night. Provide feedback to person on amount of observed sleep	Indicates their depth of depression. Most depressed people greatly underestimate the amount of sleep that they actually have. This causes great stress and reinforces their feelings of depression
15. Provide reassurance if awake at night. Observe closely at night-time	Early morning waking or disturbed sleep can leave them distressed and preoccupied with morbid thoughts. It is also a time when the risk of self-harm is greatest

Evaluation

1. Person initiates own self-care and hygiene activities.
2. Person takes an adequate diet and fluid intake unprompted.
3. Need for prompting in relation to physical needs decreases.
4. Reports that they are sleeping better. Seems more refreshed.
5. Person takes an interest in their appearance.

E. Communicate and Relate to Others

Associated problems/personal difficulties

The experience of depression may interfere with the person's ability to communicate by:

1. Damaging their self-esteem and self-worth.
2. Reducing their motivation to interact with others.
3. Impairing their concentration and judgement.
4. Keeping their mind focussed on morbid thoughts.
5. Interpreting everything in a negative and self-devaluing way.
6. Reducing verbal and non-verbal patterns of behaviour.

Assessment

1. Person's description of their communication difficulties.
2. Nurse's observation of the person's:

   (a) Communication pattern:

   - Verbal expression: tone, volume, rate, rhythm, clarity;
   - Non-verbal expression: posture, facial expression eye contact, gestures, proximity, hand movements;
   - Movement and mobility: static or move around, duration spent in particular places.

   (b) Content of speech and emotions expressed: depressive, negative, morbid, guilt, intent for self-harm, whether future- or past-orientated.

3. Interaction with others: frequency and duration of contacts with others, response to communication from others, frequency, nature and duration of self-initiated communications with others, avoidance or withdrawal demonstrated, pattern throughout the day.

4. Psychosocial environment: situations and significant others that elicit, inhibit or reinforce communication. Potential stresses in person's environment or life-style. Reactions of others in communication with person.
5. Sensory deficits: visual, auditory.

Desired outcomes

1. Person to communicate without prompting and to express their social, emotional and physical needs.
2. Person to interact with others in a more assertive way.
3. Person to make positive self-statements.

Nursing intervention	Rationale
1. Initiate therapeutic relationship	Interventions more likely to be successful in an atmosphere of trust and cooperation
2. Model skilled social and communication skills. Listen attentively and actively	Modelling by nurses has a powerful influence on the people in their care
3. Promote their autonomy and self-esteem (see **A**) Reinforce sense of self-identity	Self-belief in the person's own value and feelings of control and mastery increase confidence in dealing with others
4. Minimize the influence of automatic negative thoughts and dysfunctional perceptions (see **A**)	Dysfunctional thought patterns interfere with a person's interpretation and perception of events and cause communication misunderstandings, i.e. everything is interpreted negatively
5. Promote their feelings of security and minimize feelings of threat (see **B**)	If the person is anxious and is intent on self-harm they will tend to withdraw and to be defensive
6. Use touch and other non-verbal signals to demonstrate reassurance	Touch can be very comforting and reassuring if used with sensitivity
7. Ensure that basic needs are being met (see **D**)	Physical comfort is a prerequisite for meeting other needs. It also helps to raise self-esteem

Nursing intervention	*Rationale*
8. Advise and support relatives who may find it difficult to communicate with the person	It is very distressing for close relatives who feel unable to reach out to the depressed person and may feel rejected. They may have strong feelings of guilt, anger and rejection
9. Inform the person about their care and treatment	The person may seem withdrawn and stuporous but still has a right to know. It also reduces the possibility of unexpected and threatening interventions
10. Provide written information if required	Difficulty in concentrating and remembering when depressed. They are then able to refer back to the written details
11. Accept one-sided conversation. Accept the person's behaviour. Be non-judgemental	The person may have a communication problem which makes it difficult for them to respond. Criticism only increases feelings of guilt and stress. These are counterproductive. Withdrawal may be a sign of frustration and anger
12. Regular and short periods of interaction planned throughout the day. Gradually increase the period of time spent with them	Where people are unable or find it difficult to initiate conversation with others, prolonged periods of conversation are stressful. It is more caring to show concern throughout the day rather than focus on one period of time. The rest of the day then becomes a period of isolation
13. If they are unresponsive, periodically sit by the person. Introduce yourself and then sit quietly	If you sit by someone and say "I thought I would keep you company/come and sit with you", it is perceived even by the most withdrawn person as caring and supportive
14. Respect the person's body space and do not talk "around" them	Failure to do this shows a complete lack of respect for the person. A withdrawn person is still alert to the environment
15. Engage in physical activity as a precursor to verbal interaction, e.g. games, activities, drama, music.	Sometimes it is easier for people to talk as part of an activity or game, or afterwards

Nursing intervention	*Rationale*
Organize social and recreational activities	
16. Encourage the person to express their feelings	People who find it difficult to communicate may have pent-up emotions. It also provides the opportunity for them to practise talking about their emotions which they may have had difficulty with in the past
17. Be available, minimize role barriers and be informal	You have got to look and be approachable. More likely then for communication to occur
18. Positively reinforce self-initiated interaction and communication	Important to reward attempts by person to communicate
19. Do not reinforce withdrawn behaviour. Communicate with the person when you are engaged in caring activities	At times it is easier to do things for people than to get them to clearly ask for themselves
20. Use open-ended questions	These require multiple word answers
21. Encourage social interaction with others. Organize group activities	Social activities can be very rewarding and also provide group dynamics that the person may find therapeutic
22. Identify situations with the person in which they experience anxiety or a communication difficulty in relating to others	Many people with mental health problems are either lacking in social skills or have problems relating to others (see also Unit 3.4)
23. Role play with feedback these situations with the person. Give demonstration and guidance as required. Provide information on the nature of human interaction and the expression of feeling.	Assertiveness training helps people to develop their communication and emotional expression skills. It is a structured approach in which specific assertiveness skills are: • identified and defined; • divided into their constituent elements; • the elements are practised with feedback in role-play until

Nursing intervention	Rationale
Provide information on the principles and application of assertiveness skills	competence is achieved; • the entire skill is practised with feedback until competence is achieved; • the skill is transferred to real-life situations
24. Organize experiential exercises, e.g. drama, role-play, games, in which the person relates to others in an unstructured way and can express themselves freely	Even very withdrawn people will participate in these types of activities. They enable people to participate in a non-threatening way and to get used to being spontaneous

Evaluation

1. Person able to approach others and communicate with them of their own initiative and choice.
2. Person demonstrates raised self-esteem and confidence in the language and non-verbal communication that they use.
3. Maintains eye contact and uses extended speech in communication.

F. Facilitate the Development of the Person's and Family's Coping Skills

Associated problems/personal difficulties

The experience of depression may reveal that:

1. The family found it difficult to understand and provide emotional support to the depressed person.
2. Current life-style, expectations and relationships may be potential sources of stress.
3. Existing methods of coping may be counterproductive and maladaptive.
4. The person and their family may lack information about the resources available to help them.
5. There may be feelings of guilt in relation to their problems and asking for help.

Assessment

1. Person and their family's perception of their current situation.
2. Existing coping methods used by person and family members and their effectiveness.
3. Support available to the person and their family.
4. Accuracy of the knowledge and information given by the person and their family.
5. Statements of guilt and stigma.
6. Awareness of resources available to them.
7. Previous experience, if any, of dealing with similar problems.

Desired outcomes

1. Person and family able to make an informed choice about the resources they require.
2. Person and family able to cope better with life and personal problems.

Nursing intervention	Rationale
1. Initiate therapeutic relationship. Involve person and family in the care and planning process	Interventions more likely to be successful in an atmosphere of trust and cooperation
2. Advise that seeking help and recognition of problems are a positive step towards finding solutions	Many people feel that seeking help is a sign of weakness and failure. Also helps to reduce guilt
3. Encourage questions. Provide accurate information. Identify appropriate health care resources	May have inaccurate knowledge and expectations. Fear of the unknown. Need to know what resources are available to them
4. Advise against early correction of problems	Under stress it is sometimes easier to make short-term adaptations that only store up future problems. It takes time to help the family to work out what is best for them
5. Reassure that there are ways of improving the situation	Family may feel that the situation is hopeless
6. Advise against recrimination and	Need to focus on the present and future and to deal with anger and guilt in a

Nursing intervention	*Rationale*
focussing on past problems	more productive way
7. Advise on the need for acceptance and mutual support within their relationships	Family needs to come to terms with their situation. They are each other's primary source of support, which will need to be utilized to cope effectively
8. Explain the need to identify and recognize potentially stressful situations. Recommend methods for coping with stress	Mental health problems tend to be long-term in nature. In order to cope effectively the family needs to be taught ways of making the necessary long-term adjustments
9. Teach methods for achieving relaxation. Teach how to use problem-solving methods for coping with difficulties. Assist the family to learn new communication and coping skills. Encourage the setting of realistic goals and expectations	Most of the education needs to be directed towards coping methods. These include the way that the members of the family communicate, their expectations and the way that emotional support is given. Life-style and relationship changes may be necessary
10. Review occupational/ unemployment stresses. Encourage the development of appropriate work-related coping strategies	Work and unemployment can be major sources of stress. As these encompass such a wide range of life events it is important that the person learns how to cope constructively with these stresses
11. Encourage the setting of progressive goals in small stages. Advise the family on how to give feedback and support to one another	The re-learning needs to be done in a gradual way in which the family provides the main support and reinforcement
12. Teach the family and person to recognize the limits of their ability to cope and when it is advisable to seek help. Put family in contact with self-help and voluntary groups	The family should not over-burden itself, as this can damage relationshps and its longer-term ability to cope. Self-help groups able to offer effective and understanding help

Evaluation

1. Person and family identify and select resources they require.
2. Person and family demonstrate use of improved coping methods.

Unit Instructions

When you have researched the suggested references, have mastered the Unit Objectives and successfully answered the Self-assessment Questions, proceed with the Unit Written Test.

Suggested References

Alchin, S. and Weatherhead, R. (1976). *Psychiatric Nursing: A Practical Approach*. McGraw Hill, Sydney.

Altschul, A. and McGovern, M. (1985). *Psychiatric Nursing*, 6th edition. Baillière Tindall, London and San Diego.

Andrews, R., Jenkins, J., and Sugden, J. (1985). Origins of sadness as a response. *Nursing*, Vol. 2, No. 34, pp. 995–998.

Barker, P. J. (1985). *Patient Assessment in Psychiatric Nursing*. Croom Helm, London.

Barker, P., Hume, A. and Robertson, W. (1985). Psychological therapy in affective disorders. *Nursing Mirror*, 29 May, Vol. 160, No. 22, pp. 34–36.

Bauer, B. and Hill, S. (1986). *Essentials of Mental Health Care Planning and Interventions*. W. B. Saunders, Philadelphia.

Burnard, P. (1986). Picking up the pieces. *Nursing Times*, 23 April, Vol. 82, No. 17, pp. 37–38.

Campbell, C. (1978). *Nursing Diagnosis and Intervention in Nursing Practice*. John Wiley, New York.

Darcy, P. T. (1984). *Theory and Practice of Psychiatric Care*. Hodder and Stoughton, London.

Darcy, P. T. (1985). *Mental Health Nursing Source Book*. Baillière Tindall, London and San Diego.

Dexter, G. and Wash, M. (1986). *Psychiatric Nursing Skills: A Patient-centred Approach*. Croom Helm, London.

Doona, M. E. (1979). *Travelbee's Intervention in Psychiatric Nursing*, 2nd edition. F. A. Davis, Philadelphia.

Dunn, G. and Rosen, B. (1982). When the family must change too. *Nursing Mirror*, 1 December, Vol. 155, No. 22, pp. 28–29.

Harkness, G. and Stricklan, P. (1987). My life's not worth living, nurse. *Nursing Times*, 9 September, Vol. 83, No. 36, pp. 46–48.

Hase, S. and Douglas, A. (1986). *Human Dynamics and Nursing*. Churchill Livingstone, Melbourne.

Hawton, K. and Catalan, J. (1981). Psychiatric management of attempted suicide patients. *British Journal of Hospital Medicine*, April, Vol. 25, No. 4, pp. 365–372.

Irving, S. (1983). *Basic Psychiatric Nursing*, 3rd edition. W. B. Saunders, Philadelphia.

Kreitman, N. and Dyer, J. (1981). Suicide and parasuicide. *Nursing*, October Vol. 1, No. 30, pp. 1310–1312.

Lancaster, J. (1980). *Adult Psychiatric Nursing*. Henry Kimpton, London.

Lyttle, J. (1986). *Mental Disorder*. Baillière Tindall, London and San Diego.

McFarland, G. and Wasli, E. (1986). *Nursing Diagnoses and Process in Psychiatric Mental Health Nursing*. J. B. Lippincott, Philadelphia.

MacKay, D. (1982). Cognitive behaviour therapy. *British Journal of Hospital Medicine*, March, Vol. 27, No. 3, pp. 242–247.

Martin, P. (Ed.) (1987a). *Psychiatric Nursing: A Therapeutic Approach*. Macmillan, London.

Martin, P. (1987b). *Care of the Mentally Ill*, 2nd edition. Macmillan, London.

Moore, I. (1986). Ending it all. *Nursing Times*, 12 February, Vol. 82, No. 7, pp. 48–49.

Moores, A. (1987). Walking back to happiness. *Nursing Times*, 21 October, Vol. 83, No. 42, pp. 55–57.

Pelletier, L. (Ed.) (1987). *Psychiatric Nursing Case Studies, Nursing Diagnoses and Care Plans*. Springhouse Corporation.

Ritter, S. (1981). Nursing and depression. *Nursing*, Vol. 1, No. 30, pp. 1313–1314.

Robinson, L. (1983). *Psychiatric Nursing as a Human Experience*, 3rd edition. W. B. Saunders, Philadelphia.

Rowe, D. (1983). Helping the depressed patient. *Nursing Times*, 26 October, Vol. 79, No. 43, pp. 63–65.

Rushforth, D. (1985). Deliberate self-harm. *Nursing Times*. 18 September, Vol. 81, No. 38, pp. 51–53.

Sundeen, S. *et al.* (1981). *Nurse–client Interaction*, 2nd edition. C. V. Mosby, London.

Self-assessment Questions

SAQ 15. Identify six nursing care interventions that can help to reduce the risk of self-harm.

SAQ 16. What nursing interventions can be used to help a depressed person communicate?

SAQ 17. Describe four problems that the depressed person may experience in meeting their basic physical needs.

SAQ 18. List four interactions that can be used to facilitate an up-lift in mood.

Unit 7.4: Written Test

David Johnson, aged 46, has been transferred to an acute care ward following an overdose. He had been made redundant 9 months ago and repeated attempts to secure another job had been unsuccessful. During this period his relationship with his wife had deteriorated and just recently he discovered that she had been having an affair with another man. Following a row with her he got himself drunk and does not remember any more until he woke up in the medical ward the next day. The psychiatrist that saw him diagnosed that he was suffering from reactive depression and thought that he was still potentially suicidal. David thinks that "everything is hopeless" and feels guilt that he has "let everyone down".

1. What nursing interventions can help to restore David's self-esteem?
2. How can the staff balance the need to prevent self-injurious behaviour and yet avoid unnecessary restrictions?
3. His wife has visited and feels that she would like to give their relationship another try. However, she is very concerned about David taking an overdose. How can the couple be helped to understand what has happened to them and to learn from this experience?

TOPIC 8

Obsessional-compulsive Reactions

At the end of this Topic the learner should aim to:

1. Describe the characteristic features of obsessional-compulsive reactions.
2. Outline the range of therapeutic interventions available for people suffering from obsessional-compulsive reactions.
3. Identify the nursing care needs and interventions required for the person with obsessional-compulsive behaviour.

The Characteristics of Obsessional-compulsive Reactions

Unit Objectives

At the end of this Unit the learner should be able to:

1. Explain the relationship between obsessional thoughts and compulsive behaviour.
2. Identify the characteristic features of an obsessional-compulsive reaction.
3. Describe common presenting patterns of obsessional behaviour.

Obsessional Thoughts and Compulsive Behaviour

Obsessional-compulsive reactions are a mental health problem characterized by the persistent intrusion of unwanted thoughts and ideas into the person's awareness. These thoughts are accompanied by:

1. An overwhelming sense of compulsion to carry out and complete a specific behavioural or cognitive ritual.
2. Resistance on the part of the individual who is aware of the irrationality and absurdity of the thoughts and compulsion. However hard they try, though, they cannot ignore or resist the thoughts.
3. Severe and mounting anxiety that will not be dissipated until the ritual is completed.
4. Fear of some imagined consequence if the obsessional ritual is not completed. Performance of the ritual provides temporary relief which paradoxically acts as positive reinforcement to the obsessional thought. Within a short interval the ideas intrude again and the obsessional-compulsive cycle commences.

Obsessional-compulsive reaction is a comparatively rare diagnosis in clinical practice. The true incidence is probably higher as people tend to hide and conceal their symptoms. Obsessional behaviour may also be an early sign of schizophrenia, but can be differentiated by the presence of other significant symptoms.

Perspectives on obsessional-compulsive reactions

From the psychoanalytic perspective, the obsessional-compulsive behaviour is seen as a way of trying to displace and cope with deep-seated anxiety. The ceremonials may also be seen as self-punishing rituals for repressed guilt. Within the psychoanalytic model of human development, the symptoms are significantly associated with regression to pre-genital and anal-erotic stages. Behaviourally, the symptoms may be regarded as patterns of behaviour and thought that have been progressively reinforced and integrated into the person's everyday living.

The obsessional symptoms can also be viewed as a way that the person has of coping with stress. It may not be a very effective coping method, and in many respects is counterproductive, but it does divert their attention and provide some temporary relief.

Origins of obsessional-compulsive reactions

1. *Social modelling*: upbringing in an environment where significant role models behave in an obsessional manner and reinforce similar behaviour.
2. *Stress*: that the person is having difficulty in coping with. This may be in relation to their present circumstances or unresolved stress from earlier periods of life.
3. *Obsessive personality*: rigid, punctual, neat, meticulous and systematic. Often such a person is also insecure, has difficulty coping with changes, has a low self-esteem and suffers from doubt and indecision. Their own lives may be ordered to a strict timetable and set of standards.
4. *Organic brain disease*: cerebral trauma may produce crude obsessional behaviour.

Onset

The symptoms tend to first appear during early adulthood (early 20s), though they can develop at any age. Women tend slightly to outnumber male sufferers. The intrusive thoughts and behaviour may begin insidiously and gradually become more pronounced. In this way they can become established as part of a person's general behaviour pattern before they fully realize how they are being affected. For some people the symptoms may start suddenly with no apparent cause.

Depending upon the nature of the obsessional thoughts and accompanying ritual, the person will experience varying degrees of disruption to their everyday life. This can range from an irritating need to comply with the ritual to a totally dominating and persistent behaviour pattern. At its most extreme it can be a cycle of thoughts, ritual and stress that leaves the individual completely exhausted, demoralized and unable to carry on with everyday life. Frequently, the individual also becomes depressed as a response to the obsession and their inability to control it. At times the person may even feel that they are going "mad" as they retain insight and yet are unable to resist the overwhelming power of the compulsion.

Presentation

Obsessional thoughts or ruminations

These are intrusive, persistent ideas and impulses. They may be unremitting philosophical, religious or fantasy topics that the person is compelled to dwell upon. Sometimes the ideas and impulses are of a sexual, blasphemous, obscene, aggressive or socially inappropriate nature. Often these are at odds with the person's moral and social code and can cause considerable personal distress and misery.

Compulsive rituals

The person feels compelled to complete some very specific pattern of behaviour in a very precise way. If they are thwarted in some way or fail to follow their imposed procedure then they have to start all over again. With a very exacting ritual it may take many attempts for them to accurately complete the performance to their own satisfaction. The relief is invariably short-lived and they are soon compelled to begin once more.

Frequently, the obsessive-compulsive cycle is concerned with acts of daily living and other domestic routines. These can include:

1. *Doubts*: the person is in a state of chronic indecision, repeatedly checking everything, e.g. doors, windows, switches, gas taps. They are unable to convince themselves that they have already just done these things.
2. *Hygiene*: the person believes that either they or part of their house is contaminated with dirt and bacteria. They begin an endless round of handwashing or cleaning rituals that invariably have to be repeated each time something is touched. These rituals can be particularly exhausting and time-consuming. The constant washing can cause serious skin problems and seriously interfere with family life.
3. *Food*: food has to be prepared in a very specific way if they are to be able to eat it. The cooking, cleanliness and presentation of the food are all critical. It may have to be eaten in a certain way and chewed a specific number of times before swallowing.
4. *Dressing*: clothes have to be arranged in a certain manner and put on in a set pattern. Frequently, it involves much checking in the mirror from all angles to make sure that they look "right". The person may constantly have to check on their appearance to re-affirm that they still conform to their set standards.

5. *Touching and counting*: the person feels compelled to touch or count certain objects constantly, e.g. paving stones, cars, bricks in a wall, patterns in wallpaper, etc., as they are passed or seen.

Unit Instructions

When you have researched the suggested references, have mastered the Unit Objectives and successfully answered the Self-assessment Questions, proceed with the Unit Written Test.

Suggested References

Beech, H. R. and Vaughan, M. (1978). *Behavioural Treatment of Obsessional States*. John Wiley, Chichester.

Hughes, J. (1986). *An Outline of Modern Psychiatry*, 2nd edition. John Wiley, New York.

Lyttle, J. (1986). *Mental Disorder*. Baillière Tindall, London and San Diego.

Orme, J. E. (1984). *Abnormal and Clinical Psychology: An Introductory Text*. Croom Helm, London.

Sims, A. (1983). *Neurosis in Society*. Macmillan, London.

Sims, A. (1988). *Symptoms in the Mind*. Baillière Tindall, London and San Diego.

Snaith, P. (1981). *Clinical Neurosis*. Oxford University Press, Oxford.

Trethowan, W. and Sims, A. (1983). *Psychiatry*, 5th edition. Baillière Tindall, London and San Diego.

Willis, J. (1976). *Clinical Psychiatry*. Blackwell Scientific, Oxford.

Self-assessment Questions

SAQ 1. Identify four characteristics of obsessive-compulsive neurosis.

SAQ 2. Describe three ways that obsessional thoughts can cause stress to the individual.

SAQ 3. List four commonly occurring obsessional rituals.

SAQ 4. State four ways that one of the obsessional rituals you identified can adversely affect a person and their family.

Unit 8.1: Written Test

Jennifer Rushton, age 24, married with a young child aged 3, has referred herself to the community mental health centre. She describes a pattern of constant housekeeping, cleaning and ritualistic checking that is taking over her life.

1. What would indicate and confirm the obsessive-compulsive nature of this behaviour?
2. In what ways may her domestic rituals be·an attempt to cope with underlying stress?

Care and Treatment of the Person with an Obsessional-compulsive Reaction

---

Unit Objectives

At the end of this Unit the learner should be able to:

1. Describe the effects of obsessional behaviour and thoughts on a person's everyday life.
2. Outline the support required for the person and their family in the community.
3. Identify potential therapeutic interventions for obsessional-compulsive reactions.

Care and Treatment

A wide range of psychotherapeutic techniques may be used to help the person with an obsessional-compulsive reaction. These may focus primarily on the person's thoughts and behaviour or on more general aspects of the person's mental health. The methods chosen will depend upon the nature and severity of the person's presenting symptoms and the clinician's skills and theoretical orientation. The general approach should be an integrated programme that will support the person and their family in the community or in residential care as required.

Therapeutic aims

1. To minimize the distressing influence of obsessive-compulsive behaviour and thoughts.
2. To enable the person to regain control of their behaviour and thought processes.
3. To facilitate the development of the person and their family's coping skills.

Family and Self-care

Most people with obsessional behaviour do not necessarily regard themselves as having a mental health problem and, consequently, do not seek, and may not require, any outside intervention. They may live extremely well-regulated and ritualized lives that their families may tolerate or even participate in. In some areas of life their meticulous approach to detail and constant re-checking may be regarded as positive assets.

Aware that their behaviour may cause concern to others, they often try to conceal their problems from others. Personal difficulties begin when their obsessive demands begin to extend beyond their personal control and to interfere seriously with their own and their family's life. The person can then become a virtual slave to their own self-imposed ritualistic demands, driven to the point of distraction, despair and exhaustion, unable to continue with their normal life.

Depending upon the resolve of their support network the person's obsessive behaviour may be tolerated to quite extreme degrees. In some respects they may even unwittingly reinforce the person's symptoms. The symptoms may fluctuate over a period of time or remain relatively unchanged. Occasionally, there is a slow improvement and even spontaneous recovery. Help is sought when the person and their family become aware that a real difficulty exists and that they are no longer able to cope. At first they may present with anxiety or depression rather than obsessional-compulsive problems. Initially, the person and their family can be helped by:

1. Accurate information about the symptoms and their effect.
2. Involvement in the care and treatment process.
3. Reassurance that effective intervention is possible.
4. The opportunity to talk freely about their problems.
5. The addresses of local voluntary and contact support groups for people with similar mental health problems.
6. Advising them of the necessity of ensuring compliance with treatment programmes.
7. Teaching the family problem-solving skills and developing their ability to cope.

Community Care

Community care involves a wide range of statutory and voluntary services that aim to provide comprehensive treatment and support. Many people with obsessional-compulsive neurosis can be successfully treated and cared for at home. This will depend upon the support of the family, the severity of the symptoms and the skills available within the community mental health team. The aims of community care are:

1. To support the person and their family.

2. To minimize the influence of the obsessional rituals on the family and person.
3. To implement community-based treatment and care programmes.

The services involved include:

1. The community mental health centre: with community psychiatric nurses, social workers, psychologists, occupational therapists and consultant psychiatrists working as a team to offer skills-based therapeutic interventions.
2. General practitioners.
3. Voluntary agencies: MIND, Citizen's Advice Bureau, contact and support groups for sufferers and relatives.
4. DHSS: benefits, allowances and grants as currently available to individuals and their families.
5. Out-patient clinics and day hospitals.

Residential Care

The reasons for admission to residential facilities for care and treatment include:

1. Lack of support in the community.
2. Personal and family exhaustion.
3. Personal or physical risk due to the nature of the obsession or accompanying depression.
4. The need to remove the person from an environment that actively reinforces the obsession.
5. Detailed assessment and the need for specific types of therapy.

Therapeutic Interventions

Psychotherapeutic methods

1. *Skilled nursing care*: one of the most important factors.
2. *Individual counselling or psychotherapy*: to increase insight into their behaviour, to resolve repressed guilt and anxiety.
3. *Group therapy*: to increase insight and self-awareness.
4. *Family therapy*: to help the family cope with stress and to reorganize family life in the absence of time-consuming rituals. Obsessional behaviour may have been very disruptive of normal relationships for a considerable time.
5. *Behavioural psychotherapy*: a wide range of potential approaches that aim to teach the person to regain control of their thoughts and behaviour.

They are probably the most effective therapeutic approach for obsessional behaviour. The specific intervention will depend upon the detailed assessment of the obsession and the therapist's clinical experience:

(a) *Anxiety management training*: to control anxiety and tension. To use the relaxation skills to gradually overcome the obsession in association with other behavioural approaches.

(b) *Modelling*: the person watches the therapist model the desired behaviour and shows that they come to no harm, e.g. not washing their hands after touching something. The person is then encouraged to carry out the same behaviour and imitate the therapist – "participant modelling".

(c) *Response prevention*: the person is restrained from completing their ritual by discussion, persuasion, social reinforcement or, if appropriate, intervention. This may be used progressively with an increasing interval of response prevention until the person learns to control their anxiety.

(d) *Systematic desensitization*: the person is helped to identify a hierarchy of anxiety-provoking situations in relation to their obsession. The person is then exposed to the least anxiety-provoking situation and is encouraged to practice incompatible relaxation responses. When the person has mastered this situation they progress to the next most anxiety-provoking situation and again practice their relaxation skills. This pattern is repeated until the person is comfortable with previously stress-inducing situations.

(e) *Flooding*: the client agrees to prolonged exposure to their obsessional-producing situation. After a period of time the overwhelming anxiety subsides and the person also realizes that the feared consequences have not happened. It may require several repeated exposures for the person to regain control of their behaviours in this way.

(f) *Thought stopping*: a procedure that focusses on eliminating the unwanted distressing and repetitive thoughts. The person is encouraged to bring the obsessive thoughts into their consciousness. After a short interval the therapist may say or shout the word "stop". This is done to distract the person from their obsessive thoughts and their attention is drawn to the fact that they are now thinking about something else. This is practised until the person is able to halt the thought on the command "stop". The person is shown how to do this and further practises until they have regained control of their thoughts. After a while they no longer need to say the word "stop" audibly and can use sub-vocal speech. This approach may also be combined with progressive relaxation.

(g) *Self-regulation and self-reinforcement procedures*: all forms of therapy require the active participation of the client. If the person is given clear instructions they will be able to complete various homework assignments. It is possible to teach them specific techniques that they can use as self-administered therapy. Self-monitoring, in which the person keeps a detailed record of the frequency and duration of their unwanted thoughts, is effective in reducing the frequency of the obsessive thoughts. It also provides useful information for the therapist. Cue cards can be given which are a self-instructional aid to reinforcing positive behaviour and cognitions. Other applicable techniques can be taught to clients.

6. *Occupational therapy*: to teach activities of daily living based upon realistic and non-obsessional patterns.

Physical treatment methods

1. *Chemotherapy*: used to treat accompanying symptoms as a consequence of the obsession.

   (a) Minor tranquillizers for short-term use only where the person has severe anxiety.
   (b) Tricyclic antidepressants where the person presents as significantly depressed. Clomipramine (Anafranil) appears to be particularly effective in cases of depression associated with obsessional-compulsive neurosis.

2. *Electroconvulsive therapy (ECT)*: for accompanying depression. It has no therapeutic effect on the obsessional behaviour.
3. *Psychosurgery*: prefrontal leucotomy is performed only in very rare and exceptional cases. It is a method of last resort to reduce distressing anxiety where all other therapeutic interventions have failed and the person is extremely disabled by their obsession. It is rarely used.

Outcomes

The outcome of therapeutic interventions can be very difficult to predict. A significant proportion of people (75–80%) show some degree of improvement. This may range from complete recovery to relief from the most distressing aspects of the condition. Some people are very resistant to treatment and suffer from chronic obsessional-compulsive symptoms.

Significant factors in determining the prognosis include:

1. The history of the obsessional-compulsive reaction: in particular, the length of time that it has been established.
2. The attitude of the person and their family to the obsessive behaviour: whether there is collusion and reinforcement in the maintenance of the symptoms, their motivation to participate in treatment, whether they regard it as a problem.
3. The presence of other significant psychiatric symptoms, particularly depression.

4. The detail of the ritual, what it involves, the degree of tension and compulsion experienced, how alien it is to the person's life-style, environmental consequences.
5. Personality of the person, particularly whether they exhibit traits associated with an obsessional personality.

Unit Instructions

When you have researched the suggested references, have mastered the Unit Objectives, and successfully answered the Self-assessment Questions, proceed with the Unit Written Test.

Suggested References

Barker, P. J. (1982). *Behaviour Therapy Nursing*. Croom Helm, London.

Beech, H. R. and Vaughan, M. (1978). *Behavioural Treatment of Obsessional States*. John Wiley, Chichester.

Bloch, S. (1986). *An Introduction to the Psychotherapies*, 2nd edition. Oxford University Press, Oxford.

Hughes, J. (1986). *An Outline of Modern Psychiatry*, 2nd edition. John Wiley, New York.

Lyttle, J. (1986). *Mental Disorder*. Baillière Tindall, London and San Diego.

Mercer, S. (1984). Obsessional compulsive disorder. *Nursing Times*, 19 August, Vol. 80, No. 35, pp. 34–37.

Patterson, C. H. (1986). *Theories of Counselling and Psychotherapy*, 4th edition. Harper and Row, New York.

Simmons, S. and Brooker, C. (1986). *Community Psychiatric Nursing: A Social Perspective*. Heinemann Nursing, London.

Snaith, P. (1981). *Clinical Neurosis*. Oxford University Press, Oxford.

Trethowan, W. and Sims, A. (1983). *Psychiatry*, 5th edition. Baillière Tindall, London and San Diego.

Willis, J. (1976). *Clinical Psychiatry*. Blackwell Scientific, Oxford.

Self-assessment Questions

SAQ 4. What is meant by the term "response prevention"?

SAQ 5. Describe how the technique of thought stopping is used to overcome obsessional thoughts.

SAQ 6. How is systematic desensitization used in the treatment of obsessional-compulsive neurosis?

SAQ 7. In what ways can a person with obsessional-compulsive neurosis contribute to their own therapy?

Unit 8.2: Written Test

Roger Steadman, aged 42, has been admitted for assessment and treatment of a longstanding obsessional-compulsive problem. His life is completely dominated by rituals that involve counting and re-checking. At his job as a warehouseman, with responsibilities for safety, his qualities have been particularly useful to him.

1. What psychotherapeutic interventions may be used to help him regain control of his obsessional behaviour?

Nursing Care of the Person who is Obsessional

Mental Health Nursing Care

Each person's care needs are unique and have to be assessed individually. A range of potential care needs have been selected to illustrate the problems that the person may experience and the possible nursing interventions that may help them. For the person presenting with obsessional behaviour these may include the needs to:

A. Resist obsessional-compulsive thoughts and rituals.
B. Feel secure and free from threat.
C. Restore their self-esteem.
D. Experience relief from stress and tension.
E. Meet their basic physical needs.
F. Facilitate the development of the person's and family's coping skills.

A. Resist Obsessional-compulsive Thoughts and Rituals

Associated problems/personal difficulties

Person with obsessional behaviour may experience great difficulties in relation to:

1. An inability to resist intrusive obsessional thoughts.
2. An overwhelming compulsion to carry out behavioural or cognitive rituals.
3. Severe anxiety if ritual is not completed in a specific way.
4. Complete disruption to everyday patterns and activities of living.
5. Total pre-occupation with obsessional thoughts and behaviour to the exclusion of other needs.
6. Potential for exhaustion and damage to their physical well-being.

Assessment

1. Person's description of their obsessional-compulsive thoughts and behaviour and their effects on everyday living.
2. Family's observations of the person's obsessional behaviour.
3. Nurse's observations of the:

   (a) Specific behavioural ritual: a detailed description of what is actually done, where it takes place, frequency and duration of the ritual, pattern of ritual throughout the day, reaction to disruption of the ritual, ability to control or resist the ritual, intervals between rituals.
   (b) Obsessional thoughts: nature and content of intrusive thoughts, frequency and duration of intrusive thoughts, pattern of obsessional thoughts throughout the day, ability to resist obsessional thoughts, effectiveness of coping strategies for resisting obsessional thoughts, intervals between obsessional thoughts.
   (c) Emotional reaction to obsessional thoughts and ritualistic behaviour: intensity and duration of emotional distress experienced, emotional effects of attempting to resist rituals. Degree of relief experienced by completion of ritual.
   (d) Psychosocial environment: presence of identifiable eliciting stimuli or triggering cues, reactions of others to person's ritualistic behaviour. Potential reinforcers of obsessional behaviour and thoughts. Presence of potential stresses in the person's environment and life-style.

4. Physical consequences: potential harm arising from ritualistic behaviour, interference with attainment of physical needs.

Desired outcomes

1. Person is able to resist obsessional thoughts.
2. Person is able to resist compulsive urges.
3. Person is able to exert positive control of their behaviour.

Nursing intervention	Rationale
1. Initiate therapeutic relationship. Involve them in the care planning process	Interventions more likely to succeed in an atmosphere of trust and cooperation
2. Provide reassurance about potential for positive change and for regaining control of their thoughts and behaviour	Person may feel that their situation is hopeless after their own inability to regain control
3. Acceptance of the person. Non-judgemental and non-critical approach.	Helps to minimize distress and create the conditions for behavioural change. Person may be feeling guilty and worthless about their difficulties.
4. Promote self-esteem	Improving self-esteem helps to improve their self-image in relationships with others. Raising self-esteem also increases their commitment to regain personal control. The person is very sensitive to implied criticism
5. Provide opportunities for the person to express themselves openly and honestly	Helps to relieve tension and to demonstrate acceptance
6. Explore with the person the effects of their behaviour on their own and their family's life	Person may not be fully aware of how their behaviour is disrupting their life and relationships
7. Offer feedback on the person's behaviour and use it as a learning situation	Person may not be fully aware of how much their obsessional behaviour is dominating their life
8. Teach the person how to keep a log or diary of their obsessional thoughts and rituals	Self-recording promotes insight and helps to reduce the frequency of obsessional rituals. Also provides useful data for the therapist
9. Encourage them to identify specific factors related to the obsession, e.g. time, situation, if anything triggered off the	Can be used to identify any environmental factors that may be amenable to modification

Nursing intervention	Rationale
thought, details of the ritual, emotions experienced	
10. Assist the person to identify any environmental factors related to their obsessions	Person may not be aware of the way that environmental factors are influencing their behaviour
11. Encourage the person to modify environmental factors where possible that are contributing to obsessional thoughts and behaviour	Modification of contributing environmental factors may help to reduce stimuli that elicit obsessional thoughts
12. Negatively reinforce obsessional behaviour and cognitions. Positively reinforce non-obsessional and incompatible behaviour	Helps to decrease frequency of obsessional behaviour
13. Teach family members the skills of giving reinforcement to target behaviour	Family members may be inadvertently contributing to the maintenance of obsessional behaviour
14. Provide support when the person is attempting to resist obsessional thoughts and compulsive rituals	Resisting the compulsion is a very stressful experience. The person benefits from recognition and acceptance of this difficulty
15. Reassure about the non-harmful consequence of not completing ritualistic behaviour	Person may fear damaging consequences if unable to complete rituals
16. Model non-obsessional responses for person in situations where they respond ritualistically	Modelling can be a powerful influence for positive behaviour change
17. Role play non-obsessional responses with person. Provide guidance and feedback.	Practice in this way can be a useful stage in regaining behavioural control.

Nursing intervention	*Rationale*
18. Advise the person if their behaviour is a risk to themself or others	Promotes insight and shows that others are concerned for their welfare
19. Set limits on behaviour that is potentially self-harming. Persuade or intervene directly to stop ritual if person is at risk	Obsessional symptoms have the potential for physical harm. This may be through excessive washing, exhaustion, nutritional deficits, etc.
20. Explain the objectives of response prevention. Gain person's cooperation in a response prevention programme. Consistently implement response prevention programme. Provide feedback to the person on their attainment	Prolonged response prevention with support helps person to gradually regain control of their behaviour. Also shows that feared consequences do not happen
21. Explain the objectives of "thought stopping". Assist person to identify pattern of cognitions and triggering cues associated with their obsessional behaviour. Encourage person to focus on stated commands instead of obsessional thoughts. Rehearse thought-stopping until person is able to focus on command statements. Instruct person in skills of self-administered verbal instructions. Support person's practice until proficient. Provide feedback to the person on their attainment	Thought stopping can be an effective intervention for some people. It also serves to promote insight and to instil hope. Initially the therapist controls the programme. The skill is practised until the person is proficient. Responsibility is gradually handed over to the person

Nursing intervention	*Rationale*
22. Teach person the skills of progressive relaxation (see pp. 242–244)	An important intervention in obsessional-compulsive neurosis where anxiety plays a key part
23. Identify with person significant anxiety-provoking situations in relation to obsessional thoughts and behaviour	Person is likely to have a range of situations that cause differing degrees of anxiety
24. Assist person to rank these situations from least to most anxiety-provoking	These may be in terms of real or imagined situations. An anxiety ranking schedule or questionnaire may be helpful to achieve this
25. Expose person to least anxiety-provoking situation and at the same time encourage them to commence relaxation. Continue and practice until the person feels able to relax when exposed to least anxiety-provoking situation. Provide positive feedback on person's progress. Progressively work through hierarchy of anxiety-provoking situations. Ensure satisfactory coping at each stage	Systematic desensitization works as a process of gradual re-learning. The principle is for the person to gradually regain control and mastery of previously anxiety-provoking situations. Learning in small stages facilitates success and minimizes opportunities for failure. The physiological responses of relaxation are incompatible with being stressed by anxiety-eliciting stimuli. This also helps the person to develop more positive cognitions towards previously anxiety-provoking situations
26. Explore person's expectations and self-imposed standards	Many obsessional people have very high and unattainable expectations
27. Assist the person to acknowledge the influence of their expectations and personal standards on their behaviour. Explore alternative expectations and standards. Help person to develop	This creates a great pressure on them. The person needs to be helped to reshape their beliefs about themself and to develop more valid and realistic expectations

Nursing intervention	Rationale
more attainable expectations and standards. Encourage acceptance of self-limitations	
28. Provide appropriate written cue cards that reinforce positive cognitions and non-obsessional behaviour. Explain how to use cue cards	Cue cards provide a self-administered therapy that the person can use to regain control of their thoughts and behaviour

Evaluation

1. Occurrence of obsessional thoughts decreases.
2. Person demonstrates control of obsessional thoughts.
3. Incidence of ritualized behaviour decreases.

B. Feel Secure and Free from Threat

Associated problems/personal difficulties

Person with obsessional behaviour may feel insecure and threatened as a result of:

1. Persistent and intrusive thoughts that they are unable to resist or understand.
2. Behavioural rituals that they are unable to control.
3. Fears of the consequences if rituals are not completed.
4. Stresses that their behaviour causes in their relationships.
5. Inadequate knowledge and understanding of their care and treatment programme.

Assessment

1. Person's description of their anxieties and worries.
2. Comments made by relatives and friends.
3. Nurse's observations of the person's:

   (a) Response to questioning about their anxieties
   (b) Understanding: questions asked and statements made in relation to their health needs and treatment programme
   (c) Emotional status: concerns expressed, emotions displayed, edginess, irritability, tearfulness

(d) Non-verbal behaviour indicating anxiety: posture, gestures, tone of voice, eye movements
(e) Tension demonstrated in relation to their obsessional-compulsive behaviour.

4. Identification of potential stressors in the person's relationships, life-style and expectations.

Desired outcomes

1. Person is more relaxed and feels free from threat.
2. Person and family's understanding of their health care needs are increased.

Nursing interventions	Rationale
1. Initiate a therapeutic relationship. Spend time with them. Be available and approachable. Demonstrate active listening. Use touch. Ensure non-judgemental and non-critical approach	Interventions more likely to be successful in an atmosphere of trust and cooperation. Also shows sense of worth and acceptance which helps to increase feelings of security and safety. Being non-judgemental helps a person to deal with their guilt
2. Adopt a non-threatening, open posture and tone of voice	Reduces feelings of anxiety
3. Provide clear and understandable information about their treatment, health care and the roles of different health care workers. Encourage questions. Ask for feedback on their understanding. Clarify any misunderstandings. Enlist the person's cooperation in the planning of their health care. Promote their autonomy and self-esteem	A lot of anxiety is associated with fear of the unknown. People have a right to information about their health care. The nurse is in an ideal position to use this process to facilitate the development of the person's understanding about their health care needs. People are more likely to cooperate if they are well-informed and involved in the decision-making process

Nursing interventions	*Rationale*
4. Explain all actions in advance	Increases feelings of trust in carers
5. Ensure that significant personal items are available	Familiar objects help to increase feelings of security
6. Encourage the person to express their feelings about their behaviour and difficulties	Being labelled mentally ill is a very stigmatizing process. The person feels guilty and bewildered. There is also a sense of loss over the change of role and self-identity
7. Encourage the person to talk about their stressful feelings. Encourage them to express their feelings in an appropriate way. Provide feedback to the person on their behaviour and use it as a learning situation	Venting their feelings in this way may reduce some of the pressure experienced in relation to their obsessive-compulsive rituals. Provides an opportunity for health education in the appropriate expression of emotional stress. Helps to promote insight
8. Approach unhurriedly. Demonstrate calmness. Do not rush the person. Be aware of your own reactions and experiences of stress	Anxiety in the carer communicates itself to the person. Caring can be a stressful experience at times. This may unconsciously influence your interactions with others
9. Be patient and aware of your own feelings of frustration in dealing with the person	The person may be very demanding and resistant to interventions. Find ways of coping with your own stress
10. Facilitate the development of the person's ability to communicate and relate to others	Helps the person to express and thereby release feelings of anxiety and tension
11. Encourage diversional recreational and social activities	Helps to divert the person's attention away from obsessional thoughts. Diversional physical activity is also a beneficial channel for stress
12. Encourage the person to rest or relax if they appear to be under stress. Provide feedback on their behaviour	Person may not be aware of the effect of anxiety on their behaviour or their health needs

Nursing interventions	Rationale
13. Emphasize the importance of recognizing internal tension and external stressors. Recommend methods for reducing sensory stimulation. Teach methods for achieving relaxation. Teach how to use problem-solving methods in coping with stress. Assist the person to learn new coping skills for anxiety (see pp. 255–270)	Providing a programme of health education offers a longer-term strategy for dealing with anxiety in the person's life
14. Encourage the person to set realistic goals	Unrealistic goals cause frustration and are likely to lead to failure
15. Encourage the setting of progressive goals in small stages in relation to regaining control of thoughts and behaviour	Minimizes risk of failure
16. Provide emotionally safe experiences to increase their sense of mastery	Stress interferes with learning and can create feelings of helplessness

Evaluation

1. Person demonstrates relaxed behaviour and calmness.
2. Person demonstrates trust in their care and treatment.

C. Restore Their Self-esteem

Associated problems/personal difficulties

Person with obsessional behaviour may be experiencing a severe loss of self-esteem as a result of:

1. Feelings of hopelessness at their inability to control intrusive thoughts and ritualistic behaviour.

2. Disruption to normal patterns of living.
3. Stress caused to close relationships by their behaviour.
4. Prolonged emotional distress and demoralization.
5. Feelings of guilt and worthlessness.

Assessment

1. Person's description of their perceived self-worth at present.
2. Identify the criteria that the person uses to evaluate their self-worth in relation to others.
3. Nurse's observations of the effects of low self-esteem upon the person's:

   (a) Communication: negative self-statements, self-criticism, inferiority and inadequacy. Statements of guilt, worthlessness and hopelessness. Volume, tone, clarity and rate of speech.
   (b) Behaviour: passive, non-assertive, social anxiety, withdrawn, avoidance, submissive posture, avoiding eye contact.
   (c) Emotions expressed: sadness, failure, rejection, guilt, hopelessness.
   (d) Reactions to situations that challenge their self-esteem.
   (e) Specific activities that influence the person's self-esteem.

4. Social reinforcement available to the person: partner, friends, personal possessions, personal events, activities and interests, financial, occupational.
5. Potential stressors in the person's life and their ability to cope with them.
6. Personal experiences of success, coping and failure.

Desired outcomes

1. To assist the person to formulate a more positive self-image.
2. For the person to make positive personal statements that indicate self-worth.
3. For the person to make positive future-orientated statements.

Nursing interventions	Rationale
1. Initiate therapeutic relationship with key worker. Involve the person in the care planning process	Interventions more likely to be successful in an atmosphere of trust and cooperation. Reinforces sense of self-worth and individuality
2. Use the person's preferred name.	Personal recognition of individuality reinforces sense of identity and

Nursing interventions	*Rationale*
Facilitate the use of personal belongings. Personalize the person's intimate environment. Show recognition of person's attainments. Emphasize the person's value as an individual. Spend time with them	promotes self-esteem. This also promotes the person's feelings of security and potential for change. Helps to promote self-esteem and show concern
3. Identify and help to celebrate significant personal dates, e.g. birthdays, anniversaries. Encourage personal interests. Promote contact with relatives and personal friends. Increase opportunities for group interaction. Increase environmental stimulation	Potential situations for personal reinforcement that may also help to raise mood helps to overcome feelings of isolation and rejection. Still valued by others. Avoids boredom and increases potential distractions
4. Gradually increase personal responsibility in small stages. Set graded task assignments	Need to avoid situations of potential failure and to increase the opportunity for experience of success. This can be very reinforcing
5. Explore self-criticism. Identify criteria used to evaluate self. Assist the person to acknowledge the influence of these criteria on their self-esteem. Explore alternative ways of evaluating their self-worth. Help person to develop internal sources of self-esteem	Many obsessional people have very harsh and unattainable expectations of themselves. Inevitably, this leads to feelings of failure, guilt, self-blame and worthlessness. Hence depression is a significant aspect of an obsessional-compulsive disorder
6. Identify and work with their strengths and resources. Encourage acceptance of self-limitations	The person needs to be helped to re-shape their beliefs about themself and to develop more valid and realistic expectations
7. Offer alternative interpretations of life experiences that person	When depressed, people tend to see everything negatively and to misperceive events in a way that is

Nursing interventions	*Rationale*
uses to devalue themselves. Encourage awareness of positive responses from others. Promote a realistic assessment of situations	personally devaluing
8. Explore previous achievements and successes. Increase personal responsibility in small stages. Encourage gradual mastery of situations. Reinforce initiatives taken by person. Respect personal decisions	They tend to devalue all past attainments. Gradually need to reintroduce personal control over behaviour and life circumstances
9. Help the person to work through periods of indecisiveness. Demonstrate decision-making skills. Role play situations on decision-making and initiative. Use drama and experiential methods to promote insight and spontaneity	Indecisiveness is a common difficulty in obsessional people. It can cause great stress and prolonged vacillation that can reinforce obsessional responses. Person needs the opportunity to safely explore being spontaneous. They often lead very rigid and regulated lives
10. Teach the skills and principles of assertiveness (see Unit 3.4)	Increases personal control that can be expressed in a more effective way. Increases confidence, self-esteem and the ability to communicate
11. Identify options for work and leisure activities	Relieves boredom and helps to raise self-esteem if meaningfully employed
12. Provide factual information about the incidence of obsessional-compulsive reactions in the community	Reassuring to find that they are not "unique". Person may feel guilty and stigmatized about receiving psychiatric treatment. This can be damaging to their self-esteem
13. Encourage them to pay attention to their hygiene and appearance	Appearance and hygiene are two important factors in self-esteem. Feeling clean and looking presentable help to improve the person's self-image and the way they appear to others

Evaluation

1. Increase in the frequency of positive personal statements.
2. Decrease in the incidence of negative self-statements.
3. Demonstrates more assertive verbal and non-verbal communications.
4. Makes future-orientated statements and plans.
5. Indicates hope in their future recovery.

D. Experience Relief from Stress and Tension

Associated problems/personal difficulties

A person with obsessional behaviour may be experiencing considerable stress and tension as a result of:

1. An inability to resist distressing obsessive thoughts.
2. Attempts to resist compulsions causing great anguish.
3. Considerable apprehension if obsessive ritual is not completed.
4. Person's behaviour creating conflict with their relatives.
5. Apprehension about their future.

For assessment, desired outcomes and nursing interventions, refer to Unit 6.3.

E. Meet Their Basic Physical Needs

Associated problems/personal difficulties

The experience of obsessional-compulsive disorder may interfere with a person's ability to meet their basic physical needs by:

1. Focussing all attention on their obsessional thoughts and behaviour.
2. Interfering with their ability to rest, thereby driving them to exhaustion.
3. Ritualistic practices that can be time-consuming and damaging to the person's physical health.
4. Obsessional food preparation practices that restrict nutritional intake.
5. Elimination rituals and practices that can be time-consuming and possibly damaging.

Assessment

1. Person's statements and behaviour in regard to meeting their needs for nutrition, fluids, hygiene and rest.

2. Statements by family members in regard of the person's ability to meet their physical needs.
3. Nurse's observations of:

   (a) Person's independent activities in relation to meeting their physical needs.
   (b) Family member's interventions in helping the person to meet their needs.
   (c) Identifiable deficits in a person's physical needs.
   (d) Potential health risk factors arising from person's behaviour patterns.
   (e) Potential for regaining control.

Desired outcomes

1. Person is enabled to independently meet their own physical needs.
2. Person demonstrates a raised self-esteem in relation to regaining control of their physical needs.
3. Family members promote independence and autonomy.

Nursing intervention	Rationale
1. Initiate therapeutic relationship	Interventions more likely to be successful in an atmosphere of trust and cooperation
2. Facilitate the ability of the person to resist obsessional-compulsive thoughts and rituals (see **A.**)	Regaining control and mastery of their thoughts and behaviour is a key step in enabling them to meet their physical needs
3. Advise the person and family on the importance of meeting physical needs	May not be aware of these needs or their role in health promotion
4. Inform the family of potential health risks in person's obsessional behaviour	May not be aware of the risks inherent in obsessional practices
5. Question the person and family on knowledge of hygiene and nutritional preparation. Provide accurate information	People concerned may have inaccurate and unrealistic expectations of hygiene. Need to have an accurate knowledge base

Nursing intervention	Rationale
6. Negotiate with the person and family a programme to meet physical needs. Specify requirements for nutrition, hygiene, elimination and rest. Set clear limits on behaviour to meet physical needs	Involvement is more likely to promote compliance. Structure helps to give guidance and to meet minimum needs. Need to state boundaries on behaviour to minimize and prevent ritualistic implementation
7. Ensure compliance with programme. Reinforce compliance with programme. Monitor the implementation of the programme. Maintain observation of person's physical health status	Person will need to progressively regain control of behaviour patterns that may have been established for some time. They may need guidance, support and prompting during this period
8. Positively reinforce self-initiated and maintained compliance with programme to meet care needs. Gradually withdraw external limits and interventions	Indicates growing control of behaviour and awareness of needs. Person needs to gradually regain autonomy as they are able to cope with it
9. Ensure person gradually takes over own self-care activities	Autonomy is a positive step in health care recovery
10. Provide reassurance over periodic setbacks. Provide feedback on attainment to date	Person needs to overcome possible feelings of guilt and hopelessness

Evaluation

1. Person demonstrates non-ritualistic behaviour in regard to meeting their physical needs.
2. Person independently meets their own physical needs.
3. Behaviour patterns and thoughts no longer interfere with attainment of physical needs.

F. Facilitate the Development of the Person's and Family's Coping Skills

Associated problems/personal difficulties

The experience of obsessional behaviour may show that:

1. Existing methods of coping may be limited.
2. Current life-style expectations and relationships may be potential sources of stress.
3. Family members may find it difficult to offer emotional support to each other.
4. The person and their family may lack information about the resources available to help them.
5. There may be feelings of guilt in relation to their problems and asking for help.

Assessment

1. Person and family's description of their current situation.
2. Coping methods used and the support available.
3. Accuracy of the information given by the person and their family.
4. Statements of guilt and stigma.
5. Awareness of resources available to them.
6. Previous experience, if any, of dealing with similar problems.

Desired outcomes

1. Person and family able to make an informed choice about the resources they require.
2. Person and family able to use more appropriate coping skills for life and personal problems.

Nursing intervention	Rationale
1. Initiate therapeutic relationship	Interventions are more likely to be successful in an atmosphere of trust and cooperation
2. Advise that seeking help and recognition of problems are a positive step towards finding solutions	Many people feel that seeking help is a sign of weakness and failure. Helps to reduce guilt

Nursing interventions	*Rationale*
3. Encourage questions. Provide accurate information	May have inaccurate knowledge and expectations. Helps to promote understanding and reduce anxieties
4. Identify appropriate health care resources	Need to know what resources are available to them
5. Advise against early and unrealistic correction of problems	Under stress it is sometimes easier to make short-term adaptations that only store up future problems. It may take time to help the person work out what is best for them. Longstanding problems will also take time to resolve
6. Reassure that there are ways of improving the situation. Reassure that control of thoughts and behaviour can be regained. Advise against recrimination and focussing on past problems	Person and family may feel that it is not possible to make changes. Person and family may believe that loss of control is permanent. Need to focus on the present and future and to deal with stress in a more productive way. May be many stored-up resentments and frustrations, particularly in longstanding situations
7. Advise on the need for acceptance and mutual support within their relationships	Family needs to come to terms with their situation. They are each other's primary source of support which will need to be utilized to cope effectively
8. Explain the need to identify and recognize potentially stressful situations. Recommend methods for coping with stress	Mental health problems tend to be long-term in nature. In order to cope effectively the family need to be taught effective coping skills to deal with future stresses
9. Teach methods for achieving relaxation. Teach how to use problem-solving methods for coping with difficulties. Assist the family to learn new coping and communication skills. Encourage the setting of realistic goals and expectations. Encourage the setting up of progressive goals	Much of the education needs to be directed towards learning new coping methods. These include the way that the members of the family communicate, their expectations and the way that emotional support is given. The re-learning needs to be done in a gradual way in which the family provides the main support and reinforcement

Nursing intervention	*Rationale*
in small stages. Advise the family on how to give feedback and support to one another	
10. Encourage the use of newly acquired coping skills	Skills need to be used in order to become part of everyday living
11. Review occupational/ unemployment stresses. Encourage the development of appropriate work/non-work coping strategies	Work and unemployment can be major sources of stress. As these represent a major part of life, it is important that the person learns how to cope constructively with these stresses
12. Teach the family and person to recognize the limits of their ability to cope and when it is advisable to seek help	The family should not over-burden itself as this can damage relationships and its longer-term ability to cope
13. Put family in contact with self-help and voluntary group	Self-help groups able to offer effective and understanding practical help

Evaluation

1. Person and family identify and select resources they require.
2. Person and family able to give accurate information about their health care needs.
3. Person and family demonstrate use of improved coping methods.

Unit Instructions

When you have researched the suggested references, have mastered the Unit Objectives and successfully answered the Self-assessment Questions, proceed with the Unit Written Test.

Suggested References

Altschul, A. and McGovern, M. (1985). *Psychiatric Nursing*, 6th edition. Baillière Tindall, London and San Diego.

Barker, P. J. (1982). *Behaviour Therapy Nursing*. Croom Helm, London.

Barker, P. J. (1985). *Patient Assessment in Psychiatric Nursing*. Croom Helm, London.

Campbell, C. (1978). *Nursing Diagnosis and Intervention in Nursing Practice*. John Wiley, New York.

Darcy, P. T. (1985). *Mental Health Nursing Source Book*. Baillière Tindall, London and San Diego.

Dexter, G. and Wash, M. (1986). *Psychiatric Nursing Skills: A Patient-centred Approach*. Croom Helm, London.

Farrington, A. (1983). Obsessive-compulsive disorder. *Nursing Mirror*, 17 August, Vol. 157, No. 7, pp. vii–viii.

Irving, S. (1983). *Basic Psychiatric Nursing*, 3rd edition. W. B. Saunders, Philadelphia.

Lancaster, J. (1980). *Adult Psychiatric Nursing*. Henry Kimpton, London.

Lyttle, J. (1986). *Mental Disorder*. Baillière Tindall, London and San Diego.

McFarland, G. and Wasli, E. (1986). *Nursing Diagnoses and Process in Psychiatric Mental Health Nursing*. J. B. Lippincott, Philadelphia.

Martin, P. (Ed.) (1987a). *Psychiatric Nursing: A Therapeutic Approach*. Macmillan, London.

Martin, P. (1987b). *Care of the Mentally Ill*, 2nd edition. Macmillan, London.

Mercer, S. (1984). Obsessional-compulsive disorder. *Nursing Times*, 29 August, Vol. 80, No. 35, pp. 34–47.

Pelletier, L. (Ed.) (1987). *Psychiatric Nursing, Care Studies, Nursing Diagnoses and Care Plans*. Springhouse Corporation, Springhouse, Pennsylvania.

Robinson, L. (1983). *Psychiatric Nursing as a Human Experience*, 3rd edition. W. B. Saunders, Philadelphia.

Simmons, S. and Brooker, C. (1986). *Community Psychiatric Nursing: A Social Perspective*. Heinemann Nursing, London.

Self-assessment Questions

SAQ 9. List six observations that you would need to make in order to assess accurately a person's obsessional pattern of behaviour.

SAQ 10. Identify six possible interventions to enable a person with obsessional-compulsive neurosis to regain control of their thoughts and behaviour. ·

SAQ 11. Describe two possible objectives that would indicate a successful outcome for regaining control of their obsessional behaviour.

SAQ 12. State five ways in which obsessional-compulsive behaviour can be damaging to a person's physical health.

Unit 8.3: Written Test

Jennifer Baker, aged 24, has been experiencing increasing difficulty in coping since the birth of her son 2 years ago. Always a very meticulous and precise person, she has developed a range of domestic rituals and food preparation practices that are virtually dominating her life. She is obsessed with the idea of "dirt and germs everywhere" and attempts to keep her house spotlessly clean. The incessant cleaning has totally disrupted normal domestic life and her husband is worried about the effects upon their relationship and child. Jennifer's hands are sore with constant cleaning and she is worried about eating and drinking. She has little time for rest and experiences great anxiety if she falls behind in her cleaning schedule. Jennifer has been to her GP who originally prescribed her anxiolytics and then tricyclic antidepressants. However, these have had little effect and he has referred her to the nurse therapist at the local day hospital for assessment.

1. What observations will the nurse therapist need to make to confirm the obsessional nature of her problems?
2. Describe briefly four possible methods of intervention in obsessional behaviour patterns.
3. Describe in detail a nursing care programme designed to enable Jennifer to regain control of her obsessional thoughts and ritualistic behaviour.

TOPIC 9

Hysterical Reactions

At the end of this Topic the learner should aim to:

1. Describe the characteristic features of hysterical reactions.
2. Outline the range of therapeutic interventions available for helping people with hysterical reactions.
3. Identify the nursing care needs and interventions required for the person suffering from hysteria.

Understanding Hysterical Reactions

Unit Objectives

At the end of this Unit the learner should be able to:

1. Describe factors associated with the diagnosis of hysterical reaction.
2. Outline the theoretical role of psychological mechanisms in hysterical reactions.
3. Differentiate between the general presentation of hysterical symptoms and those with an identifiable pathology.

The Diagnosis of Hysterical Reactions

Hysterical reactions are classified as a neurotic mental disorder with a potentially infinite variety of presenting physical and mental symptoms. What is significant about hysterical reactions is that these symptoms are regarded as an unconscious attempt on the part of the individual to both cope with personal stress and to communicate their distress to others. The symptoms are psychologically generated and there is no identifiable underlying physical pathology.

In terms of current clinical practice, the diagnosis of hysterical reaction is rarely used and would appear to be decreasing. The term has become associated with derogatory and negative overtones, and to describe emotional outbursts rather than a specific mental health problem. There is also a growing school of thought who believe that the diagnosis is no longer justified. In cultural and contemporary terms, they regard the definition and use of the label "hysteria" as originating from a male-dominated and female-repressive perspective. Long-term studies have also indicated the difficulty of diagnosing hysterical reactions accurately. A number of people who were originally diagnosed as being "hysterical" have later been shown to have developed definite physical illnesses.

Nonetheless, the term is still used in clinical practice, even if only in reserved cases. Hence, it is important that the diagnosis is applied accurately to those cases where there are clear signs of personal and social stress, and physical causes and the prejudices of the diagnoser are definitely excluded.

Outside of the theoretical formulation of ego-defence mechanisms (see following section) it has been very difficult for researchers to identify significant factors in the causation of hysterical reactions. Some of the related factors appear to be:

1. *Social modelling*: early upbringing in an environment where people frequently used illness behaviour to reduce demands and to manipulate others.
2. *Hysterical personality*: with poor social and communication skills, immature, manipulative, insecure and demanding, low self-esteem, finds it difficult to face up to reality and responsibilities.
3. *Gender*: more common in women than men, possibly the effects of sex-role stereotyping and medical prejudice on female mental health problems.
4. *Limited intelligence*: with poor knowledge of the body and a lack of social and communication skills.
5. *Post-trauma*:

   - associated with head injury and brain damage;
   - where there is a possibility of financial compensation for the injury, i.e. "compensation neurosis".

6. *Heredity*: there is no identifiable genetical basis for hysteria.

The Dynamics of Hysterical Reactions

Theoretically, hysterical reactions are thought to be a classic example of the operation of certain psychological and social dynamics. It represents to the person a way of:

- coping with repressed stress and conflict, albeit in an ineffectual and maladaptive way;
- communicating with others, a plea for help and attention.

What is specific about hysterical reactions and differentiates them from malingering is that the underlying motivation is unconscious. The person is not aware of the mechanisms that are in operation and for them the symptoms are real.

In terms of psychoanalytic and social theory the person with a hysterical reaction is experiencing considerable underlying psychological or emotional stress. This stress may originate from earlier life experiences or be part of their present life circumstances. Being unable to cope with the stress effectively, the person unconsciously removes it from their awareness by repressing their feelings. However, this stress has to have an outlet and to be expressed in some way. Further psychological mechanisms then again, unconsciously, provide a means of channelling the stress.

1. *Conversion*: the expression of psychological stress through physical symptoms. Characteristically, the symptoms are seen to be symbolic of the nature of the conflict, though such a relationship may be hard to validate.
2. *Dissociation*: the expression of the stress through mental symptoms. Typically these represent an attempt to cut off from conscious awareness unpleasant and distressing feelings. Depending upon the nature and extent of the feelings being dissociated in this way, there will be a consequent disruption to mental processes. Hence mental functioning, memory and consciousness may be affected.

For the hysterical symptoms to be effective there also has to be, preferably, an illness rewarding situation. This is where the presence of physical or psychological symptoms will divert attention and also encourage support from others. Adoping a "sick role" is advantageous to the individual in terms of:

- primary gain – direct relief from the stress and tension experienced;
- secondary gain – sympathy and care, relief from responsibility and obligations.

Presentation of Hysterical Symptoms

Hysterical symptoms may present as an infinite variety of physical or mental complaints. These will depend upon:

1. The person's knowledge, experience and perceptions of physical and mental illnesses.
2. The person's cultural background, i.e. some symptoms are culturally specific.

However unrealistic the symptoms may seem to others, to the person affected they are very real. The potential for actual physical harm as a result of psychologically based symptoms should not be overlooked.

Physical presentation

1. *Sensory*: blindness, visual problems, tunnel vision, deafness, hearing problems. Localized anaesthesias: "glove and stocking" type that does not follow the anatomical distribution of sensory nerves.
2. *Motor*: partial or localized paralysis, ataxia, contractures, fits, tremors, dysphagia.
3. *General*: pain, headaches, dizziness, hyperventilation, anorexia, tachycardia, vague abdominal signs and symptoms, vomiting.

Psychological presentation

1. *Clouding of consciousness*: fugue, "disorientation" associated with wandering and flight from stress, trances, somnambulism.
2. *Memory loss*: amnesia, usually only lasting 24 hours; pseudodementia, give "approximate" answers to questions.

Differentiation of Hysterical Symptoms

Whichever signs and symptoms are presented in a hysterical reaction, there are a number of factors that differentiate them from diseases with an identifiable physical pathology:

1. There is no identifiable underlying organic pathology.
2. The symptoms do not correspond with known medical conditions. They represent the person's understanding of how their mind and body works. Hence, the presentation and combination of symptoms may not follow normal anatomical and physiological functioning and may be confused and unlikely.
3. There is a lack of anxiety and indifference to the symptoms even though they appear quite serious.
4. The person may react evasively and resist the concept that the disease has an underlying psychological cause.

As an example, the differentiation between physical fits and genuine epileptic fits is examined in Exhibit 9.1.1.

Exhibit 9.1.1 Differentiation between hysterical and epileptic fits

	Hysterical fit	*Epileptic fit (grand mal)*
Setting	Others present	May occur at any time or place
Onset	Gradual	Sudden
Risk	Chooses safe place	May suffer injury
Consciousness	Retained	Loss of consciousness
Sequence	No sequence – generalized twitching or flailing of arms and legs	Follows sequence of aura, tonic, clonic, coma and recovery stages
Movement	Increases in response to restraint	Restraint makes no difference
Pupils	Remain normal	Become dilated
Tongue	Not bitten	Risk of being bitten

Hysterical fit	Epileptic fit (grand mal)	
Response to painful stimuli	Responds to painful stimuli	No response: sensation slowly returns as recovers from seizure
Orientation	Usually well-orientated	May be confused and exhausted afterwards
Duration of fit	Dependent upon person's expectation	Varying length of time

---

Unit Instructions

When you have researched the suggested references, have mastered the Unit Objectives and successfully answered the Self-assessment Questions, proceed with the Unit Written Test.

Suggested References

Altschul, A. and McGovern, M. (1985). *Psychiatric Nursing*, 6th edition. Baillière Tindall, London and San Diego.

Dexter, G. and Wash, M. (1986). *Psychiatric Nursing Skills: A Patient-Centred Approach*. Croom Helm, London.

Hughes, J. (1986). *An Outline of Modern Psychiatry*, 2nd edition. John Wiley, Chichester.

Lancaster, J. (1980). *Adult Psychiatric Nursing*. Henry Kimpton, London.

Lyttle, J. (1986). *Mental Disorder*. Baillière Tindall, London and San Diego.

Orme, J. E. (1984). *Abnormal and Clinical Psychology: An Introductory Text*. Croom Helm, London.

Rees, L. (1982). *A Short Textbook of Psychiatry*. Hodder and Stoughton, London.

Robinson, L. (1983). *Psychiatric Nursing as a Human Experience*, 3rd edition. W. B. Saunders, Philadelphia.

Rycroft, C. (1968). *Anxiety and Neuroses*. Penguin, Harmondsworth.

Sims, A. (1988). *Symptoms in the Mind*. Baillière Tindall, London and San Diego.

Snaith, P. (1981). *Clinical Neurosis*. Oxford University Press, Oxford.

Trethowan, W. and Sims, A. (1983). *Psychiatry*, 5th edition. Baillière Tindall, London and San Diego.

Willis, J. (1976). *Clinical Psychiatry*. Blackwell Scientific, Oxford.

Self-assessment Questions

SAQ 1. Define the terms "conversion" and "dissociation".
SAQ 2. How does "secondary gain" benefit the person with hysteria?
SAQ 3. List four common psychological and physical presentations of hysteria.
SAQ 4. State four criteria that can be used to differentiate hysterical symptoms from those of a genuine physical illness.

Unit 9.1: Written Test

Janice Patterson has been in hospital for 2 weeks with a diagnosis of "hysterical reaction". Periodically she has fits and seizures, after which she wanders around apparently confused and disorientated.

1. What observations can the nursing staff make to confirm that these are hysterical and not genuine epileptic fits?
2. What underlying conscious motivation may there be for Janice to behave in this way?

Care and Treatment of the Person with a Hysterical Reaction

Unit Objectives

At the end of this Unit the learner should be able to:

1. Outline the therapeutic interventions available for the care and treatment of the person with a hysterical reaction.
2. Identify the support required for the person with a hysterical reaction and their family in the community.

Care and Treatment

There are no specific treatments for hysterical reactions. Whichever interventions are used it is important that they are implemented consistently and with confidence by the health care team. The general approach should be an integrated programme that will support the person and their family in the community or in residential care as required.

Therapeutic aims

1. To promote the person's insight and self-understanding.
2. To develop the person's ability to communicate and relate with others.
3. To facilitate the effectiveness of the person's and their family's coping skills.

Family and Self-care

The majority of people with hysterical symptoms are probably not in contact with any health care agency. Depending upon the symptoms they are experiencing and the reactions of their relatives, the majority probably exhibit a broad range of minor physical symptoms. These may become part of the individual's "personality" and family life may be built around the nature of the symptoms – someone's "deafness", "bad back", "headaches", "upset tummy", chronic pain, etc.

The individual may repeatedly attend their GP's surgery with a succession of vague and ill-defined complaints. The GP may respond to these physical symptoms or be alert to the underlying psychological problems of the person. They may become one of the many people who have repeat prescriptions for anxiolytics, antidepressants or night sedation.

If the presenting physical or psychological symptoms are particularly severe and evoke concern in the relatives, then they may insist that the person actively seeks medical intervention. This may also happen if they feel particularly stressed and are no longer able or willing to care for the person without outside support. The person, themselves, may initiate contact with health care services to validate their illness and to seek treatment.

Occasionally, the symptoms may occur as a sudden reaction to personal stress or a family crisis in order to unconsciously divert attention. The rapid onset of severe physical and psychological symptoms is likely to be effective, in the short term, of attaining this goal. Medical help is then likely to be sought as a matter of urgency.

Community Care

Community care can involve a wide range of services that are attempting to work with the person's psychological and physical problems. If the person is not at risk and their carers are able to cope, then it may be possible to initiate a community-based treatment programme. This has the advantage of not reinforcing the person's "sick role" and the legitimacy of their symptoms. Against this may have to be balanced the role of the family members in reinforcing and validating the hysterical person's behaviour. The aims of community care are:

1. To enable the person to remain in their own home.
2. To support the person and their family.
3. To implement community-based treatment and care programmes.

The services involved include:

1. The community mental health centre: with community psychiatric nurses, social workers, psychologists, occupational therapists and consultant psychiatrists working as a team to provide skills-based therapeutic interventions.
2. General practitioners.
3. Voluntary agencies: MIND, carer's support groups, Citizen's Advice Bureaux.
4. DHSS: benefits, allowances and grants as currently available to individuals and their families.

5. Department of Employment: Disablement Resettlement Officer (DRO), Register of Disabled Persons, re-training schemes.
6. Out-patient clinics and day hospitals: for individual and group therapeutic programmes.

Residential Care

Admission to a residential facility may be required in the following situations:

1. Excessive personal and family stress, especially if the support network is exhausted, frustrated and near to rejecting the affected person.
2. Family members are actively reinforcing the symptoms and dependency.
3. The need for detailed psychological assessment and for specific types of therapy not available in the community.
4. Thorough medical assessment to exclude the possibility of physical pathology. Once this has been completed and the possibility of physical illness ruled out, then the staff need to be firm and consistent in their approach. Hysteria feeds on doubt and the person will exploit situations of uncertainty.

Therapeutic Interventions

Psychotherapeutic methods

1. *Skilled nursing care*: one of the most important factors.
2. *Counselling and psychotherapy*: to promote insight and self-awareness, to raise self-esteem and autonomy.
3. *Group psychotherapy*: to develop their interpersonal understanding, communication and the way they relate to others.
4. *Behavioural psychotherapy*: to develop the person's social and communication skills and their assertiveness. Reinforcement of healthy patterns of behaviour, non-reinforcement of hysterical behaviour.
5. *Cognitive therapy*: may be appropriate in some situations to modify the person's perceptions, expectations and beliefs. Need to enhance a more reality-based model of awareness.
6. *Health education*: to develop more effective coping skills. To review lifestyle and stresses created.
7. *Occupational therapy*: life skills and activities of daily living. Diversional and recreational activities.
8. *Family or couple's therapy*: to help the partners communicate and relate more effectively. To develop their understanding of each other's needs and expectations.

Chemotherapy

Chemotherapy may be used to treat existing symptoms of anxiety or depression if these were thought to be present and significant to the person's clinical condition. The medication is not specific to the treatment of hysteria and some clinicians may be reluctant to prescribe tablets as these may reinforce the hysterical reaction. The type of medication that may be used includes:

1. *Minor tranquillizers*: diazepam, chlordiazepoxide, lorazepam.
2. *Antidepressants*: imipramine, amitriptyline, dothiepin, mianserin.

Outcomes

The outcomes for hysterical reactions are very uncertain and difficult to predict. Intervention by health care agencies may be sufficient to alter individual and family dynamics such that more healthy ways of relating and dealing with stress are developed. In some cases the person is very resistive and the symptoms intractable to treatment. It is quite possible for the symptoms to become chronic and the person to be in continuous or intermittent contact with various health care agencies.

Unit Instructions

When you have researched the suggested references, have mastered the Unit Objectives and successfully answered the Self-assessment Questions, proceed with the Unit Written Test.

Suggested References

Bloch, S. (Ed.) (1986). *An Introduction to the Psychotherapies*, 2nd edition. Oxford University Press, Oxford.

Douglas, T. (1976). *Groupwork Practice*. Tavistock, London.

Goldberg, D. and Huxley, P. (1980). *Mental Illness in the Community*. Tavistock, London.

Hughes, J. (1986). *An Outline of Modern Psychiatry*, 2nd edition. John Wiley, Chichester.

Lyttle, J. (1986). *Mental Disorder*. Baillière Tindall, London and San Diego.

Nelson-Jones, R. (1982). *The Theory and Practice of Counselling Psychology*. Holt, Rinehart and Winston, London.

Nelson-Jones, R. (1983). *Practical Counselling Skills*. 2nd Edition, Cassell, London.

Parry, R. (1983). *Basic Psychotherapy and Helping*. Churchill Livingstone, Edinburgh.

Patterson, C. H. (1986). *Theories of Counselling and Psychotherapy*, 4th edition. Harper and Row, New York.

Rees, L. (1982). *A Short Textbook of Psychiatry*. Hodder and Stoughton, London.

Snaith, P. (1981). *Clinical Neurosis*. Oxford University Press, Oxford.

Storr, A. (1979). *The Art of Psychotherapy*. Secker and Warburg Heinemann Medical, London.

Trethowan, W. and Sims, A. (1983). *Psychiatry*, 5th edition. Baillière Tindall, London and San Diego.

Trower, P., Bryant, B. and Argyle, M. *Social Skills and Mental Health*. Tavistock, London.

Willis, J. (1976). *Clinical Psychiatry*. Blackwell Scientific, Oxford.

Self-assessment Questions

SAQ 5. Identify three reasons why a person with a hysterical reaction may attend a GP's surgery.

SAQ 6. List four community services that a person with a hysterical reaction may be in contact with.

SAQ 7. Outline the clinical objectives for four methods of psychotherapeutic intervention used in the treatment of physical reactions.

SAQ 8. State three reasons why a person with hysteria might need to be admitted to hospital.

Unit 9.2: Written Test

After a history of 15 years' regular attendance at his health centre for a variety of non-specific physical complaints, Henry Patterson, age 46, has been referred to the community mental health centre. He still lives with his ageing parents who do a lot for him, and he has been unemployed for 6 years. He claims that he is unable to work due to "poor physical health". There appears to be no identifiable physical pathology and the origin of his problems appear to be psychological.

1. How could Henry have maintained such a long history of poor health and regular attendance at his health centre?

2. What community-based support services is he likely to need?

3. Describe in detail two possible methods of psychotherapeutic intervention that are likely to be helpful.

UNIT 9.3

Nursing Care of the Person with a Hysterical Reaction

Unit Objectives

At the end of this Unit the learner should be able to:

1. Identify the nursing care needs of the person with a hysterical reaction.
2. Plan an individualized care programme.
3. Select appropriate nursing care interventions for the person's needs.
4. Describe possible evaluation criteria for specific needs.

Mental Health Nursing Care

Each person's care needs are unique and have to be assessed individually. This is particularly so with hysterical reactions where the person can present with an infinite variety of physical and psychological problems. A range of potential care needs have been selected to illustrate the problems that the person may experience and the possible nursing interventions that may help them. For the person presenting with a hysterical reaction these may include the needs to:

A. Feel secure and free from threat.
B. Communicate and relate to others.
C. Increase their insight and self-awareness.
D. Meet their basic physical needs.
E. Facilitate the development of the person's and family's coping skills.

A. Feel Secure and Free from Threat

Associated problems/personal difficulties

Person may feel insecure and threatened as a result of:

1. An inability to identify and accept the source of stress in their life.
2. Unconsciously repressed stress which is expressed as physical and psychological symptoms.
3. Being challenged by others who may doubt the validity of their behaviour.
4. Potential guilt and damage to their self-esteem upon being diagnosed as suffering from a psychological rather than a physical illness.
5. Inadequate knowledge of their care and treatment programme.

Assessment

1. Person's description of their anxieties and worries.
2. Comments made by relatives and friends.
3. Nurse's observations of the person's:

   (a) Response to questioning: topics avoided, incomplete replies, willingness to supply information.
   (b) Understanding: accuracy of information given, questions asked and statements made in relation to their health and their treatment programme.
   (c) Emotional status: appropriateness in terms of severity of presenting "symptoms", indifference, lack of concern, flat, anxiety, irritability.
   (d) Non-verbal behaviour: posture, gestures, tone of voice, eye movements, edginess.
   (e) Presentation of symptoms.
   (f) Relationships with others: accepting, clinging, hostile, rejecting.

4. Identification of potential stressors in the person's relationships, life-style and expectations.

Desired outcomes

1. Person is more relaxed and feels free from threat.
2. Person's understanding of their health care is increased.

Nursing interventions	Rationale
1. Initiate a therapeutic relationship. Spend time with them. Be available and approachable. Active listening. Use touch. Non-judgemental and non-critical approach.	Interventions more likely to be successful in an atmosphere of trust and cooperation. Also, shows sense of worth and acceptance which helps to increase feelings of security and safety. Being non-judgemental helps a person to deal with any guilt. Reduces feelings of anxiety

Nursing intervention	*Rationale*
Adopt a non-threatening, open posture and tone of voice	
2. Provide clear and understandable information about their treatment, health care and the roles of different health care workers. Encourage questions. Ask for feedback on their understanding. Clarify any misunderstandings. Enlist the person's cooperation in the planning of their health care. Promote their autonomy and self-esteem. Explain all actions in advance	A lot of anxiety is associated with fear of the unknown. People have a right to information about their health care. The nurse is in an ideal position to use this process to facilitate the development of the person's understanding about their health care needs. People are more likely to cooperate if they are well-informed and involved in the decision-making process. It also increases feelings of personal control.
3. Ensure that significant personal items are available	Familiar objects help to increase feelings of security
4. Encourage the person to express their feelings about their illness and difficulties	Being labelled mentally ill is a very stigmatizing process. The person feels guilty and bewildered. There is also a sense of loss over the change of role and self-identity
5. Encourage the person to talk about their stressful feelings. Encourage them to express their feelings in a more appropriate way. Provide feedback to the person on their behaviour and use it as a learning situation	Venting their feelings in this way may reduce some of the necessity for communicating through their symptoms. Provides an opportunity for health education in the appropriate expression of emotional stress. Promotes insight (see **C.**)
6. Approach unhurriedly. Demonstrate calmness. Do not rush the person. Be aware of your own reactions and experiences of	Anxiety in the carer communicates itself to the person. Caring can be a stressful experience at times. This may unconsciously influence your interactions with others. The person may be very demanding and resistant.

Nursing intervention	*Rationale*
stress. Be patient and aware of your own feelings of frustration in dealing with the person	Find ways of coping with your own stress
7. Facilitate the development of the person's ability to communicate and relate to others	Helps the person to express and thereby release feelings of anxiety and tension
8. Encourage diversional recreational and social activities	Helps to avoid boredom and to divert the person's thoughts away from stressful topics. Physical activity is also a beneficial channel for stress
9. Encourage the person to rest or relax if they appear to be under stress. Provide feedback on their behaviour	Person may not be aware of the effect of anxiety on their behaviour
10. Advise the person if their behaviour is a risk to themselves or others. Set limits on behaviour that is potentially self-injurious. Ensure that environmental risks are minimized	Promotes insight and shows that the staff are concerned for the person's welfare. Hysterical symptoms do have the potential for physical harm through prolonged immobility, localized anaesthesias, sensory loss or accidental injury
11. Emphasize the importance of recognizing internal tension and external stressors. Recommend methods for reducing sensory stimulation. Teach methods for achieving relaxation. Teach how to use problem-solving methods in coping with stress. Assist the person to learn new coping skills for anxiety (see **E**.)	Providing a programme of health education offers a longer-term strategy for dealing with anxiety in the person's life

Nursing intervention	Rationale
12. Encourage the person to set realistic goals	Unrealistic goals cause frustration and are likely to lead to failure
13. Encourage the setting of progressive goals in small stages	Minimizes risk of failure
14. Provide emotionally safe experiences to increase their sense of mastery	Stress interferes with learning and can create feelings of helplessness

Evaluation

1. Person appears relaxed and demonstrates trust in their care.
2. Person gradually relinquishes the need to use symptoms to cope with stress.

B. Communicate and Relate to Others

Associated problems/personal difficulties

The presence of a hysterical reaction may indicate that the:

1. Person has difficulty in communicating their needs directly to others.
2. Person is using psychologically based symptoms to communicate and relate to others.
3. Method of communicating used is maladaptive and self-defeating.
4. Person is unaware of the inappropriateness of relating in this way.
5. Person lacks social and communication skills.

Assessment

1. Person's description of their communication and relationship difficulties.
2. Person's perception of their relationship needs.
3. Person's perceived self-esteem.
4. Topics that the person appears to avoid or finds difficult to talk about.
5. Nurse's observation of the person's communication pattern:

   (a) *Verbal expression*: tone, volume, rate, rhythm, clarity;
   (b) *Non-verbal expression*: posture, facial expression, eye contact, gestures, proximity, hand movements;

(c) *Emotions expressed*: appropriate, incongruous, flat, morbid, excitable, positive or negative.

6. Interaction with others: frequency and duration of contacts with others, response to communication from others, nature of exchange.
7. Psychosocial environment: reactions of others in communication with person; situations and significant others that elicit, inhibit or reinforce communication; potential stresses in person's environment or life-style.
8. Sensory deficits: visual, auditory.

Desired outcomes

1. Person able to communicate their needs verbally.
2. Person able to express their social, emotional and physical needs.
3. Person able to interact with others in a more assertive way.

Nursing interventions	Rationale
1. Initiate therapeutic relationship	Interventions more likely to be successful in an atmosphere of trust and cooperation
2. Model skilled social and communication skills. Listen attentively and actively. Promote their autonomy and self-esteem. Reinforce sense of self-identity	Modelling by nurses has a powerful influence on the people in their care
3. Promote their insight and self-awareness (see **C.**)	Psychological mechanisms interfere with a person's interpretation and perception of events and cause communication difficulties
4. Promote feelings of security and minimize feelings of threat (see **A.**)	If the person is anxious and insecure they will tend to be defensive and distrustful
5. Use touch and other non-verbal signals to demonstrate reassurance.	Touch can be very comforting and reassuring.
6. Ensure that basic physical needs are being met (see **D.**)	Physical comfort is a prerequisite for meeting other needs. Person will be unable to concentrate on

Nursing intervention	*Rationale*
	communicating if they are in physical discomfort
7. Accept the person's behaviour. Be non-judgemental	The person may be unable to communicate in any other way. Criticism increases stress and is likely to make the person withdraw
8. Engage in physical activity as a precursor to verbal interaction, e.g. games, activities, drama, music. Organize social and recreational activities	Sometimes it is easier for people to talk as part of an activity or game, or afterwards. It provides a non-threatening point of contact
9. Encourage the person to express their feelings	People who find it difficult to communicate may have pent-up emotions. It also provides the opportunity for them to practise talking about their emotions which they may have had difficulty with in the past
10. Be available. Minimize role barriers. Be informal	You have got to look and be approachable. More likely then for communication to occur
11. Positively reinforce self-initiated interaction and communication	Attempts by the person to communicate need to be encouraged
12. Communicate with the person when you are engaged in caring activities	Use all opportunities to demonstrate and encourage communication
13. Encourage social interaction with others. Organize group activities	Social activities can be very rewarding and also provide group dynamics that the person may find therapeutic
14. Identify situations with the person in which they experience anxiety or a communication difficulty in relating to others	Many people with mental health problems are either lacking in social skills or have problems relating to others
15. Role play, with feedback, these situations with the	Social skills and assertiveness training help to develop communication and emotional expression skills

Nursing intervention	Rationale
person. Give demonstration and guidance as required. Provide information on the nature of human interaction and the expression of feeling. Provide information on the principles and application of assertiveness skills	
16. Organize experiential activities, e.g. drama, role-play, games, in which the person relates to others in an unstructured way and can express themselves freely	Structured and spontaneous experiential activities can provide powerful feedback and personal learning opportunities. Can be specifically used to develop communication skills

Evaluation

1. Person able to approach others and to express their needs directly.
2. Person demonstrates raised self-esteem and confidence in the language and non-verbal communication that they use.
3. Person relinquishes the need to use symptoms to communicate with others.

C. Increase Insight and Self-awareness

Associated problems/personal difficulties

Person with hysteria may have inadequate insight and self-awareness shown by:

1. Not perceiving their behaviour as abnormal.
2. Failing to recognize their motivation in the situation.
3. Lack of corresponding anxiety in relation to severity of presenting symptoms.
4. Rejecting suggestions of a psychological basis for their presenting symptoms.
5. Inability to identify significant stressors in their life.

6. Focussing on their presenting symptoms as their primary difficulty.

Assessment

1. Identify the person's perception of their behaviour and health care needs.
2. Identify the perceptions of significant others involved with the person.
3. Compare the explanations given with normal body physiology and pathology or psychological reactions.
4. Identify significant discrepancies between person's presenting symptoms and known medical and psychological conditions.
5. Identify inappropriate use of defence mechanisms and distortions of perception.
6. Evaluate the significance of the symptoms to the person and family.

Desired outcomes

1. Person able to recognize and accept the psychological basis of their symptoms.
2. Person able to adopt more realistic ways of coping with stress and communicating with others.

Nursing interventions	Rationale
1. Initiate therapeutic relationship	Interventions more likely to be successful in an atmosphere of trust and cooperation
2. Provide reassurance and offer acceptance	To minimize distress and create the conditions for behavioural change
3. Demonstrate non-judgemental and non-critical approach	Own reactions can distance you from the person and damage their self-esteem. Criticism tends to be counterproductive
4. Do nor reinforce or encourage in any way the validity of their symptoms	Reinforcement tends to strengthen the person's belief in the validity of their symptoms
5. Reinforce person's self-esteem	Improving self-esteem helps to improve the person's self-image in relationships with others. More likely to relate to others in a "healthy" way
6. Provide opportunities for the person to express themselves	Helps to relieve tension and to demonstrate acceptance

Nursing intervention	Rationale
openly and honestly	
7. Voice doubt over basis of symptoms. Explore possibility with person of psychological basis for symptoms	The person may become aware of the fact that others do not necessarily perceive events in the same way or draw the same conclusions. Person encouraged to reconsider and re-estimate their symptoms and behaviour
8. Positively reinforce healthy behaviour and responses. Negatively reinforce presenting symptoms	Positive reinforcement of healthy behaviour is likely to increase its occurrence
9. Offer feedback on the person's behaviour. Offer feedback on the person's expressed feelings	Person may not be aware of how others perceive them. Person may benefit from reflected appraisal of their emotional experiences
10. Explore with the person the effects of their behaviour and emotions upon others	Person may not be aware of how their behaviour and emotional reactions affect others
11. Explore with the person reasons for criticisms of and by others	Person may not be aware of why others may perceive them in a negative way. This also influences how they perceive others
12. Explore with the person reasons for recurring problems	Person may not realize that their longstanding problems have a common origin
13. Encourage the use of appropriate coping mechanisms (see E.)	Need to develop and use effective ways of coping with stress
14. Encourage acceptance of self-limitations. Encourage honesty in presenting self. Support a realistic assessment of their life circumstances	Person needs to develop a more realistic image of themselves
15. Describe behaviour patterns indicating emotional maturity	Person's social experience may be limited

Nursing intervention	*Rationale*
16. Organize experiential exercises, e.g. drama, role-play, games, in which the person relates to others in an unstructured way and can express themselves freely	Structured and spontaneous experiential exercises can provide powerful feedback and personal learning opportunities. Specific exercises can be used to promote insight

Evaluation

1. Person gradually relinquishes the need for physical and psychological symptoms.
2. Person able to make reality-based statements about their behaviour.

D. Meet Their Basic Physical Needs

Associated problems/personal difficulties

The person with hysteria may have difficulty in meeting their physical needs and maintaining their physical health due to their physical and mental symptoms. These can include:

1. Risk of accidental injury arising from impaired physical, sensory or mental functioning.
2. Potential for impaired limb functioning – joint stiffening and muscle wastage – from prolonged immobility.
3. Possibility of damage to skin tissue arising from sensory impairments or from prolonged immobility.
4. Nutritional deficits arising from vomiting or anorexia.
5. Dependency for physical needs upon others due to sensory or limb impairments.

Assessment

1. Person's and family's statements and behaviour in regard to meeting their needs for nutrition, fluids, hygiene, comfort and sleep.
2. Nurse's observations of:

(a) Person's independent activities in relation to meeting their physical needs.
(b) Family members' interventions in helping person.
(c) Degree of dependence exhibited by person.
(d) History of dependence upon others.
(e) Environmental factors reinforcing dependency.
(f) Identifiable deficits in person's physical needs.
(g) Potential risk factors in person's sensory and physical deficits.
(h) Potential for promoting independence.

Desired outcomes

1. Person is enabled to meet their own physical needs independently.
2. Person demonstrates a raised self-esteem in relation to meeting their own needs independently.
3. Family members actively promote independence and autonomy.

Nursing interventions	Rationale
1. Initiate therapeutic relationship	Interventions more likely to be successful in an atmosphere of trust and cooperation
2. Accurately identify extent of exhibited dependency and baseline of current ability to meet physical needs	Nursing programme will need to be based upon progressive regaining of independence. Need to ensure consistency and to prevent regression
3. Negotiate with the person a programme of progressive regaining of independent functioning. Reassure that loss of function is recoverable	Need to work gradually with person to regain autonomy. Need to avoid creating excessive stress they cannot cope with. May choose to believe that loss of function is permanent. May strongly resist this concept
4. Ensure that negotiated programme is adhered to consistently. Never do anything for them that they are capable of themselves	Person may resist independence and cling to others. Will exploit inconsistency and doubt in carers. May regress if given the opportunity
5. Positively reinforce self-initiated attempts	Needs to perceive benefit of independence rather than dependency

Nursing intervention	Rationale
at independence and regaining lost function	
6. Gradually withdraw direct care interventions and prompting. Ensure person gradually takes over their own self-care activities	Person needs to regain autonomy gradually as they are able to cope with it
7. Monitor compliance with self-care programme and activities	When autonomy is regained, person should be able, within their own abilities, to meet their own care needs

Evaluation

1. Person and family comply with programme for regaining self-care skills.
2. Need for prompting and intervention by care staff decreases.
3. Person independently initiates actions to meet their basic physical needs and maintain their health.

E. Facilitate the Development of the Person's and Family's Coping Skills

Associated problems/personal difficulties

The experience of hysteria may show that:

1. Existing methods of coping may be counterproductive and maladaptive.
2. Current life-style, expectations and relationships may be potential sources of stress.
3. The family may find it difficult to provide emotional support to the person with hysteria.
4. Conflict and stresses are avoided and displaced.
5. The person and their family may lack information about the resources available to help them.
6. There may be feelings of guilt in relation to their problems and asking for help.

Assessment

1. Person and family's description of their current situation.
2. Coping methods used and the support available.
3. Accuracy of the knowledge and information given by the person and their family.
4. Statements of guilt and stigma.
5. Awareness of resources available to them.
6. Previous experience, if any, of dealing with similar problems.

Desired outcomes

1. Person and family able to make an informed choice about the resources they require.
2. Person and family able to use more appropriate coping skills for life and personal problems.

Nursing interventions	Rationale
1. Initiate therapeutic relationship	Interventions are more likely to be successful in an atmosphere of trust and cooperation
2. Advise that seeking help and recognition of problems are a positive step towards finding solutions	Many people feel that seeking help is a sign of weakness and failure. Helps to reduce guilt
3. Encourage questions. Provide accurate information	May have inaccurate knowledge and expectations, particularly in relation to: • their body, • ways of relating and communicating.
4. Identify appropriate health care resources	Need to know what resources are available to them
5. Advise against early and unrealistic correction of problems	Under stress it is sometimes easier to make short-term adaptations that only store up future problems. It may take time to help the person work out what is best for them. Longstanding problems will also take time to resolve
6. Reassure that there are ways of improving the situation.	Person and family may feel that it is not possible to make changes. Person and family may believe that loss of

Nursing intervention	*Rationale*
Reassure that lost physical and mental function can be restored. Advise against recriminations and focussing on past problems	function is permanent. Need to focus on the present and future and to deal with stress in a more productive way
7. Advise on the need for acceptance and mutual support within their relationships	Family needs to come to terms with their situation. They are each other's primary source of support which will need to be utilized to cope effectively
8. Explain the need to identify and recognize potentially stressful situations. Recommend methods for coping with stress	Mental health problems tend to be long-term in nature. In order to cope effectively the family need to be taught effective coping skills to deal with future stresses
9. Teach methods for achieving relaxation. Teach how to use problem-solving methods for coping with difficulties. Advise the family on how to give feedback and support to one another	Much of the education needs to be directed towards learning new coping methods. These include the way that the members of the family communicate, their expectations and the way that emotional support is given
10. Assist the family to learn new coping skills. Encourage the setting of realistic goals and expectations. Encourage the setting of progressive goals in small stages	The re-learning needs to be done in a gradual way in which the family provides the main support and reinforcement
11. Encourage the use of newly acquired coping skills	Skills need to be used in order to become part of everyday living
12. Review occupational/ employment stresses. Encourage the development of appropriate work/non-work coping strategies	Work and employment can be major sources of stress. As these represent a major part of life, it is important that the person learns how to cope constructively with these stresses

Nursing interventions	Rationale
13. Teach the family and person to recognize the limits of their ability to cope and when it is advisable to seek help	The family should not over-burden itself as this can damage relationships and its longer-term ability to cope
14. Put family in contact with self-help and voluntary groups	Self-help groups able to offer effective and understanding practical help

Evaluation

1. Person and family able to identify and select resources they require.
2. Person and family demonstrate use of improved coping methods.

Unit Instructions

When you have researched the suggested references, have mastered the Unit Objectives and successfully answered the Self-assessment Questions, proceed with the Unit Written Test.

Suggested References

Altschul, A. and McGovern, M. (1985). *Psychiatric Nursing*, 6th edition. Baillière Tindall, London and San Diego.

Barker, P. J. (1982). *Behaviour Therapy Nursing*. Croom Helm, London.

Barker, P. J. (1985). *Patient Assessment in Psychiatric Nursing*. Croom Helm, London.

Bauer, B. and Hill, S. (1986). *Essentials of Mental Health Care Planning and Interventions*. W. B. Saunders, Philadelphia.

Campbell, C. (1978). *Nursing Diagnosis and Intervention in Nursing Practice*. John Wiley, New York.

Darcy, P. T. (1985). *Mental Health Nursing Source Book*. Baillière Tindall, London and San Diego.

Dexter, G. and Wash, M. (1986). *Psychiatric Nursing Skills: A Patient-Centred Approach*. Croom Helm, London.

Hase, S. and Douglas, A. (1986). *Human Dynamics and Nursing*. Churchill Livingstone, Melbourne.

Irving, S. (1983). *Basic Psychiatric Nursing*, 3rd edition. W. B. Saunders, Philadelphia.

Lancaster, J. (1980). *Adult Psychiatric Nursing*. Henry Kimpton, London.

McFarland, G. and Wasli, E. (1986). *Nursing Diagnoses and Process in Psychiatric Mental Health Nursing*. J. B. Lippincott, Philadelphia.

Martin, P. (1987a). *Psychiatric Nursing: A Therapeutic Approach*. Macmillan, London.
Martin, P. (1987b). *Care of the Mentally Ill*, 2nd edition. Macmillan, London.
Pelletier, L. (Ed.) (1987). *Psychiatric Nursing Case Studies, Nursing Diagnoses and Care Plans*. Springhouse Corporation, Springhouse, Pennsylvania.
Robinson, L. (1983). *Psychiatric Nursing as a Human Experience*, 3rd edition. W. B. Saunders, Philadelphia.

Self-assessment Questions

SAQ 9. Identify six interventions to increase the person's feelings of security.
SAQ 10. Describe four interventions to help the person increase their insight and self-awareness.
SAQ 11. List four ways in which the person with a hysterical reaction may have difficulty in meeting their physical needs.
SAQ 12. Outline four ways that the person and their family can be helped to increase their coping and communication skills.

Unit 9.3: Written Test

David Redfern, aged 18, left school 2 years ago. His record of attainment was poor and he has been unemployed for the past 12 months. He lost his job through repeated sickness absence and claiming that he could no longer lift things in the warehouse due to a "back injury". He was not involved in any industrial injury and medical tests failed to reveal any identifiable pathology.

Over the past year he claims that his back has become increasingly worse and he has become virtually housebound as he cannot walk more than a few paces without pain. His parents, like David, believe that their son is now physically crippled and are frustrated with health care services for not treating their son. They do everything for David and their own lives have become increasingly restricted as a result.

David has been admitted to the local psychiatric unit for a thorough assessment and to try and resolve this situation.

1. As the nurse completing the initial assessment, what observations can you make to confirm the psychological nature of his presenting symptoms?
2. David appears to lack insight into his behaviour and not to be able to express his emotional needs directly. Describe in detail a nursing care programme to enable David to increase his insight and communicate more effectively.
3. One day on entering his dormitory you find David laying and moaning on the floor. He claims that his back has "completely gone" and he is unable to move or get up. Several other residents are gathered around David expressing concern and attempting to help him. What interventions would you use to deal with this situation?

TOPIC 10

Schizophrenic Reactions

At the end of this Topic the learner should aim to:

1. Describe the characteristic features of a schizophrenic reaction.
2. Discuss factors associated with the onset and development of schizophrenic reactions.
3. Outline the range of therapeutic interventions available for people suffering from a schizophrenic reaction.
4. Identify the nursing care needs and interventions required for the person who has a schizophrenic reaction.

The Nature and Origins of Schizophrenia

Unit Objectives

At the end of this Unit the learner should be able to:

1. Identify the characteristic features of schizophrenia.
2. Discuss factors associated with the onset of schizophrenia.
3. Describe the characteristic features of the early development of schizophrenia.

Definition

Schizophrenia is the name given to a group of mental illnesses characterized by disorders of thought, emotion, behaviour and perception. These concurrent psychotic disturbances commonly lead to the progressive deterioration of the person's ability to relate to others and to social withdrawal. It tends to be a chronic, life-long condition with a wide range of effects and symptoms. Its course may be insidious and unremitting or punctuated by periods of remission and acute exacerbation. Its effects vary from those of a mild disorder to one where the person is extremely disturbed and loses touch with reality. It is classed as a functional psychosis.

Typically, it is a disorder of early adult life with the majority of male sufferers being diagnosed in the early 20's. The incidence of schizophrenia for males decreases after the age of 34. Women appear to be affected less in early adulthood but the incidence for them increases from their 30's. Overall, men suffer with schizophrenia slightly more than women.

The Development of Schizophrenia

A number of factors appear to be related to the development of schizophrenia and a number of theories have been postulated to try and explain its psychopathology and presentation. Basically, its cause remains unknown and is a matter of much debate, controversy and continued research. It would appear that rather than there being one actual cause it is the result of a complex interaction of hereditary, sociological, psychological, environmental and physiological factors.

Heredity

Evidence from genetic studies indicates that hereditary factors have a high influence in a number of cases. Studies indicate that the closer the genetical relationship between two individuals the greater the likelihood of one person developing schizophrenia if their relative is diagnosed as having schizophrenia. The genetic studies undertaken are inconclusive and the findings give estimates over a wide range, for example between 50 and 90% concordance rates for twin studies.

A better perspective is gained if one appreciates that less than 10% of people with schizophrenia had parents who had this condition and less than 20% of sufferers had a schizophrenic sibling. These are important facts to remember when trying to allay the guilt of other family members.

The incidence of schizophrenia in the population is found internationally to be fairly consistent at about 0.85%. This would indicate a total of some 500 000 people in the UK who have schizophrenia. About 150 000 are affected at any one time, with possibly half this number requiring residential care. From these totals it will be seen that a large number of sufferers remain undiagnosed.

Biochemical and neurological factors

Practically every organ in the body has been investigated in terms of a possible link with schizophrenia. Much of this work is extremely theoretical and difficult to interpret. It would appear though that in schizophrenia there are some abnormalities of neurotransmission within the brain. It is thought that certain chemicals that arise from this metabolic disturbance are inducing a psychotic reaction and cause many of the symptoms complained of by schizophrenics. Whether these findings indicate a potential cause or a consequence of schizophrenia is less certain.

Family interaction theories

A large number of theories exist for the role of family life in the causation of schizophrenia. Mostly they have remained "theories" that have not been able to be duplicated in real life and suffer from severe methodological limitations. None the less, a number of ideas generated by these studies do seem to be of some interest. In principle they all propose a model in which family dynamics drive people "mad" and the schizophrenia is seen as a reaction to these stresses.

1. *Double bind theory*: in which the child is given conflicting messages by its parents and any action that it takes is wrong. The stress of the continued ambiguity causes the psychotic reaction.
2. *Disordered family communications*: members of the family communicate in incomprehensible ways. Messages are sent which do not confirm reality and there is collusion between family members. Hence the sufferer is unable to relate and is seen as deviant by the others.
3. *Parents' marital relationship*: the relationship may be "skewed" and dominated by one abnormal parent. The relationship may be one of "marital schism", in which there is conflict between the parents who compete for the child's attention. The child may also be "scapegoated" as being a cause of the parental rift.
4. *"Schizophrenic" mother*: a mother who is cold, withdrawn, has little maternal love, inconsistent and unable to understand the child's feelings. Typically the father is also indifferent to the child. These are the conditions of "maternal deprivation". The child grows up with numerous emotional and psychological difficulties.

Psychodynamic theories

Again more theories with as yet little clinical application:

1. *Sensory processing*: people with schizophrenia appear to have problems in the amount of environmental stimulation that they can process and cope with at one time. Schizophrenia is seen as a reaction to a "sensory overload", in which the sufferers' perceptions are confused, disjointed and bewildering.
2. *Ego defence mechanisms*: the world is seen as a threatening place from which the schizophrenic withdraws to a more tolerable fantasy world. He denies reality, regresses to an earlier stage of development, becomes fixated and reconstructs a less stressful internal world.

Social theories

1. *Social drift*: people with schizophrenia, in terms of social class, appear to be over-represented in social classes 4 and 5. They often live in the deprived areas of towns and to have unskilled and transient jobs. However, these seem to be more a consequence of the schizophrenic's lack of drive and motivation rather than pathologically significant.
2. *Social stress and isolation*: city life is regarded as stressful with widespread loneliness and isolation. These are social conditions which may trigger a schizophrenic episode in someone who is susceptible. However, most schizophrenics tend to become socially isolated.

Personality

A pre-morbid personality type has been described as a "schizoid personality". The person is withdrawn, isolated, indifferent and emotionally cool. They may be hypochondriacal and have a fanatical interest in unusual subjects. However, about 50% of schizophrenics show no evidence of previous personality abnormalities.

Precipitating Factors

For many people with schizophrenia there do not seem to be any identifiable precipitating events for the onset. In a certain proportion of cases there does seem to be an association with stressful life events in the period preceding the onset of relapse. Physical illness or injury, pregnancy, the puerperium, crisis in a relationship, unemployment, isolation and moving away from home can precipitate a schizophrenic reaction in some people.

Early Clinical Onset

The early stages of schizophrenia, particularly if it occurs during adolescence, are often not recognized by the family. The symptoms may come on gradually and insidiously. Adolescence is also a time when parents expect their children to be moody, challenging and to express their individuality. The symptoms may be diffuse and vague and the person may have been disturbed for a long time before being diagnosed as suffering from schizophrenia.

The changes in behaviour that the family might recognize include:

1. *Alteration in rhythms*: the person often sleeps late in the day and spends much of the night in solitary and restless wandering around the house.
2. *A change in family relationships*: they may not act towards family members as they did before. They seem "different" or "changed".
3. *The voicing of abnormal ideas*: the person may talk to him/herself in an otherwise empty room. They may express odd and strange ideas. These may be very bizarre or grandiose. They may complain that parts of their body are strange and do not belong to them or of other unusual physical symptoms.
4. *A change in behaviour*: they might be withdrawn, apathetic and shut themselves away in their room. They may appear slow in their actions and to have lost many of their interests and any concern about their appearance. Periodically, they may become restless and overactive.

In reaction to these changes the family may seek outside help or may try to cope by using unconscious defence mechanisms. These may include:

1. *Balancing*: balancing the good parts of the person's behaviour with the disturbed – "he can't be that bad, he did the shopping for me".
2. *Normalizing*: redefining abnormal behaviour as normal by saying "everyone does that, it's normal".
3. *Attenuation*: reducing the seriousness of disturbed behaviour – "it's not really all that serious".
4. *Denial*: refusing point-blank to accept that anything is at all wrong.

Unit Instructions

When you have researched the suggested references, have mastered the Unit Objectives and successfully answered the Self-assessment Questions, proceed with the Unit Written Test.

Suggested References

Clare, A. (1980). *Psychiatry in Dissent*, 2nd edition. Tavistock, London.
Davis, D. R. (1984). *An Introduction to Psychopathology*. 4th Edition. Oxford University Press, Oxford.
Hamilton, M. (Ed.) (1976). *Fish's Schizophrenia*, 2nd edition. John Wright, Bristol.
Laing, R. D. (1965). *The Divided Self*. Pelican, Harmondsworth.
Laing, R. D. and Esterson, A. (1964). *Sanity, Madness and the Family*. Pelican, Harmondsworth.
Orford, J. (1976). *The Social Psychology of Mental Disorder*. Penguin, Harmondsworth.
Sims, A. (1988). *Symptoms in the Mind*. Baillière Tindall, London and San Diego.
Szasz, T. (1973). *Ideology and Insanity*. Penguin, Harmondsworth.
Trethowan, W. and Sims, A. C. P. (1985). *Psychiatry*, 5th edition, Baillièrre Tindall, London and San Diego.
Tsuang, M. T. (1982). *Schizophrenia: The Facts*. Oxford University Press, Oxford.
Willis, J. (1976). *Clinical Psychiatry*. Blackwell Scientific, Oxford.

Self-assessment Questions

SAQ 1. What is the incidence and distribution of schizophrenia?
SAQ 2. Identify five factors thought to contribute towards the onset of schizophrenia.
SAQ 3. Describe three precipitating factors which may trigger a schizophrenic reaction.
SAQ 4. Identify three changes in behaviour that a family might notice in the early stages of schizophrenia.

Unit 10.2: Written Test

1. What do you understand by the term "schizophrenia"?
2. Describe in detail three potential factors associated with the onset of schizophrenia.
3. How might a family react in attempting to reject the fact that one of their members has schizophrenia?

Characteristics and Recognition of Schizophrenic Reactions

Unit Objectives

At the end of this Unit the learner should be able to:

1. Describe the characteristic thought disorders experienced by people with schizophrenia.
2. Outline common emotional and behavioural reactions of people with schizophrenia.
3. Define the term "delusion".
4. Describe common perceptual disturbances experienced by people with schizophrenia.

Characteristic Features

The characteristic features of schizophrenia can be considered under the following headings:

- thought disorder,
- delusions,
- emotional disturbances,
- perceptual disturbances,
- behavioural disturbances.

Thought disorder

In schizophrenia the person's thought processes are disturbed. Their conceptual thinking is impaired and they find it difficult to think in abstract terms, i.e. "concrete thinking". Their ideas seem illogical and hard to follow. They may jump from topic to topic ("flight of ideas") and talk at great length without reaching any conclusions ("circumstantiality"). Sometimes they may invent their own words ("neologisms") to express their strange ideas. The words may be spoken as a stream of meaningless words ("word salad").

Other thought disorders that may be identified include:

- poverty of ideas, i.e. lack or absence of ideas;
- thought blocking, i.e. thoughts blocked or held up;
- thought insertion, i.e. thoughts put into one's head;
- thought withdrawal, i.e. thoughts being taken out of one's mind;
- thought broadcasting, i.e. thoughts being known to others.

There is no impairment of consciousness in schizophrenia. Some may appear to be disorientated or out of touch but this is more likely to be the result of perceptual distraction, social isolation or disinterest in answering questions.

Delusions

A delusion is defined as a false, fixed belief of morbid origin which is out of context with the person's socio-cultural background and is not amenable to logical argument. They are often preoccupying and are usually irrational, absurd or impossible. The delusion tends to form out of the blue and may be preceded by a *delusional mood*, i.e. the person has a vague and apprehensive feeling that something is about to happen or is happening around him.

Many delusions consist of a "network" of ideas that are successively created to give validity to each other. There is a central or *primary delusion* from which a number of *secondary delusions* are formed:

Primary delusion	*Secondary delusions*
Delusional ideas of persecution	"My food is poisoned"
	"There are guns aimed at me"
	"All my moves are watched"
	"I cannot risk going to sleep"
	"They are trying to kill me"

Delusions influence a person's:

- behaviour: which may appear impulsive, changeable, bizarre;
- emotions: which may be intense, suddenly changeable, inappropriate;
- thought processes: particularly their interpretation and anticipation of events.

Delusions are expressed as speech and actions as the person acts on his disordered beliefs. This can lead to conflict with others who do not share those beliefs or to social isolation and rejection. The delusions can also threaten a person's basic needs, e.g. if they believe that their food is poisoned or that they can come to no harm. The thoughts can lead to impulsive action and incomprehensible behaviour.

Emotional disturbance

The schizophrenic may experience quite a fundamental emotional disturbance. This may be expressed as unpredictable mood swings in which a wide range of emotions – joy, misery, terror, love – are shown in short succession. The moods shown may be inappropriate to the situation. A person may respond with sadness at being told something pleasant. This is known as incongruity of affect.

A person suffering from schizophrenia may display a blunting or poverty of affect. Their emotional responses become shallow, dull and indifferent. They may appear as a cold, aloof and detached person with whom it is difficult to make contact or develop a relationship. The person appears uninterested in the outside world and concerned only with his inner world.

The emotional disturbance is often seen by others as a change in personality. The person is somehow "different" and not the one that they used to know. This can cause stress in close relationships, and the person may lose contact with their friends and become increasingly isolated.

Perceptual disturbances

Perceptual disturbances can occur in each sensory mode. The most common perceptual disturbance is the presence of hallucinations. These are false sensory perceptions without the presence of external stimuli. The perceptions appear real to the person experiencing them and can influence their behaviour and emotions. They may accept the delusion passively or find it very distressing behaviour in a very unpredictable way. A person may be affected with either single or multiple sensory hallucinations at the same time. The experience can be intermittent or continuous for the person. At acute stages the hallucinations may be particularly severe.

Hallucinations are identified in the following way:

1. *Auditory*: the person may hear voices commenting on their actions, speaking their own thoughts aloud, telling them what to do or a running commentary. Auditory hallucinations are the most common perceptual disturbance.
2. *Visual*: the person may see people, shapes or creatures around them when none exist. These may be very distorted and possibly distressing. Visual hallucinations are relatively rare and tend to be confined to acute phases of the illness.
3. *Tactile*: the person may experience being touched or of having things crawling over them.

4. *Gustatory*: the sense of taste is affected. There may be a strange taste in their mouth or food may taste contaminated or poisoned. The experience is nearly always unpleasant.
5. *Olfactory*: the person may complain of "gas" in the room or of other strange smells coming through the floor or walls.

For an example of the possible effects of hallucinations, see Exhibit 10.2.1.

Exhibit 10.2.1 The possible influences of hallucinations

Discrete	*Obvious*
1. Hardly visible or not show at all	Noticeable and very distracting, person very preoccupied
2. Little apparent effect on behaviour and communication, only shows in certain situations	Considerable influence on behaviour and communication, shown through movement, posture, voice pattern, eye contact
3. Person gets used to it and "screens" it out	Responding without obvious stimuli. Talking out loud to no apparent object or person

Behavioural disturbances

The person's behaviour, as described above, can be influenced by their thoughts, perceptions and the presence of delusions. There are also a number of behavioural disturbances characteristic of schizophrenia.

1. Volition (will-power)

There is a loss of motivation and initiative which is shown by apathy, disinterest, loss of energy and indecisiveness. The person shows little inclination to do anything and, if left to their own devices, will just sit around or lie in bed all day. Despite this they remain fully aware of their surroundings, memory remains intact and there is no evidence of intellectual deterioration.

2. Passivity

The person feels that he is no longer in control of his thoughts and actions. They may feel controlled by some external force or agency such as the TV. They may demonstrate automatic obedience to instructions. Extreme examples of passivity may rarely be seen in which the person's limbs may be positioned into unusual postures and maintained for long periods without apparent fatigue. They may also become immobile for long periods of time and appear to be in a "stupor", in which they remain alert but unresponsive and withdrawn. In this stupor they may neglect to eat or drink and even be incontinent.

3. Negativism

This is a strong resistance to suggestion and shows itself in stubborn behaviour or a complete refusal to do anything or to cooperate. (It may be hard to distinguish this from a person demonstrating independence and autonomy!)

4. Impulsive

In contrast to the lack of volition, the person may periodically act impulsively and become very excited and agitated. In this acute disturbance they may come into conflict with others or run the risk of injury.

5. Ritual

The person may repeat actions (echopraxia) and words (echolalia) that are demonstrated in front of them. They may repeat obsessively some action or ritual such as pointing at or touching objects. They may have mannerisms and tics. Grimacing and pursing the lips may also be seen.

Classification of Schizophrenia

The range of potential signs and symptoms seen in schizophrenia is very large. As it tends to be a chronic condition with periods of stability, remission and acute exacerbation, people may show different clinical features at different times. Clinically, people with schizophrenia are grouped into four main classifications. From a nursing viewpoint each individual should be assessed in terms of their current needs rather than their diagnostic label. The classifications are as follows.

Simple schizophrenia

This form of schizophrenia is characterized by insidious development during late adolescence. The person becomes apathetic, indifferent, socially withdrawn and detached. They may have hypochondriacal preoccupations and strange ideas. There may be conflict with their family members who are worried, concerned and perplexed by the changes they see. They tend to drift into a life-time of social isolation, aimlessness and occupational instability.

Hebephrenic schizophrenia

The motivational and emotional deficits can be similar to those of simple schizophrenia. It is differentiated by the greater degree of thought and behavioural disturbances that can occur, often with bizarre delusions and hallucinations. Severe thought disorders may be accompanied by mood swings and incongruity of affect. The presentation is of a very emotionally and behaviourally disturbed person. As the condition progresses the person becomes more withdrawn, may show mannerisms and grimaces and a fragmentation of thought and speech. The onset is usually between the ages of 15 and 30.

Catatonic schizophrenia

In catatonic schizophrenia the person may show extreme emotional, thought and behavioural disturbances. Although catatonic schizophrenia is very rare, it is primarily characterized by two extremes of behaviour. In the excitement phase the person may appear very disturbed and over-active. The mood may swing rapidly from anger and aggression to fear. The person may experience auditory hallucinations.

At the other extreme the person may be very withdrawn and seem to be in a stupor. They may appear immobile and indifferent to their surroundings but remain conscious and can clearly recall events afterwards. From this stupor the person may engage in sudden unprovoked and impulsive acts of aggression or self-injury. In this phase they are usually indifferent to personal physical needs.

Paranoid schizophrenia

Paranoid schizophrenia tends to begin later in life than the other types of schizophrenia, typically after the age of 35. The primary feature is the presence of a powerful delusional process that influences the person's perception and behaviour. The person becomes increasingly sensitive and suspicious and develops "ideas of reference" that things are being said and done with special reference to themself. These morbid suspicions become definite delusions of persecution with complaints of victimization or threats against life. The person may be litigious, threatening, aggressive and homicidal towards his supposed persecutors. Frequently, it is these hostile acts towards others that alert relatives that something is wrong.

From feelings of victimization the person may develop compensatory delusions about his own importance. He may complain that he is being victimized out of jealousy due to success or an inheritance.

Generally, the individual's personality is well-preserved and the person retains good social awareness. In these cases the person can be supported to maintain a reasonably independent life. In other cases the person may display the emotional, cognitive and behavioural disturbances characteristic of schizophrenia and may require residential care.

Suggested References

Ashton, J. R. (1980). *Everyday Psychiatry*, Update, London.

Schneider, K. (1957). *Primary and secondary symptoms in schizophrenia. In* Hirsch, S. and Shepherd, M. (Eds), *Themes and Variations in European Psychiatry*. John Wright, Bristol.

Sims, A. (1988). *Symptoms in the Mind*. Baillière Tindall, London and San Diego.

Trethowan, W. and Sims, A. C. P. (1985). *Psychiatry*, 5th edition. Baillière Tindall, London and San Diego.

Tsuang, M. T. (1982). *Schizophrenia: The Facts*. Oxford University Press, Oxford.

Vousden, M. (1987). Is there racism on the wards? *Nursing Mirror*, 21 October, Vol. 83, No. 42, p. 18.

Willis, J. (1976). *Clinical Psychiatry*. Blackwell Scientific, Oxford.

Self-assessment Questions

SAQ 5. Identify four types of thought disorder seen in schizophrenia.

SAQ 6. List five types of perceptual disturbance that may be experienced by people with schizophrenia.

SAQ 7. Define the terms "primary" and "secondary" delusion.

SAQ 8. Describe four types of schizophrenic reaction.

Unit 10.2: Written Test

David Wilson, aged 19, has been referred for mental health assessment. He was sacked from his job 6 months ago for being "slow and idle". He did not form very good relationships at work where he was noted for his strange ideas and behaviour.

His parents became concerned because he began staying up at night playing his records and sleeping during the day. He refuses to help around the house and watches television all day. He has virtually stopped talking to his parents and sister, except to ask for money for cigarettes. His parents became particularly concerned when he painted crucifixes over his bedroom walls and said that God was speaking to him.

What observations would you need to make to confirm that his behaviour and thoughts were psychotic in origin?

Care and Treatment of the Person with Schizophrenia

Unit Objectives

At the end of this Unit the learner should be able to:

1. Outline the range of therapeutic interventions available for the person with schizophrenia.
2. Identify the support required for the person and their family in the community.
3. Describe the prognosis for sufferers of schizophrenia.

Care and Treatment

There is no specific treatment for schizophrenia. The general approach should be an integrated long-term programme that will support the person and their family in the community or in residential care as required.

Therapeutic aims

1. To maintain and develop the person's positive assets.
2. To maintain the person's independence and autonomy.
3. To facilitate the development of the person and their family's coping skills.
4. To minimize the risk of relapse.

Family Care

Most of the people with schizophrenia are not in hospital and a large number of these are probably not in contact with any health care agency. In reality, most people with schizophrenia are either trying to cope alone or are being looked after by their family at great personal cost. For those not in residential care one study reported:

- 71% living with relatives,
- 17% living alone,
- 9% in a hostel,
- 3% under supervision.

The community care resources offered by health districts and local authorities barely cope with the demands made upon their services. This situation is exacerbated by the run-down and anticipated closure of many large psychiatric hospitals and there are criticisms of inadequate resources and preparation for community care alternatives (see Unit 5.3).

Schizophrenia is a distressing condition which imposes a great burden on the person and their family and, although the resources are limited, there are a number of interventions that can help:

1. Accurate information about the illness and its effects.
2. Involvement in the care and treatment process.
3. Enabling the person and family to come to terms with their guilt.
4. The opportunity to talk freely about their problems.
5. Opportunity for support and a break when suffering from exhaustion.
6. The address of a local contact support group for relatives of people with schizophrenia. This, in particular, shows that they are not alone.
7. Teaching the family problem-solving skills and developing their ability to cope.
8. Advising them of the necessity of ensuring compliance with prescribed medication to avoid a relapse.
9. Informing them of the need to maintain a balance between the demands they put upon the sufferer and the person's ability to cope. Research shows that the person's relationship with their family are crucial. There is a much higher risk of relapse if there is frequent face-to-face contact with critical and emotionally over-involved relatives. The optimum contact appears to be a maximum of 35 hours per week in a social group of three to five people. The sufferer requires a certain amount of stimulation to avoid "environmental poverty", but this needs to be given in an emotionally non-threatening way.
10. Identifying potentially stressful situations and either avoiding these or seeking help.
11. Helping the family to accept the person as they are and letting them talk openly about their experiences and fantasies without criticism and with support.

Community Care

Community care involves a wide range of services, both statutory and voluntary, that aim to provide comprehensive treatment and support. The aims of community care are:

1. To support the person and their family.
2. To enable the person to remain in their own home.
3. To monitor the person's mental and physical health.
4. To implement community-based treatment and care programmes.

The services involved include:

1. The community mental health centre: with community psychiatric nurses, social workers, psychologists, occupational therapists and consultant psychiatrists working as a team to offer skills-based therapeutic interventions.
2. General practitioners.
3. Voluntary agencies: MIND, Schizophrenia Fellowship, Richmond Fellowship, Citizen's Advice Bureaux.
4. Local authority/health authority: hostels, half-way homes, group homes, sheltered workshops.
5. DHSS: benefits, allowances and grants as currently available to individuals and their families.
6. Department of Employment: Disablement Resettlement Officer (DRO), Register of Disabled Persons, training schemes.
7. Out-patient clinics and day hospitals.

Residential Care

The reasons for admission to residential facilities for treatment include:

1. Lack of support in the community.
2. The need for intensive care when the person is acutely ill and is a potential risk to himself.
3. Detailed assessment and the need for specific types of therapy.

Therapeutic Interventions

Chemotherapy

1. *Phenothiazines*: chlorpromazine (Largactil), trifluoperazine (Stelazine).
2. *Long-acting depot injections*: flupenthixol decanoate (Depixol), fluphenazine hydrochloride (Moditen), fluphenazine decanoate (Modecate).
3. *Other major tranquillizers*: haloperidol (Serenace).
4. *Anti-Parkinsonian drugs for the side-effects of phenothiazines*: orphenadrine (Disipal), procyclidine (Kemadrin), benztropine (Cogentin), benzhexol (Artane).

Psychotherapeutic methods

1. *Skilled nursing care*: one of the most important factors.
2. *Social skills training*: to improve interpersonal skills and confidence.
3. *Behavioural psychotherapy*: for specific behavioural problems.
4. *Family therapy*: to help the family cope and to modify how they express emotion.
5. *Occupational therapy*: life skills and activities of daily living, diversional activities.
6. *Recreational and social activities*: trips, outings, holidays, social events.

The combination of social skills training and medication would appear to offer the best results and to reduce the likelihood of relapse.

Outcomes

The outcome is very uncertain and difficult to predict. About 40% of people return home free from symptoms in under 3 months, and 20% will remit sufficiently well to live in the community (some of these will require further periods of hospital care). Of the remainder, the majority will remain chronically ill but non-progressive and possibly be suitable for hostels or half-way homes. About 3–4% will require long-term residential care.

Some important prognostic indications are:

Good prognostic signs

- Acute onset;
- stable and supportive social background;
- good pre-morbid personality adjustment;
- absence of family history of schizophrenia;
- presence of identifiable psychological or physical precipitants;
- above average intelligence.

Poor prognostic signs

- Insidious onset;
- persistent thought disorder;
- social isolation and an unfavourable environment;
- past psychiatric treatment;
- presence of flattening affect;
- below average intelligence.

Suggested References

Atkinson, J. M. (1986). *Schizophrenia at Home: A Guide to Helping the Family*.
Croom Helm, London.

Cooper, G. (1987). The family way. *Nursing Times*, 6 May, Vol. 83, No. 18,
pp. 62–64.

Goldborg, D. and Huxley, P. (1980). *Mental Illness in the Community*. Tavistock,
London.

Hiller, P. (1984). Schizophrenia: An inside story. *New Society*, 14 June, Vol. 68,
pp. 439–440.

Miles, A. (1981). *The Mentally Ill in Contemporary Society*. Martin Robertson,
Oxford.

Seeman, M. V. *et al.* (1982). *Living and Working with Schizophrenia*. Open
University Press, Milton Keynes.

Silverstone, T. and Turner, P. (1982). *Drug Treatments in Psychiatry*, 3rd edition.
RKP. London.

Teasdale, K. (1986a). The withdrawn schizophrenic. *Nursing Times*, 5 February,
Vol. 82, No. 6, pp. 32–34.

Teasdale, K. (1986b). Schizophrenics and the family. *Nursing Times*, 12 February,
Vol. 82, No. 7, pp. 41–43.

Tsuang, M. T. (1982). *Schizophrenia: The Facts*. Oxford University Press, Oxford.

Willis, J. (1976). *Clinical Psychiatry*. Blackwell Scientific, Oxford.

Wing, J. K. and Brown, G. W. (1970). *Institutionalisation and Schizophrenia*.
Cambridge University Press, Cambridge.

Self-assessment Questions

SAQ 9. Describe briefly the advice and support that can be given to
the family of someone with schizophrenia.

SAQ 10. List the community services available to help people remain at
home.

SAQ 11. Identify the main elements of hospital-based treatment for
schizophrenia.

SAQ 12. List factors associated with a positive outcome in the treatment
of schizophrenia.

Unit 10.3: Written Test

David and Susan Ashworth are distressed that their only son Peter, aged
19, has been diagnosed as suffering from schizophrenia.

1. What advice and support can the community nurse give to Peter and his parents about coping with the illness at home?
2. Peter has initially been prescribed chlorpromazine 100 mg twice a day, and the parents have heard of an injection given every 2 weeks that "cures" schizophrenia. How would you deal with this situation and what information would you give to the family?

Nursing Care of the Person with Schizophrenic Reaction

Unit Objectives

' At the end of this Unit the learner should be able to:

1. Identify the nursing care needs of the person with a schizophrenic reaction.
2. Plan an individualized care programme.
3. Select appropriate nursing care interventions for the person's needs.
4. Describe possible evaluation criteria for specific problems.

Mental Health Nursing Care

Each person's care needs are unique and have to be assessed individually. A range of possible care needs have been selected to illustrate the problems that the person may experience and the possible nursing interventions that may help them. For the person suffering from schizophrenia these may include the need to:

A. Minimize the influence of perceptual distractions and delusions.
B. Maintain their autonomy and self-esteem.
C. Meet their basic physical needs.
D. Communicate and relate to others.
E. Feel secure and free from threat.
F. Facilitate the person's and family's ability to cope with problems.

A. Minimize the Influence of Perceptual Distractions and Delusions

Associated problems/personal difficulties

Person may be experiencing perceptual distractions and delusions that can.:

1. Cause him distress.
2. Distort his perception of reality.
3. Interfere with his ability to communicate.
4. Cause him to behave in an unpredictable way.
5. Interfere with his ability to meet his basic needs independently.

Assessment

1. Person's description of their sensory experiences and thoughts.
2. Nurse's observations of the effects of perceptual distortions and delusions to the person's:

   (a) Ability to communicate: content of statements made, concentration, attentiveness, relevance, volume, clarity, rate, tone.
   (b) Behaviour: appropriateness, smooth and co-ordinated, facial expression, eye movements, gestures, level of activity, mannerisms.
   (c) Emotions: congruence, appropriateness, intensity, changeability, consistency.
   (d) Own reactions to the hallucinations/delusions.
   (e) Coping strategies used and their effectiveness in attempting to resist perceptual distractions and delusional thoughts.
   (f) Which senses appear to be affected.

3. Psycho-social environment:

   (a) Place and situation.
   (b) Pattern throughout the day.
   (c) Presence of identifiable eliciting stimuli or triggering cues.
   (d) Reactions of others to person's behaviour indicating sensory distractions or delusional thoughts.
   (e) Potential reinforcers of sensory distractions and delusional thoughts.
   (f) Presence of potential stresses in person's environment or lifestyle: over-stimulation, under-stimulation, conflict resistance.

Desired outcomes

1. To reduce the influence of the hallucinations and delusions on the person's behaviour, communication and autonomy.
2. To increase the person's control over their own perceptions and behaviour.

Nursing interventions	Rationale
1. Initiate therapeutic relationship. Involve	Interventions more likely to be successful in an atmosphere of trust and

Nursing interventions	*Rationale*
in the care planning process	cooperation
2. Offer reassurance and demonstrate acceptance.	To minimize distress and create the conditions for behavioural change
3. Ensure non-judgemental and non-critical approach	Own reactions can distance you from the person and damage their self-esteem. Criticism tends to be counterproductive
4. Do not reinforce or encourage hallucinations and delusions. Do not collude with the person	Reinforcement tends to strengthen the person's belief in the validity of their thoughts and experiences. This also tends to increase their frequency and intensity
5. Encourage appropriate diversional activities	Boredom and lack of social stimulation tend to increase the occurrence of hallucinations
6. Reinforce sense of personal identity	Personal recognition and personal possessions help to reinforce contact with reality
7. Reinforce that which is real by offering alternative explanations to sensory experiences based on reality	This indicates and reinforces reality when the person misinterprets it. Indicate alternative by nurse stating her perception of the situation
8. Voice doubt over perceptions and thoughts indicating delusional thought processes or sensory distractions	The person may become aware of the fact that others do not necessarily perceive events in the same way or draw the same conclusions. Person encouraged to reconsider and re-evaluate their perceptions
9. Positively reinforce by encouragement and modelling, non-hallucinatory and healthy speech and behaviour patterns. Positively reinforce incompatible behaviour	Positive reinforcement of healthy behaviour is likely to increase its occurrence
10. Support the person to resist alien thoughts and feelings and to	May feel controlled by outside influences and needs to be helped to regain personal control. This helps to reduce

Nursing interventions	Rationale
have choice over their actions	feelings of helplessness
11. Provide opportunities for the person to express themselves openly	Helps to relieve tension and to demonstrate acceptance
12. Reinforce person's self-esteem	Improving self-esteem helps to improve the person's self-image in relationships with others. More likely to relate in a "healthy" way
13. Help to develop the person's social and communication skills. Model socially desired behaviour	Improvement of the person's ability to communicate and related to others is self-reinforcing. More likely to use appropriate means of communication
14. Identify potential stresses in the person's environment. Help the person to develop their coping skills	The experience of stress tends to exacerbate psychotic symptoms. Helping the person to cope better reduces this stress
15. Give medication as prescribed	Psychotropic medication helps to reduce the severity of psychotic symptoms

Evaluation

1. Reduction in the expression of hallucinatory and delusional experiences.
2. Appears more relaxed and less distressed.
3. Behaviour more predictable and in harmony with the environment.
4. Demonstrates evidence of self-control in his behaviour.

B. Maintain Their Autonomy and Self-esteem

Associated problems/personal difficulties

Person may be experiencing difficulties in maintaining their autonomy and self esteem due to:

1. A lack of motivation and initiative.
2. Feelings of passivity and external control.

3. Indecisiveness and indifference.
4. Poorly formed identity and low self-esteem.
5. Loss of interests.
6. Feelings of helplessness.

Assessment

1. Pattern, frequency and duration of interaction with others.
2. Nature of social contacts: self-initiated, prompted, positively or negatively reinforcing, submissive or assertive.
3. Personal choice and initiative shown.
4. External controls and environmental restrictions.
5. Social contact with family and friends.
6. Personal possessions and recognition of significant personal events.
7. Opportunities to participate in occupational and recreational activities.
8. Potential for increasing the person's autonomy.
9. Information from relatives and friends.

Desired outcomes

1. For the person to initiate their own activities and to demonstrate choice in the pattern of their everyday life-style.
2. For the person to make positive personal statements that reflect self-worth.

Nursing interventions	Rationale
1. Initiate therapeutic relationship with key worker	Interventions more likely to be successful in an atmosphere of trust and cooperation
2. Involve the person in the care planning process	Reinforces sense of self-worth and individuality
3. Use the person's preferred name. Facilitate the use of personal belongings. Personalize the person's intimate environment. Show recognition of person's attainments.	Personal recognition of individuality reinforces sense of identity and promotes self-esteem. This also promotes the person's feelings of security and potential for change

Nursing interventions	*Rationale*
4. Identify and help to celebrate significant personal dates, e.g. birthdays, anniversaries. Encourage personal interests. Promote contact with relatives and personal friends. Increase opportunities for group interaction. Increase environmental stimulation	Increases the number of potential situations that the person may find positively rewarding
5. Maintain orientation to present and contact with outside world. Remove unnecessary restrictions and rules. Increase personal responsibility in small stages. Encourage the expression of feelings	People can become "institutionalized" both in hospitals and community settings. The primary causes are external control by others and the anonymity of depersonalized living
6. Identify options for choice and opportunities to use initiative. Inform the person of the therapeutic benefit of choice and initiative. Present alternatives to the person. Facilitate the development of the person's decision-making skills. Reinforce initiatives taken by the person. Respect personal decisions. Demonstrate decision-making skills. Role play situations on decision-making and initiative. Use drama and experiential methods to promote insight and	Regaining personal control can be a very stressful process. Decision making is a skill like others that "lapses" with disease. In re-learning the skill people need opportunities to practise and to have feedback on the options chosen.

Nursing interventions	Rationale
spontaneity. Provide support during periods of stress. Give guidance and information as required.	
7. Help the person to work through periods of indecisiveness	Nurses also need to accept that "risk" is part of the process of regaining independence
8. Explore possibility of self-medication	Many people with long-term mental health problems are capable of self-medication
9. Teach the skills and principles of assertiveness	Increases personal control that can be expressed in a more effective way. Increases confidence and self-esteem
10. Identify opportunities for work-related activities	Relieves boredom which is a major problem. Raises self-esteem to be meaningfully employed

Evaluation

1. Person retains or regains initiative, control and choice over activities of daily living.
2. Behaviour indicates increased confidence and self-esteem.

C. Meet Their Basic Physical Needs

Associated problems/personal difficulties

Some of the difficulties that may interfere with the person's ability to meet their basic physical needs include:

1. Lack of volition.
2. Loss of interest and indifference.
3. Perceptual distractions.
4. Feel suspicious and threatened.
5. Lack of autonomy.
6. Disturbance of sleep pattern.

Assessment

1. Person's statements and behaviour in regard to meeting their needs for nutrition, fluids, hygiene and sleep.
2. Information available from relatives and friends.
3. Nurse's observations of:

   (a) Person's self initiated activities in relation to meeting their physical needs.
   (b) Person's skill level in meeting their physical needs.
   (c) Range of choice and options available to them.
   (d) Level of prompting required to motivate person and their reactions.
   (e) Accessibility and adequacy of cooking and hygiene facilities.
   (f) Reactions of others in the environment in relation to monitoring and non-attainment of person's physical needs.
   (g) Environmental factors reinforcing dependency and potential for promoting independence.
   (h) Identifiable physical health deficits: nutritional, hygiene, sleep, environmental.

Desired outcomes

1. Person is enabled to meet their own basic physical needs independently.
2. Person demonstrates raised self-esteem in relation to retaining autonomy for physical self-care.

Nursing intervention	Rationale
1. Initiate therapeutic relationship	Interventions more likely to be successful in an atmosphere of trust and cooperation
2. Minimize effects of sensory distractions and delusions	Person needs full awareness in order to recognize the need for nutrition, hygiene and sleep. Person needs to be in control of meeting their own needs
3. Promote their autonomy and self-esteem	Raising self-esteem increases the person's interest in their appearance and hygiene
4. Assist the person to individualize their appearance and to take an interest in how they appear to	External social feedback in the form of recognition and comment is a powerful reinforcer in an environment that is otherwise non-rewarding. Even very withdrawn and disturbed people

Nursing interventions	*Rationale*
others. Make unprompted positive comments about their appearance	can benefit from attention to their appearance
5. Encourage the person to use personalized soap, flannel, towel, toothbrush, razor, etc.	Person more likely to use items that belong to them
6. Ensure that dignity and privacy are respected and maintained	Communal dressing, washing and bathing devalue self-esteem and can cause personal distress. If you treat people in a less than respectful way they will also behave in a devalued way
7. Teach the person the skills of personal hygiene if they are lacking	If skills are not used they fade and require practice to regain mastery
8. Encourage choice and option over washing and bathing. Give positive feedback on personal initiatives	Facilitating control over their life increases motivation
9. Model and demonstrate desirable eating skills at meal-times. Encourage and give guidance on their eating skills. Facilitate choice at meal times	Nurses can exert a great influence as a role model. Person may need to re-learn skills
10. Provide opportunities for the person to take responsibility for and cook their own meals	Person will take more interest in food that they have selected and prepared
11. Encourage participation in activities during the day and evening	Prevents boredom. Reduces the likelihood of daytime sleeping
12. Encourage the person to stay up until a reasonable time	Many people go to bed too early and hence experience early morning waking. 7–9 hours sleep is a reasonable target for adults
13. Observe for drowsiness as a side-effect of medication	Over-sedation is a common side-effect of psychotropic drugs

Evaluation

1. Person complies with programme for developing self-care skills.
2. Need for prompting and guidance by carers decreases.
3. Person initiates actions to meet their basic physical needs independently.

D. Communicate and Relate to Others

Associated problems/personal difficulties

Some of the difficulties experienced by the person with schizophrenia in relation to communication include:

1. Avoidance of social contact and intimacy.
2. Lack of volition.
3. Anxiety in social situations.
4. Poor communication and social skills.
5. Thought disorders and delusions.
6. Perceptual distractions.
7. Social under-stimulation.
8. Low self-esteem.

Assessment

1. Person's description of their communication difficulties.
2. Nurse's observation of the person's:

   (a) Communication skills:
   - *Verbal skills*: tone, volume, rate, rhythm, clarity, appropriateness of content, synchronized with other speakers.
   - *Non-verbal skills*: positive, facial expression, eye contact, gestures, proximity, hand movements.
   - *Movement and mobility*: static or move around, duration spent in particular places.
   (b) Content of speech and emotions expressed: lacking, excessive, appropriate, assertive, non-assertive, intensity, changeability, consistency, morbid, negative, positive.

3. Interaction with others: frequency and duration of contacts; response to communications from others. Frequency, nature and duration of self-initiated communication with others. Avoidance or withdrawal demonstrated. Pattern throughout the day.
4. Psycho-social environment: situations and significant others that elicit, inhibit or reinforce communication. Potential stresses in the person's

environment or life-style. Reactions of others in communication with person.
5. Presence of identifiable thought or sensory distractions.
6. Sensory deficits: visual, auditory.

Desired outcomes

1. Person to initiate communication without prompting.
2. Person demonstrates appropriate and healthy speech content.
3. Person to interact with others in a more assertive way.

Nursing intervention	Rationale
1. Initiate therapeutic relationship	Interventions more likely to be successful in an atmosphere of trust and cooperation
2. Model skilled social and communication skills	Modelling by nurses has a powerful influence on the people in their care
3. Promote their autonomy and self-esteem (see **B**.) Reinforce sense of self-identity	Self-belief in the person's own value and feelings of control and mastery increase confidence in dealing with others
4. Minimize the influence of perceptual distractions and delusions (see **A**.)	Perceptual distractions interfere with a person's concentration and attention and this makes it difficult for them to communicate. Deluded thought patterns interfere with a person's interpretation and perception of events and cause communication misunderstandings
5. Promote their feelings of security and minimize feelings of threat (see **E**.)	If the person is anxious, suspicious or feels threatened, they will tend to withdraw and be defensive
6. Ensure that basic needs are being met (see **C**.)	Physical comfort is a prerequisite for meeting other needs. It also helps to raise self-esteem
7. Advise and support relatives who may find it difficult to	It is very distressing for close relatives who feel unable to reach out to the person and may feel rejected

Nursing intervention	*Rationale*
communicate with the person	
8. Inform the person about their care and treatment	The person may seem detached and aloof but still has a right to know. It also reduces the possibility of unexpected and threatening interventions
9. Provide written information if required	Person may find it difficult to concentrate. They are then able to refer back to the written details
10. Use touch and other non-verbal signals to demonstrate reassurance	Touch can be very reassuring and comforting if used with sensitivity
11. Accept one-sided conversation. Accept the person's behaviour. Be non-judgemental	The person may have a communication problem which makes it difficult for them to respond. Criticism only increases feelings of guilt and stress. These are counterproductive
12. Plan regular and short periods of interaction throughout the day	Where people are unable to find it difficult to initiate conversation with others, prolonged periods of conversation are stressful. It is more caring to show concern throughout the day rather than focus on one block of time. The rest of the day then becomes a period of isolation
13. If they are unresponsive, periodically sit by the person. Introduce yourself and then sit quietly	If you sit by someone and say "I thought I would keep you company/come and sit with you", it is perceived even by the most withdrawn person as caring and supportive
14. Respect the person's body space and do not talk "around" them	Failure to do this shows a complete lack of respect for the person. A withdrawn person is still alert to the environment
15. Engage in physical activity as a precursor to verbal interaction, e.g. games, activities, drama, music. Organize social and recreational activities	Sometimes it is easier for people to talk as part of an activity or game, or afterwards
16. Positively reinforce	Need to encourage the person to talk in

Nursing intervention	*Rationale*
appropriate and clear speech. Negatively reinforce inappropriate statements and unclear speech	a way that will facilitate communication with other people. This diminishes the likelihood of the person continuing to communicate in this way
17. Encourage the person to express their feelings	People who find it difficult to communicate may have pent-up emotions. It also provides the opportunity for them to practise talking about their emotions
18. Be available. Minimize role barriers. Be informal. Positively reinforce self-initiated interaction and communication	You have got to look and be approachable. More likely then to occur
19. Do not reinforce withdrawn behaviour. Communicate with the person when you are working with them	At times it is easier to do things for people than to get them to clearly ask for themselves
20. Use open-ended questions	These require multiple-word answers
21. Encourage social interaction with others. Organize group activities	Social activities can be very rewarding and also provide group dynamics that the person may find therapeutic
22. Identify situations with the person in which they experience anxiety or a communication difficulty	Many people with mental health problems are either lacking in social skills or have problems relating to others
23. Role play with feedback these situations with the person. Give demonstration and guidance as required. Provide information on the nature of human interaction and the expression of feeling	Social skills training helps people to develop their communication skills. It is a structured approach in which specific skills are: • identified and defined; • divided into their constituent elements; • the elements are practised with feedback in role-play until competence is achieved; • the entire skill is practised with

Nursing intervention	Rationale
	feedback until competence is achieved; • the skill is transferred to real-life situations.
24. Organize experiential exercises, e.g. drama, role-play, games, in which the person relates to others in an unstructured way and can express themselves freely	Even very withdrawn people will participate in these types of activities. They enable people to participate in a non-threatening way and to get used to being spontaneous

Evaluation

1. Person able to approach others and communicate with them of their own initiative and choice.
2. Person demonstrates raised self-esteem and confidence in the language and non-verbal communication that they use.

E. Feel Secure and Free from Threat

Associated problems/personal difficulties

Person may feel insecure and threatened as a result of:

1. Inadequate knowledge of their illness and treatment.
2. Guilt and damage to their self-esteem upon being diagnosed "schizophrenic".
3. Tension arising from their lack of control over their thoughts, feelings and behaviour.
4. Stressful and frightening sensory experiences.
5. Interpreting everything in a suspicious and distrustful way.
6. Feelings of great personal risk and malevolent intent by others.
7. Behaviour that is potentially self-injurious.

Assessment

1. Person's description of their anxieties, any feelings of threat or concerns

expressed, e.g. apprehension, specific fears, negative self-statements.
2. Nurse's observations of the person's:

(a) Response to questioning about potential anxieties.
(b) Understanding shown: questions asked and statements made in relation to their health care needs and programme.
(c) Emotions expressed: anxiety, irritability, tearfulness, dread.
(d) Verbal communication pattern: rate, tone of voice, pitch, speech errors, hesitation, thought blocking, over-talkativeness.
(e) Non-verbal behaviour indicating anxiety: positive, gestures, tremor, bodily movements, rigidity, eye movements, restlessness, pacing, fiddling, fidgeting, excessive smoking.
(f) Physiological responses: rate of respiration, perspiration, frequency of micturation, thirst, gastrointestinal upsets.

3. Support network available to the person: relationships with key people.
4. Identification of potential stressors in the person's current life situation and life-style.

Desired outcomes

1. Person is more relaxed and feels free from threat.
2. Person's understanding of their health care is increased.

Nursing intervention	Rationale
1. Provide clear and understandable information about their illness, health care and the roles of different health care workers	A lot of anxiety is associated with fear of the unknown. People have a right to information about their health care
2. Encourage questions. Ask for feedback on their understanding. Clarify any misunderstandings. Enlist the person's cooperation in the planning of their health care. Promote autonomy and self-esteem	The nurse is in an ideal position to use this process to facilitate the development of the person's understanding about their health care needs. People are more likely to cooperate if they are well-informed and involved in the decision-making process. It also increases feelings of personal control. Familiar objects help to increase feelings of security
3. Encourage the person	Being labelled mentally ill is a very

Nursing intervention	*Rationale*
to express their feelings about their situations and difficulties	stigmatizing process. The person feels guilty and bewildered. There is also a sense of loss over the change of role and self-identity
4. Initiate a therapeutic relationship. Spend time with them. Be available and approachable. Ensure non-judgemental and non-critical responses	The sense of worth and acceptance shown helps to increase feelings of security and safety. Being non-judgemental helps a person to deal with any guilt. Reduces feelings of anxiety.
5. Use touch, where appropriate	Touch can be very reassuring if used with sensitivity
6. Minimize the influence of perceptual distractions and delusions (see **A.**)	These can cause stress and make the person feel insecure
7. Facilitate the development of the person's ability to communicate and relate to others	Helps the person to express and thereby release feelings of anxiety and tension
8. Approach unhurriedly. Demonstrate calmness. Do not rush the person. Be aware of your own reactions and experiences of stress	Anxiety in the carer communicates itself to the person. Caring can be a stressful experience at times. This may unconsciously influence your interactions with others. Find ways of coping with your own stress
9. Encourage diversional recreational and social activities	Helps to avoid boredom and to divert the person's thoughts away from stressful topics. Physical activity is also a beneficial channel for stress
10. Encourage the person to rest or relax if they appear to be under stress. Provide feedback on their behaviour	Person may not be aware of the effect of anxiety on their behaviour
11. Emphasize the importance of recognizing internal tension and external stressors. Recommend methods for reducing	Providing a programme of health education offers a longer-term strategy for dealing with anxiety in the person's life

Nursing intervention	*Rationale*
sensory stimulation. Teach methods for achieving relaxation. Teach how to use problem-solving methods in coping with stress. Assist the person to learn new coping skills for anxiety	
12. Encourage the person to set realistic goals	Unrealistic goals cause frustration and are likely to lead to failure
13. Encourage the setting of progressive goals in small stages	Minimizes risk of failure
14. Provide emotionally safe experiences to increase their sense of mastery	Stress interferes with learning and can create feelings of helplessness
15. Encourage the use of newly acquired coping skills	Skills need to be used in order to become integrated into the person's everyday behaviour
16. Advise person if their behaviour is a risk to themselves or others	The person may feel that others are threatening them. They may also believe that they cannot come to any harm, that they are compelled to do some action or that parts of their body are not real. They may not realize that their actions are potentially unsafe
17. Set limits on behaviour that is potentially self-injurious. Be consistent and firm. Keep promises that you make. Get extra help	At times of fear and turmoil the nurse needs to show that they are in control of the situation and will not allow the person to harm themselves. Reduces the risk of injury to the person and to carers
18. Reassure the person of non-harmful intent	Frightened people can sometimes panic or attack the person they are fearful and suspicious of
19. Explain all actions in advance. Adopt a non-threatening, open posture and tone of	These actions help to reduce the tension

Nursing intervention	Rationale
voice. Keep calm	
20. Refrain from unnecessary actions and procedures if the person appears disturbed or agitated	These just increase the tension and are likely to be misinterpreted
21. Do not whisper to others in the presence of the person or express inappropriate emotion. Remove items which could damage the person. Remove distracting and stressful influences	This increases feelings of suspicion and threat
22. Encourage the person to talk about their hostile feelings. Encourage them to express their feelings in a more appropriate way	Venting their feelings in this way may remove the necessity for the physical expression of hostility and anger
23. Provide feedback to the person on their behaviour and use it as a learning situation	Provides an opportunity for health education in the appropriate expression of hostile feelings. Promotes insight. Nurses, too, should analyse the situation and discuss it themselves afterwards to review their practice and to learn from it
24. Co-ordinate interventions if action becomes necessary. Protect the person's safety	In order to reduce risks and to draw hostile situations to a close it is important that everyone is confident about their role in the situation
25. Use minimum restraint. Minimize period of restraint. Keep talking to the person. Provide reassurance	If people have to be held it should be in such a way that limbs and body are controlled and their airway is free. Even in these situations there is still a benefit in trying to reassure and calm the person
26. Arrange for own clinical supervision	Working with people who are suffering from schizophrenia can be very demanding. Supervision is one effective way of providing support and of personal development

Evaluation

1. Person appears relaxed and demonstrates trust in their care.
2. Person uses appropriate communication and coping skills to relate to others.

F. Facilitate the Person and Their Family's Ability to Cope with Problems

Associated problems/personal difficulties

The person's experience of schizophrenia may show that:

1. The person and their family may be presented with emotional and behavioural problems that they find difficult to understand and cope with.
2. Existing methods of coping may be counterproductive and adding to existing stress.
3. The person and their family may lack information about the resources available to help them.
4. There may be feelings of guilt in relation to their problems and asking for help.
5. The person and their family are ambivalent about working with outside agencies.
6. Current life-styles, expectations and relationships may be potential sources of stress.

Assessment

1. Person and their family's description of their current situation.
2. Accuracy of the knowledge and information given by the person and their family.
3. Statements of guilt and stigma.
4. Awareness of resources available to them.
5. Previous experience, if any, of dealing with similar problems.
6. Existing coping methods used and their effectiveness.
7. Support available to the person and their family.

Desired outcomes

1. Person and family able to make an informed choice about the resources they require.
2. Person and family able to cope better with the problems experienced.

Nursing Interventions	Rationale
1. Initiate therapeutic relationship. Involve the person and family in the care and planning process	Interventions more likely to be successful in an atmosphere of trust and cooperation
2. Advise that seeking help and recognition of problems are a positive step towards finding solutions	Many people feel that seeking help is a sign of weakness and failure. Also helps to reduce guilt
3. Encourage questions. Provide accurate information. Identify appropriate health care resources	May have inaccurate knowledge and expectations. Fear of the unknown. Need to know what resources are available to them
4. Discuss potential entitlement to financial benefits and allowances	May need and not be aware of the financial help available to them
5. Advise that highly emotional situations be avoided at first	May be pent-up feelings and stresses that need to be worked through and released in a controlled way. Sudden discharge of emotion may also increase the severity of the person's symptoms
6. Advise against early correction of problems	Under stress it is sometimes easier to make short-term adaptations that only store up future problems. It takes time to help the family to work out what is best for them
7. Reassure that there are ways of improving the situation	Family may feel that the situation is hopeless
8. Advise against recrimination and focussing on past problems	Need to focus on the present and future and to deal with anger and guilt in a more productive way
9. Advise on the need for acceptance and mutual support within their relationships	Family needs to come to terms with their situation. They are each other's primary source of support which will need to be utilized to cope effectively
10. Explain the need to identify and recognize	Mental health problems tend to be long-term in nature. In order to cope

Nursing intervention	*Rationale*
potentially stressful situations. Recommend methods for reducing sensory stimulation	effectively the family needs to be taught ways of making the necessary long-term adjustments
11. Advise on the need to maintain an optimum level of social stimulation for the person who is having difficulties	Research shows that people with schizophrenia require an environment in which they are motivated and yet not put under excessive stress. The optimum appears to be 35 hours per week social contact, given in a non-threatening way by a social group of 3–5 people
12. Teach methods for achieving relaxation. Teach how to use problem-solving methods for coping with difficulties. Assist the family to learn new coping skills. Encourage the setting of realistic goals	Most of the education needs to be directed towards coping methods. These include the way that the members of the family communicate and their expectations of the ill person
13. Encourage the setting of progressive goals in small stages. Advise the family on how to give feedback and support to one another	The re-learning needs to be done in a gradual way in which the family provides the main support and reinforcement
14. Recommend ways of setting behavioural limits. Explain the purpose of making a contract with the person	Living together is a process of negotiation. It is often useful for all concerned if the boundaries are firmly defined. Many families make implicit contracts that can be contractualized. Studies show these to be quite effective, e.g. the person must not display disturbed behaviour at meal-times/in the living room
15. Advise on the need to comply with prescribed medication. Advise on possible side-effects of	Relapse is significantly associated with failure to take medication as prescribed. This is particularly so in families where there is a lot of expressed emotion. Individuals and

Nursing intervention	Rationale
medication	their family need to be able to recognize side-effects and to communicate this to their doctor
16. Teach the family and person to recognize the limits of their ability to cope and when it is advisable to seek help	The family should not over-burden itself as this can damage relationships and its longer-term ability to cope

Evaluation

1. Person and family identify and select resources they require.
2. Person and family demonstrate use of improved coping methods.
3. Person and family able to give accurate information about their health care needs.

Unit Instructions

When you have researched the suggested references, have mastered the Unit Objectives and successfully answered the Self-assessment Questions, proceed with the Unit Written Test.

Suggested References

Altschul, A. and McGovern, M. (1985). *Psychiatric Nursing*, 6th edition. Baillière Tindall, London and San Diego.

Bauer, B. and Hill, S. (1986). *Essentials of Mental Health Care Planning and Interventions*. W. B. Saunders, Philadelphia.

Berkowitz, R. and Heinl, P. (1984). The management of schizophrenic patients. The nurse's view. *Journal of Advanced Nursing*, January Vol. 9, No. 1, pp. 23–33.

Campbell, C. (1978). *Nursing Diagnosis and Intervention in Nursing Practice*. John Wiley, New York.

Corden, A. (1988). Schizophrenia: The search for therapeutic responses. *Nursing Times*, 20 January, Vol. 84, No. 3, pp. 50–51.

Darcy, P. T. (1985). *Mental Health Nursing Source Book*. Baillière Tindall, London and San Diego.

Department of Health and Social Security (1976). *Management of the Violent and Potentially Violent Patient*. H. C. (76) 11. London, HMSO.

Dexter, G. and Wash, M. (1986). *Psychiatric Nursing Skills: A Patient-centred Approach*. Croom Helm, London.
Hase, S. and Douglas, A. (1986). *Human Dynamics and Nursing*. Churchill Livingstone, Melbourne.
Irving, S. (1983). *Basic Psychiatric Nursing*, 3rd edition. W. B. Saunders, Philadelphia.
Lancaster, J. (1980). *Adult Psychiatric Nursing*. Henry Kimpton, London.
McFarland, G. and Wasli, E. (1986). *Nursing Diagnoses and Process in Psychiatric Mental Health Nursing*. J. B. Lippincott, Philadelphia.
Martin, P. (1987a). *Psychiatric Nursing: A Therapeutic Approach*. Macmillan, London.
Martin, P. (1987b). *Care of the Mentally Ill*, 2nd edition. Macmillan, London.
Pelletier, L. (Ed.) (1987). *Psychiatric Nursing Case Studies, Nursing Diagnoses and Care Plans*. Springhouse Corporation, Springhouse, Pennsylvania.
Robinson, L. (1983). *Psychiatric Nursing as a Human Experience*, 3rd edition. W. B. Saunders, Philadelphia.
Teesdale, K. (1986). The withdrawn schizophrenic. *Nursing Times*, 5 February, Vol. 82, No. 6, pp. 32–34.

Self-assessment Questions

SAQ 13. List four potential care needs of a person suffering from schizophrenia.
SAQ 14. Describe the advice that the family may need with regard to communication and social contact with the sufferer of schizophrenia.
SAQ 15. Describe interventions for maintaining autonomy and self-esteem.
SAQ 16. Identify interventions that can be used to reduce the influence of perceptual distractions.

Unit 10.4: Written Test

Mr and Mrs Shepherd are very concerned that their 19-year-old son Peter is coming home shortly after a period of in-patient treatment for schizophrenia. They are worried about how they will cope and what will happen to their son.

1. What advice can they be given about creating the optimum domestic environment to maintain Peter's autonomy and ability to cope with stress?
2. What resources and long-term support will the family require?

TOPIC 11

Mental Health Problems Characterized by Extreme Overactivity

At the end of this Topic the learner should aim to:

1. Describe the characteristic features of mental health problems associated with extreme overactivity.
2. Outline the range of treatment interventions available and support required.
3. Identify the nursing care needs and interventions required for the overactive person.

Recognizing and Understanding Extreme Overactivity

Unit Objectives

At the end of this Unit the learner should be able to:

1. Describe the classification of mental health problems associated with extreme overactivity.
2. Outline factors associated with the onset of extreme overactivity.
3. Identify the characteristic behavioural, emotional and cognitive features of extreme overactivity.

Extreme Overactivity as a Mental Health Problem

Mania, hypomania and manic-depressive psychosis are major mental illnesses – affective psychoses – characterized by a pathological elation of mood, gross overactivity and loss of insight. They are comparatively uncommon mental health problems occurring in only about 1 in 200 people.

The first episodes tend to occur between the ages of 20 and 35 and may go unrecognized, particularly if the person is usually energetic and active. The attacks are self-limiting and most people tend to recover within a few months, even without treatment. The period between remissions tends to become shorter and the duration of the episodes becomes longer as the person becomes older. For a number of people the recurrent episodes of overactivity and its associated problems may become chronic mental health difficulties.

Clinical Classification of Extreme Overactivity

In clinical practice the person with extreme overactivity and elation may be diagnosed within one of the following categories:

1. *Hypomania.* The person is euphoric and overactive but to a lesser degree of excitement than is seen in mania. They are also less likely to be

affected by delusions and perceptual distractions. The main distinction between hypomania and mania is one of degree based upon clinical judgement.
2. *Mania*. A state of extreme elation and overactivity. Disinhibition and delusional thinking are common. The person may also experience transitory perceptual distractions.
3. *Manic-depressive psychosis*. Characterized by a cyclical pattern of mood swings, alternating between periods of over-excitement and profound depression. For some people the cyclical variations may form part of a predictable pattern, with fixed intervals between the contrasting moods. During the depressed phase of this cycle the person exhibits the characteristic signs of extreme depression (see Topic 7). In the elated phase the person shows the characteristic signs of mania or hypomania.

Origins of Overactivity

A number of factors are thought to have an influence on the occurrence of mania, hypomania and manic-depressive psychosis:

1. *Heredity*: in approximately 10% of cases, one or both parents had an episode of overactivity.
2. *Biochemical*: the cyclic pattern of overactive behaviour would seem to indicate a corresponding pattern of physiological changes. In particular, there seem to be disturbances in the person's lithium electrolyte balance. Childbirth may also precipitate a manic reaction in some mothers, possibly due to the sudden change in hormonal levels.
3. *Psychoanalytical*: in which the person is viewed as trying to deny or avoid facing up to underlying depression through excessive overactivity.
4. *Stress*: extreme stress that the person is unable to cope with may precipitate overactivity as a reaction.
5. *Behavioural*: where overactivity and elated mood are maintained by social reinforcement.
6. *Cognitive*: faulty perceptual and cognitive processes that initiate and maintain an overactive response.
7. *Personality*: a cyclothymic personality characterized by alternating cycles of sadness, normal mood and feeling "high".
8. *Gender*: women have a higher incidence than men.

Characteristic Features

Mood

From pleasant, cheerful hilarity and high spirits to elation and euphoria. Infectious humour, laughing and jovial. Extreme sense of well-being. Mood is labile and can change suddenly. Resents interference and is intolerant of others. Easily provoked and can become quarrelsome, irritable or angry if frustrated.

Behaviour

1. Continuous physical overactivity and restlessness. Boundless energy, does not feel tired. Always on the move from one thing to another, rarely finishing anything. Erratic and unruly. Interferes with other people and can be very demanding and irritating. Potentially impulsive, may be destructive towards property and aggressive with people. Rarely aware of the physical risks that their behaviour may pose for themselves or for others.
2. Socially and sexually disinhibited. Diminished social awareness and judgement. Can be offensive, crude, tactless and indiscreet. Capable of causing considerable upset to others with their comments and behaviour. Sexually provocative and erotic behaviour. Increased libido. May undress in public places without inhibition or engage in sexual activities they would not normally consider. Disinhibited about elimination. May wear excessive make-up and dress extravagantly.

Thought disturbances

1. Flight of ideas. Pressure of thought. Very distractable and constantly changing focus of interest. Short attention span and lacking in concentration. May talk very quickly, making up new words or rhyming their speech.
2. Lack of insight. Inflated self-esteem with total confidence and optimism. May make elaborate and grand plans for themselves or others. Possible delusions of grandeur and omnipotence. May believe they are wealthy and spend all their available money, incurring debts. May believe that they are very important and powerful or that they can come to no harm. Can also be very suspicious and paranoid. May have ideas of reference.
3. Perceptual distractions may occur during phases of extreme excitement and euphoria.

Physical effects

1. Exhaustion: extreme hyperactivity interferes with rest and sleep. Does not feel tired. Restless throughout the night. Preoccupied with the drive to keep active. Will stay active until they collapse with exhaustion.
2. Nutritional neglect: too active and busy to eat or drink. Risk of dehydration. May lose a considerable amount of weight.

3. Neglect of hygiene and appearance: personal habits may become very degraded. Too busy to wash or change clothes.

Differential Recognition

Initially, certain other mental health problems may appear to be similar to mania, hypomania or manic-depressive psychosis. These can be discriminated on the basis of the prolonged elevation of mood and behaviour characteristic of overactivity. Diagnostic tests may also be used to identify disorders related to physical disease or substance abuse.

1. *Schizophrenia*: during a period of elation and hyperactivity.
2. *Drug abuse*: particularly where stimulants such as amphetamines are involved.
3. *Thyrotoxicosis*: causing restless overactivity, weight loss and certain other characteristic physical signs.

Unit Instructions

When you have researched the suggested references, have mastered the Unit Objectives and successfully answered the Self-assessment Questions, proceed with the Unit Written Test.

Suggested References

Darcy, P. T. (1985). *Mental Health Nursing Source Book*. Baillière Tindall, London and San Diego.
Davis, D. R. (1984). *An Introduction to Psychopathology*, 4th edition, Oxford University Press, Oxford.
Dexter, G. and Wash, M. (1986). *Psychiatric Nursing Skills: A Patient-centred Approach*. Croom Helm, London.
Hughes, J. (1986). *An Outline of Modern Psychiatry*, 2nd edition. John Wiley, Chichester.
Lyttle, J. (1986). *Mental Disorder*. Baillière Tindall, London and San Diego.
Martin, P. (1987). *Care of the Mentally Ill*, 2nd edition. Macmillan, London.
Sims, A. (1988). *Symptoms in the Mind*. Baillière Tindall, London and San Diego.
Trethowan, W. and Sims, A. (1983). *Psychiatry*, 5th edition. Baillière Tindall, London and San Diego.
Willis, J. (1976). *Clinical Psychiatry*. Blackwell Scientific, Oxford.

Self-assessment Questions

SAQ 1. Identify four factors associated with the origins of extreme
overactivity.

SAQ 2. List five emotional characteristics of extreme overactivity.

SAQ 3. Describe five ways that a person's overactive behaviour may
cause conflict with others.

SAQ 4. Outline four characteristic thought disturbances that would
confirm a person is suffering from extreme overactivity.

Unit 11.1: Written Test

A very distressed Mrs Anderson has telephoned her community mental
health centre. She states that over the last 4 days her son John, aged 22,
has gone "mad". Apparently, he is completely overactive and is driving
everyone to distraction. She urgently pleads for a visit from someone to
help them. As the duty community psychiatric nurse you have arranged
to visit her within the next 2 hours.

What observations would you make of John's behaviour, emotional state,
thought processes and physical condition that would confirm he has a mental
health problem associated with overactivity.

Care and Treatment of the Person who Exhibits Extreme Overactivity

Unit Objectives

At the end of this Unit the learner should be able to:

1. Describe the effects of overactivity on individual and family life.
2. Describe therapeutic care and treatment interventions for people suffering from extreme overactivity.
3. Identify the support required for the person and their family in the community and in the hospital.

Care and Treatment

A wide range of therapeutic interventions may be used to help the person who is pathologically overactive. These may focus on the person's presenting behaviour, their life-style and on developing their coping skills.

The specific interventions will be based upon the person's needs, the outcomes of the assessment and the skills and resources available to the therapist. The general approach should be towards an integrated and readily accessible service that is able to support the person and their family in the community or in residential settings as required.

Therapeutic aims

1. To stabilize the person's emotional state and behaviour.
2. To minimize the risk of physical, personal or social harm to the person.
3. To facilitate the development of the person's and their family's coping skills.

Family and Self-care

The changes that occur in the person's behaviour may not, initially, be recognized as significant. The high spirits, enthusiasm and energy that tend to develop over a short period of time can be lively and entertaining. In particular, if they are usually an energetic and hardworking person or have periods of elated mood, then their overactivity and joy may not be recognized or identified as a problem. To the person, themselves, their sense of well-being and elation reinforce their own perception of feeling on top of the world. Naturally, they would tend to resist or reject any notion that they might have a severe mental health problem that may require intervention.

However, the nature of this excessive overactivity and elation is such that the person is unlikely to go unnoticed for long. For those in closest contact with the person they might recognize that the behaviour is part of a recurring cycle of behaviour or a relapse of a longstanding problem. Even if it is the person's first episode of overactivity, they are likely to find them very demanding, irritating and completely disruptive to normal family life. These may be the source of extreme domestic disagreement and distress. Eventually, the family may acknowledge that they need specialist help and support.

If those in closest contact do not recognize the person's mental health problems or they live alone, then it is quite likely that the person's disinhibited and grandiose behaviour may bring them into conflict with their neighbours or the police. This may precipitate a community-based crisis intervention or admission into care. It may be necessary to use the powers of the 1983 Mental Health Act to ensure that the person is given appropriate care and treatment.

In the longer term, the recurrent cycles of overactivity and depression, or recurrent episodes of elation, are likely to prove very damaging to the person's close relationships and employment. During these phases, the demands made on their support network may exceed the tolerance of the family and their ability to cope. Consequently, the person may be rejected by their family and close friends. They may expect to have periodic major upheavals in their life when established patterns of relationships and domestic living are completely disrupted and have to be gradually re-established.

Some people possess a degree of insight and self-awareness about their mental health problem and are able to identify when they need help. The support network can also be an invaluable source of assistance. Others can learn to recognize the early signs of forthcoming overactivity and to ensure compliance with prescribed medication. Professional help, if required, can then be sought at an early stage when it is most effective.

Initially, the person and their family can be helped considerably in coping with mania and hypomania by:

1. Accurate information about overactivity and its effects.
2. Involvement in the care and treatment process.
3. Reassurance that effective intervention is possible.
4. The opportunity to talk freely about their problems.
5. The opportunity for support and a break when suffering from exhaustion.
6. Advising them of the necessity of ensuring compliance with prescribed medication to help avoid a relapse.
7. The address of a local contact support group.

8. Developing the person's and family's coping skills.
9. Reviewing their life-style and expectations to promote their mental health.

Community Care

The behaviour and elation of the overactive person can make it very difficult for them to be cared for at home. They may require constant observation and supervision to limit their disruption, disinhibition and risk of exhaustion. Depending upon the extent and tolerance of the social support available, and the therapeutic resources available, then it may be possible to care for the overactive person at home. In reality, it would appear that a number of people and families do cope unaided. The aims of community care are:

1. To support the person and their family.
2. To enable the person to remain in their own home.
3. To monitor the person's mental and physical health.
4. To implement community-based treatment and care programmes.

The services available include:

1. The community mental health centre: with community psychiatric nurses, social workers, psychologists, occupational therapists and consultant psychiatrists working as a team to offer skills-based therapeutic interventions.
2. General practitioners.
3. Voluntary agencies: MIND, contact and support groups for sufferers and relations.
4. DHSS: benefits, allowances and grants as currently available to individuals and their families.
5. Department of Employment: Disablement Rehabilitation Officer (DRO), Register of Disabled Persons, occupational training schemes.
6. Local authority/health authority: hostels, half-way homes, group homes, sheltered workshops.
7. Out-patient clinics and day hospitals.

Residential Care

The reasons for admission to residential facilities for care and treatment include:

1. Lack of support in the community.
2. The need for intensive care when the person is extremely overactive and is a potential risk to himself.
3. Personal and family exhaustion.
4. Detailed assessment and the need for specific types of therapy.

Therapeutic Interventions

Psychotherapeutic Methods

1. *Skilled nursing care*: one of the most important therapeutic factors.
2. *Individual counselling*: to increase insight, to promote self-esteem, to release repressed emotion.
3. *Behavioural psychotherapy*: for specific behavioural problems, to reinforce non-overactive behaviour, social skills training.
4. *Health education*: to develop coping skills, to identify and modify stressors in the person's life, to facilitate recognition of early signs of overactivity, to promote compliance with treatment regimes.
5. *Family therapy*: to provide support, to help the family to find ways of coping with stress and to review their life-style, to facilitate family communications.
6. *Occupational therapy*: life skills and activities of daily living.
7. *Art therapy and psychodrama*: to help express and release feelings.
8. *Recreational and social activities*: to provide diversional activities and to meet social needs.
9. *Voluntary organizations*: self-help and support groups, MIND.

Physical treatment methods: chemotherapy

1. *Major tranquillizers*: chlorpromazine (Largactil), haloperidol (Serenace), thioridazine (Melleril), pimozide (Orap), trifluoperazine (Stelazine).
2. *Anti-Parkinsonian drugs* for side-effects of major tranquillizers: orphenadine (Disipal), benzhexol (Artane), procyclidine (Kemadrin).
3. *Lithium therapy*: a specific medication of prophylactic value in manic-depressive illness and in the treatment of mania. It may need to be taken for some years. Given orally as lithium carbonate (Priadel, Camcolit) or lithium citrate (Litarex).

   The therapeutic effect of lithium is directly related to its plasma concentration level. This has to be closely monitored as lithium has potentially very severe side-effects and may prove fatal if the serum level rises too high. In clinical practice, the dosage is regulated to maintain a blood plasma level between 0.8 and 1.5 mmol/litre.

   The specific dosage prescribed will depend upon clinical judgement and the person's individual response to lithium. The serum lithium level needs to be monitored weekly for the first 4 weeks of treatment, then monthly for 1 year, and then every 3 months thereafter. It may also need to be reviewed in the event of physical illness or if lithium toxicity is suspected.

   Lithium is contraindicated where the person has cardiac or renal impairment, thyroid disease, diabetes insipidus, Addisons disease or is taking diuretics. It should not be taken during pregnancy or where the mother is breastfeeding. Lithium should also be used with caution in combination with certain other drugs, e.g. codeine, morphine, some antirheumatic medications. Minor side-effects include nausea, mild diarrhoea, fine tremor, weight gain, oedema, exacerbation of psoriasis, polyceria and polydipsia. Some of these may disappear with continued treatment.

Signs which indicate lithium toxicity include vomiting, diarrhoea, anorexia, tinnitus, blurred vision, drowsiness, sluggishness, giddiness, ataxia, coarse tremor, lack of co-ordination, reduced ability to concentrate, muscle weakness and heaviness of limbs. If these signs are observed or reported then the medication should be ceased and immediate medical intervention sought. Signs of serious overdosage include fits, circulatory failure, syncope, oliguria and coma. These may prove fatal.

Unit Instructions

When you have researched the suggested references, have mastered the Unit Objectives and successfully answered the Self-assessment Questions, proceed with the Unit Written Test.

Suggested References

Gibbs, A. (1986). *Understanding Mental Health*. Consumers Association/Hodder and Stoughton, London.

Gillies, D. and Lader, M. (1986). *Guide to the Use of Psychotropic Drugs*. Churchill Livingstone, Edinburgh.

Hughes, J. (1986). *An Outline of Modern Psychiatry*, 2nd edition. John Wiley, New York.

Lewis, J. G. (1986). *Therapeutics*, 4th edition. Hodder and Stoughton, London.

Lunder, L. (1987). Looking back in anger. *Nursing Times*, 8 April, Vol. 83, No. 14, pp. 49–50.

Silverstone, T. and Turner, P. (1982). *Drug Treatment in Psychiatry*, 3rd edition. Routledge and Kegan Paul, London.

Sutherland, S. (1987). *Breakdown* (updated edition). Weidenfeld and Nicolson, London.

Trethowan, A. and Sims, A. (1983). *Psychiatry*, 5th edition. Baillière Tindall, London and San Diego.

Willis, J. (1976). *Clinical Psychiatry*. Blackwell Scientific, Oxford.

Self-assessment Questions

SAQ 5. Identify four ways in which an overactive person can cause disruption in their home environment or in the community.

SAQ 6. Outline the role of four agencies in providing community support for the overactive person.

SAQ 7. Describe five psychotherapeutic interventions that may be indicated in the care and treatment of pathological overactivity.

SAQ 8. List five side-effects that would indicate lithium toxicity.

Unit 11.2: Written Test

David Jarrett, aged 22, lives at home with his parents and his brother Peter, aged 17. His two married sisters live nearby. He has always been a very lively and outgoing person which has been of benefit in his job as a salesman.

Ten days ago his behaviour became even more energetic and his mood far more elated. His family were initially puzzled, but also bemused, by his constant activity, laughter and promises of grandiose schemes. However, patience began to wear thin on both sides when the family tried to put some limits on David's behaviour. They were becoming exhausted by the demands he made and the frequent arguments as they tried to confront David. Concern was rising as he was not resting, not eating or drinking very much, making bizarre and extravagant plans and appeared to lack insight into his behaviour.

The situation reached a crisis when 20 colour television sets were delivered to their house, closely followed by delivery trucks from numerous suppliers. Apparently, David had been through the *Yellow Pages* ordering vast quantities of goods. These were, fortunately, returned. However, the convoy of delivery trucks had aroused considerable interest from their neighbours.

In desperation the family contacted their GP who visited the household and after seeing David made an immediate referral to the crisis intervention team. As the CPN on duty, accompanied by an "approved" social worker (as defined by the 1983 Mental Health Act), you both have arrived at the household and have to plan your therapeutic interventions.

1. How can David and his family be immediately helped to cope with the situation?

2. What factors need to be considered in terms of deciding whether David can be cared for at home or needs admission to a hospital?

3. If David needs hospital admission but adamantly refuses to go, what sections of the 1983 Mental Health Act may be invoked to ensure that he receives appropriate care and treatment?

4. As part of his treatment David is prescribed lithium carbonate. His parents are very concerned about this and ask to talk to someone about his medication. Upon questioning it is apparent that they have a confused understanding of the drug and the need to monitor its concentration in the plasma. Briefly outline the information that they should be given in order to reassure them about the therapeutic use of lithium carbonate.

UNIT 11.3

Nursing Care of the Overactive Person

Unit Objectives

At the end of this Unit the learner should be able to:

1. Identify the nursing care needs of the person with extreme overactivity.
2. Plan an individualized care programme.
3. Select appropriate nursing care interventions for the person's needs.
4. Describe potential evaluation criteria for specific needs.

Mental Health Nursing Care

Each person's care needs are unique and have to be assessed individually. A range of potential care needs have been selected to illustrate the problems that the person may experience and the possible nursing interventions that may help them. For the person presenting with extreme overactivity these may include the needs to:

A. Moderate their overactive behaviour.
B. Feel secure in a safe environment.
C. Meet their basic physical needs.
D. Communicate and relate to others.
E. Facilitate the development of the person's and family's coping skills.

A. Moderate Their Overactive Behaviour

Associated problems/personal difficulties

Overactivity may be adversely affecting the person's health by:

1. Interfering with their awareness and ability to meet their physical needs for rest and nutrition.
2. Interfering with their ability to communicate to others.

3. Leading to conflict with others.
4. Damaging their relationships and self-esteem through disinhibition.
5. Creating situations of risk to the person's safety and those around them.
6. Precipitating unpredictable and impulsive behaviour.
7. Putting them at risk of harm.

Assessment

1. Person's description of their own behaviour patterns.
2. Information from relatives and friends.
3. Nurse's observations of the person's:

    (a) Behaviour pattern and level of activity throughout the day: frequency of contact with others, nature of specific activities, duration of particular activities, concentration span, completion and non-completion of tasks, periods of rest taken, adequacy of nutritional intake, relationship of elated behaviour to external events.
    (b) Emotional expression: intensity and duration of episode of elation, irritability, appropriateness of emotional reactions.
    (c) Thought processes: content of elated ideas, pattern and frequency of elated thoughts throughout the day, association of elated thoughts with external events.
    (d) Psychosocial environment: precence of identifiable activity stimuli or triggering ones, reactions of others to person's overactivity and elated mood, potential reinforcers of overactive behaviour and thoughts, presence of potential stresses in person's environment or life-style.
    (e) Potential risk factors arising from the person's behaviour and thoughts.

Desired outcomes

1. Person able to moderate the extent of their overactivity.
2. Occurrence of overactive behaviour decreases.
3. Person able to rest periodically and to meet their nutritional needs.
4. Person does not put themselves, or others, at risk as a result of their overactivity.

Nursing intervention	Rationale
1. Initiate therapeutic relationship. Involve them in the care planning process	Interventions more likely to succeed in an atmosphere of trust and cooperation
2. Be available and	Helps to promote calm and to create the

Nursing intervention	*Rationale*
approachable. Offer reassurance. Demonstrate acceptance. Demonstrate non-judgemental approach. Promote feelings of security and safety (see **B**.)	conditions for behavioural change. People who are overactive tend to be very sensitive to implied criticism. Overactivity can be a way of coping with stress and insecurity
3. Promote self-esteem	Improving self-esteem helps to improve their self-image in relationships with others. Raising self-esteem also increases their commitment to regain personal control
4. Reduce the number of distracting influences that the person is exposed to. Minimize contact with other disturbed or noisy people or situations	The overactive person is very alert and responsive to stimuli. Hence, reducing external stimuli helps to calm the person and to reduce the potential for distractability. Likewise, the person is very responsive to disturbed behaviour in others
5. Observe their behaviour to identify factors that contribute to overactive behaviour	Can be used to identify any environmental factors that may be amenable to modification
6. Assist the person to identify any environmental factors related to their overactivity	Person may not be aware of the way that environmental factors are influencing their behaviour
7. Encourage the person to modify environmental factors where possible that are contributing to overactive thoughts and behaviour	Modification of contributing environmental factors may help to reduce stimuli that elicit overactivity
8. Negatively reinforce overactive behaviour and cognitions. Positively reinforce healthy behaviour	Helps to decrease frequency of overactive behaviour
9. Teach family members the skills of giving reinforcement	Family members may be inadvertently contributing to the maintenance of overactivity

Nursing intervention	*Rationale*
10. Positively reinforce healthy behaviour and responses. Negatively reinforce presenting symptoms	Positive reinforcement of healthy behaviour is likely to increase its occurrence
11. Model normal paced responses for person in situations where they are overactive	Modelling can be a powerful influence for positive behaviour change. People tend to reflect the behaviour of those around them
12. Role play calm responses with person. Provide guidance and feedback	Practice in this way can be a useful stage in regaining behavioural control
13. Offer feedback on the person's behaviour. Offer feedback on the person's expressed feelings	Person may not be aware of how others perceive them. Person may benefit from reflected appraisal of their emotional experiences
14. Explore with the person the effects of their behaviour and emotions upon others	Person may not be aware of how their behaviour and emotional reactions affect others
15. Explore with the person the effects of their behaviour on their own and their family's life	Person may not be fully aware of how their behaviour is disrupting their life and relationships
16. Inform the person as to what he can realistically expect from the staff and others. Meet reasonable demands. Keep promises that you make	Promotes insight and reinforces social awareness. Shows respect for the person
17. Create a sense of awareness in others that anger and irritability may be an expression of illness and is likely to be short term	Others may reject the person during their illness and cause permanent damage to relationships
18. Protect others who may find the behaviour of the	Others may react defensively or with fear. This may create conflict situations

Nursing intervention	*Rationale*
overactive person threatening	
19. Offer feedback on the person's behaviour and use it as a learning situation	Person may not be fully aware of how much their overactive behaviour is disrupting their life and relationships
20. Explain the reasons for setting limits on their behaviour to the person	The overactive person often lacks internal controls. Initially, the carers have to set and maintain limits, which can gradually be internalized by the person as their clinical condition improves
21. Specify the boundaries of acceptable behaviour. Clearly set limits on behaviour that is: • potentially self-harmful • threatening to others • disturbing to others. Record these in detail	Overactive person lacks insight into their behaviour and may put themselves, or others, at risk. Encouraging personal responsibility helps to raise self-esteem and promote insight. This needs to be done with regard to the person's clinical condition. Also shows that others are concerned for their welfare
22. Ensure that written limits are readily accessible to carers. Give a copy to the person and family	Helps to promote consistency
23. Inform the person of the consequences of exceeding defined limits. Promote compliance with set limits. Positively reinforce compliance with limits	Person needs to know how others will react and intervene
24. Ensure that all care workers are consistent in their approach to maintaining limits	Need to ensure consistency in the limits that are set and maintained. Person will readily manipulate carers if they identify inconsistency
25. Inform the person when their behaviour is approaching set	Person may lack insight and require feedback. They may also be testing out the tolerance of others. It is

Nursing intervention	*Rationale*
limits. Inform the person when and how their behaviour and speech is disturbing others. Do not respond to taunts. Keep calm	important to retain personal control of your own feelings
26. Enforce stated limits using physical and verbal interventions as appropriate, e.g. posture, touch, tone of voice, eye contact, informing about outcomes. Be firm and consistent	Limits need to be enforced if they are to be therapeutically effective
27. Divert the person's attention, if appropriate, to more constructive activities. Encourage the person to write out their feelings	Overactive people tend to be rapidly diverted and may be tactfully guided into more appropriate ways of channelling their energy
28. Co-ordinate interventions of care staff if intervention is necessary. Use minimal force, hold non-vulnerable areas. Keep talking to the person to try and calm them. Help person overcome guilt afterwards. Be non-judgemental and respect the person	Intervention may be safer for carers and person if several people are used to enforce constraint. Needs to be done in a way that is non-threatening and assertive
29. Use seclusion or time-out if specified in limits or if others are at significant risk. Comply with organizational rules for seclusion, if used. Try to help person learn from the incident	Seclusion or time-out may be an appropriate intervention in certain situations. Needs to be used with extreme caution. Helps to promote insight if experience is analysed

Nursing intervention	*Rationale*
30. Periodically review limits that are set. Review with the person to promote learning	These are likely to change in relation to the person's clinical condition. More likely to promote compliance
31. Explore alternative ways of behaving in the situation	Helps to promote insight and learning
32. Document, in detail, necessary interventions afterwards. Document any injuries caused to person or to staff. Review staff practices afterwards to evaluate interventions and care programme	Each organization has its own rules. Important that records are kept for both review and for possible legal purposes May forget significant items if this is left for too long
33. Explore alternative and purposeful ways of directing excess energy. Encourage moderate exercise	Can channel excess energy productively. Reduces opportunity for interfering with others. Can promote self-esteem. Also helps to reduce the risk of self-harm
34. Encourage appropriate diversional activities. Suggest the person rests periodically. Identify activities that the person finds relaxing and promote rest	Divert attention from other less constructive activities and interfering with others
35. Minimize the influence of perceptual distractions and thought disorder (see Unit 10.4)	Need to reinforce contact with reality in order to promote insight and to reduce possibility of impulsive behaviour
36. Provide opportunities for the person to express themselves openly and honestly. Encourage the person to talk about any hostile feelings	Venting feelings in this way may reduce the necessity for the physical expression of hostility and anger
37. Identify situations that contribute to disinhibited speech	May be specific situations that trigger this response. To promote self-awareness. Talking may reduce the

Nursing intervention	*Rationale*
and behaviour. Teach more appropriate ways of expressing sexual feelings. Provide opportunities for the person to talk about sexual feelings. Be non-judgemental about disinhibition	need to cut out feelings. The person may try to shock carers
38. Protect from ridicule and embarrassing situations. Protect from rejection by others. Intervene tactfully. Promote dignity. Distract to more constructive topics or activities	During periods of disinhibition person may behave in ways that they would normally find embarrassing. Person needs to be protected from carrying out behaviours that are potentially damaging
39. Assist the person to acknowledge the influence of their expectations and personal standards on their behaviour. Explore alternative expectations and standards	The person needs to be helped to reshape their beliefs about themself and to develop more valid and realistic expectations
40. Help person to develop more attainable expectations and standards. Encourage acceptance of self-limitations	May be driven to attain unrealistic and overdemanding standards
41. Observe for side-effects of medication. Teach person and family how to recognize the side-effects of medication	Chemotherapy for overactivity can have unpleasant and potentially harmful side-effects if not closely monitored
42. Recognize the effects of person's behaviour on your own ability to cope. Take time out, if possible. Arrange for own clinical supervision	Caring for the overactive person can be a very demanding and draining experience. Need to maintain own mental health and to review own clinical practice to facilitate personal development.

Evaluation

1. Significant decrease in levels of overactivity.
2. Observed to rest periodically without prompting.
3. Observed to eat and drink without prompting.
4. Reduction of conflict with others.
5. Behaviour stays within stated limits.
6. Behaviour does not threaten, embarrass or result in conflict with others.

B. Feel Secure and Free from Threat

Associated problems/personal difficulties

Person may feel insecure and at risk as a result of:

1. Inadequate knowledge about their care and treatment.
2. Lack of awareness about the possibility of self-harm arising from their behaviour.
3. Frustration from limits imposed by others.
4. Stresses that their behaviour causes in their relationships.

Assessment

1. Person's description of their frustrations and concerns: feelings of threat, apprehension, specific fears.
2. Information from relatives and friends.
3. Nurse's observations of the person's:

   (a) Response to questioning about their frustrations.
   (b) Understanding shown: questions asked and statements made in relation to their health care needs and treatment programme.
   (c) Emotions expressed: anxiety, irritability, anger, hostility.
   (d) Verbal communication pattern: rate, tone of voice, speech, errors, flight of ideas, overtalkativeness.
   (e) Non-verbal behaviour indicating anxiety: eye contact, posture, gestures, restlessness, pacing, excessive smoking.
   (f) Physiological responses: rate of respiration, perspiration, thirst, gastrointestinal upsets.
   (g) Potential risks arising from the person's behaviour.
   (h) Insight and self-awareness shown.

4. Support network available to the person, i.e. relationships with key people.
5. Identification of potential stressors in the person's current life situation and life-style.

Desired outcomes

1. Person's behaviour does not cause a risk to themselves or others.
2. Person's understanding of their health care needs is increased.
3. To promote feelings of safety and security.

Nursing intervention	Rationale
1. Initiate a therapeutic relationship. Spend time with them. Be available and approachable. Demonstrate active listening. Involve person in the care planning process. Demonstrate non-judgemental and non-critical approach	Interventions more likely to be successful in an atmosphere of trust and co-operation. Also shows sense of worth and acceptance which helps to increase feelings of security and safety. Being non-judgemental helps a person to deal with guilt. Person will react with further overactivity and possible hostility if they feel threatened
2. Provide clear and understandable information about their treatment, health care and the roles of different health care workers. Encourage questions. Ask for feedback on their understanding. Clarify any misunderstandings	A lot of insecurity is associated with fear of the unknown. People have a right to information about their health care. The nurse is in an ideal position to use this process to facilitate the development of the person's understanding about their health care needs
3. Enlist the person's cooperation in the planning of their health care. Promote their autonomy and self-esteem	People are more likely to cooperate if they are well-informed and involved in the decision-making process. It also increases feelings of personal control and responsibility
4. Ensure that all carers are aware of any risk of self-harm likely to arise from person's behaviour	Carers have a responsibility to protect the person from themself
5. Set clear limits on potentially self-harmful behaviour	Person needs to be aware that others will intervene if their behaviour causes concern. This helps also to increase feelings of security if the person is shown that they will not be allowed to harm themselves

Nursing intervention	*Rationale*
6. Ensure that all potentially harmful substances and implements are removed	Reduces the possibility of accidental self-harm
7. Ensure that the person is under discreet observation at all times	The observation needs to be consistent but also non-intrusive. Person will react with hostility and irritation if they feel crowded
8. Minimize the influence of perceptual distractions and delusions, if present (see Unit 10.4)	These can cause stress and make the person feel insecure. Also more likely to behave in an impulsive way as a reaction to distractions
9. Advise person if their behaviour is a risk to themselves or others	Person may not realize that their actions are potentially unsafe
10. Reassure the person of non-harmful intent	Frightened people can sometimes panic or attack the person they are fearful and suspicious of
11. Do not whisper to others in the presence of the person or express inappropriate emotions	Likely to be misinterpreted and perceived as threatening
12. Explain all actions in advance	Interventions less likely to be seen as threatening and also less distracting. Promotes feelings of trust in carer
13. Refrain from unnecessary procedures and interventions if person is extremely agitated	Adds to potential distractions in the environment. Unnecessary interventions would add to feeings of agitation and are likely to be misinterpreted. Wait until person is calmer and more receptive
14. Ensure that significant personal items are available	Familiar objects help to increase feelings of security
15. Provide support and reassurance to relatives and carers	Stress in relatives will communicate itself to person. Reassurance in carers also communicates positively to person. Likely to have experienced great disruption and heavy demands in coping with the person
16. Encourage the person	Venting their feelings in this way may

Nursing intervention	*Rationale*
to talk about their stressful feelings. Encourage them to express their feelings in a more appropriate way. Provide feedback to the person on their behaviour and use it as a learning situation	reduce some of the necessity for communicating through their overactivity or through hostility. Provides an opportunity for health education in the appropriate expression of emotional stress. Promotes insight
17. Role model calm behaviour. Adopt a non-threatening, open posture and tone of voice	Can have a powerful calming effect as people tend to be subconsciously influenced by the behaviour of those they are with and to "mirror" their behaviour. Behaving calmly then helps to facilitate less pressure of thought
18. Use touch where appropriate	Therapeutic touch can have a very powerful calming influence and promote feelings of security and reassurance. Needs to be used with discretion as people have very different touch thresholds
19. Approach unhurriedly. Demonstrate calmness. Do not rush the person. Be aware of your own reactions and experiences of stress. Be patient and aware of your own feelings of frustration in dealing with the person. Take periodic breaks if possible	Anxiety in the carer communicates itself to the person. Caring can be a stressful experience at times. This may unconsciously influence your interactions with others. The person may be very demanding and resistant. Find ways of coping with your own stress
20. Arrange for own clinical supervision	Supervision is an effective way of providing support and of personal development. Overactive people can be very demanding
21. Facilitate the development of the person's ability to communicate and relate to others	Helps the person to express and thereby release feelings of frustrationand tension

Nursing intervention	Rationale
22. Encourage appropriate diversional, recreational and social activities	Helps to avoid boredom and to divert the person's thoughts away from interference with others. Physical activity can also be a beneficial channel for overactivity

Evaluation

1. Person demonstrates trust in their care.
2. Situations of potential conflict and harm are averted and minimized.
3. Person is able to constructively cope with feelings of frustration.

C. Meet Their Basic Physical Needs

Associated problems/personal difficulties

The overactive person may experience difficulty in meeting their basic physical needs due to:

1. Loss of insight and self-awareness in regard of physical needs.
2. Distractability and inability to focus on any activity for long.
3. Constant activity and restlessness posing a risk of exhaustion.
4. Disturbance of sleep and rest pattern.
5. Loss of interest in personal hygiene.

Assessment

1. Person's statements and behaviour in relation to meeting their needs for nutrition, fluids, hygiene and rest.
2. Information from relatives and friends in regard of the person's ability to meet their physical needs.
3. Nurse's observations of:

   (a) Person's self-initiated activities in relation to meeting their physical needs.
   (b) Present intake of fluid and food: adequacy or inadequacy, appropriateness.
   (c) Level of activity throughout the day.
   (d) Person's current sleep and rest pattern.
   (e) Potential risk factors arising from person's overactivity.

(f) Urinary and faecal elimination.
(g) Identifiable deficits in person's physical needs.
(h) Prompting required by others to focus person's attention on their physical needs: person's reaction to prompting, ability to concentrate on meeting their physical needs.

Desired outcomes

1. Person is able to maintain an adequate intake of food and fluids.
2. Person is able to re-establish an appropriate pattern of rest and sleep.
3. Person is able to identify and initiate physical health care needs independently.

Nursing intervention	Rationale
1. Initiate a therapeutic relationship. Spend time with them. Be available and approachable. Use non-judgemental and non-critical approach	Interventions more likely to be successful in an atmosphere of trust and cooperation
2. Advise the person on the importance of meeting physical needs and their roles in mental health. Specify basic physical requirements with person and family. Negotiate a programme to meet physical needs. Reinforce compliance with programme to promote physical needs	Person may not be aware of these needs or their role in health promotion. Prolonged overactivity may have disrupted normal patterns of meeting physical needs. Reintroducing a pattern helps to structure the person's day and to regain a sense of control
3. Role model calm behaviour. Approach unhurriedly. Do not rush or make sudden movements	Can have a powerful calming effect as people tend to be subconsciously influenced by the behaviour of those around them and to "mirror" this behaviour
4. Identify food preferences and previous eating	More likely to eat preferred food if it complies with previous dietary pattern. May be more prepared to eat

Nursing intervention	*Rationale*
pattern. Facilitate personal choice in regard of diet and meal-times. Provide opportunities for the person to take responsibility and cook their own meals	at certain times of the day. Person will take more interest in food that they have selected and prepared. Will need to monitor closely for safety
5. Present food in an attractive manner and in a distraction-free environment. Do not rush at meal-times	Helps to create a conducive environment and person more likely to focus attention on food. Rushing would reinforce overactivity
6. Positively reinforce self-initiated eating and drinking. Leave food and drink for person in strategic places	More likely to repeat this pattern of behaviour if experienced as rewarding. Availability of food and drink may prompt person to take it
7. Provide readily available high calorie foods and fluids. Ensure food and fluids are readily available. Respond promptly to requests for food and fluids	High calorie snacks may prove more attractive to the overactive person who is otherwise "too busy" to sit down at meal-times. High calorie intake needed to match high energy demands. Food needs to be readily available to take advantage of short lasting periods of interest in food and fluids
8. Monitor food and fluid intake. Provide periodic prompting if lack of intake is putting person at risk. Weigh periodically	Risk of dehydration and collapse if intake is insufficient. If on lithium will also need a minimum daily intake of 3–4 litres of fluid
9. Ensure adequate fibre is taken	Helps to prevent constipation
10. Monitor urinary and faecal elimination. Prompt person on the need to go to toilet periodically	Overactive person can be too preoccupied and restless to go to the toilet. Risk of faecal impaction and of urinary retention
11. Ensure that personalized soap, flannel, towel, toothbrush, etc., are	Person more likely to use items that belong to them. Profuse sweating is common in overactivity. Being clean promotes physical comfort and sense

Nursing intervention	*Rationale*
available. Encourage the person to maintain personal cleanliness and to change clothes periodically	of self-esteem
12. Encourage choice and option over washing and bathing. Give positive feedback on personal initiatives. Ecourage use of warm baths for relaxation	Facilitating control over hygiene increases potential for compliance
13. Ensure that dignity and privacy are respected and maintained during washing and bathing	Overactive people are usually disinhibited about their behaviour. Need to try to re-establish more socially approved modesty
14. Ensure that person is appropriately dressed for the prevailing climatic conditions. Advise person if their clothing is inappropriate. Positively reinforce appropriate self-initiated dressing. Dissuade person from disrobing. Distract person if they begin to disrobe. Encourage person to re-dress. Negotiate limits on approved clothing to be worn. Verbally enforce limits on clothing. Assist person to put clothes back on if disrobed	The overactive person often takes little notice of outside weather conditions. They often find clothes an unbearable incumbrance as well as being disinhibited. Hence, disrobing can be a persistent problem. This can pose a risk to physical health and comfort. Need firm limits to be set and maintained if compliance is to be attained
15. Identify with person activities that they found restful and relaxing. Explore with the person options for meeting needs for rest	These may be activities that might still have the potential to promote rest. Person more likely to cooperate if involved in identifying preferred activities. Loss of insight and sense of well-being interfere with person's

Nursing intervention	*Rationale*
and relaxation. Encourage the person to rest or relax if they appear to be tired or exhausted. Provide feedback on their behaviour. Positively reinforce attempts to rest and relax. Minimize environmental distractions. Provide periods of quiet and restfulness. Sit calmly with the person	ability to recognize their need for rest. Behaviour more likely to recur. The overactive person is readily distracted by outside events. Rest is facilitated if these distractions are minimized. Modelling can be a powerful behaviour influence
16. Assess person's need for sleep. Identify person's preferred sleep patterns	Each person's sleep is unique
17. Identify which factors promote sleep for that person. Identify factors that disturb their sleep. Promote physical comfort of their bedspace. Avoid noise at night. Switch off unnecessary light	May be environmental changes that can be made that will facilitate sleep. The overactive person is very readily distracted. It is very important that environmental distractions are kept to a minimum
18. Observe sleep pattern at night. Provide feedback to person on amount of observed sleep	Need to monitor amount of sleep that the person is actually having. Helps to promote awareness of needs for rest and sleep
19. Observe for signs of physical exhaustion	Person is unable to identify their own needs for rest and will drive themselves to the point of exhaustion

Evaluation

1. Person maintains an adequate food and fluid intake.
2. Person is observed to sleep for a minimum of 6 hours a night and to rest periodically during the day.
3. Person initiates and focusses upon own physical health care needs without prompting.

D. Communicate and Relate to Others

Associated problems/personal difficulties

Some of the communication and relationship difficulties of the overactive person may include:

1. Lack of insight.
2. Limited concentration span.
3. Distractability.
4. Rapid speech patterns.
5. Delusional beliefs and perceptual difficulties.
6. Irritability and conflict with others.
7. Longstanding social skills deficits.

Assessment

1. Person's description of their communication difficulties.
2. Nurse's observation of the person's:
   (a) Communication skills:
   - Verbal behaviour: tone, volume, rate, rhythm, clarity, appropriateness of content, synchronized with other speakers, flight of ideas.
   - Non-verbal behaviour: posture, facial expression, eye contact, gestures, proximity, hand movements.
   (b) Emotions expressed: lacking, excessive, appropriate, assertive, non-assertive, aggressive, irritability, hostility.
3. Interaction with others: frequency, nature and duration of contacts with others.
4. Psychosocial environment: situations and significant others that elicit, inhibit or reinforce communication; potential stresses in the person's environment or life-style; reactions of others to communication with person.
5. Presence of identifiable thought disorders or sensory distractions: visual, auditory.

Desired outcomes

1. Person able to communicate their needs to others.
2. Person able to maintain contact with others and to focus on specific topics.

Nursing intervention	*Rationale*
1. Initiate therapeutic relationship	Interventions more likely to be successful in an atmosphere of trust and cooperation. Person more likely to communicate with carers
2. Be available and accessible. Minimize role barriers. Open posture and non-verbal communication	You have got to look and be approachable. More likely then for communication to occur
3. Model skilled social and communication skills	Modelling by nurses has a powerful influence on the people in their care
4. Accept one-sided conversation. Accept the person's behaviour. Be non-judgemental	The person may have a communication problem due to mental and physical overactivity which makes it difficult for them to respond. Criticism only increases feelings of hostility and rejection. These are counterproductive
5. Engage person in brief, non-threatening conversations. Talk about one topic at a time. Talk in a moderate-paced, even-toned voice	Limited concentration span. Easily irritated. Limited attention span and flight of ideas. Overactive person tends to talk very rapidly
6. Positively reinforce self-initiated interaction and communication	Attempts by the person to communicate need to be encouraged
7. Reinforce normal patterns of social exchange, e.g. pauses, alternate speaking, listening. Positively reinforce appropriate and clear speech. Negatively reinforce inappropriate statements and speech	Need to encourage the person to talk in a way that will facilitate communication with other people. This diminishes the likelihood of the person continuing to communicate in an overactive way

Nursing intervention	*Rationale*
8. Identify situations with the person in which they experience anxiety or a communication difficulty	Many people with mental health problems are either lacking in social skills or have problems relating to others
9. Role play with feedback these situations with the person. Give demonstration and guidance as required. Provide information on the nature of human interaction and the expression of feeling. Provide feedback to person on their progress. Encourage the transfer of newly acquired skills to real-life situations	Social skills training helps people to develop their communication skills. It is a structured approach in which specific skills are: • identified and defined; • divided into their constituent elements; • the elements are practised with feedback in role-play until competence is achieved; • the entire skill is practised with feedback until competence is achieved; • the skill is transferred to real-life situations
10. Encourage the person to express their feelings	Reduces the need to act out their feelings. Demonstrates acceptance
11. Minimize the influence of perceptual distractions and delusions (see Unit 10.4)	Need to reinforce contact with reality in order to promote insight and to communicate more effectively. Perceptual distractions interfere with a person's concentration and attention – this makes it difficult for them to communicate. Deluded thought patterns interfere with a person's interpretation and perception of events and cause communication misunderstandings
12. Promote their feelings of security and minimize feelings of threat (see **B.**)	If the person is anxious, suspicious or feels threatened, they will tend to withdraw and be defensive
13. Promote their autonomy and self-esteem (see Unit 10.4). Reinforce sense of self-identity	Self-belief in the person's own value and feelings of control and mastery increase confidence in dealing with others

Nursing intervention	Rationale
14. Ensure that basic physical needs are being met (see C.)	Physical comfort is a prerequisite for meeting other needs. Person will be unable to concentrate on communicating if they are in physical discomfort
15. Advise and support relatives who may find it difficult to communicate with the person	It is very distressing for close relatives who feel unable to relate to the person and may feel rejected
16. Inform the person about their care and treatment	The person may seem unable to concentrate and preoccupied with other activities but still has a right to know. It also reduces the possibility of unexpected and threatening interventions
17. Provide written information if required	Difficulty in concentrating and limited attention span when overactive. May refer back to this information later
18. Engage in regular and short periods of interaction planned throughout the day	Long conversations with overactive person are likely to be experienced by them as frustrating and difficult to concentrate on. Better to have short, regular contacts that they can cope with and find a positive experience
19. Use touch and other non-verbal signals to demonstrate acceptance	Touch can be very comforting and reassuring if used with sensitivity
20. Communicate with the person when you are engaged in caring activities	Use all opportunities to demonstrate and encourage communication
21. Explore with the person reasons for criticisms by others. Explore with the person reasons for criticisms of others	Person may not be aware of why others may perceive them in a negative way. This also influences how they perceive others
22. Provide opportunities for the person to express themselves openly and honestly	Helps to relieve tension and to demonstrate acceptance. Venting their feelings in this way may reduce the necessity for the physical expression of pent-up feelings. Helps to relieve tension and to demonstrate

Nursing intervention	Rationale
	acceptance
23. Engage in constructive physical activity as a precursor to verbal interaction, e.g. games, activities, drama, music. Organize social and recreational activities	Sometimes it is easier for people to talk as part of an activity or game, or afterwards. It provides a non-threatening point of contact
24. Organize experiential exercises, e.g. drama, role-play, games, in which the person relates to others in an unstructured way and can express themselves freely	Structured and spontaneous experiential exercises can provide powerful feedback and personal learning opportunities. Specific exercises can be used to promote insight and self-awareness

Evaluation

1. Person initiates and maintains contacts with others.
2. Person uses appropriate verbal and non-verbal communication.
3. Person focusses on conversation topics.

E. Facilitate the Development of the Person's and Family's Coping Skills

Associated problems/personal difficulties

The experience of overactivity may show that:

1. The person and their family may be presented with emotional and behavioural demands that they find hard to understand and cope with.
2. Existing methods of coping may be limited, counterproductive and adding to existing stress.
3. Current life-style, expectations and relationships may be potential sources of stress.
4. The person and their family may lack information about the resources available to help them.

5. There may be feelings of guilt in relation to their problems and asking for help.

Assessment

1. Person and their family's description of their current situation.
2. Coping methods being used and their effectiveness.
3. Support available to the person and their carers.
4. Accuracy of the knowledge and information given by the person and their family.
5. Statements indicating guilt and stigma.
6. Awareness of resources available to them.
7. Previous experience, if any, of dealing with similar problems.

Desired outcomes

1. Person and family able to make an informed choice about the resources they require.
2. Person and family able to cope better with the problems experienced.

Nursing intervention	*Rationale*
1. Initiate therapeutic relationship. Involve in the care planning process	Interventions more likely to be successful in an atmosphere of trust and cooperation
2. Advise that seeking help and recognition of problems are a positive step towards finding solutions	Many people feel that seeking help is a sign of weakness and failure. Also helps to reduce guilt
3. Encourage questions. Provide accurate information	May have inaccurate knowledge and expectations. Helps to promote understanding and reduce anxieties
4. Identify appropriate health care resources	Need to know what resources are available to them
5. Advise that highly emotional situations be avoided at first	There may be pent-up feelings and stresses that need to be worked through and released in a controlled way. Sudden discharge of emotion may also increase the severity of the person's symptoms

Nursing intervention	*Rationale*
6. Advise against early correction of problems	Under stress it is sometimes easier to make short-term adaptations that only store up future problems. It takes time to help the family to work out what is best for them. Longstanding problems will also take time to resolve
7. Reassure that there are ways of improving the situation	Family may feel that the situation is hopeless
8. Advise against recrimination and focussing on past problems	Need to focus on the present and future and to deal with anger and guilt in a more productive way
9. Advise on the need for acceptance and mutual support within their relationships	Family needs to come to terms with their situation. They are each other's primary source of support which will need to be utilized to cope effectively
10. Explain the need to identify and recognize potentially stressful situations	Stress can precipitate or exacerbate episodes of overactivity. Mental health problems tend to be long-term in nature
11. Teach methods for achieving relaxation. Teach how to use problem-solving methods for coping with difficulties. Assist the family to learn new coping skills. Encourage the setting of realistic goals	In order to cope effectively the family needs to be taught ways of making the necessary long-term adjustments. Most of the education needs to be directed towards teaching effective coping methods. These include the way that the family members communicate, their expectations and the way that emotional support is given
12. Encourage the setting of progressive goals in small stages. Advise the family on how to give feedback and support to one another. Encourage the use of newly acquired coping skills. Give feedback to the person and family	The re-learning needs to be done in a gradual way in which the family provides the main support and reinforcement. Family may not be very effective at giving support or feedback to one another. Skills need to be used in order to become part of everyday life. Outside feedback helps to promote insight and to validate progress
13. Recommend ways of setting behavioural	Family may need these skills in order to deal effectively with further episodes

Nursing intervention	*Rationale*
limits. Explain the purpose of making a contract with the person	of overactivity. Living together is a process of negotiation. It is often useful for all concerned if the boundaries are firmly defined
14. Teach the person and family how to recognize signs of impending recurrence of overactivity and the actions to take	Family and person will be the main monitors of the person's mental health
15. Advise on the need to comply with prescribed medication. Advise on possible side-effects of medication	Lithium therapy is an effective prophylactic treatment if the person complies with prescribed regime. The person and their family need to be aware of potential side-effects and the signs of lithium toxicity. They also need to know what actions to take if they suspect lithium toxicity
16. Review occupational/ unemployment stresses. Encourage the development of appropriate work/ non-work coping strategies	Work and unemployment can be major sources of stress. As these represent a major part of life it is important that the person learns how to cope constructively with these stresses
17. Teach the family and person to recognize the limits of their ability to cope and when it is advisable to seek help	The family should not over-burden itself as this can damage relationships and its longer-term ability to cope
18. Put family in contact with self-help and voluntary groups	Self-help groups able to offer effective and understanding practical help

Evaluation

1. Person and family identify and select resources they require.
2. Person and family able to give accurate information about their health care needs.
3. Person and family demonstrate use of improved coping methods.

Unit Instructions

When you have researched the suggested references, have mastered the Unit Objectives and successfully answered the Self-assessment Questions, proceed with the Unit Written Test.

Suggested References

Alchin, S. and Weatherhead, R. (1976). *Psychiatric Nursing: A Practical Approach*. McGraw Hill, Sydney.

Altschul, A. and McGovern, M. (1985). *Psychiatric Nursing*, 6th edition. Baillière Tindall, London and San Diego.

Barker, P. J. (1982). *Behaviour Therapy Nursing*. Croom Helm, London.

Barker, P. J. (1985). *Patient Assessment in Psychiatric Nursing*. Croom Helm, London.

Bauer, B. B. and Hill, S. S. (1986). *Essentials of Mental Health Care Planning and Interventions*. W. B. Saunders, Philadelphia.

Campbell, C. (1978). *Nursing Diagnosis and Intervention in Nursing Practice*. John Wiley, New York.

Carr, P. J., Butterworth, C. A. and Hodges, B. E. (1980). *Community Psychiatric Nursing*. Churchill Livingstone, Edinburgh.

Darcy, P. T. (1984). *Theory and Practice of Psychiatric Care*. Hodder and Stoughton, London.

Darcy, P. T. (1985). *Mental Health Nursing Source Book*. Baillière Tindall, London and San Diego.

Dexter, G. and Wash, M. (1986). *Psychiatric Nursing Skills: A Patient-centred Approach*. Croom Helm, London.

Hammil, K. (1987). *Seclusion: inside looking out*. Nursing Times, 4 February, Vol. 83, No. 5, pp. 38–39.

Hase, S. and Douglas, A. (1986). *Human Dynamics and Nursing*. Churchill Livingstone, Melbourne.

Irving, S. (1983). *Basic Psychiatric Nursing*, 3rd edition. W. B. Saunders, Philadelphia.

Lancaster, J. (1980). *Adult Psychiatric Nursing*. Henry Kimpton, London.

Leopoldt, H. (1985). *A secure and secluded spot*. Nursing Times, 6 February, Vol. 81, No. 6, pp. 26–28.

Lyttle, J. (1986). *Mental Disorder: Its Care and Treatment*. Baillière Tindall, London and San Diego.

McFarland, G. and Wasli, E. (1986). *Nursing Diagnoses and Process in Psychiatric Mental Health Nursing*. J. B. Lippincott, Philadelphia.

Martin, P. (1987a). *Psychiatric Nursing: A Therapeutic Approach*. Macmillan, London.

Martin, P. (1987b). *Care of the Mentally Ill*, 2nd edition. Macmillan, London.

Pelletier, L. (Ed.) (1987). *Psychiatric Nursing Case Studies, Nursing Diagnoses and Care Plans*. Springhouse Corporation, Springhouse, Pennsylvania.

Pope, B. (1986). *Social Skills Training for Psychiatric Nurses*. Harper and Row, London.

Priestley, P., McGuire, J., Flegg, D., Hemsley, V. and Welham, D. (1978). *Social Skills and Personal Problem Solving*. Tavistock, London.

Rix, G. (1985). Compassion is better than conflict. *Nursing Times*, 18 September, Vol. 81, No. 38, pp. 53–55.

Robinson, L. (1983). *Psychiatric Nursing as a Human Experience*, 3rd edition. W. B. Saunders, Philadelphia.

Russell, D., Hodgkinson, P. and Hillis, T. (1986). Time out. *Nursing Times*, 26 February, Vol. 82, No. 9, pp. 47–49.

Simmons, S. and Brooker, C. (1986). *Community Psychiatric Nursing: A Social Perspective*. Heinemann Nursing, London.

Smith, L. (1978). Limit-setting. *Nursing Times*, 29 June, Vol. 74, No. 26, pp. 1074–1075.

Smith, L. (1981). Problems associated with manic depressive patients. *Nursing*, Vol. 1, No. 30, pp. 1307–1309.

Sugden, J., Bessant, A., Eastland, M. and Field, R. (1986). *A Handbook for Psychiatric Nurses*. Harper and Row, London.

Tibbles, P. (1980). Managing violent behaviour in a psychiatric ward: A psychiatric approach. *Nursing Times*, 20 November, Vol. 76, No. 47, pp. 2046–2048.

Ward, M. F. (1985). *The Nursing Process in Psychiatry*. Churchill Livingstone, Edinburgh.

Self-assessment Questions

SAQ 9. Describe six therapeutic interventions that can be used to limit the self-damaging consequences of overactivity.

SAQ 10. Outline six ways in which a person's physical health may suffer as a result of overactivity.

SAQ 11. Identify four problems that the family may face in attempting to cope with the overactive person.

SAQ 12. List six ways in which the environment can be modified in order to moderate overactivity.

Unit 11.3: Written Test

Terrance Brown, aged 26, has been admitted into care due to his extreme overactivity. On the ward his behaviour is extremely disruptive and he is in frequent conflict with the other residents. He appears to be suffering from a degree of exhaustion and yet is driven to constant activity. He is disinhibited towards the female staff and residents and believes that he is wealthy and important.

His family are shocked and baffled by his behaviour which they find difficult to accept. They are extremely concerned about whether he will ever get better and what he will be like when he comes home.

As his primary nurse you are responsible for his care and at a care planning meeting are currently discussing possible nursing interventions for his identified needs.

1. Outline the range of therapeutic interventions for moderating Terrance's overactive behaviour.

2. Some of the other nurses are unsure about the therapeutic uses of setting limits. Describe the role and process of limit setting in the management of overactive behaviour.
3. What observations should be made of Terrance's physical condition in order to monitor his health?
4. Terrance is prescribed lithium carbonate for his overactivity. A student nurse attached to the team asks for information about the use of lithium and the observations that need to be made. What information does this learner need about lithium in order to contribute towards Terrance's nursing care programme?

TOPIC 12

Mental Health and Childbirth

At the end of this Topic the learner should aim to:

1. Describe factors related to the mental health of the mother following childbirth.
2. Recognize the possible effects of childbirth on the mother's mental health.
3. Outline the range of therapeutic interventions available for a new mother with mental health problems.

The Effects of Childbirth on Maternal Mental Health

Unit Objectives

At the end of this Unit the learner should be able to:

1. Describe factors that influence the mental health of mothers after childbirth.
2. State the characteristic signs of "baby blues"/"post-natal blues".
3. Outline the main features of post-natal depression.
4. Identify features that indicate a psychotic reaction to childbirth.

Pregnancy, Childbirth and Mental Health

Pregnancy and childbirth are significant life events for a woman. The changes in role and biology transform the mother's whole life. They represent a major developmental crisis for the mother that she will have to cope with in order to maintain her mental health. Most women, often at great personal cost, are able to meet these demands and to experience the positive aspects of motherhood. However, for a significant number of mothers, the period immediately following childbirth is particularly stressful and may be associated with pronounced mental health problems.

Some of the difficulties may originate early in the pregnancy as the mother discovers that the realities are less glamorous than the image. The expectation is of a period of joy and eager anticipation. Potential problems are rarely considered. Physical discomforts such as backache, tiredness, vomiting, insomnia, varicose veins, haemorrhoids, frequent micturation, increasing girth, weight gain and restrictions can do much to negatively influence the mother's perception of her pregnancy. Pre-existing mental health problems may also pose extra demands and stress upon the mother. Problems of substance abuse and dependency may also pose potential risks to the health of the mother and foetus.

The actual birth, too, may prove to be a profound disappointment. Most deliveries (97%) now take place in hospital where the mother may have little control over the course of her delivery. Standard procedures, such as pubic shaving, enemas, induction, epidural anaesthesia, birth position and episiotomy, seriously detract from the emotional potential of birth for the mother. Some women are seriously affected by this medicalization of birth and find the whole experience unreal and intensely dissatisfying. This may make it difficult for them to adjust after the delivery and can create feelings of guilt and inadequacy for not responding like a "real woman".

Factors Influencing Maternal Mental Health after Childbirth

A number of factors are thought to be related to the mental health of the mother after childbirth. Some of these relate directly to the psychobiological effects of childbirth upon the mother, others relate to the pre-existing social and environmental conditions. In individual cases certain factors may be particularly significant.

1. *The physical and psychological stress of the delivery*: exhaustion, discomfort, pain, caesarian delivery, induced birth. Home delivery is associated with improved mental health outcomes.
2. *Endocrinal changes*: sudden fall in progesterone and oestrogen levels after delivery. Significant where the mother has a history of pronounced premenstrual tension.
3. *Expectations and attitudes towards the pregnancy*: whether the mother had doubts about having a child, reactions of the father, negative anticipation of motherhood, feeling trapped.
4. *Experience of pregnancy*: degree of discomfort, problems and complications of pregnancy.
5. *Preparation for motherhood*: past experience with own children, role models from childhood, knowledge of childrearing.
6. *Social and practical support available*: availability of a close, confiding relationship, contacts with other mothers, spouse, friends, relatives.
7. *Self-perception as a mother*: doubts and lack of confidence about own motherhood skills, negative perception of self as a capable, coping mother.
8. *Pre-existing stresses*: marital disharmony, presence of three or more young children under 14 at home, divorce, bereavement, unemployment, poor housing conditions, financial problems.
9. *Previous mental health problems*: particularly puerperal mental health problems following previous pregnancies, pre-existing or past history of other mental health problems.

Classification of Mental Health Problems Following Childbirth

The mental health problems that may occur in a mother after childbirth are poorly classified. This makes it difficult to evaluate and compare research findings. The problem for researchers has been to demonstrate the existence of specific mental health problems that have a direct causal relationship with the experience of pregnancy, childbirth and motherhood. The existence of a relationship between the period immediately following childbirth – the puerperium – and the mother's mental health is generally accepted. However, the extent to which these mental health problems are generated by the experience of motherhood or whether pre-existing problems are exacerbated or whether the problems arise independently is less clear.

There can be a wide range of generalized mental health reactions following pregnancy. These may include:

- depression,
- obsessional behaviour,
- anxiety-related problems,
- hysterical reactions.

More specific emotional and behavioural reactions after childbirth include:

- post-natal "blues"/"maternal blues"/"baby blues",
- post-natal depression,
- puerperal psychoses.

These may be seen as distinct reactions or may merge into each other.

Post-natal "blues"/"maternal blues"/"baby blues"

The "baby blues" is experienced by some 50% of all new mothers. Given the high percentage of mothers that react in this way to childbirth and the numbers that experience post-natal depression, it would appear that not to react in this way is more "abnormal".

Until recently, the "baby blues" attracted little research and medically was viewed as a relatively minor psychological reaction to childbirth. However, the subjective accounts of mothers who experience post-natal blues contrast strongly with this medical perspective. Many mothers experience high levels of distress and misery even if it is a short-term and self-limiting reaction in the majority of cases.

The first signs may be seen some 3–7 days after childbirth. The mother is very tearful, sensitive and irritable. Physically, there are the discomforts of childbirth – swollen breasts, soreness – with fatigue, exhaustion and insomnia. Attempts to rest may be interrupted by the demands of the new infant. Psychologically, the initial joy of a new infant may be replaced by feelings of flatness and disappointment. This may cause the mother further distress and guilt at her lack of joy or ability to love her new infant immediately.

Most mothers begin to recover from this period of psychological and physical exhaustion after about 10 days. However, the stress may be prolonged and spoil the first few vital months of motherhood. These feelings may persist for some 6–9 months. A significant proportion of mothers with post-natal blues (25%) go on to develop post-natal depression.

Post-natal depression

Post-natal depression is one of the most common and most severe complications after childbirth. One in 10 mothers develop a marked depressive illness which may be characterized by:

1. *Depressed mood*: initial post-natal "blues" may become more pronounced some 10–14 days after childbirth. The mother becomes very tearful, sensitive and easily upset. There is marked irritability. The mother may find it difficult to concentrate and to remember things.
2. *Sleep disturbance*: constantly tired, fatigued, exhausted.
3. *Negative self-perception*: ideas of not coping, self-blame, guilt, inadequacy.
4. *Thoughts of self-harm or fear of harming the baby*: the possibility of infanticide during post-natal depression is acknowledged by the law in that during the first year following childbirth the mother would have been deemed to have acted while the balance of her mind was disturbed. The incidence of non-accidental injury to the infant is not significantly raised during this time.
5. *Rejection of the baby*: both physically and emotionally.
6. *Anxiety*: particularly in relation to the baby.
7. Impaired, or loss of, libido.

The experience of post-natal depression may gradually lift in the months after childbirth. It may require specific therapeutic interventions in order to restore the mother's mental health and to limit the reactions. Left untreated it has the potential to last for years in some cases.

The experience of post-natal depression after childbirth will, naturally, influence the mother's attitudes towards future pregnancies. There is a significant possibility of recurrence in future pregnancies. Post-natal depression also has the potential, especially if it is not recognized, to damage seriously the mother's relationship with her partner and relatives.

Puerperal psychoses

Psychotic reactions to childbirth are relatively uncommon and constitute about 2–3 per 1000 live births (0.3%). The onset of the symptoms tends to be acute and may develop immediately after labour. A total of 50% of mothers with this reaction are admitted within 14 days of delivery. Research has failed to identify conclusively any significant differences between psychoses following childbirth and those that may occur at other periods of life.

The presenting signs and symptoms may be similar to those of schizophrenia or manic-depressive psychosis. These may include:

1. *Behavioural disturbances*: restlessness, agitation, overactivity, irrational acts, insomnia, being overdemanding.
2. *Mood disturbances*: elation, tension, depression, rejection of baby.
3. *Thought disturbances*: delusions about the baby, suspiciousness and paranoia, partial insight, threats of violence.
4. *Perceptual disturbances*: hallucinations.

Most mothers gradually recover their mental health in the months following the pregnancy. Many have limited recall or awareness of this disturbed period. However, for a significant number there may remain the possibility of longer-term problems. One research study found that, at a 4-year interval, three out of four affected mothers have a "reasonable level of recovery".

Unit Instructions

When you have researched the suggested references, have mastered the Unit Objectives and successfully answered the Self-assessment Questions, proceed with the Unit Written Test.

Suggested References

Adams, J. (1985). "I'm normal", I cried. *Nursing Times*, 16 October, Vol. 81, No. 42, pp. 44–45.

Ball, J. (1982). Stress and the postnatal care of women. *Nursing Times*, 10 November, Vol. 78, No. 45, pp. 1904–1907.

Brockington, I. F. and Kumar, B. (Eds) (1982). *Motherhood and Mental Illness*. Academic Press, London and San Diego.

Brown, G. W. and Harris, T. (1978). *Social Origins of Depression: A Study of Psychiatric Disorder in Women*. Tavistock, London.

Cox, J. (1986). *Postnatal Depression. A Guide for Health Professionals*. Churchill Livingstone, Edinburgh.

Cox, J. L., Kumar, R., Margison, F. R. and Downey, L. J. (1986). *Current Approaches to Puerperal Mental Illness*. TransMedica Europe Limited.

Cronin, C. (1983). Puerperal psychosis. *Nursing Mirror*, 7 December, Vol. 157, No. 23, pp. 43–44.

Cutrona, C. E. (1982). Nonpsychotic postpartum depression: A review of recent research. *Clinical Psychology Review*, Vol. 2, pp. 487–503.

Dalton, K. (1980). *Depression after Childbirth*. Oxford University Press, Oxford.

Davis, R. (1984). *An Introduction to Psychopathology*, 4th edition. Oxford University Press, Oxford.

Farr, P. (1985). Post-natal depression . . . and treating them. *Community Outlook*, August, pp. 6, 8, 11.

Habgood, J. (1985). Post-natal depression: Exposing the blues. . . *Community Outlook*, August, pp. 4–5.

Holden, J. (1985). Post-natal depression; Talking it out. *Community Outlook*, October, pp. 6, 10.

Holden, J. (1987). She just listened. *Community Outlook*, July, pp. 6–10.

Lyttle, J. (1986). *Mental Disorder: Its Care and Treatment*. Baillière Tindall, London and San Diego.

McConville, B. (1987). *Mad to be a Mother*. Century Paperbacks, London.

Meltzer, E. S. and Kumar, R. (1985). Puerperal mental illness, clinical features and classification: A study of 142 mother-and-baby admissions. *British Journal of Psychiatry*, Vol. 147, pp. 647–654.

Morris, B. (1979). The midwife who wanted to die. *Nursing Mirror*, 15 November, Vol. 149, No. 20, pp. 20–21.

Oates, M. R. (1983). *What is Postnatal Depression?* Central Independent Television, Birmingham.

Paykel, E. S., Emms, E. M., Fletcher, J. and Rassaby, E. (1980). Life events and social support in puerperal depression. *British Journal of Psychiatry*, Vol. 136, pp. 339–346.

Pollock, L. (1983). Women and mental illness. *Nursing Mirror*, 24 August, Vol. 157, No. 8, pp. 18–19.

Sims, A. (1988). *Symptoms in the Mind*. Baillière Tindall, London and San Diego.

Welburn, V. (1980). *Postnatal Depression*. Fontana/Collins, London.

Williams, J. (1986). Not just the baby blues. *Nursing Times*, 14 May, Vol. 82, No. 20, pp. 38–40.

Young, I. (1988). I just didn't want him. *Nursing Times*, 2 March, Vol. 84, No. 9, pp. 32–36.

Self-assessment Questions

SAQ 1. Describe six factors that may influence the mental health of a mother following childbirth.

SAQ 2. Identify four characteristics of "post-natal blues"/"baby blues".

SAQ 3. List six observations that would confirm a mother is suffering from post-natal depression.

SAQ 4. Outline five factors that would indicate a mother is having a psychotic reaction to childbirth.

Unit 12.1: Written Test

A friend that you are visiting at home, who had a child 3 months ago, confides in you that she is finding it very difficult to cope with motherhood. She appears to be under stress and her mental health is obviously suffering.

1. What observations would you need to make to confirm whether or not she has post-natal depression?

2. What factors during her pregnancy and immediately afterwards may have adversely affected her mental health?

Care and Treatment of Mothers with Mental Health Problems Following Childbirth

---

Unit Objectives

At the end of this Unit the learner should be able to:

1. Describe the range of therapeutic interventions available to help mothers with mental health problems following childbirth.
2. Identify the support required for the mother, her child and family in both community and residential settings.

Care and Treatment

The specific therapeutic approach for mental health problems after childbirth will depend upon the mother's primary presenting problems. These may range from minor emotional and behavioural difficulties requiring minimal intervention, to acute psychotic episodes or risk of self-harm when constant care may be required.

The general approach should be an integrated and readily accessible service to support the mother and family in the community or in residential settings as required.

Therapeutic aims

1. To promote the safety and welfare of the mother and baby.
2. To restore the mental health of the mother.
3. To facilitate the development of the mother's and family's coping skills.

Family and Self-care

The strains of parenthood can pose considerable demands upon the ability of the mother and father to cope. Exhausted by childbirth, the mother may find herself in a situation where she is constantly tired and drained, with little opportunity to rest. The continual activity, responsibility and restrictions deny her any individuality and a loss of previous independence. Many women, too, doubt their ability to cope and feel inadequate as "mothers". During this period they may also feel guilty and concerned by what they perceive as a failure to feel affection towards their recent offspring. The mother may not realize, or have been told, that it takes time to learn to love their child.

Faced with these normal difficulties of adjustment and coping with a new infant, the mother, or significant others, may fail to recognize that the mother is experiencing real mental health problems. Even quite severe emotional and behavioural problems may be put down to the stress of recent motherhood, with the expectation that everything will soon be "right".

However, should these problems persist, then the outcomes are likely to be prolonged misery for the mother and damage to close relationships. Particularly significant may be the influence that the mother's mental health problems have on her ability to bond with the child. The mother and child may be deprived of a key opportunity to develop their relationship.

Therapeutic intervention may be initiated at an early stage of the mother's difficulties if it is identified by key primary health workers or by the relatives as an atypical reaction to childbirth. However, research studies indicate a wide discrepancy between the incidence of post-natal mental health problems in the community and those mothers who receive care and treatment. This would indicate that there are many mothers in the community who are suffering unaided when they could be supported through this difficult time. Left untreated the problems may in fact gradually improve with time. However, some mothers may suffer for years. Written accounts by health care workers who failed to recognize their own mental health problems after childbirth are particularly telling.

Mothers can be helped considerably in coping with their difficulties by:

1. Recognition and acknowledgement of their difficulties.
2. Accurate information about post-natal mental health problems.
3. Involvement in the care and treatment process.
4. Reassurance that effective intervention is possible.
5. The opportunity to talk freely about their problems.
6. The address of a local contact support group for mothers with mental health problems following childbirth.
7. Developing the mother's and family's parenthood and coping skills.

Community Care

Most mothers with mental health problems after pregnancy are cared for in the community. Community care involves a wide range of statutory and voluntary services that aim to provide comprehensive treatment and support. An accurate assessment needs to be made of the mother's support network, potential for self-harm and ability to care for her child. The aims of community care are to:

1. To support the mother, child and family at home.
2. To monitor the mental and physical well-being of the mother and child.
3. To implement community-based treatment and care programmes.

The services involved include:

1. Primary health care team: midwives, health visitors and general practitioners. Each offering specific interventions based upon their specialist skills and statutory responsibilities.
2. The community mental health centre: with community psychiatric nurses, social workers, psychologists, occupational therapists and consultant psychiatrists working as a team to offer skills-based therapeutic interventions.
3. Social Services: nursery facilities, home aids.
4. Voluntary agencies: The Association for Post-natal Illness, Meet-a-Mum Association, Caesarian Support Groups, The National Childbirth Trust, Organization for Parents Under Stress, National Marriage Guidance Council.
5. Out-patient clinics and day hospitals.
6. DHSS: allowances and benefits as currently available, e.g. child benefit, family income support.

Residential Care

The reasons for admission to residential facilities for care and treatment include:

1. Lack of support in the community.
2. Potential for physical harm to the mother or child due to the nature of her mental health problems.
3. The need for intensive care where the mother is very distressed or disturbed.
4. To implement specialist residential-based therapeutic programmes or facilities, e.g. mother and baby unit.

Therapeutic Interventions

The specific treatment interventions and approaches will depend upon the mother's needs and the presenting clinical problems. Readers are advised to cross-refer to the appropriate Topics and Study Units. The range of interventions may include the following.

Psychotherapeutic

1. Skilled nursing care.
2. Individual counselling or psychotherapy.
3. Group work.
4. Family therapy.
5. Health education: particularly on childrearing skills.
6. Behavioural psychotherapy.
7. Cognitive therapy.
8. Development of coping and stress management skills.
9. Occupational therapy.
10. Recreational and social activities.

Physical treatment methods

1. Chemotherapy: specific to the mother's clinical condition. Particular caution will have to be taken if the mother is breastfeeding, which may be contraindicated.
2. ECT.
3. Hormonal therapy.

Mental Health Nursing Care

The mother's specific care needs will depend upon the nature of her mental health problems. (Readers should cross-refer to the appropriate Topics and Units.) The psychiatric nursing care programme may incorporate the needs for:

1. A safe environment for the mother and child.
2. Promoting the physical welfare of the mother and child.
3. Developing the mother's relationship with her child.
4. Facilitating the development of the mother's/father's childrearing skills.
5. Improving the mother's/father's coping and communication skills.

Unit Instructions

When you have researched the suggested references, have mastered the Unit Objectives and successfully answered the Self-assessment Questions, proceed with the Unit Written Test.

Suggested References

Adams, J. (1985). "I'm normal", I cried. *Nursing Times*, 16 October, Vol. 81, No. 42, pp. 44–45.

Ball, J. (1982). Stress and the postnatal care of women. *Nursing Times*, 10 November, Vol. 78, No. 45, pp. 1904–1907.

Brockington, I. F. and Kumar, R. (Eds) (1982). *Motherhood and Mental Illness*. Academic Press, London and San Diego.

Brown, G. W. and Harris, T. (1978). *Social Origins of Depression: A Study of Psychiatric Disorder in Women*. Tavistock, London.

Cox, J. (1986). *Postnatal Depression. A Guide for Health Professionals*. Churchill Livingstone, Edinburgh.

Cox, J. L., Kumar, R., Margison, F. R. and Downey, L. J. (1986). *Current Approaches to Puerperal Mental Illness*. TransMedica Europe Limited, London.

Cronin, C. (1983). Puerperal psychosis. *Nursing Mirror*, 7 December, Vol. 157, No. 23, pp. 43–44.

Cutrona, C. E. (1982). Nonpsychotic postpartum depression: A review of recent research. *Clinical Psychology Review*, Vol. 2, pp. 487–503.

Dalton, K. (1980). *Depression after Childbirth*. Oxford University Press, Oxford.

Davis, R. (1984). *An Introduction to Psychopathology*, 4th edition. Oxford University Press, Oxford.

Farr, P. (1985). Postnatal depression . . . and treating them. *Community Outlook*, August, pp. 6, 8, 11.

Habgood, J. (1985). Exposing the blues. . . . *Community Outlook*, August, pp. 4–5.

Holden, J. (1985). Talking it out. *Community Outlook*, October, pp. 6, 10.

Lyttle, J. (1986). *Mental Disorder: Its Care and Treatment*. Baillière Tindall, London and San Diego.

Meltzer, E. S. and Kumar, R. (1985). Puerperal mental illness, clinical features and classification: A study of 142 mother-and-baby admissions. *British Journal of Psychiatry*, Vol. 147, pp. 647–654.

Morris, B. (1979). The midwife who wanted to die. *Nursing Mirror*, 15 November, Vol. 149, No. 20, pp. 20–21.

Oates, M. R. (1983). *What is Postnatal Depression?* Central Independent Television, Birmingham.

Paykel, E. S., Emms, E. M., Fletcher, J. and Rassaby, E. (1980). Life events and social support in puerperal depression. *British Journal of Psychiatry*, Vol. 136, pp. 339–346.

Pollock, L. (1983). Women and mental illness. *Nursing Mirror*, 24 August, Vol. 157, No. 8, pp. 18–19.

Simmons, S. and Brooker, C. (1986). *Community Psychiatric Nursing: A Social Perspective*. Heinemann Nursing, London.

Welburn, V. (1980). *Postnatal Depression*. Fontana/Collins, London.

Williams, J. (1986). Not just the baby blues. *Nursing Times*, 14 May, Vol. 82, No. 20, pp. 38–40.

Note: Readers are advised to cross-refer to appropriate Topics elsewhere in this book for references in relation to therapeutic interventions for specific mental health problems exhibited by the mother.

Self-assessment Questions

SAQ 5. List six stresses that the new mother may face in the first few weeks after her pregnancy.

SAQ 6. Outline the roles of the members of the primary health care team in relation to the mother with post-natal mental health problems.

SAQ 7. State five ways in which the mother with mental health problems can initially be helped in the community.

SAQ 8. Identify five potential care needs of the mother with post-natal mental health problems.

Unit 12.2: Written Test

Jennifer Evans, aged 19, gave birth to a healthy girl, named Suzette, 9 weeks ago. Physically she has recovered well from the birth but her health visitor is concerned at the psychological effects upon Jennifer's mental health and her difficulty in coping. Jennifer is very tearful and appears to demonstrate only rudimentary knowledge about childrearing. She repeatedly seeks guidance and reassurance and says that she feels hopeless and inadequate as a mother. The general condition of her home has deteriorated and Jennifer has made little attempt to get organized. She states that everything is an effort, she feels constantly tired and is sleeping poorly. Of particular concern is the fact that Jennifer lives on her own and has been deserted recently by her ex-boyfriend. Jennifer does not appear to have any relatives or friends nearby. She has missed several appointments at the baby clinic and the health visitor is finding it increasingly difficult to gain entry into her flat.

At the health centre the health visitor has consulted the community psychiatric nurse for a professional opinion and to consider a joint approach.

1. What community-based support services may prove helpful to Jennifer?
2. What factors would the health visitor and CPN need to consider in identifying the potential for risk to the mother and child?
3. How could the health visitor and community psychiatric nurse co-ordinate their roles to provide the mental health support that Jennifer requires?

TOPIC 13

Confusion in Later Life

At the end of this Topic the learner should aim to:

1. Describe factors that influence mental health in later life.
2. Recognize the effects of confusion upon a person's behaviour and emotions.
3. Outline the range of therapeutic interventions and support facilities available for the confused elderly person and their carers.
4. Identify the nursing care needs and interventions required for the confused elderly person.

UNIT 13.1

Mental Health in Later Life

Unit Objectives

At the end of this Unit the learner should be able to:

1. Describe how ageing and other factors influence mental health in later life.
2. Outline the origins and presentation of acute confusional states.
3. Describe the onset of chronic confusion.
4. Identify the characteristic cognitive and behavioural effects of chronic confusional states.

Ageing and Health

The process of ageing has direct consequences for physical, social and mental health. Biologically, the physical aspects of ageing are genetically programmed and individuals vary widely at the rate at which they age. People of the same chronological age can differ considerably as to how they have been affected by and responded to the demands of ageing.

For most people, ageing is a slow and variable process that only periodically impinges upon a person's consciousness. This may include situations in which the person actively compares themselves with others or with their perceived previous self, particularly at times when their age has significant consequences – retirement, bereavement, being excluded or feeling out of place for being "too old".

Ageing is not a passive process purely dictated by a person's heredity or chronological age. A person's self-perception, lifestyle, health choices and occupation can significantly influence the course that ageing takes, their personal experience of ageing and their ability to cope with it.

Aspects of Ageing

Social aspects of ageing

In Western culture ageing and being old are viewed unfavourably. Many people dread the thought of becoming old. There are many negative stereotypes and prejudices towards the elderly that tend to isolate them from the mainstream of social activity. These attitudes can exert a powerful influence on an elderly person's self-perception and reinforce low self-esteem and confine them to "age-appropriate" activities. Attempts to move outside of these confines may be treated with ridicule or contempt – "you're too old", "dirty old man", "at your age?" Such "ageism" is implicit in many dealings that elderly people have with younger lay people and health care workers. As people age their social needs do tend to change and to become more settled and orientated to established relationships. This withdrawal or "disengagement" from a hectic pace of life may be viewed as a deliberate life choice or as a consequence of exclusion by younger people. Right to the end of their days, elderly people have the potential, frequently unrealized, to continue their social life, develop relationships and to make a worthwhile contribution to their family and the community.

Psychological aspects of ageing

Some mental functions do appear to decline with age; in particular, there is an increase in the amount of time that a person takes to respond. However, if an allowance is made for this and an age-appropriate and relevant measure is used, then it would appear that the cognitive decline associated with old age has been greatly over-estimated. Many elderly people continue their intellectual development to the end of their days through attending Adult Education classes and the Open University. Four out of five people over the age of 85 experience no problems with their memory. The cognitive potential of many elderly people remains sadly neglected, frequently as a result of negative self-perception: "I'm too old to learn that", "you can't teach an old dog new tricks".

Physical aspects of ageing

After the growth and development of early life there is a slow and progressive decline in physical function and performance. This is most marked after the age of 75. The physical effects of normal ageing are considerably influenced by a person's lifestyle and health habits. Unhealthy patterns of living during a person's middle years can compound the adverse effects of both ageing and of physical health problems. As we age there is an increase in the incidence of health problems – both acute and chronic – and a decrease in the body's ability to cope and respond to these stresses. Unfortunately, many elderly people tend to accept physical health problems that are amenable to intervention in the mistaken belief that these are "inevitable". The response of health care professionals also, unfortunately, tends to reinforce such beliefs – "what can you expect at your age?"

However, much can be done to promote physical health in later life. Sensible dieting, regular exercise, positive health choices, information and periodic screening are measures that can contribute to good health in later life. Most people under the age of 75 do not consider themselves to be elderly and the majority are in good health and able to get about.

The Incidence of Mental Health Problems in the Elderly

Life expectancy has increased considerably this century, primarily as a result of improved nutrition, public health measures and housing conditions. As a consequence, there are profound demographic changes taking place in the age structure of the population. The proportion of elderly people in the population is increasing in relation to the number of younger people. This has considerable implications for the incidence of mental health problems in later life and also for the availability of carers for the elderly.

There are currently some 8 million people – about 15% of the population – over the age of 65 in the UK. Of these, just over one-third are aged over 75. The incidence of all mental illnesses increases with age and the first admission rate for mental health problems in those aged over 75 is more than twice that of middle life.

It is estimated that about 1 in 10 of those aged over 65 are suffering from some degree of confusion or dementia; half of these are moderately to severely confused. Overall, it would seem that there are about 500 000 people over 65 who are confused to a degree that noticeably affects their ability to meet their needs. However, a significant number of people who are confused (some 50%) are not known to health care agencies or their GPs.

In comparison, depression is a much more common mental health problem in later life than confusional states. Many of the factors associated with the causation of depression (see Unit 7.1) are most prominent in later life. However, although depression in the elderly may present in a similar way to a confusional state, it is readily treatable if accurately diagnosed.

The full range of mental health problems may be seen in later life. These may represent continuation or recurrence of mental health difficulties earlier in life or be a recent experience.

Factors Influencing Mental Health in Later Life

1. *Physical health*: the presence of chronic and painful conditions, particularly those that limit mobility and increase dependency. Good physical health is related to good mental health.

2. *Social contact*: the presence of supportive relationships, and regular contact with others. Loneliness and social isolation have negative effects on mental health.
3. *Personal interests*: ability to meet leisure needs, meaningful activity and sense of purpose, avoidance of boredom. Inability to continue activities that give meaning to life leads to frustration and despair.
4. *Housing conditions*: the elderly tend to live in the poorest housing conditions, i.e. cold, poorly maintained and with limited hygiene facilities. A warm, safe and clean environment gives a sense of security and promotes physical and mental health.
5. *Income*: the elderly are the poorest members of the community. Financial security is an important resource that helps to avoid money worries and to give a sense of freedom, control and choice.
6. *Stresses experienced*: bereavement, specific worries and difficulties, adverse life events, losses experienced. The ability to resolve and cope with stresses is particularly important in the maintenance of mental health.
7. *Self-esteem*: negatively influenced by low perception of self-worth and usefulness, loss of active work and social role, stigmatized group. Important for the older person to develop strong internalized sources of self-worth and to realistically perceive and come to terms with their own ageing.

Orientation, Confusion and Mental Health

The maintenance of orientation involves a complex interaction of cognitive processes. Perceptual stimuli and environmental cues are actively processed and matched with existing memories to reinforce our sense of identity, location, time and purpose. The sense of continuity of existence that orientation provides is important in promoting feelings of security and in enabling people to relate to their immediate environment in a meaningful way. Disturbances of cognitive functioning, severe stress, unexpected events and strange surroundings can interfere with the processes of orientation and create confusion. As a consequence, a person's ability to communicate, behave and respond appropriately and meet their physical needs becomes increasingly disrupted. If the experience of confusion continues, then a person is faced with very severe mental health difficulties that have profound consequences for all aspects of living.

The Classification of Confusional States

Confusion is a collective term used to describe a wide range of behavioural, emotional and cognitive disturbances. In mental health practice, confusional states are primarily classified in terms of their underlying pathology and prognosis. They are described as "organic psychoses", because the disorders tend to have an identifiable physical pathology. During periods of confusion the sufferer will tend to lose insight into their behaviour and their perception of the environment. In terms of their potential outcomes they are categorized as to whether they are short-term ("acute") or long-term ("chronic") confusional states.

Acute confusional states (delirium)

Acute confusional states are transient in nature. They occur as a response to systemic bodily or cerebral disturbances that temporarily disrupt the fragile physiology of the brain. As a consequence, the person experiences the characteristic signs of acute confusion. A similar reaction may also occur as a reaction to severe psychological stress.

Characteristic signs of acute confusion

1. Rapid onset, often over the preceding 24–48 hours.
2. Disorientation to time, place and person.
3. Fluctuating severity with lucid intervals, often worse in the evening.
4. Labile moods – suspiciousness and irritability.
5. Restlessness and agitation.
6. Distractability and limited concentration.
7. Clouding of consciousness.
8. Hallucinations and delusions.
9. Signs and symptoms of underlying systemic or cerebral disorder.

Potential causes of an acute confusional state

1. Infections: particularly chest and bladder infections, septicaemia, cellulitis.
2. Toxins: alcohol, chemical agents; iatrogenic – reaction to medication, particularly hypnotics and other psychoactive drugs.
3. Malnutrition and dehydration.
4. Cardiovascular disease.
5. Metabolic disorder: hepatic and renal failure.
6. Trauma: physical injury from an accident or fall.
7. Severe psychological stress: bereavement, life crisis, chronic pain and discomfort, physical exhaustion.
8. Endocrine disorder: diabetes, thyroid over- or under-activity.
9. Epilepsy.

Treatment of acute confusional states

1. Identification and treatment of underlying physical causes.

2. Rest and reassurance.
3. Nourishment and hydration.
4. Reality orientation.
5. Information and health education.

It is important to differentiate between an acute and reversible confusional state and one which is longer-term. Detailed physical and mental assessment should facilitate discrimination. It is also necessary to be aware that an acute confusional state can be superimposed on an underlying chronic confusional state.

Chronic confusional states (dementia)

Chronic confusional states are the result of an underlying pathological process that causes progressive and irreversible brain damage. As a consequence, there is gradual and severe impairment in all aspects of cognitive functioning, behaviour and independence.

The course of this process may be moderately rapid or very slow with long periods of little cognitive deterioration. This will depend in part upon the degree and rapidity of the underlying pathology, but also upon environmental conditions that are favourable towards the maintenance of mental health and orientation.

In the early stages the effects may be subtle and insidious. They may be so global and diffuse that those close to the person may not be very aware that a serious mental health problem is developing. Others may be aware that the person seems "different", "changed" or a "bit absent-minded", but only realize that these were early signs of confusion in retrospect.

A deterioration in short-term memory is one of the most noticeable and early signs for many people that has profound implications for their behaviour, relationships and independent living.

Frequent memory lapses may cause difficulties for the person and may bring them into conflict with others. Others may be accused of moving the person's possessions and of not keeping them fully informed. The person may initially be aware that their memory is not very reliable and develop strategies to cope or compensate for this. As their forgetfulness worsens, they may not be able to find their way back home and may become lost in previously familiar places.

With the loss of short-term memory the person finds it increasingly difficult to stay focussed on an activity for any length of time. Numerous activities are started – housework, cooking, eating, socializing – only for the person to forget what they are doing and to wander on to another unrelated activity. This may create safety hazards in the home with unlit gas fires, food burning on the cooker or burning cigarettes left about the home. There is a loss of continuity and purpose in their activities and behaviour which becomes more fragmented and erratic.

Personality and emotional changes may also be prominent. Certain personality traits may become more pronounced or the person may behave in a way that is increasingly out of character. Relationships with others may become increasingly strained with the person behaving and reacting unpredictably. Concern expressed by others may evoke a strong and hostile reaction. Pronounced mood changes may happen without any obvious external cause. The person themselves may be worried in the early stages at these changes happening to them which they cannot comprehend or control. This may give rise to feelings of anxiety, fear, frustration or depression. This is particularly so if they have lucid intervals and are periodically aware of their growing difficulties. Suicide can be a risk at such times.

As the confusion worsens, then the person's behaviour can become even more divorced from external events and this begins to have serious implications for their ability to meet their basic needs. Self-neglect of nutrition, hygiene and their environment can have consequences for their physical health and safety.

In the later stages, the person may become progressively less able to relate and communicate with others. Close relatives may not be recognized, their names and the nature of their relationship forgotten; their conversation becomes rambling, incoherent and vague; they fail to understand what is said to them and seem to be locked into their own internal world. Ultimately, the sufferer loses sense not only of time and place but also of their own identity and existence.

Eventually, motor functions may also become affected. Co-ordination, skilled movement, balance and mobility gradually deteriorate and the person becomes physically helpless and reliant upon others. Death usually intervenes after several years of progressive and advanced deterioration from physical causes.

The pathology and classification of chronic confusional states

1. *Alzheimer's disease* (senile dementia) forms the majority (some 65%) of cases of chronic confusion in the elderly. It is a progressive irreversible condition that involves the premature degeneration and death of brain cells with shrinkage and loss of brain substance. The cause of this condition is unknown. A number of potential causes have been suggested, e.g. heredity, toxins.
2. *Multi-infarct type* (arteriosclerotic dementia) forms about 30% of cases of chronic confusion in the elderly. Typically, the onset tends to be sudden with clouding of consciousness from which the person may make a limited recovery. The disease progresses in a step-like and episodic fashion, often with lucid intervals, until an advanced stage is reached. The degenerative changes take the form of small areas of softening in the brain (infarcts) as a result of repeated emboli disrupting the fragile blood supply. Other arteriosclerotic changes may likewise interfere with the blood and hence oxygen supply to the brain.

3. *Jakob-Creutzfeldt disease* is a diffuse degeneration of brain tissue caused by a slow virus that progressively destroys brain tissue. This is a very rare condition. Fortunately, the virus is not particularly contagious. The disease may begin in middle age or later and once established leads to death within 1 year or so.

4. *Pick's disease* is a progressive, premature degeneration of brain cells characterized by personality changes, with disorders of conduct being prominent.

5. *Other causes*

   - degenerative disease – Huntington's chorea;
   - trauma – head injury;
   - toxins – industrial accidents, prolonged alcohol or drug abuse.
   - infections – human immunodeficiency virus (HIV), acquired immune deficiency syndrome (AIDS).

Characteristic signs of chronic confusional states

1. Slow and progressive onset.
2. Disorientation to time, place and person, with eventual complete loss of insight.
3. Progressive memory loss: initially short-term memory tends to be mainly affected with an inability to learn or to store new information. This tends to be progressive and eventually earlier memories, too, are lost. Many sufferers appear to live in a permanent world of their past.
4. Impaired cognitive functioning: all cognitive functions are affected. Poor concentration, diminished problem-solving, judgement, abstraction and discrimination.
5. Restlessness and wandering: particularly so in people who were previously active. There appears to be some difference between daytime and night-time patterns of restlessness, with the latter more marked by nocturnal confusion.
6. Emotional lability: sudden and unpredictable mood changes. This may include anxiety, fear, belligerence and aggression.
7. Impaired ability to communicate with others: rambling speech, repetitive statements, confabulation, inappropriate replies.
8. Self-neglect of nutrition and hygiene: other physical problems may arise from the confusion such as incontinence or weight loss.
9. Deterioration in social behaviour: inability to perceive and to respond appropriately to social situations, disinhibition, loss of awareness of appearance and clothing, regressive eating habits.
10. Profound changes in personality: may seem like a different person to relatives who may no longer be able to identify with them.

Suggested References

Anderson, F. (1984). Retirement can damage your health. *Nursing Mirror*, 1 August, Vol. 159, No. 3, pp. 25–26.

Barrowclough, F. and Pinel, C. (1981). The process of ageing. *Journal of Advanced Nursing*, Vol. 6, No. 4, pp. 319–325.

Bromley, D. B. (Ed.) (1984). *Gerontology: Social and Behavioural Perspectives*. Croom Helm, London.

Carver, V. and Liddiard, P. (1978). *An Ageing Population*. Hodder and Stoughton/ Open University, London.

Church, M. (1985). Forgotten something? *Nursing Times*, 24 July, Vol. 91, No. 30, pp. 23–24.

Clarke, C. (1987). Reaching for reality. *Nursing Times*, 19 July, 83, No. 30, pp. 24–27.

Cowl, N., Davison, W. and Webster, S. (1984). *Ageing: The Facts*. Oxford University Press, Oxford.

Davis, D. R. (1984). *An Introduction to Psychopathology*, 4th edition. Oxford University Press, Oxford.

French, S. (1986). The rejuvenation of geriatrics. *New Society*, 12 December, Vol. 78, No. 1250, pp. 16–18.

Garrett, G. (1984). Caught and not taught? *Nursing Times*, 24 October, Vol. 80, No. 43, pp. 48–51.

Garrett, G. (1985). Ageing and individuals. *Nursing*, September Vol. 2, No. 41, p. 1230.

Gibbs, A. (1986). *Understanding Mental Health*. Consumer's Association/Hodder and Stoughton, London.

Gilleard, C. J. (1984). *Living with Dementia: Community Care of the Elderly Mentally Infirm*. Croom Helm, London.

Goodwin, S. and Mangen, P. (1985). Do old people come from outer space? *Nursing Times*, 10 July, Vol. 81, No. 28, pp. 52–53.

Gray, B. and Isaacs, B. (1979). *Care of the Elderly Mentally Infirm*. Tavistock, London.

Gray, M. (1985). Biological ageing and screening. *Nursing*, September, Vol. 2, No. 41, pp. 1227–1229.

Griffiths, E. (1988). No sex please, we're over 60. *Nursing Times*, 6 January, Vol. 84, No. 1, pp. 34–35.

Hughes, J. (1986). *An Outline of Modern Psychiatry*, 2nd edition. John Wiley, Chichester.

Kingston, B. (1987). *Psychological Approaches in Psychiatric Nursing*. Croom Helm, London.

Kirby, D. and Kay, P. (1987). Support for the silent sufferers. *Nursing Times*, 13 May, Vol. 83, No. 19, pp. 43–44.

Mace, N. L., Rabins, P. W. with Castleton, V., Clarke, C. and McEwen, E. (1985). *The 36-hour Day: Caring at Home for Confused Elderly People* (UK edition). Hodder and Stoughton/Age Concern, London.

Mahendra, B. (1985). The diagnosis trap. *Nursing Times*, 24 July, Vol. 81, No. 30, pp. 25–26.

Mitchell, R. (1983). Confusion. *Nursing Times*, 13 April, Vol. 79, No. 15, pp. 62–64.

Murphy, E. (1986). *Dementia and Mental Illness in the Old*. Papermac, London.

Norman, A. (1986). The challenge of dementia. *Self Health*, September, No. 12, pp. 16–17.

Pitt, B. (1982). *Psychogeriatrics: An Introduction to the Psychiatry of Old Age*, 2nd edition. Churchill Livingstone, Edinburgh.

Pitt, B. (1985). Brain failure in old age. *Nursing*, September, Vol. 2, No. 41, pp. 1219–1221.

Roberts, A. (1986a). Senior systems 1. *Nursing Times*, 16 April, Vol. 82, No. 16, pp. 39–42. Systems of life, No. 136.

Roberts, A. (1986b). Senior systems 2. *Nursing Times*, 21 May, Vol. 82, No. 21, pp. 43–46. Systems of Life, No. 137.

Roberts, A. (1986c). Senior systems 3. *Nursing Times*, 11 June, Vol. 82, No. 24, pp. 43–46. Systems of life, No. 138.

Shaw, M. W. (1984). *The Challenge of Ageing: A Multidisciplinary Approach to Extended Care*. Churchill Livingstone, Edinburgh.

Skeet, M. (1982). *The Third Age*. Darton, Longman and Todd, London, in association with Age Concern, England and the Disabled Living Foundation.

Skeet, M. (1985). Some international concepts of old age. *Nursing*, September, Vol. 2, No. 41, pp. 1206–1208.

Stott, M. (1985). A personal experience of ageing. *Nursing*, September, Vol. 2, No. 41, pp. 1203–1205.

Taylor, B. (1987). A living bereavement. *Nursing Times*, 19 July, Vol. 83, No. 30, pp. 27–30.

Tinker, A. (1984). Health and housing. *Nursing Times*, 2 May, Vol. 80, No. 18, pp. 57–59.

Trethowan, W. and Sims, A. (1983). *Psychiatry*, 5th edition. Baillière Tindall, London and San Diego.

Wattis, J. P. and Church, M. (1986). *Practical Psychiatry of Old Age*. Croom Helm, London.

Willis, J. (1976). *Clinical Psychiatry*. Blackwell Scientific, Oxford.

Wilson, B. A. and Moffat, N. (Eds) (1984). *Clinical Management of Memory Problems*. Croom Helm, London.

Wolanin, M. and Phillips, L. (1981). *Confusion, Prevention and Care*. C. V. Mosby, London.

Self-assessment Questions

SAQ 1. List five factors that influence mental health in later life.

SAQ 2. Identify five potential causes of acute confusion.

SAQ 3. List five characteristics of chronic confusion.

SAQ 4. State four differences between acute and chronic confusional states.

Unit 13.1: Written Test

Albert King, aged 84, was found wandering and confused at 6 a.m. by his local policeman who returned him to his home. When the constable went inside, he found the house to be in a state of squalor, and Albert had obviously been neglecting himself for some time. The policeman contacted Albert's GP who arranged for the duty team from the local community mental health centre to make an urgent assessment visit later that morning.

1. What observations would the team make to confirm that Albert was suffering from a confusional state?
2. What observations would they need to make to confirm whether this was likely to be an acute or chronic confusional state?
3. What factors in Albert's life-style may have contributed towards the development of self-neglect and a loss of interest in his home environment?

Care and Support of the Confused Elderly Person

Care and Treatment

A wide range of practical approaches and therapeutic interventions may be used to help the confused person and their family. The general approach should be towards an integrated and readily accessible service to support the confused person and their family in the community or in residential settings as required.

Therapeutic aims

1. To promote orientation and independence.
2. To maintain the person's physical and mental health.
3. To facilitate the development of the person's and their family's coping skills.

Family and Self-care

The vast majority of confused elderly people are cared for at home. Of those in care about one in five are cared for in an old people's home, part three accommodation or in voluntary or private nursing homes. Hospital and residential services are only able to cope with about 3% of the elderly confused at one time. This is in stark contrast to the widespread belief that the elderly have been "abandoned" by their relatives. In reality the family is the main source of help for elderly people. It is only comparatively recently that families have been faced with the great numbers of people living to a great age.

About 30% of elderly people live on their own and look after themselves. Naturally, as their confusion increases, their ability to meet their needs effectively decreases. Even this group receives fairly regular assistance and contact from relatives – one-third are seen every day, one-third two or three times a week and one-quarter once a week. Only 3% have no contact with their family and 10% no contact with their neighbours.

Some 30% of the elderly confused are cared for by their spouse, often elderly and with some difficulties themselves. Partners often try to cover up for the disabilities of their spouse. The majority (75%) of carers in this category are women. It would appear that where elderly men are looking after a female spouse they receive more help from health and social services than elderly women in a similar situation.

Families and single children care for about one-third of elderly confused people. In reality, this aspect of family care, like that of care by a married partner, means care by a woman. Other members of the family often only provide peripheral support. There are currently more women caring for old people than are caring for babies. There are now about 1 million elderly dependent people in the community who require help with shopping, collecting pensions, etc. Over the age of 85, levels of physical dependency also increase dramatically.

Caring for a confused elderly person is an extremely demanding and stressful experience. It poses a severe strain upon the carer and their family – 40% report some burden, 40% report a severe degree of burden. Some carers are very resourceful at coping with these demands and develop a range of effective psychological and behavioural strategies. Other carers are less able to cope. Even those who cope well are likely to find their tolerance decreasing over time and to experience profound changes of life-style.

A wide range of behavioural and physical problems are reported. These can mount up and become continuous sources of stress. Those most frequently encountered include wandering, restlessness, carelessness, destructiveness, obstinacy, troublesome behaviour, over-talkativeness, withdrawal, mood disturbances, communication difficulties, incontinence, assistance with dressing and mobility, disinhibition, embarrassing behaviour, nocturnal confusion, safety hazards, non-recognition of carer, and making threats.

The mental disturbances often create more strain to carers than the physical difficulties. Damage to the caring relationship primarily arises from the lack of affectional responses and difficulty in communicating with the confused person.

The presence of a confused, dependent elderly person who requires constant attention can cause severe difficulties within the family. Problems reported include guilt, embarrassment, stress, grief, anger, frustration, resignation, social isolation, loss of contact with friends and relatives, strain on family relationships, and resentment towards the sufferer.

In theory, a wide range of health care and social services exist to help the elderly confused and to support carers. However, there exists a large shortfall in the resources available for the elderly and the ever-growing demand for services. Additionally, many carers find it difficult to gain access to services or to understand the roles of the various agencies involved. They often feel that their difficulties are not fully acknowledged and that they are left unsupported to cope with an intolerable burden.

Abuse of elderly dependent relatives by carers

Coping with the formidable demands of a confused, dependent, elderly relative can sometimes drive the carer beyond their "breaking point". Frustrated, angry and feeling trapped, they may vent their feelings on what they perceive to be the source of their problems. Abuse is primarily the response of someone who is unable to cope or express their feelings in any other way. The abuse may be by the spouse, daughter or son or by a grandchild who is looking after them. The person needs as much support and sympathy as the elderly person in their care. Careful assessment and observation should alert health care workers to situations of potential abuse and facilitate effective intervention.

Types of abuse by carers

1. Psychological abuse: taunting, ridicule, threats, shouting.
2. Physical abuse: hitting, punching, cutting, physical constraints, burns, assault.
3. Sexual abuse: indecent assault, rape, embarrassment.
4. Emotional abuse: rejection, ambivalence.
5. Physical neglect: malnutrition, dehydration, cold, excessive heat.
6. Exploitation: financial, housing.

Warning signs of potential abuse by carers

1. Heavy dependency on one carer.
2. Carer also responsible for other dependents.
3. Multiple stress of carer: family conflict, divorce, alcohol abuse, unemployment, financial problems, cramped housing conditions.
4. Physical injuries to dependent person with vague or unconvincing explanations by carer.
5. History of mental health problems in carer.
6. Low self-esteem of carer: feelings of desperation, hopelessness, helplessness.
7. Triggering condition or situation: incontinence, screaming.
8. Inadequate health and social service provision.

Providing family support

Initially, the person and their carers can be helped considerably in coping with confusion by:

1. Accurate information about confusion and its management.
2. Involvement in the care and therapeutic programme.
3. The opportunity to talk freely about their problems.
4. The address of a local contact and support group.
5. Developing the person's and family's coping skills and strategies.
6. Reviewing their needs for practical help and assistance from welfare agencies.
7. The opportunity for support and a break when suffering from stress and exhaustion.

Community Care

The vast majority of confused people are cared for at home. Their needs may range from periodic support and reassurance to constant attendance and care. Depending upon the extent and tolerance of the social support network and the health care resources available, it is possible to care for even the most confused person at home. The aims of community care are:

1. To support the person and their family.
2. To enable the person to remain in their own home.
3. To monitor and promote the person's mental and physical health.
4. To implement community-based support and care programmes.

The services available include:

1. The community mental health centre: with community psychiatric nurses, social workers, psychologists, occupational therapists and consultant psychiatrists working as a team to offer skills-based therapeutic interventions.
2. Intensive domiciliary support schemes: some health districts have established multidisciplinary teams and services to provide integrated and intensive support for the elderly confused in their own homes.
3. General practitioners.
4. Primary health care team: health visitors, district nurses.
5. Voluntary agencies: Age Concern England, Help the Aged, Alzheimer's Disease Society, MIND, Association of Carers, volunteer visitors and sitters.
6. DHSS: benefits, allowances and grants as currently available to individuals and carers.
7. Local authority/health authority: Meals on Wheels, home helps, inconti-

nence laundry, chiropody, night watch/sitters. Provision of aids for mobility, dressing, eating and incontinence.
8. Day hospitals, homes and centres for the elderly confused: these may be organized by social services, health authorities or voluntary agencies.

Residential Care

Residential care is appropriate when:

1. There is a lack of support in the community.
2. There is a need for intensive and skilled care when the person is very confused and it is difficult for the family to cope.
3. The care and family network is exhausted and requires a temporary break, e.g. respite care, holiday relief admission.
4. Detailed assessment for specific types of therapy are required.

The settings may include:

1. Homes for the elderly confused which provide a locality-based health care resource for the elderly confused.
2. Assessment units which have the resources for detailed mental and physical assessments.
3. Psychiatric hospital or unit with full care and treatment services for the elderly confused.
4. Private or voluntary nursing homes: in some areas of the country these provide a significant part of the care for the elderly confused.

Most carers feel a sense of guilt at having an elderly relative admitted into full-time care. Even short-term or relief admissions can add greatly to the level of confusion and distress experienced by the sufferer.

Therapeutic Interventions

Psychotherapeutic approaches

1. *Skilled nursing care*: one of the most important therapeutic factors.
2. *Individual counselling*: in the early stages of confusion for the sufferer. To promote self-esteem, insight and to release repressed emotion in the carer.
3. *Health education*: to develop coping skills, to identify and modify stressors in the person's and family's life-style. To facilitate recognition and understanding of the signs of confusion. To develop practical strategies, to promote orientation and to meet physical health care needs.

4. *Family therapy*: to help the family to find ways of coping with stresses arising from caring. To facilitate family communications.
5. *Voluntary organizations*: self-help and constant support groups. To share experiences and ways of coping. To offer mutual support and practical help.
6. *Occupational therapy*: to maintain life and domestic skills.
7. *Recreational and social activities*: to provide diversional activities, to promote orientation, to provide physical activities.
8. *Art, music and drama*: to help express and release feelings, to promote orientation, to provide physical activities.
9. *Behavioural psychotherapy*: for specific behavioural problems, to reinforce existing positive behaviour, social skills' training.
10. *Reality orientation*.

Reality orientation

The disorientation that is characteristic of chronic confusional states is primarily the result of underlying pathological processes in the brain. However, there is evidence that the degree of confusion is also influenced by environmental and social factors. "Reality orientation" (RO) is the name given to a broad range of therapeutic approaches that attempt to purposefully modify these factors to promote the confused person's contact with reality. The immediate environment and the interactions between clients and care-givers are structured to help the confused person:

- become more aware of everyday events;
- regain and maintain contact with their environment;
- function as independently as possible.

Reality orientation builds upon existing good care practices: therapeutic relationships (Unit 1.2), therapeutic communication (Unit 1.3) and the care environment (Unit 4.4). Effective programmes require that:

- all care givers are given training in the techniques that are used;
- staff attitudes and expectations towards the elderly are positive;
- programmes are consistently implemented by all those involved.

The techniques that are used include:

1. *Modification of the physical environment*:
   - Large orientation board that states the day, date, weather and special events in bold, visible print. This needs to be updated daily.
   - Large print calendar.
   - Large, bold-faced clocks.
   - Large print signs in the care environment to identify significant places, e.g. toilets, bedrooms, kitchen.

2. *Orientation cues*

- Each contact with a client is used to reinforce the time, place, person's identity, carer's name and the immediate activity.
- Clear, brief communications are used – the person is only spoken to when they can see the speaker.
- Positive reinforcement – a smile, nod or touch is given immediately to correct responses.
- Repetition is used to reinforce orientation.
- Incorrect responses are tactfully corrected – situations of potential frustration are minimized or avoided.
- Firm, gentle limits are set on confused behaviour.
- Clients are encouraged to find their own way around the care environment.
- Clients are encouraged to identify their own bed, chair, clothes and possessions.
- Clients are encouraged to participate in activities of daily living, domestic activities, and social events that serve to reinforce orientation.
- Meaningful choice and decision making is encouraged.
- Routine is used to provide a sense of security and structure.
- Social events are regularly organized with age-appropriate activities encouraged – boredom is avoided.

Reality orientation often forms part of the philosophy of care of centres that specialize in the care of the elderly confused person. The approaches may be described as:

1. *"Informal" or "24-hour" reality orientation*: in which the entire environment and all interactions with care givers are used to promote orientation. A wide range of activities may also be used as further opportunities to promote orientation, e.g. gardening, housekeeping, cooking, music, art and crafts, sport and games, pets, special events, religion, video films of the 1930s–1950s.
2. *"Classroom" or "formal" reality orientation*: intensive sessions several times a week that focus upon orientation or recall of past events. Such sessions may be used as a form of therapy in their own right or may be a periodic supplement to 24-hour reality orientation.

Some groups are established to focus upon past events and to stimulate long-term memories that may remain relatively unaffected and accessible. These approaches may be called "reminiscence therapy", "recall groups" or "bibliotherapy". Books, pictures, newspapers, films, music, clothing, artefacts, etc., from the client group's past are used. Additional reinforcement may be given if the group is held in a setting that reflects this era. Some centres have set aside rooms that are furnished in the style of the 1930s or 1940s, or as a bar-room of the period. Elderly confused people often respond to such stimulation and attempts are then encouraged to share reminiscences and to try and relate their past experiences to the present.

Reality orientation has been the subject of some research and attempts to validate this approach appear to be inconclusive. Some clients do respond very favourably during sessions or specific interactions. The primary difficulty is differentiating whether it is the specific techniques or reality orientation that reduce confusion or whether having motivated staff who interact purposefully in an optimistic and stimulating environment with clients is the therapeutic influence. Nevertheless, both staff and clients do appear to benefit from a programme that encourages interaction, develops relationships and promotes hope.

Chemotherapy

No currently available drug can influence the degree of confusion or rate of cerebral deterioration. Attempts to influence chemically cerebral blood flow or the level of neurotransmitters in the brain have been tried but do not at present appear to have any clinical application.

The use of any form of medication for the confused elderly person has to be very carefully considered and monitored. As we age the ability of our bodies to detoxify potent medicines decreases. There is a very real risk that drugs prescribed for mental or physical symptoms may add to the degree of disorientation by imposing a toxic reaction upon a pre-existing organic confusional state. In someone who is only mildly or moderately confused this can precipitate severe disorientation.

If the person is suffering from agitation, severe anxiety or restlessness, then appropriate medications may be indicated for short-term use only. However, the use of medication to control troublesome behaviour should not become a substitute for effective and skilled care interventions.

Unit Instructions

When you have researched the suggested references, have mastered the Unit Objectives and successfully answered the Self-assessment Questions, proceed with the Unit Written Test.

Suggested References

Adams, T. (1987). Dementia is a family affair. *Community Outlook*, February, pp. 7–9.

Bailey, E. A., Browns, S., Goble, R. E. A. and Holden, U. P. (1986). Twenty four hour reality orientation: changes for staff and patients. *Journal of Advanced Nursing*, Vol. 11, No. 2, pp. 145–151.

Barker, P. J. (1982). *Behaviour Therapy Nursing*. Croom Helm, London.

Black, S. and Simon, R. (1980). The specialist nurse, support care and the elderly mentally infirm. *Community Outlook*, 14 February, pp. 45–46.

Bloomfield, K. (1986). Ask the family. *Nursing Times*, 12 March, Vol. 82, No. 11, pp. 29–30.

Burton, M. (1982). Reality orientation for the elderly: A critique. *Journal of Advanced Nursing*, Vol. 7, No. 5, pp. 427–433.

Carr, P. J., Butterworth, C. A. and Hodges, B. E. (1980). *Community Psychiatric Nursing*. Churchill Livingstone, Edinburgh.

Clarke, L. (1984). *Domiciliary Services for the Elderly*. Croom Helm, London.

Clough, N. (1984). A short answer to long-term care. *Nursing Times*, 5 December, Vol. 80, No. 49, pp. 40–42.

Cormack, D. (Ed.) (1984). *Geriatric Nursing. A Conceptual Approach*. Blackwell Scientific, Oxford.

Daniels, E. (1985). Trapped in the caring net. *Community Outlook*, February, pp. 22–24.

Davis, A. (1983). Behavioural techniques for elderly patients 2. *Nursing Times*, 26 October, Vol. 79, No. 43, pp. 26–27.

Duffy, H., Leeming, D. and Bracey, R. (1988). Checking on skills. *Nursing Times*, Vol. 84, No. 6, pp. 31–32.

Eastman, M. (1984). Abusing the elderly. *Nursing Mirror*, 24 October, Vol. 159, No. 15, pp. 19–20.

Fitton, J. M. (1984). Health visiting the elderly: Nurse manager's views. *Nursing Times*, 18 April, Vol. 80, No. 10, pp. 59–61.

Ford, M., Fox, J., Fitch, S. and Donovan, A. (1987). Light in the darkness. *Nursing Times*, 7 January, Vol. 83, No. 1, pp. 26–28.

Fry, J. (1984). Relative support. *Nursing Mirror*, 23 May, Vol. 158, No. 21, pp. 25–26.

Garrett, G. (1985). Family care and the elderly. *Nursing*, Vol. 2, No. 36, pp. 1061–1063.

Garrett, G. (1986). Old age abuse by carers. *The Professional Nurse*, August, Vol. 1, No. 11, pp. 304–305.

Georghiou, G. (1986). Home service. *Nursing Times*, 19 March, Vol. 82, No. 12, pp. 57–58.

Gilleard, C. J. (1984). *Living with Dementia: Community Care of the Elderly Mentally Infirm*. Croom Helm, London.

Gilleard, C., Mitchell, R. G. and Riordan, J. (1981). Ward orientation training with psychogeriatric patients. *Journal of Advanced Nursing*, Vol. 6, No. 2, pp. 95–98.

Godber, C. (1979). Don't overwhelm the family! *Nursing Mirror*, 26 July, Vol. 149, No. 4, pp. 30–32.

Gray, B. and Isaacs, B. (1979). *Care of the Elderly Mentally Infirm*. Tavistock, London.

Gray, J. A. M. (1984). Prevention of family breakdown. *Nursing Mirror*, 13 June, Vol. 158, No. 23, pp. 16–17.

Hanley, I. and Gilhooly, M. (1986). *Psychological Therapies for the Elderly*. Croom Helm, London.

Holden, U. P. and Woods, R. T. (1982). *Reality Orientation: Psychological Approaches to the "Confused" Elderly*. Churchill Livingstone, Edinburgh.

Keller, J. F. and Houghston, G. A. (1981). *Counselling the Elderly: A Systems Approach*. Harper and Row, New York.

Kempton, M. (1984). Family involvement. *Nursing Mirror*, 14 November, Vol. 159, No. 18. Psychiatry Forum Supplement (vii)–(viii).

Kingston, B. (1987). *Psychological Approaches in Psychiatric Nursing*. Croom Helm, London.

Lilof, V. (1983). Keeping them out of hospital. *Nursing Mirror*, 30 November, Vol. 157, No. 22, pp. 36–38.

Lyttle, J. (1986). *Mental Disorder: Its Care and Treatment*. Baillière Tindall, London and San Diego.

Lyttle, P. (1985). A supportive network. *Nursing Mirror*, 12 June, Vol. 160, No. 24, pp. 36–37.

Mace, N. L., Rabins, P. W. with Castleton, B., Clarke, C. and McEwen, E. (1985). *The 36-hour Day: Caring at Home for Confused Elderly People* (UK edition). Hodder and Stoughton/Age Concern, London.

Mathieson, A. (1986). Old people and drugs. *Nursing Times*, 8 January, Vol. 82, No. 2, pp. 22–25.

May, D., McKeganey, N. and Field, M. (1986). Extra hands or extra problems. *Nursing Times*, 3 September, Vol. 82, No. 36, pp. 35–38.

McKay, B., North, N. and Murray-Sykes, K. (1983). The effect on carers of hospital admission of the elderly. *Nursing Times*, 30 November, Vol. 79, No. 48, pp. 42–43.

McMichael, I. (1983). Reality orientation 2. Feeling at home. *Nursing Times*, 9 November, Vol. 79, No. 45, pp. 53–56.

Morris, M. (1986). Music and movement for the elderly. *Nursing Times*, 19 February, Vol. 82, No. 8, pp. 44–45.

Morton, I. (1988). Reality orientation. Does it matter whether it's Tuesday or Friday? *Nursing Times*, Vol. 84, No. 6, pp. 25–27.

Murphy, E. (1986). *Dementia and Mental Illness in the Old*. Papermac.

Norman, A. (1987). The old: Who cares? *New Society*, 13 March, Vol. 79, No. 1263, p. 19.

North, S. (1985). Breaking point. *Nursing Mirror*, 18 September, Vol. 161, No. 12, pp. 42–43.

Phillips, L. R. (1983). Abuse and neglect of the frail elderly at home: An exploration of theoretical relationships. *Journal of Advanced Nursing*, Vol. 8, No. 5, pp. 379–392.

Pitt, B. (1982). *Psychogeriatrics: An Introduction to the Psychiatry of Old Age*, 2nd edition. Churchill Livingstone, Edinburgh.

Pope, B. (1986). *Social Skills Training for Psychiatric Nurses*. Harper and Row, London.

Potterton, D. (1984). Drugging the elderly *Nursing Times*, 15 February, Vol. 80, No. 7, pp. 20–21.

Ratcliffe, J. (1988). Worth a try. *Nursing Times*, Vol. 84, No. 6, pp. 29–30.

Robertson, C. (1984). Health visitors and preventive care. *Nursing Times*, 22 August, Vol. 80, No. 34, pp. 29–31.

Saddington, N. (1986). Training the carers. *Nursing Times*, 22 January, Vol. 82, No. 4, pp. 42–43.

Shaw, M. W. (1984). *The Challenge of Ageing: A Multidisciplinary Approach to Extended Care*. Churchill Livingstone, Edinburgh.

Simmons, S. and Brooker, C. (1986). *Community Psychiatric Nursing: A Social Perspective*. Heinemann Nursing, London.

Skeet, M. (1982). *The Third Age*. Darton, Longman and Todd, London, in association with Age Concern, England and the Disabled Living Foundation.

Sterenborg, Y. (1982). From home to home. *Nursing Times*, 22/29 December, Vol. 78, No. 51, pp. 2191–2193.

Teasdale, K. (1983). Reality orientation 1. A programme for the elderly. *Nursing Times*, 9 November, Vol. 79, No. 45, pp. 49–52.

Wade, B. (1983). Different models of care for the elderly. *Nursing Times*, 25 May, Vol. 79, No. 12, pp. 33–36.

Wade, B. and Finlayson, J. (1983). Drugs and the elderly. *Nursing Mirror*, 4 May, Vol. 156, No. 18, pp. 17–21.

Watt, G. M. (1982). A family orientated approach to community care for the elderly mentally infirm. *Nursing Times*, 15 September, Vol. 78, No. 37, pp. 1545–1548.

Wattis, J. P. and Church, M. (1986). *Practical Psychiatry of Old Age*. Croom Helm, London.

Whitehead, T. (1983). Battered old people. *Nursing Times*, 16 November, Vol. 79, No. 46, pp. 32–33.

Willis, J. (1976). *Clinical Psychiatry*. Blackwell Scientific, Oxford.

Wilson, B. A. and Moffat, N. (Eds) (1984). *Clinical Management of Memory Problems*. Croom Helm, London.

Wolanin, M. and Phillips, L. (1981). *Confusion, Prevention and Care*. C. V. Mosby, London.

Self-assessment Questions

SAQ 5. List six problems commonly encountered by carers of elderly confused people.

SAQ 6. Identify four types of potential abuse of elderly confused people by stressed carers.

SAQ 7. Recall six agencies or services that provide support to the elderly confused people in the community.

SAQ 8. Describe four characteristics of an effective reality orientation programme.

Unit 13.2: Written Test

Joan Freeman, aged 45, has approached her local mental health centre in desperation. For some years she has provided support to her elderly mother, Agnes Farrow, a widow of 77, who lives nearby. However, over the last 6 months her mother has become increasingly confused and Joan is worried about her safety and ability to meet her physical needs. Joan's husband and family had initially provided some extra support but are becoming resentful of the increasing demands on their time. They think that Joan should spend more time with them and less with her confused mother who they think should be admitted into hospital. Joan is very reluctant to consider this alternative unless no other option is available. A subsequent joint assessment visit by the GP and CPN confirmed that Agnes has a moderately advanced chronic confusional state.

1. From the details given above, identify what services may be needed to provide community support for Agnes Farrow.
2. What therapeutic interventions may be necessary to help Agnes Farrow to live at home and to facilitate the support and care given by her daughter?

Nursing Care of the Confused Elderly Person

Unit Objectives

At the end of this Unit the learner should be able to:

1. Identify the nursing care needs of the confused elderly client.
2. Plan an individualized care programme.
3. Select appropriate nursing care interventions for the person's needs.
4. Describe possible evaluation criteria for specific needs.

Mental Health Nursing Care

Each person's care needs are unique and have to be assessed individually. For the confused elderly client a wide range of potential needs may be identified. It is also possible that the person may have physical health problems. A range of potential care needs have been selected to illustrate some of the problems that the person and their family may experience and the potential nursing interventions that may help them. For the elderly confused person these may include the needs to:

A. Promote their orientation to time, place and person.
B. Feel secure in a safe environment.
C. Meet their physical needs.
D. Facilitate the development of the person's and family's coping skills.

A. Promote Their Orientation to Time, Place and Person

Associated problems/personal difficulties

The experience of disorientation and memory lapses may interfere with a person's ability to meet their needs by:

1. Reducing their awareness and ability to meet their physical needs.
2. Diminishing their awareness of risks arising from their behaviour or in the environment.
3. Interfering with their ability to communicate and relate to others.
4. Causing feelings of insecurity and non-comprehension of external events.
5. Behaving and responding inappropriately.
6. Reducing their self-esteem.
7. Causing stress in relationships with carers.

Assessment

1. Statements made by person indicating disorientation to time, place and person.
2. Information from relatives and friends.
3. Nurse's observation of the person's:

   (a) cognitive function: memory and recall of significant details of personal history; concentration, alertness and distractability; ability to identify and recognize carers; recall of current events.
   (b) Orientation: ability to locate places and find their way around care environment and nearby locality; awareness of date, time, place, season and weather; pattern of orientation and confusion throughout the day and night; wandering.
   (c) Self-awareness and insight: understanding of health care needs; strategies used for confusion and their effectiveness.
   (d) Emotional reactions to their own confusion: irritability, frustration, indifference, accepting, anger, suspicion.

4. Psychosocial environment: presence of identifiable eliciting stimuli or triggering uses that influence confusion and orientation. Relationship of confused behaviour to external events. Reactions of others to person's behaviour.
5. Presence of potential stresses in the person's environment or life-style.
6. Completion of locally used/commercially prepared tests of orientation and memory function.

Desired outcomes

1. Person will be able to find their way around the care environment.
2. Person will be able to identify family members and carers.
3. Person will be able to supply relevant orientation information in relation to self, time, day, month and season.

Nursing intervention	Rationale
1. Initiate therapeutic relationship. Involve person and family in the care planning process	Interventions more likely to succeed in an atmosphere of trust and cooperation. Helps to reduce tension and to create the conditions for behavioural change
2. Demonstrate active listening. Be available and approachable. Demonstrate acceptance and non-judgemental responses. Offer reassurance	Interventions to promote orientation need to be based upon sound communication and relationship practices
3. Allocate person to key worker. Introduce person to members of care team	Orientation is facilitated if person can identify with primary carers
4. Show person around the care environment	Facilitates orientation
5. Give necessary verbal and written information about care programme and environment	Written information can be referred to by clients with memory problems. Clients have a right to have information about their care programme
6. Promote feelings of security and safety (see B.)	Interventions to promote orientation will not be successful if the person feels anxious and insecure
7. Ensure basic physical needs are being met (see C.)	Need to ensure that their needs are being met before able to focus on dealing with person's confusion. Can also use physical care interventions to promote orientation
8. Role model social and communication skills	Modelling by nurses has a powerful influence on the people in their care. Provides a baseline of orientated behaviour for the confused person to model upon
9. Positively reinforce self-esteem. Encourage acceptance of self-limitations. Avoid situations that are beyond the person's capabilities	Can be helpful to identify areas in which the person can cope effectively and enhance self-esteem, rather than attempting activities outside of their capabilities. This can cause frustration and stress, both of which increase confusion and a negative self-image

Nursing intervention	Rationale
10. Ensure that all care workers are consistent in their approach to maintain orientation	For reality orientation to be effective, it has to be implemented consistently by all care workers. Research into the implementation of reality orientation indicates that this is rarely done
11. Reassure family members that memory loss is not deliberate. Provide information to relatives on the nature of memory loss	At times the person may be very difficult to cope with. Carers may attribute the problems to personality factors or awkwardness. Relatives need this information in order to begin to understand and cope with confusion
12. Advise that person will become lost in unfamiliar environments	Person has limited ability to orientate to unfamiliar surroundings
13. Teach family members and carers the skills of reality orientation	They will be the main agents of reality orientation if it is to be effective
14. Teach family members strategies for dealing with confused and inappropriate behaviour	Enables them to cope with confused behaviour effectively
15. Promote contact with relatives and personal friends	Helps to overcome feelings of isolation and rejection. Still valued by others
16. Recognize the effects of the person's behaviour upon yourself. Arrange for own clinical supervision	Caring for the confused elderly person can be a very demanding and frustrating experience. Need to maintain own mental health and to review own clinical practice and to facilitate professional development
17. Ensure that the care environment is clearly signposted	All significant areas should be indicated and signposted – toilets, bedroom, kitchen, sitting room, etc. This facilitates orientation and autonomy. The signs act as prompts to remind the person where they are and the function of that area
18. Provide visual stimuli which continually orientate the person to time (large bold face clocks), date,	Research indicates that orientation boards and signs do help to reduce confusion. They need to provide a framework of information that serve as cues to orientate the confused

Nursing intervention	*Rationale*
place, weather, daily activities, significant forthcoming events.	person. Need to be readily legible. Symbols may also be usefully employed to complement written details
19. Ensure orientation details are updated and accurate	Becomes counterproductive if details are outdated
20. Reinforce sense of personal identity through recognition and personal possessions. Personalize an area of the care environment. Put person's name in large print on their bedroom. Ensure personal possessions are accessible and used	Personal recognition and personal possessions help to reinforce contact with reality. Also increases feelings of security. Personal possessions, clothes, pictures, photographs, bed, pet, etc., may all help in this. Possessions have to be visible to person to promote orientation
21. Ensure that sensory deficits are corrected. Ensure aids work properly and are used	About 30% of elderly people have some degree of hearing loss. Visual problems are even more common. Fortunately glasses and hearing aids can do much to overcome these problems. These are vital sources of sensory input if the person is to remain orientated and be responsive to efforts to promote orientation
22. Ensure that dentures fit and are worn	Promotes communication, comfort and self-esteem
23. Ensure regular planned interaction throughout the day	Orientation information requires repeated reinforcement to be effective. The confused person may have little awareness of time and the intervals may seem prolonged and isolating
24. State name and relationship with person at each contact. Remind person of their own name, the time and place during each contact	This basic orientation information is required at each contact. Serves to reinforce sense of identity and orientation to time and place

Nursing intervention	Rationale
25. Use contacts to reinforce reality orientation	Each contact needs to be used productively. Research indicates that many contacts between carers and the elderly confused are not used to reinforce orientation
26. Reduce distracting background noise and activities when communicating with person	Helps to focus on presenting material. Background noise distracts and can be stressful
27. Position self in person's line of vision. Ensure face is well lit. Look directly at the person during interaction. Use person's preferred name. Gain and maintain person's attention by using touch. Ensure only one carer speaks to person at a time	The confused person presents particular communication difficulties. The nurse needs to be particularly aware of all aspects of verbal and non-verbal communication and to use these to facilitate communication
28. Lower pitch of voice	Helps to compensate for high pitch hearing loss which is a common consequence of ageing
29. Ask one question or make one statement at a time. Ask questions that the person is likely to be able to answer	Need to stay focussed on one area at a time. Minimizes frustration
30. Use short words and simple sentences. Speak slowly and clearly, leave pauses	Helps person with limited attention span and recall to stay focussed on topic
31. Use non-verbal communication and words to facilitate communication. Be aware of own non-verbal communication during interaction	Although their verbal memory may be affected they may be quite receptive to non-verbal cues. This awareness should be used in communications
32. Allow time for the person to respond.	If the person feels pressured or stressed then their ability to respond is

Nursing intervention	*Rationale*
Keep calm, be patient. Pace the interview to the person's responses	impaired. They can also become agitated and confused
33. Observe person's non-verbal communication	Person may communicate non-verbally things that they are unable to say verbally
34. Reward appropriate responses with praise and touch. If inappropriate, reward and acknowledge the effort made by person	Positive reinforcement needs to be given to maintain orientated responses. All responses should be acknowledged
35. Repeat statement and try again for a correct response. Gently correct mistakes	Repetition and reinforcement are basic techniques of reality orientation. Should not argue or disagree with confused person as this increases disorientation
36. Use repetition to confirm understanding and to reinforce orientation	Need to ensure understanding as well as recall
37. Do not allow to ramble incoherently. Seek clarification of statements	To be effective the person has to be brought into contact with reality at each interaction
38. Supply missing words for person if they are unable to identify words or express themselves	Generally, attempts should be made to help the person find the words themselves. If they are unable and appear to be becoming more agitated as a consequence, then it may be appropriate to attempt to supply missing words and to reinforce their meaning
39. Do not reinforce or encourage disorientated misperceptions or behaviour. Provide accurate information	Reinforcement tends to strengthen the person's belief in the validity of their thoughts and experiences. This makes it more difficult to promote orientation
40. If person has forgotten recent events, gently remind them. Protect person from embarrassment	The person may react defensively if they feel criticized by others over their memory lapses. This can cause agitation and insecurity. Confabulation may also be used in an

Nursing intervention	Rationale
over memory lapses. Accept periodic lapses of memory	attempt to compensate for memory difficulties
41. Minimize the complexity of new information	For the person with a memory problem new information needs to be presented in such a way as to promote understanding and recall
42. Discuss events from the past that the person can share	Stimulates long-term recall and provides a point of social contact with others
43. Use person's experiences and recall of past to help orientate him to the present	Provides a point of contact from the person's past to the present day
44. Assist individual in ordering recent events according to time	Time sequencing is useful in promoting orientation and an understanding of recent events
45. Use external climatic conditions and observable view to reinforce orientation	External weather conditions, light and dark, vegetation, can be used to reinforce orientation to time of day, month and season
46. Give stimulation to as many senses as possible to stimulate recall	Memory is a very complex cognitive function. Deterioration is not global and some areas may be responsive to a broad range of sensory stimulation, e.g. touch, taste, smell, texture, colour
47. Encourage the use of a diary to record daily events and as a reminder	Can be used to promote orientation
48. Provide cue cards or lists to person to aid memory or task completion	Can help person to work through and complete tasks. This can be useful in promoting esteem and autonomy
49. Give person simple written instructions to support verbal instructions. Prompt person to follow written instructions. Give verbal reminders if person refuses or forgets to perform a task	Can be used to reinforce verbal information that the person may forget. Also helps to promote security if they feel anxious about forgetting

Nursing intervention	*Rationale*
50. Simplify activities if possible to within person's capabilities	Many activities of daily living can be adapted or modified to make them easier to perform
51. Inform person before carrying out activities or procedures	Facilitates orientation and shows respect to the person
52. Provide memory card to person with simple instructions on what to do if they become lost. Ensure person wears an identity bracelet, securely fastened with significant personal details, e.g. name, address, telephone number. Alternatively, details can be put on the back of a watch	This may help the person or those trying to assist. It should advise the person to stay calm, not to wander any further, and instructions on getting help, e.g. 'phone number of home or hospital. Can state that the person has a memory problem
53. Help person to compile a scrapbook of their significant family and life events	Can act as a very individualized memory aid
54. Provide daily newspapers, magazines, radio and TV programmes. Encourage residents to use these resources. Discuss significant news items and daily activities with residents	A further source of sensory input that helps to orientate person to the present. To be effective the television, radio, papers, etc., need to be actively used with residents and not just be background noise or decoration
55. Graduate orientation and recall activities to person's responses	As the person becomes aware of basic orientation – time, place, person, carers' names – then can move to more complex recall and recognition situations
56. Promote autonomy	Need to avoid feelings of helplessness. Promotes positive mental health
57. Offer choice over alternative activities. Discuss options with person	Can use the discussion to promote orientation and a sense of personal control
58. Promote responsibility for their own	Within limits of safety, person needs to experience the outcomes of their

Nursing intervention	*Rationale*
decisions and actions. Respect personal decisions	decisions. Person has a right to have their decisions respected
59. Reduce demands and expectations made of the person in the evening if they become more confused later in the day	Some people appear to have a pattern of confusion that becomes worse with failing light and as the day wears on. Carers need to be alert to this and adjust their interventions and expectations accordingly
60. Use subdued lighting to reduce agitation.	Research indicates that low-level lighting contributes to the reduction of agitation. It also makes carers feel calmer. Other effects are a reduction in noise levels and eating more quickly by people.
61. Use colour contrasts on signs and environment	Colour can be used to emphasize visual discrimination
62. Observe for signs of frustration and stress. Adopt a non-threatening tone and posture during agitation. Role model calm behaviour	Agitation is a common sign of confusion. Need to intervene skilfully to calm the person
63. Advise person if their behaviour is perceived as distressing or threatening to others	Confused person may not be aware that their behaviour is upsetting to others. May be disinhibited or easily irritated
64. Set and enforce behavioural limits on undesirable behaviour	Part of the process of making person's behaviour more reality-based
65. Distract person's attention to other incompatible activities. Ignore inappropriate behaviour. Keep calm. Correct incorrect behavioural and social responses	The confused person can be easily distracted if their behaviour is inappropriate. Need to use the principles of social skills training to modify and direct person's behaviour
66. Encourage personal interests and hobbies	Person may still be able to cope with previous activities. Stimulation of longer-term memories helps to promote orientation. Personal hobbies also enjoyable and help to prevent boredom

Nursing intervention	*Rationale*
67. Allow person to participate in household and physical tasks	Activities serve to stimulate memories and orientation. Help to maintain existing capabilities and to provide purposeful activity
68. Organize daily recall or reminiscence groups (see Unit 13.2)	Within an environment of informal or ongoing reality orientation, formal approaches can be used to reinforce orientation on specific topics and to meet social needs
69. Organize age-related social and recreational activities	Social activities help to meet social needs. Help to promote orientation and enjoyment. Activities need to be selected in terms of their relevance to the age group concerned to achieve these objectives, e.g. films and music from the 1930s–1940s
70. Make changes in care environment and routine gradually. Prepare the person in advance for changes, if possible. Reorientate them to care environment after changes are made	Takes time for the confused person to reorientate themselves to change. Can cause stress and increase short-term confusion
71. Maintain even lighting in care area. Avoid glare	Lighting levels are an important factor in maintaining visual orientation. In conditions of falling light or glare the person is less able to respond to visual cues
72. Ensure night lights are available and used	Assists visual orientation if the person wakes up during the night
73. Moderate the level of environmental stimulation	A certain level of stimulation is necessary to avoid monotony and to provide interest. However, if this becomes excessive, then it becomes sensory overload and adds to confusion

Evaluation

1. Person is able to find their way around the care environment unaided.
2. Person is able to demonstrate recognition of family members and carers.

3. Person is able to supply appropriate orientation details in respect of self, time, day, month and season.

B. Feel Secure in a Safe Environment

Associated problems/personal difficulties

Person may feel insecure and be at risk as a result of:

1. Disorientation in time, place and person.
2. An inability to comprehend what is happening around them.
3. The difficulty of attempting to cope with a failing memory.
4. Periodic lucid intervals in which they gain insight into their memory loss.
5. Diminished awareness of risks in the environment or arising from their behaviour.
6. Restlessness and agitation.
7. Inadequate knowledge and understanding of their health care programme.

Assessment

1. Statements made by person indicating insecurity, anxiety, apprehension or specific fears.
2. Information from relatives and friends.
3. Nurse's observations of the person's:

    (a) Degree of confusion and disorientation.
    (b) Ability to identify and react to risks.
    (c) Ability to safely cope with activities of daily living and self-care.
    (d) Verbal and non-verbal behaviour indicating anxiety: restlessness, pacing, agitation, gestures, eye contact, tearfulness, physiological response.
    (e) Needs for supervision and guidance.
    (f) Home/care environment in relation to safety factors and potential risks.

4. History of any accidents or situations of risk arising from their confused behaviour.
5. Support network available to the person: extent of supervision available and required.
6. Identification of potential stressors in the person's environment and life-style.

Desired outcomes

1. Person appears settled and indicates trust in carers.
2. Person is able to maintain maximum autonomy.
3. The potential for accidents or self-harm is minimized.

Nursing intervention	Rationale
1. Initiate a therapeutic relationship. Spend time with person. Be available and approachable. Demonstrate active listening	Interventions more likely to be successful in an atmosphere of trust and cooperation. Also shows sense of worth and acceptance which helps to increase feelings of security and safety
2. Adopt a non-judgemental and non-critical approach	Being non-judgemental helps a person to deal with any guilt and feel accepted
3. Empathize with their difficulties. Adopt a non-threatening, open posture and tone of voice. Use touch and other non-verbal signals to convey reassurance and to reduce anxiety	Reduces feelings of anxiety and threat. The confused person often feels very anxious at losing their sense of continuity and understanding. Skilled interventions are required to reduce anxiety and distress. Non-verbal interventions are often effective in helping people with cognitive impairments. Their verbal memory may be affected but they may still be responsive to non-verbal interventions. Hugging and gentle rocking may prove effective interventions. Touch can be very comforting and reassuring
4. Role model calm behaviour	Can have a powerful calming effect as people are subconsciously influenced by the behaviour of those around them
5. Approach unhurriedly. Demonstrate calmness. Do not rush the person. Be aware of your own reactions and experiences of stress	Anxiety in the carer communicates itself to the person. Caring can be a stressful experience at times. This may unconsciously influence your interactions with others
6. Be patient and aware of your own feelings	Caring for the confused person is a very demanding experience. They may be

Confusion in Later Life

Nursing intervention	*Rationale*
of frustration in dealing with the person. Take periodic breaks if possible	very resistant and seemingly uncooperative. Takes extreme patience and tolerance to remain calm
7. Arrange for own clinical supervision	Supervision is an effective way of coping with the stress of caring and for professional development
8. Provide clear and understandable information about their treatment, health care and the roles of different health care workers. Encourage questions. Ask for feedback on their understanding. Clarify any misunderstandings	A lot of anxiety is associated with fear of the unknown. People have a right to information about their health care. The nurse is in an ideal position to use this process to facilitate the development of the person's understanding about their health care needs
9. Provide written information that the person and carers can refer to. Identify appropriate written and audio-visual resource material	The confused person may later refer back to this. There is a growing amount of resource material on confusion that is specifically for lay people and carers
10. Enlist the person's cooperation in the planning of their health care	People are more likely to cooperate if they are well-informed and involved in the decision-making process. The person may have difficulty understanding but has a right to participate in their individualized care planning. Can also use this process to facilitate the development of the person's understanding about their health care needs
11. Encourage the person to express their feelings and to talk about their difficulties	Venting feelings in this way reduces stress and tension. These may be contributing to the degree of confusion that the person experiences. Also demonstrates acceptance
12. Promote orientation (see **A.**)	Disorientation can be a very distressing experience. Promoting orientation enhances feelings of security
13. Provide support and reassurance to	Anxiety in relatives will communicate itself to person. Reassurance of carers

Nursing intervention	*Rationale*
relatives and carers. Encourage carers to express their feelings and to share their difficulties. Observe for signs of stress in carers	also communicates positively to person. Caring for the confused person is a very demanding experience. Carer's mental health needs should also be considered in trying to provide a safe and secure environment
14. Observe for signs of mental and physical abuse of confused elderly person by carers	Stress and frustration may be directed towards the confused elderly person. Nurse needs to be alert to risk factors associated with abuse of the elderly person by carers
15. Initiate appropriate action if concerned for welfare and safety of confused elderly person	The nurse has a professional responsibility to act as an advocate for vulnerable clients. The action to be taken will depend upon the nurses' skills, their relationship with the carers and the nature of the abuse. If detected early, then the nurse may be able to resolve the situation and facilitate more appropriate coping in future. Serious abuse may require the involvement of other agencies
16. Ensure that significant personal items are available and used	Familiar objects help to increase feelings of security. These may include clothing, pictures, ornaments, personal possessions, bedding, furniture and pets
17. Explain all actions in advance	Interventions do not then come as an anxiety-provoking surprise. Promotes feelings of security and of trust in carers
18. Communicate with the person when you are engaged in caring activities	Promotes orientation and feelings of security
19. Reassure the person of non-harmful intent	Person may be fearful and suspicious
20. Refrain from unnecessary procedures and interventions if person appears agitated or distressed	Interventions at this time would be threatening and possibly add to disorientation. Wait until person is calmer and more receptive

Nursing intervention	*Rationale*
21. Promote autonomy. Offer choice wherever possible	Increases feelings of personal control. Important in helping to overcome feelings of helplessness and in promoting positive mental health
22. Ensure that basic physical needs are being met (see **C.**)	Physical comfort is a prerequisite for meeting other needs. Person will be unable to relax if they feel physically uncomfortable
23. Do not whisper to others in the presence of the person or express inappropriate emotion	This increases feelings of suspicion and threat
24. Ensure that all carers are aware of any risk of self-harm likely to arise from person's confused behaviour	Carers have a responsibility to protect the person and others who may be at risk from the behaviour of confused person
25. Advise person if their behaviour is a risk to themselves or others. Directly intervene if person appears to be at risk	Person may not realize that their actions are potentially unsafe. This may be necessary to protect the safety of the person or of others in the immediate environment
26. Ensure that the person is observed and monitored during situations where there is a degree of risk	Carers need to balance the needs for protection with the needs to take risks. Over-protection can lead to dependence and loss of initiative. It is important to enable the confused person to function at the limits of their abilities – "use it or lose it".
27. Engage in physical activity as a precursor to verbal interaction, e.g. games, activities, drama, music. Organize social and recreational activities	Sometimes it is easier for people to talk as part of an activity or game, or afterwards. It provides a non-threatening point of contact, promotes orientation, gives physical exercise and meets social needs. These are important in helping the person to feel settled and secure
28. Ensure that the prson has an identification bracelet that details their name, address, telephone number and that they have a memory problem	If the person wanders, then others are able to respond sympathetically and to return them home promptly. Bracelet needs to have a firm clasp to make removal difficult by confused person

Nursing intervention	*Rationale*
29. Modify the environment to allow as much freedom and safety as possible within external boundaries	Restlessness and wandering are major problems in the care of the confused person. This can be very demanding on carers and poses risks to the confused person from wandering
30. Modify exit door handles to require skilled opening	To prevent undue frustration and the need for constant observation it usually helps to modify exits, so that others who are not suffering from cognitive impairment are able to gain entry/exit whereas the confused person finds it difficult
31. Ensure that the layout of the care environment is kept relatively constant	Helps the confused person to become orientated and to know their way around. This promotes feelings of security. Environmental changes can be very disruptive
32. Ensure that the care environment is kept tidy and organized. Make changes in layout gradually	Enables the confused person to locate items. Helps to promote autonomy and security
33. Explore the possibility of making modifications to household fitments and utensils to promote safety and utility. Contact public utilities for advice (electricity, gas and water boards)	More accidents happen in the house than in any other setting. The confused person has particular difficulties and can benefit from the steps taken to promote home safety. Steps required may include fitting fire guards, keeping stairways clear, non-slip mats, stable chairs and furniture, padding hard edges, locking away potential toxins, child-proof lids, keeping electric flexes out of the way. Adaptations can be made to cookers, fires and taps to promote safety and ease of use
34. Check that levels of daytime and evening lighting are adequate. Ensure that night lights are available and used	Lighting needs to be adequate both from a safety viewpoint and for orientation purposes. Failing light and darkness and particularly disorientating and increase the risk of an accident
35. Observe and monitor when confused person is engaged in tasks	Important to maintain autonomy, promote safety and yet not to be over-protective. A degree of risk

Nursing intervention	*Rationale*
that have an element of risk. Observe when person is smoking cigarettes. Remove matches or lighters. Ensure they are only used under supervision	taking may be necessary to achieve these objectives. The risk of fire arising from unattended or discarded cigarette butts is very high. Hence the need for sensible precautions
36. Promote access and mobility around the home/care environment and in outside paths and gardens. Arrange for necessary alterations and fitments. Ensure mobility aids are available if required. Check on stability of furniture. Keep stairways and passages clear	Promotes both autonomy and safety. Careful placing of hand-rails, bath-rails, non-slip floor coverings, good lighting and firm chairs with a high centre of gravity are all potentially useful
37. Check the suitability of footwear and health of person's feet. Arrange for chiropody services if required	Well-fitted shoes aid mobility and reduce the risk of a fall. Painful feet can seriously impede mobility
38. Ensure regular exercise and practice at walking. Provide positive reinforcement for active mobility	Important to maintain health and also to retain confidence when walking. Many falls are associated with anxiety and loss of confidence in the older person

Evaluation

1. Person's behaviour indicates calmness.
2. Person demonstrates trust in their care and treatment.
3. Person does not suffer any unnecessary accidents.

C. Meet Their Basic Physical Needs

Associated problems/personal difficulties

The confused person may experience difficulty in meeting their basic physical needs due to:

1. Disorientation and confusion.
2. Loss of insight and self-awareness in regard of physical needs.
3. Distractability and limited attention span.
4. Loss of interest in personal hygiene.
5. Physical health deficits: sensory impairment, mobility.

Assessment

1. Person's statements and behaviour in relation to meeting their needs for nutrition, fluids, hygiene and rest.
2. Information from carers in regard of the person's ability to meet their physical needs.
3. Nurse's observations of:

   (a) Person's independent activities and competence in relation to meeting their physical needs.
   (b) Adequacy of present intake of fluid and food: current weight, history of weight loss or gain, balance and appropriateness of diet taken.
   (c) Personal mobility: limited, require aids, fully mobile.
   (d) Pattern of rest and sleep.
   (e) Prompting required to focus person's attention on their physical needs and the person's response to prompting.
   (f) Patterns of continence or incontinence.
   (g) Person's awareness of environmental conditions and their ability to respond appropriately.
   (h) Identifiable physical health deficits.
   (j) Adequacy and suitability of self-care facilities: hygiene, toilet, kitchen.
   (k) Environmental limitations and their potential for modification: furniture, cooking facilities, stairways, handles.

Desired outcomes

1. Person is able to identify their physical health care needs independently.
2. Person is able to initiate or participate in activities to meet their physical needs.
3. Person is able to maintain their physical health.

Nursing intervention	Rationale
1. Initiate therapeutic relationship	Interventions more likely to be successful in an atmosphere of trust and cooperation
2. Advise the person and carers on the importance of meeting physical needs and their role in mental health. Specify basic physical requirements with person and family. Negotiate a programme to meet physical needs. Reinforce compliance with programme to promote physical needs attainment	May not be aware of these needs or their role in health promotion. Prolonged confusion may have disrupted normal patterns of meeting physical needs. Reintroducing a pattern helps to structure the person's day and to regain a sense of control
3. Promote orientation (see **A.**)	Disorientation is a prime factor in the person's inability to meet their basic physical needs
4. Accurately identify extent of dependency and baseline of current ability to meet physical needs	Care programme will need to be directed towards maintaining autonomy and increasing the person's self-help skills. Need to ensure consistency and to prevent regression
5. Advise on the importance of a regular healthy diet. Ensure adequate roughage is taken. Encourage regular activity. Add fibre to diet, if necessary. Monitor nutritional intake. Periodically weigh	Important for mental and physical health. Roughage helps to prevent constipation which can be very discomforting. Need to ensure that adequate nutrition is being taken
6. Identify food preferences and previous eating pattern. Facilitate personal choice in regard of diet and meal-times. Provide	More likely to eat preferred food if it complies with previous dietary pattern. May be more prepared to eat at certain times of the day. Person will take more interest in food that they have selected and prepared. May need to monitor closely for safety

Nursing intervention	*Rationale*
opportunities for the person to take responsibility and cook their own meals	
7. Present food in an attractive manner and in a distraction-free environment. Do not rush at meal-times	Helps to create a conducive environment and person more likely to focus attention on food. Rushing may cause agitation. Confused person is easily distracted away from meal
8. Model and demonstrate desirable eating skills at meal-times. Encourage and give guidance on their eating skills. Facilitate choice at meal-times	Nurses can exert a great influence as a role model. Person may need to re-learn skills and to have existing abilities reinforced
9. Monitor person's ability to feed themselves using ordinary utensils. Explore the possibility of utilizing appropriate eating aids, if required	The provision of certain aids may enable the person to feed themselves independently at meal-times, e.g. non-slip pads or suction, hemi-dishes, large handled cutlery, bowls with edging
10. Provide only the cutlery required at meal-times. Remove salt, vinegar and sauces after use	More likely to use the appropriate utensils. Extra items may cause confusion. Prevents repeated and excessive use. Taste diminishes in later life
11. Protect person's clothing, if required, at meal-times.	Need to protect clothing yet not harm self-esteem
12. Give prompting to eat meal, if required	May forget that they are sat at the table to eat
13. Hold hand round person's and guide to mouth. Remind them to swallow, if required	May require this level of active guidance if they have severe cognitive impairment
14. Remind person to return to their meal if they wander away. Focus person's attention on their meal	May be easily distracted and wander off before they have completed their meal

Nursing intervention	*Rationale*
15. Advise person and family on clothing and alterations that may facilitate ease of dressing	Loose fitting clothes that stretch, slip on shoes, velcro fasteners, etc., can help considerably both in terms of the person dressing themself and in ease of dressing by carers
16. Ensure clothes are clean and well-fitting	Helps to raise self-esteem.
17. Put out clean clothes in the order that the person will require to put them on	Helps to guide the confused person
18. Remove unnecessary clothes from sight	Distracting influence
19. Provide prompting and guidance during dressing, if required. Be patient	Simple instructions may enable the person to dress themselves. Dressing may take some time but it is important that the person maintains any skills that they have for self-care
20. Ensure that person is appropriately dressed for the prevailing climatic conditions. Advise person if their clothing is inappropriate	The confused person may take little notice of outside weather conditions
21. Advise that a simple, short, attractive hairstyle facilitates grooming and hygiene	Easier for person and carers to cope with
22. Encourage their interest in how they appear to others. Make unprompted positive comments about their appearance	External social feedback in the form of recognition and comment is a powerful reinforcer. Even confused people can benefit from attention to their appearance
23. Periodically monitor environmental conditions of care area and take corrective action if required	Confused person may not be aware of the need to take corrective action if it is too hot, cold, draughty, etc.
24. Encourage participation in activities during the day and evening	Prevents boredom, promotes orientation and can help to meet social and recreational needs

Nursing intervention	*Rationale*
25. Ensure person does not sleep during the daytime. Encourage the person to stay up until a reasonable time	Reduces the need for sleep at night-time. This can contribute to nocturnal wandering and confusion. Better for person to go to bed later and to sleep through until the morning. The need for sleep tends to decrease with ageing
26. Assess person's need for sleep. Identify person's preferred sleep patterns	Each person's pattern is unique
27. Personalize bed-space. Make bed-space visually distinctive	Helps to orientate person to bed-space and to facilitate recognition
28. Identify which factors promote sleep for that person	May be environmental changes that can be made that will facilitate sleep
29. Identify factors that disturb their sleep. Promote physical comfort of their bed-space	The confused person is very readily distracted. It is very important that environmental distractions are kept to a minimum
30. Ensure person goes to toilet before bedtime	Reduces possibility of incontinence and nocturnal wandering
31. Avoid noise at night. Switch off unnecessary lights. Switch on night light	Promotes orientation if they wake up at night. Reduces risk of accidents
32. Observe sleep pattern at night	Need to monitor amount of sleep that the person is actually having
33. Provide reassurance if they wake up at night	May be confused and distressed. Disorientation is often worse at night-time
34. Identify if there are any factors distracting them or making them uncomfortable. Take corrective action. Speak to them softly and quietly. Gently guide them back to bed. Orientate to time and place. Suggest they go back to sleep	May be simple actions that can be taken to promote their comfort. May respond to prompting to return to bed and to sleep

Nursing intervention	*Rationale*
35. Observe for drowsiness, particularly in the morning as a side-effect of medication	Often the time when this side-effect is most prominent. It adds to confusion and also the risk of an accident. Medication may need to be reviewed
36. Identify with client and family activities that person found restful and relaxing. Explore with the person options for meeting needs for rest and relaxation. Encourage the person to rest or relax if they appear to be tired or exhausted. Positively reinforce attempts to rest and relax	These may be activities that might still have the potential to promote rest. Person more likely to cooperate if involved in identifying preferred activities. Loss of insight and disorientation interfere with person's ability to meet their needs for rest
37. Minimize environmental distractions. Provide periods of quiet and restfulness. Sit calmly with the person	Rest is facilitated if these distractions are minimized. Confused person is easily distracted. Modelling can be a powerful behaviour influence
38. Ensure that personalized soap, flannel, towel, toothbrush, etc., are available and used	Person more likely to use items that belong to them
39. Encourage the person to maintain personal cleanliness and to change clothes periodically. Encourage choice and option over washing and bathing. Give positive feedback on personal initiatives	Person may need prompting due to loss of insight. Facilitating personal choice increases the person's sense of well-being and is more likely to gain their cooperation
40. Ensure that dignity and privacy are respected and maintained during washing and bathing	Person may be embarrassed or distressed by dependency on others. Need to be aware of their feelings. Alternatively, the confused person may appear disinhibited about disrobing. May need to moderate their disinhibition

Nursing intervention	*Rationale*

41. Promote oral hygiene. Check that dentures are labelled and fit well. Ensure dentures are regularly cleaned

Important to maintain oral hygiene. Even a few of the person's own teeth can increase the effectiveness of dentures. Dentures can promote both eating and communication. Need to be kept clean in order to promote comfort in the mouth

42. Ensure regular exercise and practice at walking. Provide positive reinforcement for active mobility

Important to maintain health and also to retain confidence when walking. Many falls in later life are associated with anxiety and loss of confidence

43. Ensure person has a daily fluid intake of 1.5–2 litres. Allocate majority of fluid intake to morning and afternoon rather than evening

This is the minimum range of fluid intake required for health. Helps to reduce the occurrence of nocturnal incontinence and to promote daytime continence

44. Ensure good access to toilets. Provide visual cues on location of toilet

In later life the interval between the sensation and need to void can be very short. Hence the need for ready access to toilets to prevent incontinence. These may prompt the confused person to locate and use toilet

45. Identify pattern of urinary/faecal elimination. Use pattern to promote continence. Observe behaviour to identify verbal and non-verbal signals associated with the need to go to the toilet. Direct person to the toilet. Give prompting, if necessary. Give positive reinforcement

This information is the first step in identifying appropriate interventions. Much can be done to reduce the frequency and occurrence of incontinence in the confused elderly person. Elimination involves a complex sensory and behavioural sequence. This has to be followed accurately for "successful" elimination. The confused person may not be able to express their need for elimination or able to co-ordinate their behaviour. Carers may, over time, learn to recognize key signals early on in this sequence and to take prompt action

46. Provide tactful assistance if required. Maintain person's dignity. Clean person

Confused person may be very embarrassed and distressed. Need to respect their feelings and to ensure help is given promptly and

Nursing intervention	Rationale
and change aids or clothes, if required. Check on condition of skin	sympathetically. Can easily develop rashes which are uncomfortable and sore
47. Arrange for adaptations to toilet to facilitate use by confused elderly person	Aids such as raised toilet seat, padded toilet seat and hand-rails promote ease of use and independent use
48. Explore whether the use of incontinence aids is appropriate for the person	Incontinence aids need to be carefully matched to the person's needs. They should be used as a means of helping to regain both control and confidence. Incontinence can be very distressing and some people find the wearing of an aid reassuring
49. Promote access and mobility around the home/care environment and in outside paths and garden. Arrange for necessary alterations and fitments. Ensure mobility aids are available, if required	Promotes independent mobility. Careful planning of hand-rails, bath-rails, non-slip floor coverings, good lighting and firm chairs with a high centre of gravity are all potentially useful
50. Check the suitability of footwear and health of person's feet. Arrange for chiropody services if necessary. Periodically check toe and finger nails to see if they require trimming	Well-fitted shoes aid mobility and reduce the risk of a fall. Painful feet are uncomfortable and can seriously impede mobility
51. Organize appropriate recreational and social activities, e.g. singing, dancing, physical activity group, walking	Helps to keep person awake during daytime. Provides the opportunity for physical exercise. Promotes mobility
52. Ensure person exercises daily	Need to maintain suppleness and fitness. Much can be done to promote physical health in later life through exercise

Nursing intervention	*Rationale*
53. Participate in exercises and activities with clients	Participation by carers facilitates involvement

Evaluation

1. Person's physical health is maintained.
2. Person/carers are able to identify and initiate action to meet physical health care needs.

D. Facilitate the Development of the Person's and Family's Coping Skills

Associated problems/personal difficulties

The experience of confusion may show that:

1. Existing methods of coping may be counterproductive and maladaptive.
2. Current life-style, expectations and relationships may be potential sources of stress and contributing to the degree of confusion.
3. The family may find it difficult to provide emotional support to the confused person.
4. The person and their family may lack information about the resources available to help them.
5. The person and their family may lack information about practical approaches towards coping with confusion.
6. There may be feelings of guilt in relation to their problems and asking for help.

Assessment

1. Person and family's perceptions of their current difficulties and needs.
2. Existing coping methods used and their effectiveness.
3. Support available to the person and family.
4. Accuracy of the knowledge and information given by the person and their family.
5. Statements of guilt and stigma.
6. Awareness of resources available to them.
7. Previous experience, if any, of dealing with similar problems.
8. Approaches being used to cope with confused behaviour by person and carers.
9. Identification of potential stressors in the person's current environment and life-style.

Desired outcomes

1. Person and family able to make an informed choice about the resources they require.
2. Person and family able to cope better with the personal and practical problems posed by confusion.

Nursing intervention	Rationale
1. Initiate therapeutic relationship with person and their family	Interventions more likely to be successful in an atmosphere of trust and cooperation. The family is the main source of support for the elderly and a good relationship with them is essential
2. Advise that seeking help and recognition of problems are a positive step towards finding solutions	Many people feel that seeking help is a sign of weakness and failure. Also helps to reduce guilt. This is a common problem of close relatives of elderly people who feel a considerable obligation towards caring for them
3. Encourage questions. Provide accurate information	May have inaccurate knowledge and expectations. Fear of the unknown
4. Provide appropriate written information. Advise on suitable self-help publications and audio-visual aids	There is an increasing number of useful learning resources for carers of elderly confused relatives
5. Identify appropriate health care resources	Need to know what resources are available to them
6. Identify practical services that may help to support the person and their family. Make appropriate arrangements for the provision of support services	A wide range of statutory and voluntary agencies may be able to offer practical assistance that the family needs, e.g. home sitters, home helps, incontinence laundry and aids, visiting, social activities, Meals on Wheels, physical care
7. Put family in contact with self-help and voluntary groups	Self-help groups are able to offer effective and understanding help
8. Ensure that carers have positive and realistic attitudes towards the elderly	Negative attitudes in carers communicate themselves to dependents and influence how they approach their caring activities

Nursing intervention	*Rationale*
9. Reassure that there are ways of improving the situation	Family may feel that the situation is hopeless, especially if they have been under considerable strain for a long time
10. Advise against recrimination and focussing on past problems. Assist family members to resolve conflicts	Need to focus on the present and future and to deal with anger and guilt in a more productive way. May be many unresolved conflicts within family as a result of the long-term burden of caring for confused person
11. Advise against early correction of problems	Under stress it is sometimes easier to make short-term adaptations that only store up future problems. It takes time to help the family to work out what is best for them, Long-term adjustments may be required
12. Encourage the person and family to express their concerns and difficulties	Problems need to be brought out into the open to facilitate solutions and to reduce emotional tension
13. Advise on the need for acceptance and mutual support within their relationships. Advise the family on how to give feedback and support to one another	Family needs to come to terms with their situation. They are each other's primary source of support which will need to be utilized in order to cope effectively. May need to consider the way that they communicate, their expectations and the way that emotional support is given
14. Reassure that memory loss is not deliberate	Family members may be mis-attributing some of the confused person's behaviour to personality factors or deliberate awkwardness. Under stress and frustration it can be easy to assume this motivation
15. Advise the family members on methods of coping with the stress of caring. Advise carers to rest periodically. Advise carers to reward themselves periodically. Teach methods for achieving relaxation. Assist the family to learn new coping skills	It is important to maintain the mental health of the carers. There may be many practical strategies that they can use to minimize stress. Life-style and relationship changes may be necessary

Nursing intervention	*Rationale*
16. Emphasize the importance of maintaining social contacts and of avoiding isolation	Social contacts are valuable sources of support. They also help the confused person to maintain their orientation. Under the strain of caring, relatives may withdraw from social contacts
17. Ensure that the needs of younger family members are considered and are being met	Younger household members may feel neglected by parents and resentful towards the confused person
18. Promote the orientation of the confused person (see **A.**)	The more orientated the confused person is, the easier it is for carers to help them meet their physical and mental needs
19. Teach the family members/carers the practical skills of promoting orientation	As they have the most contact with the confused person they are in the best position to promote on-going orientation
20. Teach family members strategies for dealing with confused behaviour. Explain the need to identify and recognize situations that increase confusion	Existing interventions may be counterproductive. Carers need to feel that they are making effective interventions. Helps carers to plan ahead to minimize or avoid confusing situations
21. Advise the person to always carry a pocket calendar and personal details when outside the house	If the person becomes lost outside of their house, then the information may be sufficient to help them to return or for others to quickly help them
22. Ensure that the person has an identification bracelet that details their name, address, telephone number and that they have a memory problem	Enables others to respond sympathetically to confusion and to return them home promptly. Bracelet needs to have a firm clasp to make removal difficult by confused person
23. Establish the environment to allow as much freedom as possible within external boundaries. Modify exit door handles to require skilled opening	Continual restrictions within the internal environment can be a source of major frustration to carers and the confused person. It is usually better to ensure secure boundaries within which the confused person can wander safely and without restriction

Nursing intervention	*Rationale*
24. Ensure that the home is kept neat. Remove valuable items. Check through bins before emptying them. Label and identify significant personal items. Check through chairs, sofas, drawers, cupboards, etc., periodically.	Keeping the care environment organized promotes orientation. Items can be located readily and missing items readily identified. The loss of key personal items is a common problem with confused people. Carers need to monitor and check unlikely places where items may be discarded or hoarded
25. Explore whether the fitting of a house alarm is appropriate	A house alarm to raise help may be useful for the confused person on their own or where they are dependent on another elderly carer
26. Explore the possibility of making modifications to common household fitments to promote safety and utility	Modifications can be made to many items to promote their ease of use and safety for people with handicaps. Some of these may also be useful for the confused person, e.g. adaptations to taps so that the cold tap has to be turned on first, fitments to prevent unlit gas cookers and fires being left on. Public utilities can provide further advice
27. Recommend ways of setting and maintaining behavioural limits	Family may need these skills in order to deal effectively with specific behavioural problems
28. Explain the need to promote and maintain the autonomy and independence of the confused person	Feelings of choice and personal control are important factors in the maintenance of positive mental health
29. Reinforce initiatives taken by person. Ensure that carers are not being over-protective	Need to take some risks in caring. Over-protectiveness can lead to over-dependence and apathy
30. Focus on attainable activities that the person can cope with. Simplify activities, if possible, to keep them within person's capabilities. Provide emotionally safe experiences to increase sense of mastery	Promotes esteem of the person, minimizes frustration and facilitates autonomy. Creative solutions to activities of everyday living can promote independence. Need the opportunity to practice new skills in sympathetic environment

Nursing intervention	*Rationale*
31. Teach how to use problem-solving methods for coping with difficulties. Focus on solving one problem at a time. Encourage the setting of progressive goals in small stages	Existing approaches to problem solving may be ineffective and vague. People need to be taught how to define difficulties so that they can be progressively tackled
32. Encourage the setting of realistic goals and expectations	The attainment of realistic goals promotes a positive outlook. Unrealistic goals lead to failure and are likely to cause resentment
33. Teach the family and person to recognize the limits of their ability to cope and when it is advisable to seek help	The family should not over-burden itself as this can damage relationships and its longer-term ability to cope
34. Advise family members on any physical care skills that they may require	The family is the main source of care. Having the requisite skills helps them to cope and to promote the physical health of the confused person
35. Advise on possible side-effects of any prescribed medication	Individuals and their family need to be able to recognize side-effects, particularly those that contribute towards confusion

Evaluation

1. Person and family able to identify their health care needs.
2. Person and family identify and select resources they require.
3. Person and family demonstrate use of improved coping methods.
4. Confused person is able to maintain their autonomy.

Unit Instructions

When you have researched the suggested references, have mastered the Unit Objectives and successfully answered the Self-assessment Questions, proceed with the Unit Written Test.

Suggested References

Adams, S. (1987). The relationship of clothing to self-esteem in elderly patients. *Nursing Times* 9 September, Vol. 83, No. 36, pp. 42–45.

Altschul, A. and McGovern, M. (1985). *Psychiatric Nursing*, 6th edition. Baillière Tindall, London and San Diego.

Armstrong-Esther, C. A. and Hawkins, L. H. (1982). Day for night circadian rhythms in the elderly. *Nursing Times*, 28 July, Vol. 78, No. 30, pp. 1263–1265.

Ashwell, G. (1986). An independent mind. *Nursing Times*, 8 January, Vol. 82, No. 2, pp. 25–27.

Bailey, E. A., Brown, S., Goble, R. E. A. and Holden, U. P. (1986). Twenty four hour reality orientation: Changes for staff and patients. *Journal of Advanced Nursing*, Vol. 11, No. 2, pp. 145–151.

Bailey, R. D. (1985). *Coping with Stress in Caring*. Blackwell Scientific, Oxford.

Barker, P. J. (1982). *Behaviour Therapy Nursing*. Croom Helm, London.

Barker, P. J. (1985). *Patient Assessment in Psychiatric Nursing*. Croom Helm, London.

Barrowclough, C. and Fleming, I. (1986). *Goal Planning with Elderly People*. Manchester University Press, Manchester.

Bauer, B. B. and Hill, S. S. (1986). *Essentials of Mental Health Care Planning and Interventions*. W. B. Saunders, Philadelphia.

Black, S. and Simon, R. (1980). The specialist nurse, support care and the elderly mentally infirm. *Community Outlook*, February, pp. 45–46.

Bloomfield, K. (1986). Ask the family. *Nursing Times*, 12 March, Vol. 82, No. 11, pp. 28–30.

Burton, M. (1982). Reality orientation for the elderly: A critique. *Journal of Advanced Nursing*, Vol. 7, No. 5, pp. 427–433.

Campbell, C. (1978). *Nursing Diagnosis and Intervention in Nursing Practice*. John Wiley, New York.

Carr, P. J., Butterworth, C. A. and Hodges, B. E. (1980). *Community Psychiatric Nursing*. Churchill Livingstone, Edinburgh.

Castledine, G. (1982). Sorry I haven't got time. *Nursing Mirror*, 29 September, Vol. 155, No. 13, pp. 17–20.

Chadwick, P. (1984). Social stimulation and the elderly. *Nursing Times*, 7 March, Vol. 80, No. 10, pp. 41–42.

Church, M. (1985). Cues to clarity. *Nursing Times*, 31 July, Vol. 81, No. 31, pp. 35–36.

Copp, L. A. (1986). The nurse as advocate for vulnerable persons. *Journal of Advanced Nursing*, Vol. 11, No. 3, pp. 255–263.

Cormack, D. (Ed.) (1984). *Geriatric Nursing. A Conceptual Approach*. Blackwell Scientific, Oxford.

Cross, J. N. (1983). Caring for a demented patient. *Nursing Times*, 2 November, Vol. 79, No. 44, pp. 57–60.

Cullen, A. (1984). 2. The nurse practitioner's view. *Nursing Times*, 26 September, Vol. 80, No. 39, p. 60.

Darcy, P. T. (1985). *Mental Health Nursing Source Book*. Baillière Tindall, London and San Diego.

Dexter, G. and Wash, M. (1986). *Psychiatric Nursing Skills: A Patient-centred Approach*. Croom Helm, London.

Ekberg, J. Y. (1986). Spouse burn out syndrome. *Journal of Advanced Nursing*, Vol. 11, No. 2, pp. 161–165.

Ford, M., Fox, J., Fitch, S. and Donovan, A. (1987). Light in the darkness. *Nursing Times*, 7 January, Vol. 83, No. 1, pp. 26–28.

Garrett, G. (1986). Old age abuse by carers. *The Professional Nurse*, August, Vol. 1, No. 11, pp. 304–305.

Gilleard, C., Mitchell, R. G. and Riordan, J. (1981). Ward orientation training with psychogeriatric patients. *Journal of Advanced Nursing*, Vol. 6, No. 2, pp. 95–98.

Hanley, I. and Gilhooly, M. (1986). *Psychological Therapies for the Elderly*. Croom Helm, London.

Hargie, D. and McCartan, P. (1986). *Social Skills Training and Psychiatric Nursing*. Croom Helm, London.

Hase, S. and Douglas, A. (1986). *Human Dynamics and Nursing*. Churchill Livingstone, Melbourne.

Holden, U. P. and Woods, R. T. (1982). *Reality Orientation: Psychological Approaches to the 'Confused' Elderly*. Churchill Livingstone, Edinburgh.

King, M. R. (1979). A study on incontinence in a psychiatric hospital. *Nursing Times*, 5 July, Vol. 75, No. 26, pp. 1133–1135.

Kingston, B. (1987). *Psychological Approaches in Psychiatric Nursing*. Croom Helm, London.

Lego, S. (1984). *The American Handbook of Psychiatric Nursing*. J. B. Lippincott, Philadelphia.

Lyttle, J. (1986). *Mental Disorder: Its Care and Treatment*. Baillière Tindall, London and San Diego.

Mace, N. L., Rabins, P. W. with Castleton, B., Clarke, C. and McEwen, E. (1985). *The 36-hour Day: Caring at Home for Confused Elderly People* (UK edition). Hodder and Stoughton/Age Concern, London.

Marr, J. (1983). The capacity for joy. *Nursing Times*, 21 September, Vol. 79, No. 38, pp. 58–61.

Martin, P. (1987a). *Psychiatric Nursing: A Therapeutic Approach*. Macmillan, London.

Martin, P. (1987b). *Care of the Mentally Ill*, 2nd edition. Macmillan, London.

Mawson, D. (1983a). Assessment of the mental state. *Nursing Times*, 15 June, Vol. 79, No. 24, pp. 41–42.

Mawson, D. (1983b). Extended cognitive state examination. *Nursing Times*, 22 June, Vol. 79, No. 25, pp. 28–32.

McFarland, G. and Wasli, E. (1986). *Nursing Diagnoses and Process in Psychiatric Mental Health Nursing*. J. B. Lippincott, Philadelphia.

McMichael, I. (1983). Feeling at home. *Nursing Times*, 9 November, Vol. 79, No. 45, pp. 53–56.

Miller, S. (1986). A lesson for the learning. *Nursing Times*, 19 March, Vol. 82, No. 12, pp. 55–56.

Morris, M. (1986). Music and movement for the elderly. *Nursing Times*, 19 February, Vol. 82, No. 8, pp. 44–45.

North, S. (1985). Breaking point. *Nursing Mirror*, 18 September, Vol. 161, No. 12, pp. 42–43.

Pelletier, L. (Ed.) (1987). *Psychiatric Nursing Case Studies, Nursing Diagnoses and Care Plans*. Springhouse Corporation, Springhouse, Pennsylvania.

Phillips, L. R. (1983). Abuse and neglect of the frail elderly at home: An exploration of theoretical relationships. *Journal of Advanced Nursing*, Vol. 8, No. 5, pp. 379–392.

Pope, B. (1986). *Social Skills Training for Psychiatric Nurses*. Harper and Row, London.

Poulton, K. (1984). A measure of independence. *Nursing Times*, 22 August, Vol. 80, No. 34, pp. 32–35.

Robertson, I. (1986). Learned helplessness. *Nursing Times*, 17/24 December, Vol. 82, No. 51, pp. 28–30.

Robinson, L. (1983). *Psychiatric Nursing as a Human Experience*, 3rd edition. W. B. Saunders, Philadelphia.

Seers, C. (1986). Talking to the elderly and its relevance to care. *Nursing Times*, 8 January, Vol. 82, No. 1, pp. 51–54.

Shives, L. R. (1986). *Basic Concepts in Psychiatric Mental Health Nursing*. J. B. Lippincott, Philadelphia.

Simmons, S. and Brooker, C. (1986). *Community Psychiatric Nursing: A Social Perspective*. Heinemann Nursing, London.

Skeet, M. (1982). *The Third Age*. Darton, Longman and Todd, London, in association with Age Concern, England and the Disabled Living Foundation.

Stevens, P. (1983). Mary, Mary, quite contrary. *Nursing Times*, 1 June, Vol. 79, No. 22, pp. 50–53.

Sugden, J. and Saxby, P. J. (1985). The confused elderly patient. *Nursing*, March, Vol. 2, No. 35, pp. 1022–1025.

Ward, M. F. (1985). *The Nursing Process in Psychiatry*. Churchill Livingstone, Edinburgh.

Ward, W. (1987). A new life for Emily. *Nursing Times*, 25 March, Vol. 83, No. 12, pp. 40–41.

Watt, G. M. (1982). A family-orientated approach to community care for the elderly mentally infirm. *Nursing Times*, 15 September, Vol. 78, No. 37, pp. 1545–1548.

Wolanin, M. and Phillips, L. (1981). *Confusion, Prevention and Care*. C. V. Mosby, London.

Wright, S. (1985). Tearing down walls. *Nursing Mirror*, 10 July, Vol. 161, No. 2, pp. 48–49.

Self-assessment Questions

SAQ 9. Describe four nursing interventions that are used to promote orientation.

SAQ 10. Identify four nursing interventions that can be used to help the confused elderly person feel secure.

SAQ 11. List four observations that may be required to assess the confused person's physical needs.

SAQ 12. Describe four strategies that can be used to help carers cope with a confused elderly person in their home environment.

Unit 13.3: Written Test

Elsie Chadwick, 73, has been admitted for 2 weeks while her daughter and family go on a well-earned holiday. In the unit Elsie is very restless and agitated. She continually wanders around, going into every possible room where she empties the contents of drawers, lockers, shelves and bins on the floor. When she is questioned she states that she is looking for the "rent book". Detailed assessment shows that she is disorientated in time and place. However, with guidance and prompting she can cope with most activities of daily living. Physically she is in good health.

1. What strategies can the nurses use to promote Elsie's orientation?
2. How can staff direct Elsie's daytime activities more constructively?
3. From an evaluation of Elsie's short-term stay, it is apparent that more could have been done to prepare her for this experience. What actions and arrangements could the family and care staff make in future to minimize the disorientating effects of relief admission?

TOPIC 14

Alcohol and Drug Dependency

At the end of this Topic the learner should aim to:

1. Describe factors that contribute to the onset of misuse and dependency upon alcohol/drugs.
2. Recognize the effects of dependency upon a person's mental, physical and social health.
3. Outline the range of therapeutic interventions and support facilities for the person who is dependent on alcohol/drugs.
4. Identify the nursing care needs and interventions required for the person who is dependent on alcohol/drugs.

Alcohol Misuse and Dependency

Alcohol and Mental Health

Alcohol dependency and alcohol-related problems are currently one of our major health problems. Alcohol is the most abused drug in the UK. Although the history of alcohol abuse spans many centuries, it is only comparatively recently that it has received serious scientific study and intervention.

Used sensibly, alcohol can enhance many pleasant and enjoyable social situations. However, it also has the potential to be a very destructive influence that can cause great psychological, social and physical suffering.

In 1952, the World Health Organization defined alcoholics as:

"those excessive drinkers whose dependence on alcohol has attained such a degree that it shows a notable mental disturbance or an interference with their bodily and mental health, their interpersonal relations and their smooth social and economic functioning: or who show the prodromal signs of such development. They therefore require treatment."

There are a number of other definitions. What they have in common are the concepts of:

- excessive and damaging drinking behaviour;
- physical, social and mental harm to the individual and those in contact with them.

Underlying any attempt to define alcohol dependency as a "disease" are the widely held perceptions of drinking problems as a moral issue. In this context, the alcohol dependent person is "irresponsible", his sufferings are "self-inflicted" and they lack "moral fibre". As such, the person is regarded as being deserving of little sympathy or assistance. These attitudes influence the person with a drinking problem, those around them and those trying to help. Research studies have shown that even health care workers often have negative and moral-based attitudes towards those with alcohol problems that influence their interventions.

While it is useful to have definitions of alcohol dependency (a term now used in preference to "alcoholism"), attention is increasingly being focussed on those who are experiencing the early effects of harm from their drinking behaviour. Identifying people who have "drinking problems" or "alcohol-related problems" is important in influencing their current drinking behaviour and preventing the serious consequences of chronic alcohol abuse.

The Effects of Alcohol

Alcohol is a very potent drug that has a wide range of psychological and physical effects. The effects will depend upon:

1. *The total amount of alcohol consumed* (number of units): the greater the quantity the more potent the effects. The actual type of drink has primarily a psychological effect upon the individual.
2. *Previous habituation*: tolerance to alcohol increases during a person's early drinking experience. With moderate drinking tolerance tends to stabilize. In the later stages of chronic heavy drinking tolerance decreases due to liver impairment. Periods of abstinence tend to reduce tolerance.
3. *Gender*: women are affected more than men due to physiological differences that give a blood alcohol level 25–30% higher than men for a given quantity of alcohol.
4. *Person's perception and expectations*: the immediate social environment and expectations have a significant influence upon the person's response to alcohol.
5. *Psychological needs and problems*: the person's pre-existing mood tends to be reinforced and exaggerated.
6. *Body weight and size*: this influences the blood alcohol concentration.

Physical effects of alcohol

Alcohol is readily digested and spread throughout the body. The rate of absorption is dependent upon the relative concentration of alcohol in the drink and whether there is food in the stomach.

In the body alcohol is detoxified by the liver and excreted relatively slowly. It takes approximately 1 hour for the body to eliminate the alcohol in one standard drink. (See Section on "Alcoholic beverages".) This is significant because individuals who rapidly consume great quantities of alcohol may have high levels of blood alcohol concentration many hours after their initial consumption.

Physiologically, alcohol has a depressant effect upon the central nervous system. Impairment of motor functions – co-ordination, balance, rate of performance, response times – begins with the first drink. Alongside this is a parallel increase in confidence, even though judgement is progressively impaired. Other physical effects of alcohol include irritation of the lining of the stomach, peripheral vasodilation, suppression of antidiuretic hormone, which contributes to dehydration, and impairment of sexual responses.

Excessive consumption of alcohol in a short period leads to the classic effects of intoxication, i.e. staggering, blurred vision, memory loss, sleepiness, nausea and vomiting. This may subsequently give rise to the unpleasant effects associated with heavy drinking – a "hangover" – which is basically due to the toxic effects of the alcoholic drink, dehydration and gastritis.

At very high levels of blood alcohol concentration exceeding 800 mg/100 ml – death is possible from suppression of the respiratory centre or inhalation of vomit. This would equate to drinking one bottle of spirits in a short space of time.

Psychological effects of alcohol

Alcohol is a very potent anxiolytic. People feel more relaxed, cheerful, friendly and talkative. There is a subjective experience of well-being and a glow of satisfaction. In moderation the consumption of alcohol can be a very pleasant experience that enhances many social experiences. However, in greater quantities the effects become more pronounced. Alcohol tends to accentuate the drinker's existing mood. If the person already feels unhappy then they are likely to become more morose and depressed. If their existing mood is positive then they are likely to become joyful and merry.

As the level of alcohol rises then the person tends to lose insight and to become more disinhibited. Judgement is impaired and the person may become more impulsive and reckless. Irritability and aggression are easily evoked in response to perceived slights. The person may behave in ways that they would find unacceptable if they were sober. Recollection of events is likely to be seriously impaired.

Alcoholic Beverages

Alcoholic drinks come in a variety of presentations. Although each type has a distinctive flavour, aroma and appearance due to the method of preparation and additives, the nature of the alcohol is identical. This is significant because many myths and misperceptions exist as to the relative potency and harm that can arise from the consumption of certain alcoholic drinks.

In terms of the relative alcohol concentration of different types of drink and as an aid to health education and therapy, the concept of "units of alcohol" is used as a reference point. Using this method of assessment the following drinks equate to "one unit of alcohol":

- $\frac{1}{2}$ pint of beer,
- 1 glass of table wine,
- 1 glass of sherry,
- 1 single whisky.

In terms of these units an assessment can then be made between levels of alcohol consumption and the potential risk of harm, irrespective of the type of drink consumed. Sensible limits for men and women are as follows:

- men: 2–3 pints of beer or equivalent 2–3 times per week, i.e. approximately 20 units per week;
- women: 2 or 3 standard units 2–3 times per week, i.e. approximately 13 units per week.

The risk of alcohol-related problems increases directly in relation to the quantity of alcohol consumed. The figures for men are:

- 21–30 units of alcohol per week – an increased health risk;
- 31–50 units of alcohol per week – some harm is apparent;
- 50+ units of alcohol per week – definite harm from alcohol;
- 8 units daily, i.e. 4 pints of beer or equivalent – definite harm.

Due to physiological differences the corresponding levels for women are about half those for men.

The significance of these figures are that levels of alcohol consumption that are known to cause harm and to put people at risk are below widely held beliefs about safe drinking levels. Health education messages about moderating alcohol intake are then viewed with scepticism and derision, especially if they challenge what is regarded as one of life's "pleasures".

Social Aspects of Alcohol Consumption

Alcohol is a readily available drug. It can be purchased from a wide range of outlets and there are few restrictions on its sale. Increasing amounts are purchased from retail outlets for consumption in the home.

Alcohol features prominently at many significant social events – parties, weddings, christenings, celebrations, funerals – where it serves both symbolic functions and to facilitate participation. In most social situations there is a definite pressure and expectation on people to drink. Moderate drinking is socially encouraged and over 90% of adults drink alcohol. Each week 75%

of men and 50% of women consume alcohol. By implication, not to drink is perceived of as unusual and refusal is often interpreted as an insult. Such pressures have significant implications for those who are trying to restrict or give up alcohol.

Drinking patterns are also closely related to gender. There are distinct patterns of male and female drinking that influence the type, quantity and frequency of alcohol intake. Within our complex network of contradictory sexual stereotypes, male intoxication and drunkenness is tolerated far more than in women. Male drinking patterns are closely equated with perceptions of masculinity. Women who are perceived as having drunk "too much" attract high social and moral disapproval.

Environmentally, alcohol has a very high profile with numerous public houses, wine bars, off-licences, posters and television advertising. An image is fostered that reinforces drinking alcohol as a friendly and sociable activity. The risks of unpleasant or harmful consequences are never mentioned. This high profile given to alcohol is significant in influencing consumption patterns and perceptions of its potential for harm.

The Incidence of Alcohol-related Problems

Excessive alcohol consumption is now one of our major health problems. Like many affluent Western nations, sales of alcoholic drink have virtually doubled over the past 20 years in the UK. Contrary to common belief the relative cost of alcoholic drinks has continued to decline. The increase in consumption is alarming, as there is a direct correlation between levels of alcohol consumption in the community and the frequency of alcohol-related problems. Levels of consumption have recently stabilized but this is thought to be more due to economic recession than an increase in public awareness of drinking problems.

It is estimated that about 0.5–1.0 million people are currently experiencing harmful physical and psychological effects as a result of their drinking habits. Of these some 300 000 are alcohol dependent. This figure is based upon estimates related to total sales of alcohol and indices of the harm that are directly associated with alcohol consumption (see p. 562). A particular difficulty in attempting to research alcohol abuse is the stigma attached to the label "alcoholic", the reluctance of people to admit to a drinking problem and the difficulty of detecting problem drinkers.

In terms of alcohol consumption levels 1 in 12 men and 1 in 24 women have heavy drinking patterns. The incidence of alcohol-related problems in women would appear to be increasing. This is of a cause concern because women appear to be more damaged socially and physically by alcohol and to be less responsive to intervention.

Another group in which alcohol problems are increasing rapidly are younger people, who often start drinking excessively in their early teens and are heavy drinkers by their late teens.

Social Consequences of Alcohol Abuse

1. *Road traffic accidents*. One in five car drivers and one in four pedestrians that are killed in road accidents have blood levels of alcohol that exceed the legal limit for driving – 80 mg per 100 ml of blood. (This equates with approximately 2 pints of beer or equivalent for men, less for women.) In 1984 over 113 000 drivers were guilty of drunken driving in mainland UK.

2. *Work place and industry*. About 14 million working days are lost each year due to sickness and absenteeism due to excessive alcohol consumption. Some 2% of any work-force suffer problems related to alcohol or drug abuse. Frequently, though, they are "carried" by their work-mates. At work their output is low and they have a very high accident rate.

3. *Suicide risk*. Alcohol is frequently associated with acts of self-harm and suicide. The alcohol may feature as part of the attempt to induce oblivion or may trigger off a depressive mood. People with chronic drinking problems also have a much higher suicide risk rate.

4. *Physical ill-health*. Alcohol is generally known to be associated with cirrhosis of the liver. However, it is also associated with a wide range of other serious physical ill-health problems. These include peptic ulceration, pancreatitis, cancer of the mouth, throat, liver and stomach, and peripheral neuropathy. General ill-health is common due to poor diet, smoking and life-style.

5. *Admissions to residential health care facilities*. In 1983 there were some 5000 first admissions to mental care facilities for alcohol dependency. There were many more readmissions. Additionally, some 10% of people admitted to general hospitals are estimated to have alcohol-related problems without their alcohol dependency being recognized.

6. *Family and personal suffering*. Chronic alcohol dependency causes much suffering and misery to the person and their family. Alcohol often plays a significant role in family violence, sexual abuse, divorce and separation.

7. *Convictions for drunkenness*. Convictions for drunkenness exceed 110 000 per year. There is a high re-conviction rate with some people being charged repeatedly. Alcohol is often involved with many other crimes of violence and assault.

Factors Influencing Drinking Behaviour and Attitudes to Alcohol

Over 20 million people in this country drink alcohol and for the majority of them it is a pleasurable and harm-free experience. However, a significant proportion of these do experience problems with alcohol. The difficulty is in identifying factors that contribute towards taking alcohol from a relatively safe experience to a destructive dependency. There is no one factor that predominates. For each person it is a complex interaction between themselves, those around them and their environment. Anyone can be at risk. Significant factors that appear to influence an individual's alcohol consumption and suceptibility to harm include:

1. *Family role models who drink excessively*: 45% of problem drinkers parents are or have been alcohol abusers.
2. *Gender*: men with a serious alcohol-related problem outnumber women by four to one. The ability to consume vast quantities of alcohol is associated with stereotypes of masculinity. The prohibitions against male public displays of drunkenness are far less than those applied to women. Men are able to drink openly on their own without attracting undue attention in a way that is not readily available to women. Once established though, women appear to suffer far more damaging physical and social consequences from heavy drinking than do men.
3. *Occupation*: some occupations have a particularly high incidence of problem drinkers. These include barmen, merchant seamen, doctors, travelling salesmen and accountants. At particular risk are people who work in a job where alcohol is made or sold, there are high stress levels, alcohol is used in the course of business, the person is repeatedly away for long periods, there is a strong drinking tradition, or the work group regularly meet in social activities.
4. *Accessibility and availability*: alcohol is widely and readily available. There are few restrictions on its sale and these are often flouted.
5. *Relative cost*: contrary to popular belief the actual cost of alcohol has actually declined. Increased standards of living and higher disposable incomes have contributed towards doubling the sales of alcohol over the past 20 years.
6. *Culture*: cultural and regional factors influence consumption levels and prohibitions in relation to the quantity and appropriateness of drinking in certain situations.
7. *Religion*: some religions have very strong prohibitions on the use and consumption of alcohol. Strong adherents to these beliefs are likely to avoid alcohol.
8. *Peer groups*: these establish and reinforce approved drinking levels and patterns among members. They may reinforce excessive and harmful drinking patterns.
9. *Prolonged stress*: in which alcohol is used as a way of coping and for relief of tension.
10. *Personal factors*: feelings of low self-esteem, inadequacy and social anxiety which alcohol helps to overcome.
11. *Self-medication*: alcohol has a powerful anxiolytic effect and may be used by those who experience chronic anxiety, depression or other mental health problems.
12. *Self-appraisal*: of own drinking levels and whether this is perceived as harmful. Public awareness of harmful drinking levels tends to be limited and many people would be shocked to find out that their drinking pattern is potentially damaging.

The Development of Dependency upon Alcohol

The onset of dependency upon alcohol and the experience of alcohol-related problems tends to be a progressive and insidious process. Often, it is only in retrospect that a person's changes in behaviour, personality and health can be understood as the consequence of increasing harm from alcohol. The drinking pattern of the person can be viewed as a series of stages of increasing harm that may take anything from a few to many years to pass through.

Early phase

Initially, the person's drinking behaviour is determined by their own social experience. This will define the boundaries within which the person's drinking is moderated. However, the person may find that they need to drink greater quantities for the same effect and that alcohol is an effective short-term coping method for reducing stress or for making life's problems more bearable. Their drinking becomes both more frequent and heavier. Previous personal and external constraints on their drinking becomes less effective.

Established phase

Alcohol and drinking become a significant part of their life and take precedence over other activities. Strategies are adopted to ensure alcohol is readily available and to disguise their level of consumption. Although the person does not acknowledge any difficulties associated with their drinking they become very defensive and aggressive to any implied criticism. Early difficulties may be experienced in relationships and at work. There is evidence of harm from alcohol. The person may experience "blackouts" or amnesia associated with drinking which initially may cause great concern and lead to short-term abstinence. Any awareness of the difficulties they are experiencing are outweighed by the immediate gratification they can gain from alcohol.

Crucial phase

The person loses control over their drinking and once they start drinking are unable to stop until they are too intoxicated or nauseated to drink any more. Such a pattern is impossible to disguise and causes serious disruption to relationships and their ability to work. As personal difficulties mount the person begins to rationalize and to blame others for his problems. The only way they have of coping is to drink more alcohol which causes further difficulties. Physical health deficits due to the effects of alcohol, malnutrition and life-style are experienced.

Chronic phase

The person is completely dominated by alcohol. Periods of intoxication may extend over several days. They may go on prolonged "benders" of which they have no recollection. The person suffers severe psychological, social and physical damage and yet will do anything to obtain alcohol. A wide variety of substances, cheap but potentially very harmful, may be used to become intoxicated – polishes, cleaning agents, after-shave, meths. By this stage the person's tolerance begins to fall markedly as a result of extensive liver damage from dietary deficiencies and alcohol. Even small smounts of drink can cause gross intoxication. Severe withdrawal effects – delirium tremens – an acute confusional state with fears, tremors and hallucinations, may be experienced. By this stage even the person may admit that they need help.

Alcohol Dependency Syndrome

Alcohol is a very potent drug that can lead to both physical and psychological dependency. Prolonged and excessive consumption of alcohol is associated with the development of the characteristic signs of a dependency state:

1. *Narrowing of drinking repertoire*: the person adopts a drinking pattern characterized by excessive consumption at an increased rate. The person is unable to limit their consumption once they have started drinking.
2. *Primacy of drinking over other goals*: the person focusses on activities that are associated with alcohol. Other interests and aspects of living are of secondary importance.
3. *Increased tolerance to alcohol*: the need to consume increasing quantities of alcohol for the same desired effect. In advanced stages the tolerance decreases due to liver damage.
4. *Craving*: a subjective awareness of a compulsion and drive to drink alcohol for its effects and to avoid or obtain relief from withdrawal symptoms.
5. *Withdrawal syndrome*: a physiological and behavioural response to falling blood alcohol levels. The effects are basically those of the body being freed from the depressant effects of alcohol. The signs are:
   - physical: agitation, tremor, shakes, dry mouth, perspiration, cramps, headaches, malaise, diarrhoea, vomiting, tachycardia, possibility of fits.
   - psychological: restlessness, insomnia, anxiety, irritability, desire for alcohol, tension, smoking excessively.
6. *Rapid reinstatement of the syndrome following a period of abstinence*: many problem drinkers find it relatively easy in the short-term to maintain abstinence. This especially applies if they are in an environment, like a hospital, where the normal cues that trigger and maintain their drinking behaviour are absent. However, once re-exposed to alcohol the person soon returns to their previous excessive drinking patterns.

Recognizing the Person with Alcohol-related Problems

Psychological and behavioural

1. *Warning signs*

- Increase in the rate and amount of alcohol consumed.
- Relationship problems at home: arguments, stress, sexual difficulties, morbid jealousy, fights, family violence.
- Occupational problems: loss of job due to drunkenness. Seeking employment which offers ready access to alcohol.
- Social relationships become more strained.
- Mounting financial problems: debt and difficulty in paying bills. Increased percentage of income spent on alcohol.
- Frequent car accidents or injuries around the house or work-place.
- Defensive attitude about drinking: irritable, rationalize, denial, aggressive.
- Drinking on their own.

2. *High risk*

- Craving for alcohol at certain times, with morning drinking in particular.
- Loss of control: inability to abstain once they have started drinking.
- Concealing and disguising their alcohol intake: hiding alcohol about the house.
- Blackouts: the person remains conscious but experiences memory loss of drinking episodes.
- Repeated unsuccessful attempts to limit drinking: changing drink, making promises.
- Loss of interest in activities and relationships not associated with alcohol.
- Drinking for relief of tension and as a way of coping.
- Severe relationship difficulties: divorce, separation, constant arguments, nagging.
- Outbursts of rage and anger: family violence, involved in fights.
- Threats of suicide and self-injurious behaviour: drinking to drown sorrows.

3. *Definite harm*

- High consumption of alcohol: over 50 units of alcohol per week.
- Indiscriminate use of alcohol: social constraints are ineffective.
- Persistent drinking despite obvious personal social and physical damage.

Physical

1. *Warning signs*

   - Repeated sickness absence and unexplained absences from work.
   - Repeated attendances at GP's surgery for the physical effects of heavy drinking: chronic gastritis and other "stomach upsets", malaise, loss of appetite.
   - Dietary deficiencies: weight loss, imbalanced diet, anaemia, vitamin deficiencies.
   - Impaired eyesight: may prompt them to visit an optician.
   - Nocturnal sweating, especially in the early hours of the morning.
   - Bruising, cuts and cigarette burns on body and limbs due to falls and accidents.
   - Cardiac irregularities: ECG changes, increased incidence of cardiovascular disease and atherosclerosis.
   - Decreased tolerance to alcohol: liver less able to detoxify alcohol.

2. *High· risk*

   - Increased infections, particularly respiratory, as heavy drinkers also tend to be heavy smokers.
   - Pancreatitis: often the association with heavy drinking is not recognized.
   - Cirrhosis of the liver due to toxic effects of alcohol and dietary deficiencies. Occurs in some 10–15% of people with alcohol problems.
   - Peripheral neuropathy which affects longest nerves first. Toxic effects of alcohol and lack of thiamine (vitamin B_{12}).
   - Alcoholic cerebral effects: concentration and memory impaired. About 50% have a degree of shrinkage in their brain substance.
   - Alcoholic myopathy and cardiomyopathy.

3. *Definite harm*

   - Withdrawal symptoms on stopping alcohol.
   - Delirium tremens: acute alcoholic psychosis characterized by disorientation, coarse tremor, risk of fits, hallucinations, paranoia and panic attacks. Symptoms start 24–72 hours after cessation of alcohol and person usually recovers within 5–7 days. This is quite a rare reaction to alcohol withdrawal.

Alcohol and Pregnancy

There is increasing evidence of the harmful effects that alcohol can have upon foetal health during pregnancy. Apart from an increased risk of midterm abortion or stillbirth, alcohol consumption during pregnancy is also associated with a specific syndrome of congenital abnormalities – "fetal alcohol syndrome". The main physical and mental signs include low birth weight, poor physical development, intellectual impairment, fractiousness, tremulousness, feeble sucking, slow development, small head size, minor abnormalities of facial characteristics, crossed eyes, heart defects, abnormal kidneys, slightly malformed genitals, abnormalities of joints and palmar creases.

The degree of potential harm to the infant would appear to be directly related to the amount of alcohol consumed by the mother during pregnancy. The period of most risk is during the first trimester. In extreme cases there is also the possibility of the birth of an alcohol-dependent child. Additional harm is caused if the mother smokes excessively, takes tranquillizers or drugs, neglects her own health or nutrition and does not attend antenatal clinics.

It is uncertain as to whether there is any safe level of alcohol consumption during pregnancy. There would appear to be definite benefits in reducing alcohol consumption during this period, especially in the early stages. As most mothers learn to drink before they become pregnant, it requires concerted effort on their part and that of health educators to achieve the desired behavioural change.

After the birth of the child the consumption of alcohol also interferes with breastfeeding by inhibiting the expulsion of milk from the breast.

Alcoholic Dementias

Very heavy drinking over many years along with vitamin and dietary deficiencies can give rise to a form of alcoholic dementia. The two main syndromes are Korsakoff's psychosis and Wernicke's encephalopathy. They are differentiated by the specific areas of brain damage caused. They are comparatively rare in the UK. The primary signs are:

1. Cognitive impairment: diminished abstraction, poor problem-solving ability, difficulty in abstract thinking.
2. Severe memory loss: especially for recent events. Disorientation and marked confabulation may be present.
3. Emotional lability and blunting: often the person is suspicious, ambivalent and critical.
4. Lack of motivation.
5. Cerebellar ataxia: varying degrees of difficulty in movement and co-ordination.

Unit Instructions

When you have researched the suggested references, have mastered the Unit Objectives and successfully answered the Self-assessment Questions, proceed with the Unit Written Test.

Suggested References

Allison, B. (1987). How alcohol affects the memory. *Nursing Times*, 23 September, Vol. 83, No. 38, pp. 42–44.

Black, J. (1983). Drinking habits during pregnancy. *Nursing Times*, 31 August, Vol. 79, No. 35, pp. 25–26.

Davies, I. and Raistrick, D. (1981). *Dealing with Drink*. BBC Publications, London.

Dowdell, P. M. (1981). Alcohol and pregnancy. A review of the literature 1968–1980. *Nursing Times*, 21 October, Vol. 77, No. 43, pp. 1825–1831.

Eastman, C. (1984). *Drink and Drinking Problems*. Longman, London.

Edwards, G. (1982). *The Treatment of Drinking Problems. A Guide for the Helping Professions*. Grant McIntyre, London.

Gibbs, A. (1986). *Understanding Mental Health*. Consumer's Association/Hodder and Stoughton, London.

Grant, M. (1984). *Same Again. A Guide to Safer Drinking*. Penguin, Harmondsworth.

Heath, T. (1984). Know your poison. *Nursing Times*, 19 September, Vol. 80, No. 38, pp. 38–39.

Heather, N. and Robertson, I. (1986). Is alcoholism a disease? *New Society*, 21 February, Vol. 75, No. 1208, pp. 318–320.

Hughes, J. (1986). *An Outline of Modern Psychiatry*, 2nd edition. John Wiley, Chichester.

Kennedy, J. and Rogers, C. (1985). How much do you drink? *Nursing Mirror*, 30 October, Vol. 161, No. 18, pp. 35–37.

Lyttle, J. (1986). *Mental Disorder: Its Care and Treatment*. Baillière Tindall, London and San Diego.

McConville, B. (1983). *Women Under the Influence*. Virago, London.

Madden, J. S. (1984). *A Guide to Alcohol and Drug Dependence*, 2nd edition. Wright, Bristol.

Minshull, D. (1985). Sick or self-indulgent? *Nursing Mirror*, 3 July, Vol. 161, No. 1, pp. 15–18.

Paton, A. (Ed.) (1985). *Handbook on Alcoholism for Health Professionals*. William Heinemann, London.

Rix, K. (1983). Predicting blood alcohol concentrations. *Nursing Times*, 5 October, Vol. 79, No. 40, pp. 55–56.

Royal College of Psychiatrists (1986). *Alcohol, Our Favourite Drug*. Tavistock, London.

Sims, A. (1988). *Symptoms in the Mind*. Baillière Tindall, London and San Diego.

Trethowan, W. and Sims, A. (1983). *Psychiatry*, 5th edition. Baillière Tindall, London and San Diego.

Waterson, J. (1985). Alcohol and pregnancy. *Nursing Times*, 28 August, Vol. 81, No. 35, pp. 38–40.

Willis, J. (1976). *Clinical Psychiatry*. Blackwell Scientific, Oxford.
Wilson, M. (1981). Fetal alcohol syndrome – the American scene. *Nursing Times*, 21 October, Vol. 77, No. 43, pp. 1832–1835.
Wright, J. (1986). Fetal alcohol syndrome. *Nursing Times*, 26 March, Vol. 82, No. 13, pp. 34–35.

Self-assessment Questions

SAQ 1. Identify five factors that influence a person's drinking behaviour.
SAQ 2. Describe briefly the four stages of dependency upon alcohol.
SAQ 3. Outline five psychological and behavioural signs that would indicate a person has an alcohol-related problem.
SAQ 4. List five harmful physical consequencs of alcohol dependency.

Unit 14.1: Written Test

David Bragg, aged 47, has a long history of heavy drinking. From a somewhat deprived early life he joined the merchant navy and was at sea for over 20 years. Attempts to settle down were very problematic and he had repeated changes of occupation. He has referred himself to the community alcohol centre as he is aware that many of his difficulties are related to his drinking. As the alcohol counsellor on duty you have to interview David to assess his needs and to plan a care programme.

1. What type of drinking pattern would indicate that David's problems were related to alcohol?
2. What behavioural and social problems is David likely to describe and demonstrate?
3. What are the physical consequences of prolonged heavy drinking that David is at risk of experiencing?

Care and Treatment of the Person with Alcohol-related Problems

---

Unit Objectives

At the end of this Unit the learner should be able to:

1. Describe the range of therapeutic interventions used to help people with alcohol-related problems.
2. Identify the support required for the person and their family in the community.
3. Outline the principles of controlled and harm-free drinking.

Care and Treatment

A wide range of therapeutic interventions may be used to help the person with an alcohol-related problem. These may focus on both the presenting symptoms and the person's life-style and coping skills. The specific interventions will depend upon the assessment undertaken by the therapist, the resources available and the client's motivation. The client's ability to accept that they have a problem with their drinking and their willingness to cooperate are a key factor in any therapeutic programme. Likewise, the client has to feel that the therapists are accepting, non-judgemental and positive.

The general approach should be towards developing an integrated and readily accessible service that is able to support the person and their family in the community and in residential settings as appropriate.

Therapeutic aims

1. To minimize the extent of any harm and distress.
2. To enable the person to regain control of their drinking behaviour.
3. To facilitate the development of the person's and their family's coping skills.

Family and Self-care

Alcohol-related problems, from minor to severe difficulties, directly affect several million people. For each of the 0.5–1.0 million people who drink excessively are many more family members, friends and work-mates who are also likely to experience the consequences of an alcohol-related problem.

The insidious nature of alcohol problems are such that the person is rarely consciously aware of their increasing alcohol consumption or of the effect that it is having upon themselves or their relationships. Initially, a broad range of minor difficulties may cause general resentment that they can find solace from in drinking. As conflicts and difficulties mount so does the quantity of alcohol. Drinking becomes their main coping response to most difficulties.

The priority that is given to alcohol means that other areas of their life have to suffer. Requests by their spouse to limit their drinking are bitterly resented. Subterfuges, cheating and lying may be used to disguise the extent of their drinking or to account for missing money. Alcohol may be hidden around the house or garden to ensure its ready accessibility. Constant arguments, deceit and debt frequently bring an end to many relationships, often after a protracted period in which the spouse and children suffer.

Inefficiency and repeated absences may lead to problems at work. Paradoxically, despite the difficulties they cause, it is not uncommon for work-mates to cover up for them. Ultimately, though, the person's drinking may be so excessive that they are dismissed for drunkenness. Other jobs may be sought that are less demanding and often well below the person's occupational skills.

Attempts may be made by the person to change their preferred alcoholic drink in the mistaken belief that this will reduce the harm they will experience. The early experience of blackouts may also be enough to scare them into restricting their alcohol for a short time. Invariably, though, they return to their previous levels of consumption.

Approaches may be made to their GP for symptomatic relief of the physical consequencs of excessive drinking – malaise, gastritis, insomnia. Often the sufferer repeatedly attends the surgery with a succession of complaints without the underlying alcohol-related nature of the problem being recognized. Many sufferers, though, do not give very accurate or honest information to their GP. It is estimated that only about 20% of people with alcohol problems are known to their GP.

In some cases the individual may be able to acknowledge the nature of their difficulties and to seek help and support from voluntary or community agencies that deal with alcohol problems. In other cases the individual may have suffered quite severe harm before they seek help.

Initially, the person and their family can be helped considerably in coping with alcohol-related problems by:

1. Accurate information about alcohol problems and their effects.
2. Involvement in the care and treatment process.

3. Reassurance that effective intervention is possible.
4. The opportunity to talk freely about their problems.
5. The address of local contact support groups.
6. Developing the person's and family's coping skills.
7. Reviewing their life-style and expectations to promote their mental health.

Community Care

The majority of people with alcohol-related problems do not seek help. They attempt in their own way to deal with the problems they experience. In clinical practice most people with drinking problems can be treated successfully and cared for at home. This will depend upon the person's motivation, the support available to them, the severity of their symptoms and the community resources available. The aims of community care are:

1. To support the person and their family.
2. To monitor the person's mental and physical health.
3. To facilitate regaining control of their drinking behaviour.
4. To implement community-based treatment and care programmes.

The services available include:

1. The community mental health centre: with community psychiatric nurses, social workers, psychologists, occupational therapists and consultant psychiatrists working as a team to offer skills-based therapeutic interventions.
2. The community alcohol team/community alcohol centre: a centre or resource base from which a team of multidisciplinary health care workers operate, who specialize in alcohol-related problems. They can usually offer both domiciliary and centre-based support programmes. Often they work in close collaboration with local voluntary agencies.
3. Voluntary agencies: AA, Al-Anon, Al-teen, Councils on Alcoholism, Drink-watchers, Salvation Army, local contact and support groups for sufferers and relatives (80% of alcohol services are organized by voluntary services), CAB, marriage guidance.
4. Probation and after-care services.
5. General practitioners.
6. Primary health care teams: particularly health visitors if children are involved.
7. DHSS: benefits, allowances and grants as currently available to individuals and their families.
8. Local authority/health authority: hostels, half-way homes, group homes.
9. Out-patient clinics and day hospitals.

Residential Care

There are some 14 500 admissions annually for treatment for alcohol dependency. However, with a prevalence rate of some 500 000, it would appear that residential services are only dealing with a relatively small proportion of potential clients. Residential care may be indicated where there is:

1. A lack of support in the community.
2. Personal and family exhaustion.
3. The need for specialized treatment programmes and therapy.
4. The need for detailed physical assessment where the person is experiencing or at risk of the physical complications of chronic alcohol abuse.

The residential settings may include:

1. Regional or local Alcohol Treatment Units (ATU): a centre specializing in alcohol-related problems.
2. Detoxification unit: a centre specializing in the short-term care and treatment of the habitually drunk person. A limited number of centres were opened in the 1970s as a joint Home Office/DHSS project.
3. Hostels run by voluntary or statutory agencies for the person with alcohol problems.
4. Psychiatric unit or hospital.

Therapeutic Goals

The objectives in the treatment of alcohol-related problems and alcohol dependency have been primarily towards the attainment and maintenance of complete abstinence. This philosophy has been influential in directing the approaches taken by many statutory and voluntary agencies, notably Alcoholics Anonymous. The reformed drinker is perceived of as someone who has a continual struggle within themselves and with others to resist alcohol and is only one drink away from lapsing. This reformist zeal and approach has been very successful in helping many people with drink problems over the years. However, a number of other approaches are now being developed that advocate "controlled" and "sensible" drinking.

These perspectives, based upon behavioural and health education approaches, focus primarily on the person continuing to drink but regaining control of and limiting their alcohol consumption. The advantages claimed by this approach are that:

1. Effective forms of therapy need to consider the kind of behaviour that is encouraged socially, which moderate drinking is.
2. It does not require a complete change of life-style.
3. Most people with a drinking problem do not permanently abstain.

4. Problem drinkers may prefer this as a treatment goal and be more likely to seek help if there is the prospect of being able to continue drinking, albeit in a modified way. This is especially relevant to both the young and those who are at the early stages of developing alcohol-related problems.
5. There are opportunities for practice and reinforcement in a natural environment.

The two approaches have been viewed as being mutually incompatible. However, if the therapist considers the client's preferred choice, their motivation, the support available, the degree of dependence and the harm experienced, then a suitable objective can be identified. Many clients may express a strong preference though their intentions may not always be very realistic.

In practice, those who are highly motivated, have support and are least damaged may be suitable candidates for controlled drinking. Those with severe harm, expecially liver damage, may need to consider complete abstinence.

Whichever treatment approach is adopted, it has to be accepted that it may take many years for an effective recovery. A drink problem of some 10 years or more standing is not going to be resolved quickly. The rate of relapse is high and workers in this field need to be both realistic and yet hopeful.

Therapeutic Interventions

Detoxification

Detoxification or "drying out" is often one of the first stages in treatment programmes. The aim is to help the person to cope with the psychological and physical effects of withdrawal from alcohol and to resist their craving for more drink.

The first psychological effects of withdrawal may be experienced from the beginning of detoxification. The physical signs may take 3–4 days to manifest themselves and may last for 7–10 days. The reaction is self-limiting and the majority do not experience great distress.

Detoxification may be carried out either in a residential or home setting. The main considerations are the person's commitment, the resources and support available and the person's safety. The advantages of residential settings are that the person is removed from an environment that could be contributing to their drinking and that the transfer of responsibility to the care staff helps to reduce their craving for alcohol. Very close monitoring is possible and skilled intervention is available for any serious complications.

Home-based detoxification is increasingly being used and, provided there is adequate support and supervision, can usually be carried out successfully.

In one study of over 1000 people undergoing detoxification there was only one instance of delirium tremens, six people experienced one convulsion and six people more than one fit.

A successful detoxification programme requires:

1. Preparation of the person and others who may be providing support. Written information may be useful.
2. Health education on the nature of alcohol withdrawal.
3. Supervision: to restrict access to alcohol and to monitor the person's safety.
4. Reassurance: empathy, acceptance, trust.
5. Tranquillizers: to overcome the effects of withdrawal from alcohol. Initially, quite high dosages may be given, progressively reduced over a short period and then withdrawn. The dosage prescribed will depend upon the severity of withdrawal symptoms and the clinician's judgement. The most commonly used medications are:

   - Chlordiazepoxide (Librium) in starting doses of 10–20 mg three times a day. In severe reactions much higher levels may be given – 40–60 mg three times a day. Because of their potential for dependency, benzodiazepines should not be used for more than 2 weeks.
   - Chlormethiazole (Heminevrin) starting from 3–4 capsules given three or four times a day; the dosage is progressively reduced over 6–9 days. Chlormethiazole is used less frequently now as it has a higher risk of dependency.

In the rare occurrence of delirium tremens as a reaction to alcohol withdrawal, the person may also need bed rest to prevent exhaustion, a quiet environment to prevent over-stimulation and promote calm, constant supervision to prevent danger to themselves, sedation, adequate nutrition and fluids.

Psychotherapeutic approaches

1. *Skilled nursing care*: one of the most important therapeutic factors in residential settings. A number of CPNs also work as clinical specialists with people who have alcohol-related problems in the community.
2. *Individual counselling and psychotherapy*: to increase insight and promote understanding of their motivation to drink excessively. To develop coping skills.
3. *Group therapy*: to increase insight and self-awareness, to share personal experiences, to provide opportunities for social learning.
4. *Self-help*: to share difficulties and strategies for problem solving, to provide empathy and non-judgemental acceptance.
5. *Family or couple's therapy*: to enable couples to be more supportive and to communicate more effectively. To help the family find ways of

coping with the problems caused by alcohol. To rebuild damaged relationships.

6. *Social skills and assertiveness training*: to raise confidence and self-esteem. Many people with alcohol problems find social situations difficult to cope with. Of particular use is learning how to say "no" to an offer of a drink assertively without giving offence. Helps to increase feelings of personal control and mastery.

7. *Anxiety management and relaxation skills*: the consumption of alcohol is often related to feelings of stress and anxiety. Learning anxiety management skills helps to increase personal control and reduce the need for drink as an anxiolytic.

8. *Self-confrontation on video*: in which the person is given video feedback of themselves when intoxicated. The video is used as a basis for counselling and therapy to promote insight and facilitate behavioural change.

9. *Role modelling of sensible drinking*: the person with a drinking problem is assigned to go drinking with a role model who demonstrates moderate drinking behaviour.

10. *Cognitive aversion therapy*: in which the person visualizes the unpleasant effects of intoxication as an aversive outcome.

11. *Art therapy and psychodrama*: to help express and release feelings, to promote insight.

12. *Occupational therapy*: to develop life skills.

13. *Recreational and social activities*: to meet social needs, overcome isolation and to provide positively rewarding experiences.

14. *Minimal contact therapy*: after a brief initial contact and assessment interview the person is given printed guidelines on how to control their drinking. The follow-up, often by telephone, is focussed primarily on maintaining the drinking goals set. For some people this is all they require.

Controlled and Sensible Drinking Behaviour

Drinking alcohol is a complex learned behaviour. It involves a network of cognitive processes (perceptions, needs, choices) and behavioural strategies (obtaining a drink, holding the glass, swallowing, ordering another drink). There are also a number of personal and environmental factors that tend to reinforce and maintain the person's drinking behaviour – the pub environment, the company they keep, the effects of the alcohol.

The aim of controlled drinking is to demonstrate to the person with an alcohol problem that they are in control of their drinking and not at the mercy of alcohol. They can re-learn the skills of sensible drinking in order to moderate their intake and, just as importantly, enhance their self-esteem and develop a more positive approach to living.

Controlled drinking is not a suitable approach for everyone with an alcohol problem. People have to be carefully selected in terms of their motivation, support, personality and degree of dependence. Those who have severe physical damage as a result of their drinking may need to consider abstinence. However, there is evidence that many people with a drinking problem, even a long-term difficulty, are able to achieve moderate controlled drinking patterns and maintain them over a long period of time.

The approach to controlled drinking may be pursued as an individual programme or in a group format, as used by "Drinkwatchers". Other therapeutic approaches may be used in parallel to facilitate the controlled drinking programme and to resolve other problems, e.g. assertiveness, anxiety management, marriage guidance, physical health promotion.

Initially, the processes and objectives of the programme are explained. Participants are also given health education on alcohol and the nature of alcohol-related problems. This will explore the difficulties that people have experienced and the potential benefits from limiting their alcohol consumption.

People are shown how to keep a diary or log of their drinking behaviour. This facilitates assessment and analysis of their drinking. It also helps to reduce the quantity consumed and to increase control. Factors that contribute towards the maintenance of excessive drinking are identified, as are factors that promote moderation. Details may be kept of day, quantity, time, place, company, thoughts and feelings.

Strategies that facilitate control and moderation are explored and may be rehearsed in role play or in real-life situations (see below). An important skill is learning how to refuse a drink. New leisure activities are considered, especially those that are incompatible with drinking.

Programmes may need to run over a period of time in order to facilitate the development of new drinking skills and to provide emotional support. Participants may find it useful to join a peer group programme such as "Drinkwatchers" to provide long-term support.

A controlled drinking programme may begin with a period of abstinence. From this the person is gradually enabled, with support and guidance, to increase their alcohol intake and to keep within their identified limits.

Approaches to Regaining Control and Limiting Alcohol Consumption

1. Do not drink every day of the week, have two or three alcohol-free days per week.
2. Set and monitor weekly limit on consumption.
3. Plan drinking sessions ahead, do not go drinking on impulse.
4. Identify and be aware of drinking cues.
5. Do not drink when taking other drugs.
6. Do not drink and drive, operate machinery or make important decisions.
7. Arrange alternative activities instead of going to the pub, especially relaxing and enjoyable pursuits.
8. Eat before drinking.

9. Set a limit on consumption each night, and monitor and record intake.
10. Set a time limit.
11. Arrive at the pub later.
12. Limit the money that you take.
13. Do not drink alone, choose people you like and who have moderate and sensible drinking habits.
14. Do not drink at lunch time.
15. Order a non-alcoholic drink when thirsty.
16. Order singles or half-pints.
17. Dilute spirits to reduce rate of absorption.
18. Alternate with soft drinks.
19. Do not get caught up with rounds.
20. Learn to refuse drinks.
21. Make alcoholic drinks last at least 30 minutes.
22. Sip drink, do not gulp.
23. Put glass down between sips.
24. Do something else with your hands, e.g. read a paper, play cards or dominoes.
25. Attend to own reactions to alcohol, do not get intoxicated.
26. Reward yourself for compliance and successes.
27. Set yourself some penalties for lapses, e.g. money to charity, unfinished tasks, etc.

Chemotherapeutic Approaches to Drinking Problems

Disulfiram (Antabuse) and citrated calcium carbonate (Abstem) are both medications that are used to maintain abstinence in people with drinking problems. Both of these cause an extremely unpleasant reaction in the person if they ingest alcohol while taking the medication. The effects will vary according to the person, the dose of medication and the amount of alcohol consumed and include nausea, vomiting, hot flushes, palpitations, pallor, perspiration, malaise, feelings of constriction in the head and chest.

Potential clients have to be carefully selected in terms of their motivation and sound physical health. People who are pregnant, have heart, respiratory, renal or hepatic disease, or who are psychotic are not suitable candidates. The sequence of therapy is as follows:

1. Informed consent and explanation of the programme.
2. Health education about the effects of alcohol and its interaction with the medication.
3. Detoxification to ensure that alcohol is cleared from their body. This may take from 3 to 7 days depending upon their previous alcohol consumption.
4. Disulfiram (Antabuse), as an example, is given in a high initial dose of 800 mg. This is then progressively reduced over 4–5 days to a single daily dose of 100–200 mg. The equivalent daily dose of citrated calcium carbonate is 50–100 mg.

5. On the fifth day the person may be given a supervised test dose of some 10–15 ml of alcohol to evoke the unpleasant reaction. If the response is minimal a further dose of alcohol is given to gain the desired response that may last some 45–60 minutes. The intention is to make this a powerful learning situation and to demonstrate the need to avoid alcohol while taking the medication. During this experience the person's pulse and blood pressure are closely monitored in case of collapse. Rarely, a short-term psychotic reaction occurs that clears in a few days.

As a treatment, these types of deterrent drugs need to be used as part of a comprehensive therapeutic approach that includes counselling and support. They do not stop the desire for alcohol, they make the consequences of drinking sufficiently unpleasant to deter people. For many people it facilitates abstinence, while other therapeutic interventions can be made to promote positive personal change. Some people have been taking these medications for many years with great effect. It requires only one conscious decision to take the tablet each day rather than a constant struggle to resist alcohol.

Some people find that if they stop taking the medication they can usually start drinking again within a week. Some have even attempted to drink through the effects, even though this is a very dangerous practice. The side-effects include gastrointestinal upsets, body odour, bad breath, unpleasant taste, drowsiness, headache, impotence, peripheral and optic neuritis, malaise, depression and psychotic reaction.

Physical Care and Treatment

Physical health problems may exist as a direct result of alcohol upon the body, prolonged malnutrition, excessive smoking and personal neglect. The physical care and treatment required will depend upon the specific harm caused by prolonged drinking. Physical care interventions may include:

1. Detoxification and abstinence to prevent further harm.
2. Vitamin replacements: high doses of vitamin B_1, particularly thiamine, and vitamin C. Intramuscular injections of Parentravite may be given.
3. Nutrition: diet high in carbohydrates and protein.
4. Hydration: plentiful fluids to avoid dehydration.
5. Attention to personal hygiene.
6. Rest.
7. Specific treatment:

    • Infections: antibiotics. Chronic drinkers have a low resistance to infection. Chest infections in particular are common.
    • Polyneuritis or peripheral neuritis: analgesia, physical comfort and physiotherapy may be required.
    • Gastric ulcers: medication, rest and diet.
    • Pancreatitis or cirrhosis of the liver: diet, rest and medication.

Therapeutic Outcomes

The outcome is more successful when the client is motivated, has insight, adequate support and where the degree of social, physical and psychological harm is minimal. Where there is little motivation or support and extensive harm the outcome is less hopeful. In particular, women and younger drinkers who have a serious drink problem are particularly difficult to treat. In terms of differing therapeutic approaches it would seem that a wide range of interventions that are actively applied are more likely to be successful.

Due to the very long-term nature of alcohol problems the need for prolonged support and a high relapse rate it is difficult to give accurate figures about the outcomes. As a crude approximation about one-third recover, for one-third there is little change and about one-third deteriorate. Those involved with providing long-term support for the problem drinker need to be aware of potential stresses in the person's life – relationships, occupational, financial – that may precipitate a relapse. Christmas and New Year present particular difficulties to the abstinent and those trying to limit their consumption. There is a high risk of self-harm or suicide.

Ultimately, the problems of alcohol abuse are not going to be solved by therapy alone. It will require a huge will of political and social effort to make significant changes in the way that we perceive and use alcohol – legal controls, licensing restrictions, advertising controls, expansion of health education and a change in the perception of alcohol as a drug of potential abuse that needs to always be used carefully.

Health Education and Alcohol

With alcohol abuse forming one of today's major public health problems it is a natural target for health education programmes. However, the resources available to health education compared with those of the drink industry are minimal. Such restrictions as there are on the advertising of alcoholic drinks are easily circumvented by skilful advertisers. Especially at Christmas and New Year, when the warnings on drink and driving are at their most frequent, the alcohol adverts increase considerably. Additionally, the health education message has to compete with well-established social beliefs and perceptions that regard alcohol as one of life's "pleasures".

In competition with these forces the health education message seems to be relatively ineffective in altering drinking behaviour. However, in certain areas there is a growing awareness of the potential for harm that excessive and indiscriminate drinking can cause. By identifying and directing information at specific target groups the health education message has been more successful. Two examples are drinking in pregnancy and in developing company employee alcohol policies. There are also attempts to increase alcohol awareness and education among schoolchildren. Even relatively young children have developed attitudes and perceptions towards alcohol.

The primary health education messages are concerned with increasing public awareness about the limits of safe alcohol consumption, developing harm-free drinking habits and identifying potential risk groups. It is often found that those with drinking problems are surprisingly ignorant of the effects of alcohol and the relative alcohol content of different drinks.

Unit Instructions

When you have researched the suggested references, have mastered the Unit Objectives and successfully answered the Self-assessment Questions, proceed with the Unit Written Test.

Suggested References

Allsop, D. (1987). Battle of the bottle. *Nursing Times*, 22 April, Vol. 83, No. 16, pp. 49–50.

Bellamy, N. (1982). On the rocks. *Nursing Mirror*, 1 December, Vol. 155, No. 22, pp. 41–43.

Booth, P. (1985). Back on the rails. *Nursing Times*, 28 August, Vol. 81, No. 35, pp. 16–17.

Brewer C. (1986). Controlling the demon. *Nursing Times*, 2 July, Vol. 82, No. 27, pp. 46–47.

Cyster, R. (1986). Setting limits. *Nursing Times*, 7 May, Vol. 82, No. 19, pp. 51–52.

Dally, P. and Watkins, M. J. (1986). *Psychology and Psychiatry*, 6th edition. Hodder and Stoughton, London.

Davies, I. and Raistrick, D. (1981). *Dealing with Drink*. BBC Publications, London.

Dodd, T. (1985). Drinkers respond to the CAT. *Nursing Times*, 27 February, Vol. 81, No. 9, pp. 48–49.

Eastman, C. (1984). *Drink and Drinking Problems*. Longman, London.

Edwards, G. (1982). *The Treatment of Drinking Problems*. Grant McIntyre, London.

Ewles, L. and Simnett, I. (1985). *Promoting Health: A Practical Guide to Health Education*. John Wiley, New York.

Fulton, A. (1985). Alcohol: how much is too much? *Nursing Mirror*, 8 May, Vol. 160, No. 19, pp. 32–33.

Gillies, D. and Lader, M. (1986). *Guide to the Use of Psychotropic Drugs*. Churchill Livingstone, Edinburgh.

Grant, M. (1984). *Same Again: A Guide to Safer Drinking*. Penguin, Harmondsworth.

Jacobson, S. (1983). Coping without alcohol. *Nursing Mirror*, 9 February, Vol. 156, No. 6, pp. 53–55.

Kennedy, J. (1986). Sobering thoughts. *Nursing Times*, 23 July, Vol. 82, No. 30, pp. 38–39.

Kennedy, J. and Rogers, C. (1985). How much do you drink? *Nursing Mirror*, 30 October, Vol. 161, No. 18, pp. 35–37.

Lyttle, J. (1986). *Mental Disorder: Its Care and Treatment*. Baillière Tindall, London and San Diego.

McConville, B. (1983). *Women Under the Influence*. Virago, London.

Madden, J. S. (1984). *A Guide to Alcohol and Drug Dependence*, 2nd edition. John Wright, Bristol.

Minardi, H. (1986). One day at a time. *Nursing Times*, 5 March, Vol. 82, No. 10, pp. 34–36.

Mitchell, D. (1985). Defeating the demon. *Nursing Mirror*, 3 July, Vol. 161, No. 1, pp. 18–20.

Mitchell, R. (1982). Breakdown. Common sense psychiatry for nurses 1. Alcohol. *Nursing Times*, 13 October, Vol. 78, No. 41, pp. 1704–1706.

Morris, P. (1985). The dependent spirit. *Nursing Times*, 6 February, Vol. 81, No. 6, pp. 12–13.

Paton, A. (Ed.) (1985). *Handbook on Alcoholism for Health Professionals*. William Heinemann, London.

Plant, M. (1985). Sights that are set too high. *Nursing Times*, 23 October, Vol. 81, No. 43, p. 39.

Rix, K. (1983). Alcohol intoxication: Diagnostic pitfalls. *Nursing Times*, 28 September, Vol. 79, No. 39, pp. 58–61.

Robinson, D. (1979). *Talking out of Alcoholism. The Self-help Process of Alcoholics Anonymous*. Croom Helm, London.

Royal College of Psychiatrists (1986). *Alcohol, Our Favourite Drug*. Tavistock, London.

Ruzek, J. (1982). *Drinkwatcher's Handbook*. ACCEPT Publications.

Silverstone, T. and Turner, P. (1982). *Drug Treatment in Psychiatry*, 3rd edition. Routledge and Kegan Paul, London.

Trethowan, W. and Sims, A. (1983). *Psychiatry*, 5th edition. Baillière Tindall, London and San Diego.

Willis, J. (1976). *Clinical Psychiatry*. Blackwell Scientific, Oxford.

Self-assessment Questions

SAQ 5. Describe three therapeutic interventions that can be used to support a person during alcohol detoxification.

SAQ 6. List eight ways of promoting sensible drinking.

SAQ 7. State five reactions that may occur if a person who is taking disulfiram (Antabuse) consumes alcohol.

SAQ 8. Identify four factors that influence the outcome for helping people with alcohol-related problems.

Unit 14.2: Written Test

Peter Blair, aged 32, has referred himself to the local community alcohol centre for advice on his drinking. During the assessment interview it becomes apparent that he has a long drinking history since the age of 17. He is a self-employed plumber and his business has begun to suffer as a result of missing appointments and extensive lunch-time drinking. His wife has become concerned at both the damage to their relationship and the effect his drinking is having on the children. They have become hostile towards their father and their school work is suffering. His wife has threatened to throw him out unless he seeks help for his drinking problem.

Peter has some vague knowledge on the treatment and support approaches used for alcohol problems and has come along with plenty of questions.

1. Peter has heard of "controlled drinking" and wants further information on this approach. How would you explain how controlled drinking is used? Briefly, what factors might determine Peter's suitability for such a programme?
2. Peter also believes that there are "tablets that stop you drinking". Describe how you would explain the use of disulfiram (Antabuse) in the maintenance of abstinence.

Drug Misuse and Dependency

Unit Objectives

At the end of this Unit the learner should be able to:

1. Describe the characteristic signs of physical and psychological dependency on drugs.
2. Identify factors that contribute towards dependency on or the misuse of drugs.
3. State how various routes of administration influence the effects and potential for harm of various substances.
4. Differentiate between the harmful potential of different drugs.

Social Aspects of Drug Misuse

Throughout history a wide variety of substances have been taken that have the potential to stimulate, relax, enhance pleasure or to distort perception of self or the world. Within each culture strong prohibitions and rules exist as to the use or restrictions that are applied to these substances and a recognition of their potential for harm if misused.

As a current health problem, drug misuse is a very controversial topic and invariably draws in a wide range of political, moral and legal opinions. Very strong perceptions and stereotypes exist as to what constitutes a "drug", the inevitability of harm and the draconian penalties that should be applied. Such perspectives can make it very difficult for both health care workers or users to gain a tolerant and understanding response from the public in attempting to deal with drug-related problems.

Interestingly in this debate, the substances that actually cause the most harm to individuals and society – alcohol, tobacco and minor tranquillizers – are rarely thought of as "drugs". Nonetheless, in relation to the broad range of other substances that people misuse, there does exist a major public health problem.

Drug Dependency

Certain drugs, if repeatedly taken in appropriate dosages, have the potential to cause dependency. Drugs vary considerably in their potential for users to become dependent and it is possible, if several different drugs are being taken regularly, for a person to be dependent upon each of them. Dependency can be both physical and psychological and is recognized by the following.

Psychological dependence

A compulsion or craving to take the drug on a continuous or periodic basis in order to experience their effects or to avoid the consequences of its absence. A person can be psychologically dependent upon any substance. The powerful psycho-active effects of many drugs means that in their absence people experience a pronounced flatness of mood that is only relieved by further dosage of the drug. The degree of psychological dependence can vary from an intermittent desire to a powerful all-consuming drive.

The signs of psychological dependency include restlessness, anxiety, tension, irritability, insomnia, preoccupation with the drug, craving for the drug and poor concentration.

Physical dependence

Falling levels or an absence of the drug in the body lead to a range of physical symptoms. These are characteristic for the specific drug that the person is using. Only certain drugs cause physical dependency, i.e. alcohol, barbiturates, amphetamines, heroin and other opioids.

The severity of the withdrawal that the person experiences – "abstinence syndrome" – is dependent upon the quantity that they have been taking and the duration of the effects of the drug. Characteristically, the shorter the period of action the more rapidly the withdrawal syndrome develops and the more severe its consequences. Hence, to avoid withdrawal, the user has to take repeat dosages regularly.

Tolerance

A phenomenon of repeated drug use is the need to take increasing amounts of the drug to achieve the same effect. Users either have to take more to meet their needs or find that with a period of abstinence the tolerance level begins to decrease. The mechanisms for this are not fully understood and may involve effects on neurotransmitters or drug receptor sites.

The potential for tolerance varies enormously between drugs. For some drugs it is only a small multiple of initial dosages, for others it can be several hundred times, up to levels that would be fatal for non-users.

Another phenomenon is that of cross-tolerance, whereby the tolerance developed for one drug also influences the user's tolerance for other related drugs. This principle is used in the treatment of opiate dependency when other drugs can be substituted for a similar effect. Users often become aware of other similar drugs that they can take to achieve the desired effects and to avert withdrawal symptoms.

The Development of Dependency

The development of harm or dependency arising from drug misuse is not automatic. A number of factors – personal, social, environmental, the drug – will influence an individual's potential to become "hooked". Not all drugs are as dependency-forming as others and some people become dependent far easier than others.

Many people experiment with drugs for a short period of time either out of curiosity or from peer group pressure and then give up. Large numbers even refuse to try them. For both groups the potential pleasures of drug misuse are outweighed by the social, personal and physical costs. Many people report a very unfavourable initial experience that subsequently deters them.

Large numbers of people use "soft" drugs for recreational purposes and suffer relatively little harm. Their intake may be fairly regulated and the drugs are used in a moderate way, e.g. at weekends and time off.

As with alcohol, a large number of people are not dependent but, nonetheless, may experience many harmful consequences as a result of their indiscriminate use. This may be a persistent pattern of deteriorating physical, mental and social health that is ultimately as damaging as dependency can be. Frequently, those who use drugs in this way and those who are dependent will take a variety of drugs to meet their needs. This pattern of "polydrug" misuse is one of the most common presentations. It is not known what percentage of irregular users go on to develop dependency.

The onset of dependency upon harder drugs tends to be a more progressive and insidious process. Most users, often at their suppliers' prompting, tend to believe themselves to be firmly in control and to deny any potential for harm. Even at advanced stages of harm these beliefs may still persist.

One controversy that surrounds the topic of drug misuse is that of "escalation" from soft to harder drugs. An assumption is made that as people tire of the effects of soft drugs they will seek the more potent "kicks" to be had from more powerful drugs. Despite widespread research and study this concept of progression has not been validated. Each drug has different effects and is taken by individuals for very specific reasons in preferred circumstances. Users tend to want more of the same drug, not to switch to other substances.

Incidence of Drug Misuse

In 1984 there were 5850 registered addicts notified to the Home Office. However, it is also estimated that there are about 60 000 regular users of heroin and many more casual users. As drug misuse is essentially an illegal activity, the majority of users are not known and estimates are based upon:

- the number of convictions for illegal drugs' activities, i.e. dealing, possession;
- the quantity of drugs confiscated by customs officers or by the police;
- research studies into known addicts and potential risk groups.

All of these indicate that for any given drug the official estimate is only the "tip of the iceberg" and can be multiplied at least 10 times. For some of the "soft" drugs, especially cannabis, their use is very widespread.

As a health problem, the majority of users are primarily in the 18–30 age group of whom 70–80% are male and 20–30% are female.

Factors Influencing Drug Misuse and Attitudes Towards Drugs

It is difficult to identify factors that definitely contribute towards the onset of dependency or patterns of misuse for an individual. For each user it is a complex interaction of personal, social and environmental factors. Anyone can be at risk. Significant factors that appear to influence an individual's potential for drug misuse include:

1. *Accessibility and availability*: despite being illegal, the majority of drugs of misuse can be readily obtained if the person has the right contacts. Patterns of drug misuse appear to be particularly prevalent in areas of inner-city deprivation.
2. *Relative cost*: the cost of drugs is dictated by powerful market forces. As an illegal trade the mark up from source to user is very high and prices can fluctuate widely. The relative costs of drugs also vary considerably. Cocaine and heroin are usually the most expensive. The cost to the user is determined by the drug they wish to take, the quantity they require and their contacts. Someone who is dependent upon heroin could expect to pay about £40 a day or £300 a week at current prices to support their habit. A wide range of other drugs can be obtained relatively cheaply, e.g. cannabis, barbiturates, amphetamines and solvents, and if they are used periodically for "recreational purposes", it may be a comparatively inexpensive habit.
3. *Gender*: males who misuse drugs outnumber women by about three or four to one. Male adolescents and young adults seem to be particularly attracted to acts of social rebellion and illegal activities. Once established though, women appear to suffer far more damaging physical and social consequences from drug dependency than do men. Women form the majority of those who are therapeutically dependent upon benzodiazepines. (see p. 248)
4. *Peer group*: the majority of users are introduced to drugs by a friend

or a known acquaintance, not by a "pusher". Peer groups exert a powerful influence upon patterns of drug misuse. Some drugs are primarily used in a social context and are used to reinforce group membership and relationships, e.g. passing round a joint, sharing a hookah, sharing syringes.

5. *Age*: some drugs appear to be particularly significant within certain age groups, solvents are primarily misused by 11–16 year olds, the majority of heroin users are aged 16–30; benzodiazepines are seen among the over 25s.

6. *Prolonged stress*: for which the drugs are used as a way of coping and of relieving tension. Most drugs are potent anxiolytics. Stresses identified with drug misuse include unemployment, overcrowding, single parents, boredom, family disharmony.

7. *Personal factors*: feelings of low self-esteem, inadequacy and social anxiety which the drugs help them to overcome. Problems often seem related to poor early childhood experiences, especially deprivation.

8. *Occupation*: those in medical professions who had access to drugs used to be a high-risk group. With increasing awareness and controls the risks of this group becoming dependent have decreased but are still present.

9. *Therapeutic use*: in the past a significant proportion of those dependent upon narcotics and barbiturates were the result of poorly monitored therapeutic programmes. For both of these drugs this is now a minimal risk. However, if anxiolytics are included then there are some 250 000 at risk of benzodiazepine dependency.

10. *Self-appraisal* of one's drug habit and whether this is perceived as being potentially harmful. The nature of dependency is such, however, that users rarely acknowledge any harmful consequences. Knowledge among users about the potential for harm is often limited.

11. *Media portrayal*: drugs are invariably presented in a negative context. However, there is often an undercurrent of glamour and mystique about drug misuse among the famous that may influence those who are impressionable.

Routes of Administration

The route of administration influences the rate of action of a substance and its concentration in the body. These will both determine the subjective experience of the user. For some drugs there is a traditional method of administration. Use is also influenced by personal preference or by current fashion.

Inhalation

The inhalation of smoke or fumes is quite a potent route. It ensures a very rapid action that tends to be relatively short-lived. Substances may be smoked on their own or mixed with tobacco. Fumes may be inhaled directly, sucked in through a tube or inhaled from a bag. There is a risk of potential harm to the respiratory system and from sudden intoxication. Used for cannabis, opium and solvents.

Sniffing

The sniffing of powders is slightly less effective than inhalation. A fairly rapid effect that tends to be relatively short-lived. The nasal mucosa has a rich blood supply to facilitate absorption but tends to be damaged by repeated administration. Used for cocaine and heroine.

Oral

Oral administration is generally slower in onset and the effects are less pronounced; however, the duration is increased. Some drugs are less effective by this route. The influence also depends on whether the stomach is empty or full. Used for barbiturates, amphetamines, LSD, any drug in tablet form, cannabis cooked into food, and mushrooms.

Subcutaneous ("popping"), intramuscular or intravenous injection ("mainlining")

Very rapid and potent effects that can give a powerful "high" result from these routes, though there is a relatively short duration. The potential for harm arises primarily from unhygienic practices, unskilled injection techniques and impurities in drugs. Of particular concern is the repeated use of disposable needles and syringes by the same or several people sharing. Drugs that can be injected include heroin, barbiturates and cocaine.

Potential harm from injections

1. Abscesses: chronic infection at sites of repeated administration.
2. Scarring and damage to local tissues, tendons, muscles and nerves.
3. Local infections: cellulitis, phlebitis.
4. Systemic infections: septicaemia, endocarditis, pulmonary complications.

Of particular concern to drug misusers and carers are:

- Acute hepatitis B: a virulent and potentially fatal infection transmitted through body secretions.
- Acquired Immune Deficiency Syndrome (AIDS): a potentially fatal infection spread through blood products. With the sharing of needles and syringes among drug misusers a common practice, they are a very high-risk group for AIDS.

For both of the above infections there is a long symptomless incubation period. Carers should therefore exercise maximum caution.

Dosages Taken

Identifying the dosages taken by drug misusers is often an important part in assessing the person's therapeutic needs. However, it is also very problematic. Coming from an illegal source, often from illicit manufacturers, the basic constituents are of variable purity. Steps are taken at each stage of production and distribution to maximize the potential for profit and extravagant claims may be made as to the drug's potency.

Apart from many drugs of unknown potency, supplies are also often:

1. Mixed with other substances to bulk out the quantity: lactose, sucrose, starch, baking soda, chalk, flour
2. Mixed with other drugs to give it a boost, particularly stimulants.
3. Mixtures of unknown composition, i.e. "cocktails", taken for kicks.

Adulterating drugs in this manner can cause particular problems for users. These include:

- a high risk of accidental overdose as a consequence of extremely variable dosages;
- an increased risk of tissue damage or injections from inappropriate additives.

The dosage of a drug taken is only one factor that influences how a person responds. The response is very subjective and also influenced by:

1. *The placebo effect*: the trust and anticipation that a user has in respect of the effects of the drug.
2. *Previous experience of the drug*: if the person is familiar with the effects of the drug then they will respond more favourably to its effects. If they are anxious they will tend to resist its effects.
3. *Social setting*: being with others who approve or are also participating promotes a more positive experience.

Drug Misuse and Pregnancy

Many therapeutic drugs are known to have adverse effects upon the growth and development of the foetus and to be present in breast milk. It is not unreasonable, therefore, to expect that drugs that are being misused may also be having harmful effects. Further complications are likely to arise from heavy smoking, poor nutrition and unhygienic administration where drugs are injected. These can all contribute to miscarriage, prematurity, increased morbidity, malnutrition and low birth weight. Depending upon the drugs being misused, particularly heroin, it is also possible for the infant to experience physical withdrawal symptoms after birth.

Recognizing the Person with Drug-related Problems

The effects of each drug and their potential for harm are specific. However, there are a number of characteristic signs that can indicate that a person is experiencing harm as a consequence of misusing drugs. These may include:

1. *Relationship problems*: arguments, conflict, loss of trust, lying, deceit, sexual difficulties, unreliability, separation, leaving signs of drug use around the house (needles, syringes, burnt foil, drugs, empty crisp packets and polythene bags, stains on clothes, concealing their intake), harmful effects on children.
2. *Psychological problems*: anxiety, low self-esteem, misery, despair, hopelessness, helplessness, irritability, tension, uncharacteristic behaviour and mood swings, suspicion, defensiveness, restlessness at certain times contrasted by apathy and indifference, repeated unsuccessful attempts at abstinence, signs of psychological withdrawal.
3. *Social problems*: loss of established friendships, mixing with people who use drugs, indiscriminate use of drugs, loss of interests, concealing their level of intake.
4. *Occupational problems*: repeated sickness and absences, poor productivity, stealing, arguments, unreliability, lying, accidents at work.
5. *Academic problems*: poor attainment, lack of concentration, poor attendance, truancy, stealing from fellow students, offering drugs to others in school or college.
6. *Financial problems*: increasing amounts of money are required to pay for drugs, which may lead to selling personal possessions, stealing, buildup of unpaid bills, debt, fraud, dealing in drugs to finance dependency, prostitution.
7. *Legal problems*: fines or conviction for possession or dealing in drugs, reckless behaviour while under the influence of drugs, stealing, fraud, debts.
8. *Physical health problems*: these are often more dangerous than the drug itself – malaise, tiredness, anorexia, gastrointestinal upsets, nausea, vomiting, weight loss, pallor, anaemia, malnourishment, vitamin deficiencies, systemic and local infections, tissue damage, bruising, scarring, abscesses, tremor, physical withdrawal symptoms.

Commonly Misused Drugs

Heroin and other opioids

Dependency upon opioids, particularly heroin and morphine, and synthetically manufactured equivalents (methadone and pethidine) are particularly associated with the stereotypes that surround drug addicts. In clinical use they are powerful analgesics; however, they also have the potential to be seriously abused.

The most potent effects are experienced from intravenous use. They have poor effects orally. Opium can be smoked or sniffed through the nasal mucosa. Many heroin users prefer to inhale the smoke through a tube or directly from heroin that is being burned on silver foil, i.e. "chasing the dragon".

When "mainlined", the user experiences almost instantaneous intense bodily and mental pleasure. There is also a wide range of secondary physical effects, e.g. reduced peristalsis, hypotension, sense of warmth as blood vessels in the skin dilate, depressant effect on many activities of the brain, especially pain, respiration, cough and vomiting reflexes. Tolerance develops to a very marked degree and regular users may be taking dosages that would be lethal to others. Cross-tolerance and dependence for other opioids also develops. Tolerance also subsides rapidly over a few weeks of abstinence and has been associated with accidental overdoses by users. The brain seems to be very sensitive to even small doses of heroin and this may in part account for its strong dependence qualities. Users become both physically and psychologically dependent upon opioids and withdrawal effects are experienced some 4–12 hours after the last "fix". For longer-acting drugs, such as methadone, the effects may be slower in onset, less intense and of a longer duration. Therefore, users need a regular supply to avoid withdrawal. Opioid abstinence syndrome is recognized by:

1. *Psychological signs*: restlessness, irritability, agitation, depression, craving, fatigue, insomnia, malaise.
2. *Physical signs*: aching pains in muscles, bones and joints, pain and cramp in the abdomen, diarrhoea, nausea and vomiting, increase in nasal secretions, sniffing and sneezing, watery eyes, increase in salivation and bronchial fluids, sensations of hot and cold, gooseflesh, shivering and perspiration ("cold turkey"), raised blood pressure, pulse raised or lowered.

These signs and symptoms peak by the end of the second day and are mostly resolved within 3–4 days, though there may be minor discomforts for several weeks. The intensity of this unpleasant experience is difficult to evaluate. Users cite it as a major motivation to obtain further "fixes". To outsiders it appears similar to severe influenza. Subjective research found prolonged opioid use a mainly depressing and miserable experience in which the participants felt chronically unwell.

Cannabis

Cannabis is known under a variety of slang names, e.g. hash, weed, grass, ganja and dope. It comes in a variety of presentations – grass, oil, resin, leaves, blocks – and is usually smoked either on its own or with tobacco in a "joint". The effects are variable and depend upon the user's expectations, mood and the social setting. Generally, users feel more relaxed, cheerful, talkative ("laid back") and ultimately sleepy. They may also experience degrees of depersonalization and derealization. In large doses the user may experience anxiety, hallucinations and paranoid delusions, though these are rare.

There is no evidence of physical dependency and its potential for long-term harm seems minimal. It is dangerous to drive or operate machinery while under its effects. Its use is widespread in the UK – several million people have tried it apparently – and many are regular or intermittent users. It is probably one of the most widely used psychoactive drugs in the world after alcohol.

Benzodiazepines

A major mental health problem that has only recently been recognized and acknowledged. Users can become dependent upon benzodiazepines and experience withdrawal symptoms following abstinence (see p. 248).

Cocaine

Cocaine is a powerful stimulant that has a long history of misuse. It leads to feelings of great well-being and euphoria, reduces anxiety, relieves fatigue and hunger and has stimulant effects on the brain and central nervous system. These effects, and the fact that it causes little physical damage, have always made it a "high-class" drug, i.e. it is expensive and used by "top people" – stars, executives.

Cocaine leads to psychological dependency and in the increasing dosages that users need to take can be a very expensive habit to support. Cocaine is usually sniffed and repeated use ulcerates the nasal septum. It can also be taken intravenously.

A new form of cocaine, known as "crack", has recently become widespread in the USA. It is a highly refined preparation that is very potent and addictive. It can be smoked and is very cheap and plentiful. It has the potential to be a major problem in this country, too.

Solvents

Abuse of inhalants and volatile solvents is not a new problem; it is one that tends to re-emerge periodically. It involves the misuse of an extensive range of products that are easily available and in themselves are not illegal: industrial solvents, glues, paint thinners, paint removers, lighter fluid and fuel, antifreeze, petrol, aerosol propellents, hair sprays, perfumes, nail polish, etc. The effects last from a few minutes up to half an hour. The substances are poured or sprayed into a plastic bag, poured on to a rag or collar or directly inhaled. Typically, they are taken in out-of-the-way places, e.g. railway lines, river banks, disused buildings. They give rise to a transient intoxication, marked euphoria, exhilaration, light-headedness, dizziness and floating, and feelings of omnipotence. They can also give rise to intense nausea and headaches.

The primary users are adolescent boys aged 11–16, often as part of a short-term passing phase. Most stop when they can pass for 18 in pubs and start drinking alcohol. A small number progress to other forms of drug misuse. There is no evidence of physical dependency, although tolerance develops with frequent use. The solvents can cause widespread systemic damage to the lungs, liver, kidneys, pancreas, heart, bone marrow and the central nervous system. A particular risk is of sudden death due to asphyxiation, from their tongue obstructing the airway, clinging bag over their head, inhalation of vomit, or from cardiac arrest or failure. In 1982 there were 66 deaths associated with solvent abuse, in 1983 there were 77.

Barbiturates

Barbiturates are one of the most potentially dangerous drugs to misuse. They have a powerful intoxicating effect similar to alcohol and lead to widespread depression of the central nervous system. Initially, there is impairment of motor co-ordination, thought and speech are slowed down, and attention and concentration are affected. Often users stagger about in a haze until the drugs wear off or they fall asleep. In larger doses it induces coma and respiratory depression that can prove fatal, especially if taken with alcohol. Barbiturates tend to be a part of poly-drug abuse where they are taken to counter the effect of amphetamines or to cope with opiate withdrawal symptoms.

Tolerance is limited and is not much more than therapeutic dosages. An abstinence syndrome develops within 1–3 days depending upon the type of barbiturate taken. The main signs are of a rebound anxiety, restlessness, insomnia, anorexia and tremors. Users may also experience nausea and vomiting and hallucinations when falling asleep or waking. There is a risk of delirium and epileptic convulsions.

Barbiturates are usually taken orally. Some users attempt to dissolve tablets and to "mainline" the drug, often under very unhygienic conditions and with pronounced local tissue damage.

Amphetamines

Amphetamines ("speed") have a powerful stimulant effect. Users experience an increase in energy, confidence, alertness, wakefulness and a great sense of well-being or euphoria. They can move quicker, speak faster and thoughts are speeded up. There is an increase in pulse and blood pressure, pupils are dilated and there is a loss of appetite. However, when these effects wear off there is a profound sense of flatness and fatigue.

Amphetamines are usually taken orally although they can also be injected. Tolerance is very pronounced and develops rapidly. From a therapeutic dose of 5–10 mg, abusers may take 100 mg in a day. Abstinence leads to physical and psychological effects of withdrawal that are usually over in a few days. Signs include restlessness, irritability, tiredness, fatigue, depression and an increase in appetite. Taken in excess, a toxic confusional state can develop that is marked by paranoid delusions, visual and tactile hallucinations, restlessness, tension and irritability. This amphetamine psychosis takes a benign course and usually passes within a few days to 1 week.

Hallucinogens

Hallucinogenic drugs (psilocybin, mescalin and LSD) can exert powerful effects on the mental, sensory and emotional processes. They distort perception of the self, the world, colours, sounds, smells, touch, perspective and time. Thoughts may seem very profound and the person's emotions may change very rapidly. Physically, there is an increase in pulse and blood pressure, pupils are dilated and there may be a mild tremor. Some users experience muscle weakness, nausea and vertigo.

Overall, depending upon the drug, the effects may last up to 24 hours. The expectations of the user seem to be particularly important in influencing the effects. For many it is an interesting and enjoyable experience, for others it can seem like a terrifying nightmare – "a bad trip".

There is no evidence of physical dependency and the greatest risk is of the person putting themselves at harm during the "trip" due to loss of awareness of potential dangers. Some users experience "flash backs" or brief hallucinatory experiences for some weeks or months afterwards.

Designer drugs

"Designer drugs", as they are known, have been specifically designed and manufactured as equivalents to existing drugs of known pharmacological action. In this sophisticated process, some extremely powerful new drugs have been illegally produced that are literally hundreds of times stronger than known chemicals. For example, fentanyl, which is a powerful narcotic, about 100 times stronger than morphine, has been modified to make it 3000 times the strength of morphine. This can then be readily sold to narcotics' users.

These types of drugs are currently restricted to the USA, although there is no reason to believe that they will not become available in the UK. They can have some very unpleasant side-effects due to faults in production and arising from the nature of the drugs.

Unit Instructions

When you have researched the suggested references, have mastered the Unit Objectives and successfully answered the Self-assessment Questions, proceed with the Unit Written Test.

Suggested References

Anon (1987). There but for the grace. . .? *Nursing Times*, 30 December, Vol. 83, No. 51, pp. 29–30.

Blank, M. (1985). Addictive attitudes. *Nursing Times*, 27 November, Vol. 81, No. 48, p. 64.

Cameron, J. (1985). Solvent abuse in Glasgow. *Nursing Mirror*, 15 May, Vol. 160, No. 20, pp. 25–26.

Cameron, J. (1986). Hidden dangers. *Nursing Times*, 19 March, Vol. 83, No. 11, pp. 59–60.

Dally, A. (1987). Drug addiction and dependence. *In* Dally, P. J. and Watkins, M. (Eds), *Psychology and Psychiatry: An Integrated Approach*, 6th edition. Hodder and Stoughton, London.

Dalton, S. (1985). Heroin abuse. *Nursing Mirror*, 6 February, Vol. 160, No. 6, pp. 15–19.

Dixon, A. (1987). *Dealing with Drugs*. BBC Publications, London.

Gay, M. (1986). Drug and solvent abuse in adolescents. *Nursing Times*, 29 January, Vol. 82, No. 5, pp. 34–35.

Gibbs, A. (1986). *Understanding Mental Health*. Consumer's Association/Hodder and Stoughton, London.

Gillies, D. and Lader, M. (1986). *Guide to the Use of Psychotropic Drugs*. Churchill Livingstone, Edinburgh.

Hodgkinson, L. (1986). *Addictions*. Thomson's Publishing Group, Wellingborough.

Hoffman, F. G. (1975). *A Handbook on Drug and Alcohol Abuse. The Biomedical Aspects*. Open University Press, Milton Keynes.

Hughes, J. (1986). *An Outline of Modern Psychiatry*, 2nd edition. John Wiley, New York.

Kohn, M. (1986). The virus in Edinburgh. *New Society*, 2 May, Vol. 76, No. 1218, pp. 11–13.

Lyttle, J. (1986). *Mental Disorder: Its Care and Treatment*. Baillière Tindall, London and San Diego.

McKerlie, L., Hodgson, A., McCulloch, K. and MacDonald, A. (1983). Solvent abuse. *Nursing Mirror*, 14 December, Vol. 157, No. 24, Community Forum 10 (ii)–(iv).

MacLennan, A. (1986). Taken over by heroin. *Nursing Times*, 12 February, Vol. 82, No. 7, pp. 45–47.

Madden, J. S. (1984). *A Guide to Alcohol and Drug Dependence*, 2nd edition. John Wright, Bristol.

Merrill, E. (1986). *Sniffing Solvents*. PEPAR Publications, Birmingham.

Morton, A. (1983). Transitory thrills or lasting lows. *Nursing Mirror*, 14 December, Vol. 157, No. 24, Community Forum 10 (viii).

Morton, A. (1984). The nurse addict – a state of emotional bankruptcy? *Nursing Mirror*, 22 August, Vol. 159, No. 6, pp. 16–20.

Parker, H., Bakx, K. and Newcombe, R. (1986). Heroin and the young. *New Society*, 24 January, Vol. 75, No. 1204, pp. 142–143.

Patterson, M. A. (1979). Addictions and neurolectric therapy. *Nursing Times*, 29 November, Vol. 75, No. 48, pp. 2080–2083.

Peers, I. S. (1981). *Solvent Abuse: Educational Implications*. TACADE, Manchester.

Phillips, K. (1986). Neonatal drug addicts. *Nursing Times*, 19 March, Vol. 83, No. 11, pp. 36–38.

Power, R. (1988). Drug scenes. *New Society*, 4 March, Vol. 83, No. 1314, pp. 15–17.

Reed, M. T. (1983). The dependent nurse. *Nursing Times*, 19 January, Vol. 79, No. 3, pp. 12–13.

Silverstone, T. and Turner, P. (1982). *Drug Treatment in Psychiatry*, 3rd edition. Routledge and Kegan Paul, London.

Standing Committee on Drug Abuse (1986). *AIDS: How Drug Users Can Avoid It*. SCODA, London.

Stimson, G. (1986). Off the peg drugs. *New Society*, 7 February, Vol. 75, No. 1206, pp. 224–225.

Terrance Higgins Trust (1986). *Facts about AIDS for Drug Users*. Terrance Higgins Trust, London.

Trethowan, W. and Sims, A. (1983). *Psychiatry*, 5th edition. Baillière Tindall, London and San Diego.

Watson, J. (1987). *Solvent Abuse: The Adolescent Epidemic*. Croom Helm, London.

Willis, J. (1976). *Clinical Psychiatry*. Blackwell Scientific, Oxford.

Woollatt, B. (1984). Changes in drug dependency. *Nursing Times*, 21 November, Vol. 80, No. 47, p. 61.

Note: Readers are advised to refer to Unit 6.2 for references on benzodiazepine dependency.

Self-assessment Questions

SAQ 9. List six factors associated with drug misuse and dependency.

SAQ 10. Identify four routes of administration and their potential for harm.

SAQ 11. Describe four characteristics of physical and psychological dependency.

SAQ 12. Outline the effects of four drugs that are commonly misused.

Unit 14.3: Written Test

You have been invited to a local sixth form college to give a talk on "Drug Dependency and Drug Misuse". As part of your talk you have been asked to cover a number of areas in relation to the sixth formers' syllabus. These topics include:

- factors that are associated with drug misuse and dependency;
- the nature of physical and psychological dependency; and
- commonly misused drugs, and their potential for harm and dependency.

Describe briefly the details that you would need to include in each area to ensure that the sixth formers are well-informed.

Care and Treatment of the Person with Drug-related Problems

Unit Objectives

At the end of this Unit the learner should be able to:

1. Describe the range of therapeutic interventions used to help the person with drug-related problems.
2. Outline the interventions required to help a person withdraw from dependency producing drugs.
3. Identify the support required for the person and their family in the community.
4. State factors associated with the therapeutic outcomes for drug-related problems.

Care and Treatment

A wide range of therapeutic interventions may be used to help the person with a drug-related problem. These may focus on both the presenting symptoms and the person's life-style and coping skills. The specific interventions will depend upon the assessment undertaken by the therapist, the resources available and the client's motivation. A key factor in any treatment programme is the client's willingness to accept that they have a drug-related problem and their motivation to adopt a drug-free or minimal harm life-style.

Also, the client must feel that the therapists are accepting, non-judgemental and hopeful. The general approach should be towards developing an integrated and readily accessible service that is able to support the person and their family in the community or in residential settings as appropriate.

Therapeutic aims

1. To minimize the extent of any harm and distress.
2. To enable the person to safely overcome their dependency.

3. To facilitate the development of the person's and their family's coping skills.

Family and Self-care

Drug-related problems, from minor to severe difficulties, directly affect many people. For each individual who misuses drugs there are many more family members, friends and work-mates who are also likely to experience the negative consequences of a drugs-related problem.

The many users of soft drugs who control their intake are unlikely to suffer much harm. Taking their drugs in very circumscribed situations and company, their low profile habit can remain undetected indefinitely. There is evidence, too, that not all users of hard drugs are necessarily severely harmed. Some heroin addicts are able to remain employed and to lead a satisfactory family life. The main factors in minimizing harm for such users are being able to support their habit financially, having access to a regular source of supply and sterile administration (if injected).

Others, however, may experience far more destructive consequences. Initially, using drugs for "kicks" or to promote group acceptance, they may find that their need becomes more pervasive and demanding. What was taken originally for pleasure has to be taken in order to avoid the unpleasant effects of withdrawal. Their peer group, too, may advocate the excessive and indiscriminate use of potentially harmful substances.

At this stage of dependency others cannot but fail to notice. What may initially have been perceived as a "troubled adolescence" or a "phase that they are going through" becomes viewed in a very different way. Families can be torn apart in the desperate and frustrating struggle to try and understand why a member is taking drugs and to get them to stop. Arguments, threats, broken promises, lying and stealing may become part of everyday life. All may suffer in this process as the user visibly declines physically, mentally and socially.

Life for the user becomes a constant struggle to finance their habit, obtain further supplies and avoid arrest. Living a rootless and miserable existence they may be driven to desperate lengths to support their habit. Despite the high costs of dependency they rarely regard themselves as needing help and bitterly resent any intrusion.

In some cases the individual may be able to acknowledge that they have a problem and seek help and support from voluntary or other agencies that deal with drug-related problems. Families may be able for a short while to enforce abstinence or to force an adolescent to have treatment. However, such coercion is rarely effective in the long-term. Often an individual may have suffered quite severe harm before they can accept that they have a problem and are able to acknowledge that they need help.

Initially, the person and their family can be helped considerably in coping with drug-related problems by:

1. Accurate information about drug-related problems.
2. Involvement in the care and treatment process.
3. Reassurance that effective intervention is possible.
4. The opportunity to talk freely about their problems.
5. The address of local contact support groups.
6. Developing the person's and family's coping skills.
7. Reviewing their life-style and expectations to promote their mental health.

Community Care

The majority of people with drug-related problems do not actively seek help. They attempt in their own way to deal with the problems they experience. Most people with drug-related problems can be successfully treated and cared for in the community. This will depend upon the person's motivation, the support available to them, the severity of their symptoms and the community resources available. Clients with drug-related problems tend to prefer non-residential treatment. The aims of community care are:

1. To support the person and their family.
2. To monitor the person's mental and physical health.
3. To facilitate withdrawal and prolonged abstinence.
4. To implement community-based treatment and care programmes.

The services available include:

1. The community mental health centre: with community psychiatric nurses, social workers, psychologists, occupational therapists and consultant psychiatrists working as a team to offer skills-based therapeutic interventions.
2. Local drug advice and counselling centres: a centre or resource base from which a team of multidisciplinary health care workers who specialize in drug-related problems are based. They can usually offer both domiciliary and centre-based therapeutic programmes. The centre may be run by the health district, local authority or voluntary agencies often working in close collaboration. Some centres work specifically with certain client groups, e.g. Solvent Abuse Centres.
3. Voluntary agencies: Narcotics Anonymous, Release, DAWN (Drugs Alcohol Women Nationally), Families Anonymous, Citizen's Advice Bureaux, local contact and support groups. The voluntary sector in relation to drugs-related problems is not well-developed. Only one group, Narcotics Anonymous, currently offers a national network. Other drug-related agencies tend to operate on a local level.
4. Social services: personal and family social workers.
5. General practitioners.

6. Educational welfare services: educational psychologists, school nurses, youth workers.
7. Legal agencies: police, juvenile courts, probation and after-care services.
8. Out-patient clinics and day hospitals: in drug treatment centres or attached to a psychiatric hospital.
9. Needle and syringe exchanges; conditional upon; use of this facility may be people receiving counselling and treatment. Some centres offer non-conditional and readily accessible service. May be operated from counselling centres, pharmacists, clinics etc.

Residential Care

People with drug-related problems are not popular clients with most generic treatment centres. They tend to do better in specialist treatment centres where expert help is available and they have the peer support of other users. Residential care may be indicated where there is:

1. A lack of support in the community.
2. Personal and family exhaustion.
3. The need for specialized treatment programmes and therapy.
4. The need for detailed physical assessment where the person is experiencing, or at risk of, the physical complications of chronic drug misuse.

The residential settings may include:

1. Regional or local drug treatment clinics specializing in drug-related problems and their treatment.
2. Psychiatric unit or hospital.
3. Therapeutic communities that specialize in helping people with drug-related problems. These may be run by health authorities or by voluntary or private agencies, e.g. Broadreach House, Phoenix House, Suffolk House, Blenheim Project, Concept House.

Therapeutic Goals

The preferred goal in the treatment of drug misuse and dependency is complete and permanent abstinence. However, this requires a high degree of motivation and cooperation from drug users that they may find difficult. Many users are convinced that they will never be able to give up their drugs and are appalled by the prospect of not being able to continue their habit. As a consequence, they often do not seek treatment or participate reluctantly. As with most therapeutic programmes the client's commitment is crucial.

Another more controversial approach used in narcotic dependency is that of maintenance: the medical supply of their drug to the user. The advantages are that the person does not have to rely on illegal sources, does not have to resort to criminal activities to finance their habit and can be stabilized on a monitored dose. During maintenance, efforts can then be made towards improving the user's mental and physical health in the hope that abstinence can become a realistic objective.

The Misuse of Drugs Act 1971 requires that all doctors must notify the Home Office Central Register of any person whom they consider or suspect is dependent upon cocaine, diamorphine, opium, pethidine, morphine or related drugs. Only specially licensed doctors are able to prescribe these drugs; other doctors must refer any person who requires these drugs to a specialist treatment centre.

Therapeutic Interventions

Withdrawal and abstinence

Withdrawal for those who are dependent or a period of abstinence for those who misuse drugs is a main feature of most treatment approaches. This may be required at the commencement of therapy or at a suitable stage when the user's trust and commitment have been gained. Most people require a lot of careful preparation for this process, or else they may abruptly leave therapy.

The initial aim is to help the person to cope with the psychological and physical effects of withdrawal or abstinence and to resist any craving or temptation for further supplies of their drug. The first psychological signs of abstinence – restlessness, irritability, tension, anxiety, preoccupation, desire for the drug – may be experienced from the start of withdrawal. The period and extent of discomfort will depend upon the drug they have been misusing, the period of misuse and their commitment to succeed. The physical signs shown will depend upon the nature of the drug that they have been misusing, the dosages taken and the period of misuse.

With careful management and, where appropriate, the use of specific medication, both the physical and mental distress of withdrawal can be minimized and completed within a few days. Chronic minor withdrawal symptoms may be experienced for up to 6 months as the body and person gradually adapt to a drug-free life-style. In reality, short periods of abstinence and withdrawal may be relatively easy to attain. The difficulty is in trying to minimize the very high risk of subsequent relapse.

Withdrawal may be carried out either in a residential or community setting. The main considerations are the person's commitment, the resources and support available and the person's safety. The advantages of residential settings are that the person is removed from an environment that could be actively reinforcing their drug-taking and that the transfer of responsibility on to others helps to reduce their craving. Also, very close monitoring is possible and skilled intervention is available for any serious complications. Particular caution has to be taken when dealing with people who are dependent upon barbiturates as there is a risk of severe epileptic fits.

A successful withdrawal or abstinence programmes requires:

1. *Preparation* of the person and others who may be providing support. Contact with others who have successfully overcome their dependency and written information may be useful.
2. *Health* education on the nature of withdrawal and the symptoms they are likely to experience.
3. *Supervision* to restrict access to their drug and to monitor the person's safety.
4. *Reassurance*: empathy, acceptance, trust, non-judgemental perspective.
5. *Medication* where appropriate. This may include:

   • Tranquillization: using minor tranquillizers to reduce anxiety and tension and to overcome some of the stress of withdrawal. The drugs used and the dosages will depend upon clinical judgement.
   • Substitution and gradual withdrawal of drugs with a similar chemical action (see Chemotherapeutic interventions, p. 607).
   • Antagonists that block the effects of the misused drug and minimize the physical effects of withdrawal (see Chemotherapeutic interventions, p. 607).

Psychotherapeutic approaches

1. *Skilled nursing care*: one of the most important therapeutic factors in residential settings. A number of CPNs also work as clinical specialists with people who have drugs-related problems in the community.
2. *Individual counselling and psychotherapy*: to increase insight and promote understanding of their motivation to misuse drugs. To develop more effective coping skills.
3. *Group therapy*: to increase insight and self-awareness, to share personal experiences, to provide opportunities for social learning.
4. *Self-help*: to share difficulties and strategies for problem solving, to provide empathy, support and non-judgemental acceptance.
5. *Family or couple's therapy*: to enable couples to be more supportive and to communicate more effectively, to help the family to find ways of coping with the problems caused by drugs, to rebuild damaged relationships.
6. *Social skills and assertiveness training*: to promote confidence and self-esteem. Helps to increase feelings of personal control and mastery after a period when many have felt at the mercy of their dependency or need for drugs.
7. *Anxiety management and relaxation skills*: the consumption of drugs is often related to feelings of stress and anxiety. Learning anxiety management skills helps to increase personal control and reduce the need for drugs as an anxiolytic.
8. *Contract therapy*: negotiating on a therapeutic programme that is confirmed as a "contract" with rewards for compliance and penalties for non-compliance.

9. *Milieu therapy/therapeutic community*: in which residents are given a high degree of control over the care environment and have to take full responsibility for their actions. Reality confrontation, peer support and the development of more mature and realistic attitudes are a prominent part of this approach.
10. *Hypnotherapy*: appears to help some people.
11. *Art therapy and psychodrama*: to help express and release feelings, to promote insight.
12. *Occupational therapy*: to develop life skills.
13. *Recreational and social activities*: to meet social needs, overcome isolation and to provide positively rewarding experiences. Of particular importance may be the need to develop a new drug-free social network.
14. *Acupuncture or electroacupuncture*: the mode of action is uncertain. Practitioners claim that it encourages the release of natural endorphins in the brain that have a similar effect to heroin. There also appears to be a significant psychological effect. For some clients this approach has been very effective.

Chemotherapeutic interventions

Methadone

Methadone has a similar chemical effect to that of heroin or related opioids. It is given in oral form by licensed doctors as a substitute for these drugs and is used in the following ways:

1. *Maintenance*: the dependent user is supplied with methadone in order to avoid the necessity of the person using illegal sources. They can also be monitored and offered counselling services.
2. *Reduction programmes*: where the methadone is given in gradually decreasing dosages over a short period of time (often 10–21 days) in order to wean the person off opioid-type drugs. This approach helps to minimize the distressing effects of withdrawal. Small dosages of methadone may be given with clonidine, an efficient opiate antagonist, to reduce the effects of withdrawal.

Opiate antagonists

Certain drugs act as antagonists to opiates and are able to block their effect without any dependency forming properties themselves. They need to be used under medical supervision as there is a small risk of hypotension. Otherwise, they have relatively few other side-effects. Naltrexone and clonidine can be used in combination to suppress the withdrawal effects of heroin and other opiates with the worst symptoms passing within 2–3 days.

On the first day of therapy, within 24 hours of the last dose of opiates, the person is given 10–20 mg of naltrexone every 4 hours. On the second day 25–50 mg is given depending upon the response. Each of these doses is preceded by 0.1–0.4 mg of clonidine. By the third day the person is given the normal daily dose of 50 mg naltrexone. This is often taken, for example, as 100 mg on Mondays, Wednesdays and Fridays. Once the person is established on the full dose of naltrexone the physical symptoms of withdrawal quickly fade. By this stage the naltrexone can be safely withdrawn itself.

Physical Care and Treatment

Physical health problems may exist as a direct result of the effects of the drug upon the body, the route of administration, impurities, unhygienic administration, malnourishment and personal neglect. The physical care and treatment required will depend upon an assessment of the person's physical health care needs. Interventions may include:

1. Withdrawal and abstinence: to prevent further harm.
2. Dietary correction: well-balanced diet with roughage and vitamin supplements.
3. Attention to personal hygiene.
4. Rest.
5. Specific interventions, where required:

   - treatment for abscesses or other tissue damage;
   - physiotherapy for damaged muscles and tendons;
   - antibiotics for systemic infections;
   - infection control measures where acute hepatitis B or AIDS is suspected or confirmed.

Health Education and Drug Misuse

Drug misuse is a major public health problem. The dilemma is how to present messages that can both dissuade people from taking drugs without increasing their awareness on how to misuse them. Health education programmes have become more explicit and direct, especially since the added threat of AIDS. However, these approaches are not without their critics, who often complain that the message is too negative or mistargeted upon potential risk groups.

The primary health education messages are concerned with increasing awareness about the potential danger of drug misuse and how to recognize their effects. Attempts have been made to identify those at most risk and to direct health education programmes at them, particularly among schoolchildren.

The Prevention of Drug Misuse

The problem of drug misuse involves a large number of social agencies as it is more than just a health care problem. The steps needed include:

1. *Health education*: nationally and aimed at specific risk groups.
2. *Medical education*: to reduce indiscriminate prescription of potentially harmful drugs.
3. *Medical control*: to limit the practitioners who can legally prescribe potentially harmful drugs.
4. *Security*: of chemists' premises, health centres, GPs' surgeries.
5. *Customs*: to detect the large number of drugs smuggled into this country.
6. *Police*: to detect those who illegally manufacture, distribute and deal with drugs.
7. *Legal penalties*: to deter those who engage in criminal activities, e.g. sequestration of assets, periods of imprisonment.

Therapeutic Outcomes

The outcomes will depend upon a variety of factors, including the user's motivation, the specific drugs being misused, the route of administration, social environment and the support available. Abstinence is more likely where there is:

- short-term use,
- non-injection rather than injection of drugs,
- contact with relatives and good social integration.

Within such a diverse group of users and potential drugs to misuse it is difficult to generalize about outcomes. What is important to always bear in mind is that it is possible, though by no means easy, for people who have been dependent upon drugs to give them up and lead a drug-free life. There is much professional and client pessimism about this.

Those who remain dependent, particularly upon injected narcotics, have a reduced life expectancy and a high risk of mortality from accidental overdoses or physical health complications. It is estimated that the mortality rate for this group is about 19 per 1000 per year. The longer-term impact of AIDS upon those who inject drugs is likely to be significant.

Various studies based upon differing client groups, patterns of drug misuse and length of review find differing outcomes. Long-term studies indicate that the figures tend to be in the range:

- 40–50% not known to be using drugs,
- 25–30% still using drugs,
- 25% died.

Unit Instructions

When you have researched the suggested references, have mastered the Unit Objectives and successfully answered the Self-assessment Questions, proceed with the Unit Written Test.

Suggested References

Blank, M. (1986). Hannah's family. *Nursing Times*, 18 March, Vol. 83, No. 11, pp. 61–62.

Brewer, C. (1986). Tailor made for the job? *Nursing Times*, 27 August, Vol. 82, No. 35, pp. 42–43.

Carr, J. (1987). An injection of common sense. *Nursing Times*, 17 July, Vol. 83, No. 24, pp. 19–20.

Childs-Clarke, A. and Cottrell, D. (1984). An 11-year follow-up of drug clinic attenders. *Nursing Times*, 12 December, Vol. 80, No. 20, pp. 52–53.

Cohen, D. (1986). Hope for heroin addicts. *Nursing Times*, 9 April, Vol. 82, No. 15, p. 40.

Dally, A. (1987). Drug addiction and dependence. *In* Dally, P. J. and Watkins, M. (Eds), *Psychology and Psychiatry: An Integrated Approach*, 6th edition. Hodder and Stoughton, London.

Dixon, A. (1987). *Dealing with Drugs*. BBC Publications, London.

Dobson, M. (1984). Responding to problem drug users. *Nursing Times*, 21 November, Vol. 80, No. 47, pp. 57–58.

Donnellan, V. and Agerholm, L. (1984). Care in the community. *Nursing Times*, 21 November, Vol. 80, No. 47, pp. 58–60.

Faugier, J. (1985). Money well spent? *Nursing Times*, 10 July, Vol. 81, No. 28, p. 56.

Gibbs, A. (1986). *Understanding Mental Health*. Consumer's Association/Hodder and Stoughton, London.

Hase, S. and Douglas, A. (1986). *Human Dynamics and Nursing*. Churchill Livingstone, Melbourne.

Hoffman, F. G. (1975). *A Handbook on Drug and Alcohol Abuse. The Biomedical Aspects*. Open University Press, Milton Keynes.

Hughes, J. (1986). *An Outline of Modern Psychiatry*, 2nd edition. John Wiley, New York.

Laurence, J. (1987a). Racketeer or rescuer? *New Society*, 23 January, Vol. 79, No. 1256, pp. 18–19.

Laurence, J. (1987b). The happy addict. *New Society*, 24 April, Vol. 80, No. 1269, pp. 9–10.

Lyttle, J. (1986). *Mental Disorder: Its Care and Treatment*. Baillière Tindall, London and San Diego.

Madden, J. S. (1984). *A Guide to Alcohol and Drug Dependence*, 2nd edition. John Wright, Bristol.

Merrill, E. (1986). *Sniffing Solvents*. PEPAR Publications. Birmingham.

Morton, A. (1983). Ronnie's story. *Nursing Mirror*, 14 December, Vol. 157, No. 24. Community Forum 10 (vi)–(vii).

Patterson, M. A. (1979). Addictions and neurolectric therapy. *Nursing Times*, 29 November, Vol. 75, No. 48, pp. 2080–2083.

Platt, S. (1986). Kicking the habit – and staying off. *New Society*, 11 April, Vol. 76, No. 1215, pp. 17–18.

Robertson, R. (1987). *Heroin, AIDS and Society*. Hodder and Stoughton, London.

Sadler, C. (1984). Breaking down the barrier. *Nursing Mirror*, 14 March, Vol. 158, No. 11, pp. 21–24.

Stimson, G. (1985). Can a war on drugs succeed? *New Society*, 15 November, Vol. 74, No. 1194, pp. 275–277.

Trethowan, W. and Sims, A. (1983). *Psychiatry*, 5th edition. Baillière Tindall, London and San Diego.

Willis, J. (1976). *Clinical Psychiatry*. Blackwell Scientific, Oxford.

Self-assessment Questions

SAQ 13. List five problems that the family may experience as a result of drug misuse by a teenage member.

SAQ 14. Outline four interventions that can help a user safely withdraw from drug dependency.

SAQ 15. Select four psychotherapeutic interventions for drug misuse and describe their role in treatment.

SAQ 16. Describe briefly how methadone and opiate antagonists can be used in the treatment of heroin withdrawal.

Unit 14.4: Written Test

Robert Harris, aged 27, has a long history of drug misuse and dependency. He has taken a broad range of drugs and is currently "mainlining" heroin. He has suffered severe social, mental and physical harm from drugs. In the past, Robert has had repeated contact with little success with a wide range of voluntary and statutory treatment services. Short-term abstinence was invariably followed by relapse and further damage.

Following the recent death of his long-term girlfriend from an accidental overdose, Robert has come to his local drug treatment centre for help. He appears to be highly motivated and states that his only options are to "get out or die".

Describe the range of therapeutic interventions that may be helpful in resolving Robert's dependency upon heroin and in facilitating a drug-free life-style.

UNIT 14.5

Nursing Care of the Person who is Dependent upon Drugs/Alcohol

---

Unit Objectives

At the end of this Unit the learner should be able to:

1. Identify the nursing care needs of a person who is dependent upon drugs/alcohol.
2. Plan an individualized care programme.
3. Select appropriate nursing care interventions for the person's needs.
4. Describe possible evaluation criteria for specific needs.

Mental Health Nursing Care

Each person's care needs are unique and have to be assessed individually. For the client who abuses or is dependent upon drugs or alcohol a wide range of potential needs may be identified. These will depend upon the nature of the substances being misused, the period of misuse, the harm suffered and their current difficulties. It is also possible that the person may have other physical health care problems as a result of their dependency. A range of potential care needs have been selected to illustrate some of the problems that the person may experience and the potential nursing interventions that may help them.

For the person who is dependent upon alcohol or drugs these may include the needs to:

A. Acknowledge the harmful effects of their dependency.
B. Overcome their dependency.
C. Promote their physical health.
D. Facilitate the development of the person's and family's coping skills.

A. Acknowledge the Harmful Effects of Their Dependency

Associated problems/personal difficulties

Person with dependency problems may have difficulty acknowledging the harmful effects of substance misuse shown by:

1. Denying and rationalizing any harmful consequences experienced as a result of dependency.
2. Blaming others and life circumstances for any difficulties.
3. Insisting that dependency can be halted whenever the abuser desires.
4. Anger and defensiveness at suggestions that the substance is potentially harmful.
5. Inability to accept the need to stop or reduce patterns of misuse.
6. Ambivalent attitudes towards therapy.

Assessment

1. Person's perception of the consequences of their dependency.
2. Information from relatives and friends.
3. Nurse's observations of the person's:

   (a) Response to questioning about their dependency.
   (b) Understanding and awareness of motivation to abuse substances.
   (c) Accuracy of knowledge about potential harm arising from substance abuse.
   (d) Concerns expressed about the future: positive, negative, hopeful, pessimistic
   (e) Emotional condition: anxious, depressed, guilt, helplessness, low self-esteem.
   (f) Descriptions of attempts to limit intake of substance and their effectiveness.
   (g) Expressed desire to abstain or limit substance misuse: degree of motivation and realism

4. History of substance abuse: when and how they started, types of substances taken, frequency and quantity, route of administration.
5. Role of substance in person's life: supportive, peer group, key relationships, personal identity.
6. Previous attempts to attain abstinence and factors contributing to relapse.
7. Identifiable physical harm arising from substance abuse.
8. Identification of potential stresses in the person's life situation and lifestyle.

Desired outcomes

1. Person able to acknowledge the harmful consequences of dependency.
2. Person able to accept the need to restrict substance misuse.
3. Person able to acknowledge the benefits of abstinence/harm reduction.

Nursing intervention	Rationale
1. Initiate therapeutic relationship. Involve the person in the care planning process	Interventions more likely to succeed in an atmosphere of trust and cooperation
2. Be available and approachable. Demonstrate non-judgemental responses. Demonstrate acceptance	Need to develop trust in order to work effectively with client and to create the conditions for behavioural change. People who are dependent are very sensitive to implied criticism
3. Promote feelings of security and freedom from threat (see Unit 6.3, pp. 251–255)	If the person feels insecure they will tend to be defensive and distrustful
4. Advise that seeking help and recognition of problems are a positive step towards finding solutions	May feel that seeking help is a sign of weakness and failure. Helps to reduce guilt
5. Reassure that there are ways of improving the situation	May feel trapped in pattern of dependency and that the situation is hopeless
6. Introduce to people who have successfully acknowledged the harm of substance dependency/misuse	May believe that it is impossible to give up their dependency. High source credibility from people who are making progress in therapy
7. Explore with the person the effects of their dependency upon themselves and others	Person may not be aware of how their dependency is influencing their own life and that of others
8. Explore with the person reasons for criticisms by others and stress in relationships	Person may not be aware of why others may perceive them in a negative way. This also influences how they perceive others

Nursing intervention	Rationale
9. Identify if the person has experienced any sexual difficulties since commencing substance misuse	Sexual problems often arise following substance misuse
10. Explain relationship between sexual problems and drug misuse	Person may not realize that there is a link
11. Explore with person reasons for recurring problems related to habituation	Person may not be willing or able to associate persistent difficulties with dependency or substance misuse
12. Encourage the person to identify specific harmful consequencs arising as a result of dependency	May not be fully aware or willing to accept that their dependency is harmful. Many people who have dependency/misuse problems find this difficult to do
13. Assist the person to recognize the association of negative or harmful experiences and dependency habituation	Tend to project blame on everything else rather than their dependency. Need to promote and demonstrate the relationship between substance misuse and personal harm
14. Inform the person, as required, of the harmful consequences that can arise from substance misuse/ dependency. Correct misinformation. Explain the need to achieve abstinence/ reduced intake in order to halt further harm	Person may be misinformed or have inadequate knowledge base about the potential harm from substance misuse/ dependency. Need to emphasize the health care advantages of halting/ limiting substance misuse
15. Advise person on the health benefits of abstinence/restricted substance misuse	Person may not be aware of the potential for restoring their health. May perceive a substance-free life as negative and unstimulating
16. Instruct the person in how to keep a diary or "log" of their pattern of substance misuse and associated factors	A record of specific details – where, when, how much, situation, place, etc. – provides useful information. The ability to keep this record and to begin to identify related factors is an important start to regaining control and promoting insight

Nursing intervention	*Rationale*
17. Assist person to identify environmental factors that contribute to their dependency	Person may be unaware of factors that are contributing towards and maintaining their dependency. Promotes understanding and insight into their dependency
18. Encourage the person to modify environmental factors, where possible, that are contributing to dependency	Modification of these factors may help in the initial steps towards abstinence/control. Helps to promote an understanding of the relationship between environment, life-style and dependency
19. Identify and give feedback on person's inappropriate defence mechanisms concerning substance misuse/dependency	May not be aware of the defences that they habitually use to ward off threats and to protect their integrity
20. Differentiate between realistic and unrealistic perceptions of their difficulties	Many people who misuse substances have very unrealistic expectations about the future role of alcohol/drugs in their life. Many wish to continue with their substance dependency and will find all sorts of excuses to continue
21. Challenge distorted perceptions and expectations	The person who is dependent constructs very powerful and effective defences that need to be challenged if they are to be overcome
22. Positively reinforce reality-based perceptions of their dependency problems	Helps to reinforce and promote a realistic perception of their dependency problems
23. Encourage the person to accept the need to limit/stop substance misuse	This is one of the most fundamental requirements for the successful resolution of dependency problems. Frequently, they will admit the need to abstain to others while not accepting it themselves
24. Arrange for own clinical supervision	Working with people who have dependency problems can be very demanding. They tend to have very elaborate defences and are resistant to change. The therapist will need guidance and support during their client contact

Nursing intervention	*Rationale*
25. Organize experiential exercises, e.g. drama, role play, games, in which the person relates to others in an unstructured way and can express themselves freely	Structured and spontaneous experiential exercises can provide powerful feedback and personal learning opportunities. Specific exercises can be used to promote insight

Evaluation

1. Person can state the benefits of abstinence/controlled use.
2. Person complies with therapeutic programme.
3. Person demonstrates motivation towards establishing a drug-free or harm reduction life-style.

B. Overcome Their Dependency

Associated problems/personal difficulties

Person may be experiencing problems in relation to their dependency due to:

1. A continuous, overwhelming desire for the effects of the substance.
2. The development of withdrawal symptoms following abstinence.
3. Difficulty in moderating their use of substances.
4. Feelings of hopelessness and helplessness in overcoming their habituation.
5. The harmful physical consequences of substance misuse.
6. Disruption to patterns of everyday living.
7. Psychological harm and stress arising from dependency.

Assessment

1. Information from relatives and friends.
2. Person's description of their dependency/misuse:

   (a) Specific substances misused: potential for habituation, degree of tolerance, dependency forming characteristics.
   (b) Frequency and pattern of use: daily, weekends, evenings, mornings.
   (c) Quantity/dosage taken: as far as can be ascertained.

(d) Rate of use: quantity taken within a specified time.
(e) Route of administration: oral, injection, smoked, sniffed.
(f) Place where substance is taken: openly taken, secrecy, public, private.
(g) Social situation and others present: condone, encourage, negative responses, friends, other activities.
(h) Physical and psychological effects of substance on person: relief, joy, "high", duration of effects.

3. History of misuse/dependency:

(a) When person first used substances: who introduced them, initial expectations and effects.
(b) Reasons for taking substance: social, experimentation.
(c) Onset of tolerance and withdrawal: early experiences and reaction.
(d) Experience of physical, social and psychological harm: identifiable physical harm, damage to relationships, effects on occupation, debt.
(e) Person's description of effects of withdrawal: cognitive, behavioural, physical, emotional, intensity, duration of reaction.

4. History of previous attempts to reduce or cease substance use: coping methods used and their effectiveness, factors that contributed towards abstinence and subsequent relapse, periods of time able to abstain.
5. Current motivation to overcome dependency or limit use: realistic or unrealistic expectations, positive and negative factors.
6. Potential reinforcers of dependency behaviour: peer group, social circumstances, identifiable triggering cues.
7. Presence of potential stresses in person's environment and life-style.

Desired outcomes

1. Person is able to control their desire for substance.
2. Person is able to overcome their dependency/misuse of substance.
3. Person is able to maintain a substance-free harm-reduction life-style (as appropriate).

Nursing intervention	Rationale
1. Initiate therapeutic relationship. Involve person and family in the care planning process	Interventions more likely to succeed in an atmosphere of trust and cooperation. This promotes compliance

Nursing intervention	*Rationale*
2. Demonstrate active listening. Be available and approachable. Minimize role barriers. Offer reassurance. Demonstrate acceptance and non-judgemental responses	Helps to reduce tension and to create the conditions for behavioural change. Facilitates the development of a therapeutic relationship. Likely to be very sensitive to implied criticism. May cause them to reject help
3. Promote feelings of personal security and safety (see Unit 6.3)	Person needs to feel secure in order to overcome dependency. Often substances are used to enhance feelings of personal security
4. Promote attainment of physical health care needs (see C.)	Physical health needs to be optimized to promote personal comfort and well-being, which also reinforce the benefits of abstinence
5. Introduce to people, if possible, who have successfully overcome their dependency and misuse	Many people who are dependent or misuse substances believe that abstinence/controlled use is impossible. They feel trapped, hopeless and helpless. Former users are able to demonstrate that success is possible. They can be a useful source of information and support that has a high credibility
6. Explain the objectives of the therapeutic programme. Ask for feedback and check the person's understanding. Correct misunderstandings	Person needs to be aware of these in order to participate actively and to understand the purposes of therapeutic interventions
7. Explain the difficulties they may encounter in attempting to overcome their dependency	Person needs to be aware of the difficulties that they may face in order to prepare and cope with them effectively
8. Differentiate between realistic and unrealistic expectations	Many people who misuse substances have unrealistic expectations about the future role of drugs in their life. Often they want only short-term help and intend to return to substance misuse after their immediate crisis is resolved. Many are ambivalent about their commitment and find it hard to envisage a substance-free or harm reduction life-style

Nursing intervention	*Rationale*
9. Explore with the person methods of overcoming the desire for the substance. Identify which approaches are most suitable for client's needs	Person may not be aware of the range of options open to them. Increases hope and motivation
10. Supply written material to support verbal information	Person can refer to this
11. Educate the person on the psychological and physical effects of abstinence	Person's own understanding may be inaccurate or faulty
12. Explain that craving is most intense during early phases and will gradually decrease in intensity and frequency as abstinence continues	Prepares person for the experience and encourages hope. Reinforces to person that they can regain mastery and control
13. Support self-initiated ideas and positive attempts to maintain abstinence or regain control of dependency	Personal initiatives should be rewarded and supported
14. Make a contract with the person to abstain from substance misuse during initial stages of therapeutic programme	Need to establish a short-term substance-free interval in order to proceed to either abstinence or controlled use as appropriate
15. Advise person and relatives on the need to abstain from substance misuse during withdrawal/ detoxification	May attempt to obtain further supplies in the mistaken belief that the periodic use of the substance during this time will do no harm
16. Observe for physical and psychological signs of withdrawal. Give feedback to the person on these signs to facilitate insight and understanding	Person may not be aware of how their behaviour and emotions are affected by withdrawal. Can use this experience to facilitate learning

Nursing intervention	*Rationale*
17. Observe for continued abstinence during detoxification/ withdrawal. Ensure others do not supply alcohol/drugs to person	Person may be surreptitiously taking further supplies of the substance to overcome effects of abstinence
18. Acknowledge the difficulty and efforts made by person to overcome their dependency	Overcoming a dependency requires considerable effort and motivation. Person needs this feedback to maintain their motivation
19. Help person to identify factors that contribute towards misuse and dependency. Help person to modify, where possible, factors that contribute towards dependency/ misuse	Problems of misuse and dependency tend to exist in an environmental context in which the person's relationships and life-style may be actively involved in maintaining habituation
20. Give feedback to the person on their progress in overcoming dependency	To the person this period may seem endless and they may not be able to identify any progress they are making
21. Encourage positive thinking about potential for success. Encourage person to remind themselves periodically about the goals of therapy	Person may feel from past experience that it will be impossible for them to resist their desire for the substance
22. Discourage preoccupation with causes and consequences of dependency	Person may dwell on past at the expense of dealing with the main present problems of overcoming dependency
23. Teach the person how to use the skills of thought-stopping to resist craving	This may prove useful for some people. Everyone who is trying to alter an established habituation finds themselves constantly preoccupied by it

Nursing intervention	*Rationale*
24. Encourage the use of alternative coping methods (see **D.**)	Person may be using the substances as an inappropriate method of coping
25. Explain the role of medication in facilitating detoxification and overcoming withdrawal. Give medication as prescribed	Important that medication is viewed as a short-term therapeutic measure and not a long-term alternative. Helps to reduce the effects of withdrawal and feelings of stress. Facilitates person overcoming despondency
26. Positively reinforce compliance with care programme	Promotes compliance
27. Teach person the skills of relaxation and anxiety management. Encourage the person to use and practise these skills	Many substances that are misused have anxiolytic properties and may be used as an inappropriate way of coping with stress. Abstinence creates tension and anxiety. Person needs to re-learn more healthy ways of dealing with stress and anxiety in their life
28. Encourage the person to talk about difficulties and to express their feelings and frustrations	Abstinence and regaining control are very stressful experiences. People need to be able to express these feelings and to reduce tension
29. Take threats of self-harm seriously. Promote safety in the care environment. Minimize risks. Alert carers to risk of self-harm. Observe for signs of potential self-harm (see Unit 7.4, **B.**)	During this stressful time feelings of hopelessness, helplessness and low self-esteem may precipitate self-harmful behaviour. Careful assessment of a person's potential for self-harm is essential as it is a real risk
30. Negotiate and set clear limits on expectations and the consequences of non-compliance. Ensure that limits are consistently	The person may become manipulative and demanding under the stress of withdrawal. Clear behavioural limits need to be maintained in order to demonstrate to the person that the carers are firm in their commitment towards the attainment of abstinence.

Nursing intervention	*Rationale*
maintained by carers. Inform the person if their behaviour is close to limits set. Explore set limits and consequences if person does not comply with stated boundaries. Provide educative feedback to person when their behaviour exceeds stated limits. Reinforce positive healthy behaviour. Negatively reinforce undesirable behaviour	More healthy ways of meeting their needs and communicating can be explored to facilitate personal growth
31. Identify and encourage participation in appropriate diversional activities	Helps to distract person from constant preoccupation and effects of abstinence.
32. Provide on-going support so that person is able to consistently maintain substance-free/limited use life-style	Overcoming problems of dependency and misuse are long-term targets. Hence long-term support is required

Evaluation

1. Person is able to maintain a period of abstinence.
2. Person successfully overcomes the effects of withdrawal.
3. Person maintains a substance-free/harm-reduction life-style (as appropriate).

C. Promote Their Physical Health

Associated problems/personal difficulties

Person with dependency problems may have physical health problems due to:

1. Neglect of personal hygiene.
2. Prolonged inadequate nutritional intake.
3. Physical stress and tension from withdrawal.
4. Effects of substances on normal body physiology.
5. Pathological effects of substances on body tissues.
6. Harm arising from route and manner of administration.
7. Primacy of dependency over physical health needs.

Assessment

1. Person's statements and behaviour in regard of meeting their physical needs.
2. Person's understanding of their physical health needs.
3. Information from relatives and friends.
4. Nurse's observations of person's:

   (a) Appearance and hygiene: maintained, neglected, adequacy.
   (b) Non-verbal behaviour indicating drug use or withdrawal: alertness, speech patterns, restlessness, agitation, perspiration, respiration.
   (c) Nutritional status: adequacy and balance of diet, evidence of weight loss.
   (d) Skin and body condition: clear, healthy looking, emaciated, bruised, cigarette burns and stains, abscesses, needle marks.
   (e) Living conditions: adequate, facilities available, homeless.

5. Route of administration: oral, injection, sniffed, smoked.
6. Source of income: state benefits, dealing with drugs, prostitution, crime.
7. Identifiable physical harm resulting from drug misuse: abscesses, infections, scarring, tissue damage, liver damage, chronic gastritis, respiratory.
8. Identifiable physical health deficits: nutritional, rest and sleep.
9. Results of medical investigations: blood tests, urine tests, liver and renal function.
10. Presence of potential stresses in person's environment and life-style.

Desired outcomes

1. Person able to identify own physical health care needs.
2. Person can acknowledge the importance of maintaining physical health.
3. Person able to acknowledge the relationship between substance abuse and their physical health.
4. Person's physical discomfort during withdrawal is minimized.

Nursing intervention	Rationale
1. Initiate therapeutic relationship. Involve the person in the care planning process	Interventions more likely to succeed in an atmosphere of trust and cooperation
2. Evaluate the person's understanding of their physical health care needs. Provide accurate information. Clarify any misunderstandings	Person may have inaccurate or unrealistic expectations in relation to physical health needs
3. Negotiate with the person a programme to meet their physical needs	Structure helps to give guidance and to ensure that minimum physical health care needs are met
4. Specify requirements for nutrition, hygiene, elimination and rest	Also serves a useful educational purpose
5. Advise the person and relatives on the importance of meeting physical health needs	May not be aware of these needs or their role in health promotion. Many people with dependency/misuse problems experience chronic malaise and poor physical health
6. Encourage person to acknowledge the relationship between physical harm and substance misuse/dependency (see **B**.)	Person may not be able to relate substance misuse to the experience of physical harm
7. Encourage person to accept the need to stop/limit substance misuse to promote physical health	Person needs to be aware of the need to stop/limit substance abuse to maintain physical health
8. Monitor compliance with programme to meet physical health care needs. Positively reinforce compliance with programme	Programme needs to be consistently implemented to promote physical health effectively
9. Advise person to inform carers if experiencing distress or discomfort	Important that person feels able to communicate any problems to carers

Nursing intervention	Rationale
10. Encourage person to talk about any difficulties experienced	Helps to relieve tension and enables carers to monitor closely signs that may not be readily observable
11. Observe for physical signs of withdrawal	Person may be experiencing signs that they do not associate with withdrawal. Need to observe and monitor progress of withdrawal in case of serious complications, e.g. fits, collapse
12. Monitor vital physical signs if indicated by nature of person's dependency	Depending upon the nature of the person's dependency and their health care needs, a wide range of observations may be indicated to monitor the person's health, e.g. pulse, blood pressure, temperature
13. Give medication as prescribed to overcome physical effects of withdrawal	Tranquillizers, substitutes or antagonist drugs may be prescribed depending upon the substance's misuse. They are a short-term measure to minimize physical withdrawal symptoms
14. Give medication as prescribed for physical health care problems	A wide range of physical health care problems may be present, e.g. vitamin deficiencies, anaemia, infections, constipation, diarrhoea
15. Take action to relive physical feelings of stress and tension (see Unit 6.3)	The process of withdrawal can be a very stressful experience. Reducing stress and tension helps the person to overcome this and to reduce the need for medication to be used. Can also be used to facilitate the development of the person's ability to relax
16. Promote the maintenance of personal hygiene	Person may have neglected their hygiene for some time. Also promotes physical comfort
17. Ensure that personal hygiene facilities are available	Personalized items are more likely to be used by person
18. Encourage the person to take an interest in their appearance. Provide positive feedback on their appearance	Person may have neglected their appearance for some time. Also promotes self-esteem
19. Advise people who inject substances on the particular risks associated with this	Injection of substances that are misused carries particular risks. Needles and syringes may be non-sterile, substances may be impure or

Nursing intervention	*Rationale*
route of administration. Advise people who inject substances on the need to maintain sterility. Emphasize the importance of not sharing own or using other people's needles and syringes	adulterated with harmful substances, equipment may be shared with other users. Apart from systemic and local damage there is a particular risk of hepatitis B and a growing risk of AIDS
20. Take necessary hygiene precautions where person is suspected of having a contagious infection arising from dependency. Advise relatives on the precautions that need to be taken	If the person is suspected of having hepatitis B or AIDS, then carers will need to take particular precautions to avoid the risk of infection
21. Assist the person to formulate new budgeting habits giving priority to nutrition and to accommodation	People who are dependent often spend their income on drugs/alcohol rather than on the physical necessities of life
22. Identify food preferences. Monitor dietary and fluid intake. Ensure person takes a balanced diet. Weigh periodically. Encourage person to eat. Monitor for feelings of nausea or loss of appetite. Promote oral hygiene. Monitor elimination.	Important to re-establish healthy eating patterns. Person may have problems of anorexia or nausea during withdrawal that make it difficult for them to eat. May have neglected oral hygiene. Irregular diet and effects of substances misused can disrupt bowel activity resulting in diarrhoea or constipation
23. Give nutritional supplements as prescribed	Person may require supplements to compensate for prolonged malnutrition
24. Advise person on approaches to improve sleeping (see Unit 6.3)	Sleeping disturbances are common as a result of withdrawal

Nursing intervention	Rationale
25. Advise on the need to avoid excessive tea, coffee or cigarettes	High levels of caffeine or nicotine may be habitually used to help cope with withdrawal. Howver, these also can produce physical dependency and increase feelings of agitation and restlessness.
26. Monitor person's physical health status	Need to monitor person's health care progress
27. Provide feedback to person on attainment of physical health needs	Person may not be aware of the progress that they are making in meeting their physical needs

Evaluation

1. Person is able to meet own physical health care needs unaided.
2. Person is able to acknowledge the importance of maintaining their physical health.
3. Person's physical discomfort during withdrawal is minimized.

D. Facilitate the Development of the Person's and Family's Coping Skills

Associated problems/personal difficulties

The experience of misuse and dependency problems may indicate that:

1. Existing methods of coping may be counterproductive and adding to existing stress.
2. Current life-style, expectations and relationships may be potential sources of stress and reinforcing misuse/dependency.
3. Patterns of misuse/dependency may be causing personal and relationship problems.
4. Person and their family may lack information about the resources available to them.
5. There may be feelings of guilt in relation to their problems and asking for help.
6. Person may reject outside help even though under stress.

Assessment

1. Person and family's perception of their current difficulties.
2. Existing coping methods used and their effectiveness.
3. Role of misused substances in person's life.
4. Support available to the person and family.
5. Accuracy of the knowledge and information given by the person and their family.
6. Statements of guilt and stigma.
7. Awareness of resources available to them.
8. Previous experience, if any, of dealing with similar problems.

Desired outcomes

1. Person and family able to make an informed choice about the resources they require.
2. Person and family able to cope better with life and personal problems.
3. Person able to cope with difficulties without using drugs/alcohol.

Nursing intervention	Rationale
1. Initiate therapeutic relationship. Involve person in the care planning process	Interventions more likely to be successful in an atmosphere of trust and cooperation
2. Advise that seeking help and recognition of problems are a positive step towards finding solutions	Many people feel that seeking help is a sign of weakness and failure. Also helps to reduce guilt
3. Encourage questions. Provide accurate information. Identify appropriate health care resources	May have inaccurate knowledge and expectations. Need to know what resources are available to them
4. Advise against early correction of problems	Many problems associated with drug misuse tend to be long-term in nature. Under stress it is sometimes easier to make short-term compromises that only store up future problems. It will take time to help those involved to work out what is best for them
5. Reassure that there are ways of improving the situation	Person and family may feel that the situation is hopeless
6. Advise against recrimination and focussing on past problems	Need to focus on the present and future and to deal with anger and guilt in a more productive way

Nursing intervention	*Rationale*
7. Advise on the need for acceptance and mutual support within their relationship. Advise the family on how to give feedback and support to one another	Family needs to come to terms with their situation. They are each other's primary source of support which will need to be utilized to cope effectively
8. Explore the role of the substances in the person's life and life-style	Substances that are misused have a central role in the person's life that needs to be explored and understood
9. Explore with the person ways in which their life-style contributes towards their drug and alcohol misuse. Identify with the person changes which are necessary to help overcome dependency/misuse. Support person in the implementation of these changes	Long-term patterns of misuse become integrated into a person's life-style. For them to overcome their problems of misuse/dependency often requires a complete change of life-style. This is a major change that many find very difficult to implement
10. Encourage the setting of progressive goals in small stages	The changes that the person may need to make need to be done gradually to facilitate readaptation
11. Identify potential risk situations with person that may precipitate drug misuse	Person needs to be able to recognize these situations in order to prepare how to deal with them
12. Explore with the person strategies for dealing with risk situations	Person needs to develop a wide range of strategies in order to deal with potential situations that may arise
13. Promote their self-esteem	Long-term misuse can readily damage a person's self-esteem. Often the substance becomes a source of esteem in its own right, from having a social life and friendships built around it. Person needs to develop more healthy sources of esteem
14. Develop the person's assertiveness. Role play situations in which the person can develop and be given feedback on these skills	Alcohol and drugs are often used to enhance confidence and to give "Dutch courage". Person needs to practise these skills, particularly in refusing drinks or alcohol, in order to promote control/abstinence
15. Explore with the person more appropriate means of need gratification	Misused substances become the person's major source of pleasure against which other sources may appear insignificant. Need to refocus person's perceptions towards more healthy means of need gratification

Nursing intervention	*Rationale*
16. Teach how to use problem-solving methods for coping with difficulties	Long-term dependency/misuse tends to lead to a narrowing of coping strategies
17. Recommend more appropriate ways of coping with stress and anxiety in the person's life (see Unit 6.3)	Substances are frequently used to cope with anxiety and stress. The person needs to develop more healthy alternative ways of coping
18. Assist the person to acknowledge the influence of their expectations and perceptions in maintaining their patterns of misuse/dependency. Differentiate between realistic and unrealistic expectations	Person may be perceiving the world in an unrealistic and immature way that influences their patterns of drug misuse. Long-term drug misuse also distorts how users both see themselves and the outside world
19. Help person to develop more realistic and attainable expectations. Encourage acceptance of self-limitations	Need to develop more realistic and attainable expectations that are self-fulfilling. Unrealistic goals cause frustration and are likely to lead to failure
20. Encourage the setting of realistic goals and expectations in overcoming problems of drug misuse	Many people who misuse substances have unrealistic expectations about overcoming their drug misuse. Many want the incompatible goals of continued patterns of misuse and minimal harm
21. Review occupational/unemployment stresses. Encourage the development of appropriate work/non-work related coping strategies	Work and unemployment can be major sources of stress. They are frequently implicated in dependency/misuse problems. It is important that the person learns how to cope with these stresses constructively.
22. Teach the family and person to recognize the limits of their ability to cope and when it is advisable to seek help	The family should not over-burden itself as this can damage relationships and its longer-term ability to cope
23. Put person and family in contact with self-help and voluntary groups	Self-help groups are able to offer effective and understanding help. Have high credibility in helping clients with misuse/dependency problems
24. Emphasize that relapse should not be regarded as failure	Relapse may be interpreted by the person that freedom from drug use is impossible and that seeking further help is useless. Need to stress that it is a short-term setback from which something can be learned to prevent future relapses

Nursing intervention	*Rationale*
25. Provide long-term support to person. Ensure person knows how to contact agencies if experiencing an alcohol/drug problem in the future	Problems of drug misuse tend to be long-term. Need to ensure that adequate support is available and accessible to person

Evaluation

1. Person and family able to identify their health care needs.
2. Person and family identify and select resources they require.
3. Person and family demonstrate use of improved coping methods.
4. Person able to maintain an abstinent harm reduction life-style.

Unit Instructions

When you have researched the suggested references, have mastered the Unit Objectives and successfully answered the Self-assessment Questions, proceed with the Unit Written Test.

Suggested References

Altshul, A. and McGovern, M. (1985). *Psychiatric Nursing*, 6th edition. Baillière Tindall, London and San Diego.

Barker, P. J. (1982). *Behaviour Therapy Nursing*. Croom Helm, London.

Barker, P. J. (1985). *Patient Assessment in Psychiatric Nursing*. Croom Helm, London.

Bauer, B. B. and Hill, S. S. (1986). *Essentials of Mental Health Care Planning and Interventions*. W. B. Saunders, Philadelphia.

Briggs, K. and Stewart, A. (1987). *Case Studies in Mental Health Nursing*. Churchill Livingstone, Edinburgh.

Campbell, C. (1978). *Nursing Diagnosis and Intervention in Nursing Practice*. John Wiley, New York.

Dally, P. and Watkins, M. J. (1986). *Psychology and Psychiatry: An Integrated Approach*, 6th edition. Hodder and Stoughton, London.

Darcy, P. T. (1985). *Mental Health Nursing Source Book*. Baillière Tindall, London and San Diego.

Dexter, G. and Wash, M. (1986). *Psychiatric Nursing Skills: A Patient-centred Approach*. Croom Helm, London.

Estes, N. J., Smith-Dijulio, K. and Henemann, M. E. (1980). *Nursing Diagnosis of the Alcoholic Person.* C. V. Mosby, St. Louis.

Hargie, O. and McCartan, P. J. (1986). *Social Skills Training and Psychiatric Nursing.* Croom Helm, London.

Hase, S. and Douglas, A. J. (1986). *Human Dynamics and Nursing.* Churchill Livingstone, Melbourne.

Irving, S. (1983). *Basic Psychiatric Nursing,* 3rd edition. W. B. Saunders, Philadelphia.

Lancaster, J. (1980). *Adult Psychiatric Nursing.* Henry Kimpton, London.

Lyttle, J. (1986). *Mental Disorder: Its Care and Treatment.* Baillière Tindall, London and San Diego.

McFarland, G. and Wasli, E. (1986). *Nursing Diagnoses and Process in Psychiatric Mental Health Nursing.* J. B. Lippincott, Philadelphia.

MacLennan, A. (1986). Taken over by heroin. *Nursing Times,* 12 February, Vol. 82, No. 7, pp. 45–47.

Martin, P. (1987a). *Psychiatric Nursing: A Therapeutic Approach.* Macmillan, London.

Martin, P. (1987b). *Care of the Mentally Ill,* 2nd edition. Macmillan, London.

Minardi, H. (1986). One day at a time. *Nursing Times,* 5 March, Vol. 82, No. 10, pp. 34–36.

Pelletier, L. (Ed.) (1987). *Psychiatric Nursing Case Studies, Nursing Diagnoses and Care Plans.* Springhouse Corporation, Springhouse, Pennsylvania.

Pope, B. (1986). *Social Skills Training for Psychiatric Nurses.* Harper and Row, London.

Priestly, P., McGuire, J., Flegg, D., Hemsley, V. and Welham, D. (1978). *Social Skills and Personal Problem Solving.* Tavistock, London.

Robinson, L. (1983). *Psychiatric Nursing as a Human Experience,* 3rd edition. W. B. Saunders, Philadelphia.

Royal College of Nursing (1986). Nursing guidelines on the management of patients in hospital and in the community suffering from AIDS.

Simmons, S. and Brooker, C. (1986). *Community Psychiatric Nursing: A Social Perspective.* Heinemann Nursing, London.

Ward, M. F. (1985). *The Nursing Process in Psychiatry.* Churchill Livingstone, Edinburgh.

Ward, R. (1983). A prisoner of herself. *Nursing Mirror,* 27 July, Vol. 57, No. 4. Mental Health Forum 7, pp. iii–v.

Self-assessment Questions

SAQ 17. Outline four interventions that may facilitate a person acknowledging that they have a dependency problem.

SAQ 18. List six interventions that can help a person overcome their dependency.

SAQ 19. Identify four factors that need to be assessed in order to evaluate a person's physical health status.

SAQ 20. Describe four interventions that may help a person and their family to improve their coping skills.

Unit 14.5: Written Test

Jonathan Long, aged 27, has a long history of drug and alcohol abuse. He has suffered considerable harm and yet he seems reluctant to acknowledge any relationship between his alcohol and drug intake and his current problems. He has been unemployed for 4 years and relies on the proceeds of petty crime to supplement his benefits and to buy his drugs and alcohol. He is currently living in a squalid bed-sit that he shares with his girlfriend who also drinks excessively and takes drugs.

At present he is an in-patient in an acute care ward in a psychiatric unit following an accidental overdose of heroin. He appears to have adapted well to hospitalization and is already able to manipulate cigarettes and some money out of the other residents.

1. Describe in detail how you would encourage Jonathan to acknowledge the harmful effects of his dependency and drug misuse.
2. What nursing interventions may prove useful in enabling Jonathan to resist his constant desire to take more heroin and overcome the effects of withdrawal?
3. How can Jonathan be helped to break out of his pattern of misuse and to adopt healthier alternative coping methods?

TOPIC 15

Eating Problems

At the end of this Topic the learner should aim to:

1. Describe factors associated with the onset of eating problems.
2. Differentiate between anorexic and bulimic eating patterns.
3. Outline the range of therapeutic interventions available.
4. Identify the nursing care needs and interventions required for the person with an anorectic eating pattern.

The Origins and Recognition of Eating Problems

Unit Objectives

At the end of this Unit the learner should be able to:

1. Outline the influence of upbringing, gender and body image in eating problems.
2. Describe factors associated with the onset of eating problems.
3. Identify the behavioural characteristics of anorexia and bulimia.
4. List the physical consequences of prolonged nutritional abuse.

Social and Psychological Factors in Diet and Nutrition

We live in a society where most people are able to meet their basic nutritional requirements. However, the activities and perceptions involved in eating involve far more complex processes than merely meeting our physiological needs. Food has a powerful symbolic value both to the individual and to the family. Time, effort and care are invested in the preparation and choice of food and strong expectations exist as to how the food should be prepared and eaten.

People develop highly personalized preferences and habits in regard to their diet and can react strongly if these are interfered with in any way. The way we choose to eat is also an expression of both our personality and of our autonomy. Having control and feeling secure about our food intake are very basic needs.

Meal-times often act as a focus for family life and relationships. Strong feelings can be expressed or implied from the way that food is accepted or rejected. Food in its various forms is often used as an incentive for children who may be rewarded by sweets etc. for parentally desired behaviour. Children are also rewarded for eating all of their food at meal-times. Conversely, the witholding of "treats" or refusal to eat can also be used as a way of expressing displeasure, anger or frustration. Refusal can evoke very strong feelings of guilt and anxiety in parents who may find themselves being manipulated by a determined child.

Food can also take on other symbolic uses in everyday life. The strong feelings of oral gratification that arise from eating mean that food can also be used as a "comforter" in times of stress. In the short term it can relieve feelings of anxiety or loneliness and act as a distraction for persistent worries. Additionally, the purchase and eating of specially favoured foods can be used as a means of self-reward when external social reinforcement is lacking.

Gender and Culture

Food has a special significance for women. Within the stereotyped role of the "woman" or "mother" is usually an assumption that they will be responsible for the purchase and preparation of food. It is potentially a powerful source of emotional exchange and her success as a "woman" or "mother" may be judged upon her ability to meet these demands.

It is especially significant that within our culture the majority of sufferers from food disorders are women. Women within Western culture are brought up to be very aware of their physical shape and appearance. Very powerful images are continually projected of what is defined as the desirable female body shape. Typically, this is of a slim narrow-hipped, sometimes large-breasted woman who appears to be physically perfect in every respect. Men focus very readily upon such images and the sexually attractive woman is expected to comply with this anatomically atypical type. Nonetheless, many women feel a need to comply with this image if they are to appear attractive to men. Dissatisfaction with their own body shape, low physical self-esteem and chronic dieting are a way of life to many women, who strive unsuccessfully to achieve this unattainable goal.

Body Image and Mental Health

We all develop an internalized awareness of our own body. From sensory feedback, visual feedback, the comments of others, comparison with those around us and media images, we judge how much our body conforms to the "normal". The larger the perceived difference between our own "body image" and the way that we think we should be, the greater the sense of dissatisfaction. Even small differences between our physical appearance and what we perceive as desirable, can generate powerful negative feelings and stress.

Satisfaction with our body image is also important in the development of self-esteem and social confidence. People who are dissatisfied with their body image tend to be self-conscious and insecure. Efforts can then be made, where possible, through clothing, cosmetics, dieting, exercise and social strategies, to manipulate the presentation of their body image to maximum advantage. If necessary, aids, prostheses or cosmetic surgery may be necessary to facilitate a more secure body image.

The Origins of Eating Problems

A number of theories have been proposed to attempt to explain the onset and maintenance of disordered eating patterns. Alongside the theoretical perspectives, a number of more practical explanations have also been offered. These include:

1. *Early childhood eating difficulties*: in which the eating of food was used to manipulate and reward, setting a precedent for later life.
2. *Family and parental stress*: depression in the mother, broken home, divorce, separation. Conflicts over autonomy and independence. In some situations the person may become the focus of such stress within the family.
3. *Sexual abuse as a child*: causing profound loss of self-esteem, guilt, extreme problems of psychosexual development.
4. *Extreme perfectionism on the part of the person*: such that their own attainments and life itself are profoundly disappointing. This can be especially frustrating and cause low self-esteem if the person is also unable to live up to high family expectations.
5. *Psychosexual regression or conflict*: the starvation is viewed as an attempt to resist the physical development of secondary sexual characteristics. The sufferer has often made a poor sexual adjustment.
6. *Distorted body image*: in which the person perceives themself to be grossly overweight despite visual feedback and comments from others that affirms their actual size. Hence vigorous dieting is pursued despite obvious malnutrition.
7. *Feeling of not being in control of their own lives*: a passive perception of control in which others make decisions for them, direct their lives and where they have little influence. The rigid dietary regime is seen as an attempt to regain control over at least some part of their life and to develop their self-esteem from this control.
8. *Stressful life events*: examinations, prolonged physical illness, bereavement, starting a new school, separation from family.
9. *Social class*: the majority of sufferers would appear to come from the middle and upper classes. This may be due to a variety of explanations such as high expectations to achieve or affluence, or it may be more related to the recognition of the anorexia. There would appear to be an increase in the incidence of anorexia from people of a working-class background.
10. *Dieting*: the person initially diets as an attempt to lose weight. However, the dieting apparently gets out of control and is pursued despite the harmful consequences. There is often a history of weight problems and dieting in other family members.

Mental Health and Eating Problems

In mental health practice nutritional deficits or excesses may be seen as a consequence of other emotional, behavioural or cognitive disorders. When people become distressed their appetite frequently suffers. However, there are two mental health problems in which the person's behaviour and perceptions significantly involve their eating habits, their self-perception and related behaviour. These are

- anorexia nervosa, and
- bulimia nervosa.

Anorexia Nervosa

Anorexia nervosa is the medical term used to describe an eating pattern characterized by the person's:

1. Pathological drive to lose weight despite potentially harmful physical consequences.
2. Behaviour and strategies adopted to promote and disguise their weight loss.
3. Distorted body image of themselves and their distorted attitudes towards food and eating.

Anorexia often begins with the person pursuing a rigorous diet in order to lose weight. Initially, this may be triggered off by growing self-consciousness about their body size and weight or for being teased for being plump. Often, too, there is a background of family stress, pressure on the person to achieve high standards or the experience of loss.

The dieting is pursued with a fanatical drive well beyond the needs of just losing excess weight. The early experience and success of weight loss acts as a powerful reinforcement to continue dieting. During this period the person appears to undergo a significant psychological shift. Their motivation to lose weight becomes all consuming and despite their falling weight and evident thinness they persist in perceiving themself as being grossly overweight.

As they continue to lose weight successfully their behaviour becomes more secretive and a range of strategies are adopted to facilitate further dieting. The behavioural changes are intended to both increase their rate of weight loss and to ensure that their thinness is hidden from others. It is significant at this stage that the person is aware that others would intervene to prevent further weight loss and would react in alarm at the person's emaciation if it were recognized.

Periodically, they may be overcome by extreme hunger, which for much of the time they are able to suppress. This may result in bingeing of large amounts of easily ingested food. Invariably, this is followed by feelings of self-disgust and shame at having "given in". To reassert control and to minimize the risk of weight gain the person might begin vigorous exercise or attempt to purge themselves by self-induced vomiting or laxative abuse.

The anorexic pursues their dieting even at the risk of serious physical consequences. In the longer term they may begin to experience the physical effects of starvation and nutritional deficits. They are at risk of literally starving themselves to death despite the ready availability of food. Some 5–10% of anorexics die from starvation or from related physical complications despite medical intervention.

The person is often remarkably successful at hiding their weight loss from their family. Others may identify that the person seems "tense" or "difficult" in some way and be quite shocked to discover the degree of emaciation. For some sufferers the anorexia becomes a way of life and they may pursue their dieting and vomiting for many years, maintaining a perilous balance between survival and starvation.

As a mental health problem anorexia nervosa occurs primarily in young women from middle- and upper-class families. The incidence of anorexia in males would appear to be increasing but the current ratio of female to male is approximately 10 to 1. The clinical incidence of anorexia is difficult to establish as it is estimated that only half of those affected actually seek professional help. A number of cases appear to be self-limiting and the person makes a spontaneous recovery. Whether the incidence of anorexia is actually on the increase or whether recognition of potential cases has improved is difficult to establish.

The diagnosis of anorexia is made when the person is identified as having the characteristic behavioural and psychological patterns associated with the condition. Physical illness, depression, schizophrenia and hypothalamic lesions have to be excluded.

Psychological characteristics of anorexia nervosa

1. *Morbid fear of weight gain*: the person is terrified of becoming overweight. Even their normal weight may arouse feelings of tension and panic.
2. *Distorted body image*: the person grossly overestimates their body size, seeing themself as enormously fat despite visual evidence to the contrary. They may spend excessive periods of time gazing at their reflection in mirrors.
3. *Denial of having an eating disorder*: the person cannot see what all the fuss is about and rejects any notion that they have a problem. They may state that they have "never felt better".
4. *Fear of losing control*: the person has a constant struggle to control their hunger. They live in fear that they will lose control and eat an excessive amount of food. This creates constant stress and tension. Periodically, the urge to eat becomes overpowering and the person binges excessive amounts of food. Such episodes are invariably followed by guilt and purging.
5. *Distorted perception of food*: all food is seen as potentially fattening, far in excess of its calorific content.
6. *Narrowing of interests*: attention becomes exclusively focussed on their diet. Other interests are neglected.

7. *Guilt and loss of self-esteem*: the deceptions and secrecy involved in excessive weight loss often result in feelings of shame and depression. Combined with feelings of helplessness and hopelessness there may be a risk of self-harm.

Behavioural strategies of the anorexic person

1. *Very strict dieting*: avoidance of fattening foods, food "fads", bizarre diets. All intake, including fluids, is very strictly regulated. The person is obsessed with food calories and recipes and gains a vicarious pleasure from watching others eat food that they have prepared themselves.
2. *Missing meals*: getting up later to miss breakfast, going out early in the evening, pretending to have eaten while out, avoiding eating with others.
3. *Eating very slowly*: taking a long time at meals, covering food with salt or vinegar to prevent eating too much, cutting the food up very small and moving it around the plate, chewing the food excessively.
4. *Secretly disposing of food*: emptying food into bins when others not looking, giving food to others, putting food into pockets, handbag, etc.
5. *Wearing loose clothes*: to disguise the extent of the weight loss, to present a loose, flowing body outline.
6. *Excessive concern with privacy*: avoiding situations or activities in which they might have to show their body. Obsessive privacy in the home.
7. *Laxative abuse*: to speed up weight loss and excretion of food from the body. Excessive quantities may be secretly taken.
8. *Self-induced vomiting*: to regurgitate recently eaten food. This may form part of a strategy, whereby they can appear to eat normally in front of others and can secretly induce vomiting afterwards. With repeated practice the person is readily able to vomit rapidly without noticeable distress.
9. *Excessive activity and exercise*: to increase weight loss, to show that they are alright to others, to divert attention from food. Housework and cooking may form part of these activities which tend to be positively reinforced by the family.

Physical effects of prolonged starvation in anorexia nervosa

1. *Severe emaciation and weight loss*: this may be life-threatening unless the person returns to normal eating habits. May also be chronically dehydrated.
2. *Mild hypothermia*: constantly feeling cold despite warm weather or thick clothing. This is due to the loss of subcutaneous fat from under the skin.
3. *Low blood pressure and a slow pulse*: as a consequence of starvation. The person may also suffer from giddiness and ankle oedema.
4. *Chronic diarrhoea and/or constipation*: from lack of roughage in diet and prolonged abuse of laxatives.
5. *Lanugo hair*: a fine downy growth of hair on the back and arms. This is a consequence of prolonged starvation.
6. *Damage to teeth enamel*: from the effects of stomach acid due to frequent

self-induced vomiting.
7. *Sleep disturbance*: this is directly related to the degree of weight loss. As the person's weight is restored their sleep improves.
8. *Hair, skin and nails*: dry, brittle and deteriorated condition. A yellow tinge may be seen in the hands that is specific to anorexia.
9. *Cessation of menstruation*: menstruation often ceases prior to the attainment of significant weight loss. This is thought to be due to psychological stress. Amenorrhoea is then maintained by starvation and does not return until some 75% of ideal body weight is regained. Menstruation may, however, continue if the person is on oral contraception.

Bulimia nervosa

Bulimia nervosa has only recently been recognized as a separate eating pattern from anorexia with which it shares certain characteristics. In particular, the cycles of bingeing and vomiting which are characteristic of bulimia are also found in anorexia, and a number of bulimics go on to develop anorexia. Bulimia nervosa is characterized by:

1. *Powerful and uncontrollable urges to eat which precipitate periodic excessive bingeing of food*: enormous quantities of easily ingested food are consumed until the person is full, nauseated, discovered or the urge diminishes. Binges are often triggered by stress, tension, loneliness or having eaten "forbidden" foods. The eating initially represents a comfort and coping method which becomes an uncontrollable urge. Strategies may be developed to try and cope with these urges, e.g. diversion, driving, not keeping food in the house, taking exercises, telephoning someone.
2. *Action to prevent weight gain*: to regain control and to avoid weight gain the binge is often followed by self-induced vomiting or by consumption of enormous quantities of laxatives. In this way the person can keep their weight within normal limits despite frequent bingeing. Often the sufferer also pursues other strategies to keep their weight under control, e.g. strict dieting, exercise, fasting.
3. *Strategies to avoid detection*: the binges take place in secrecy and the person attempts to avoid detection. Strategies are developed to cope with social situations in which the person is required to eat in public. Food may be hoarded in advance of any intended binge. Deception may be required to account for the large sums of money that may be involved. Often the person will visit different shops to disguise the amount that they are buying or make excuses that they are buying for friends or a "party".
4. *Guilt and loss of self-esteem*: the deceptions involved and the shame over the binges often result in depression, self-condemnation and a loss of self-respect. Underlying these feelings is a morbid fear of becoming fat.

Sufferers are predominantly female. They tend to be slightly older than those with anorexia and 25–50% have a past history of anorexia. About 20% also abuse alcohol and drugs. This pattern of eating is apparently much more common than previously realized and it is estimated that a minimum of 1–2% of young women are affected. One-quarter of sufferers are married. The real incidence is probably much higher as bingeing, vomiting and laxative abuse appear to be quite widespread, if somewhat episodic practices, among teenage women. Most people with this behaviour pattern would probably not recognize themselves as having an eating disorder. The potential long-term physical consequences of bulimia include hypokalaemia, fits, cardiac arrhythmias, renal damage, menstrual irregularity and acute dilatation of the stomach.

Unit Instructions

When you have researched the suggested references, have mastered the Unit Objectives and successfully answered the Self-assessment Questions, proceed with the Unit Written Test.

Suggested References

Abraham, S. and Llewellyn-Jones, D. (1984). *Eating Disorders: The Facts.* Oxford University Press, Oxford.

Aniskowitz, S. (1984). Anorexia nervosa. *Nursing Mirror*, 11 April, Vol. 158, No. 15, pp. 42–43.

Beard, P. (1984). A cry for help. *Nursing Mirror*, 5 September, Vol. 159, No. 8, pp. 27–28.

Brown, M. S., King, C. N., Kleeman, K. and Short-Tomlinson, P. (1977). *Distortions in Body Image in Illness and Disability.* John Wiley, New York.

Chudley, P. (1986). An unhealthy obsession. *Nursing Times*, 26 March, Vol. 82, No. 13, pp. 50–52.

Crisp, A. H. (1980). *Anorexia Nervosa: Let Me Be.* Academic Press/Grune and Stratton, London and San Diego.

Dally, P. (1981). Treatment of anorexia nervosa. *British Journal of Hospital Medicine*, May, Vol. 25, No. 5, pp. 434–440.

Dally, P. and Gomez, J. (1979). *Anorexia Nervosa.* Heinemann Medical, London.

Dexter, J. M. (1980). Anorexia nervosa. *Nursing Times*, 21 February, Vol. 76, No. 8, pp. 325–327.

Gibbs, A. (1986). *Understanding Mental Health.* Consumer's Association/Hodder and Stoughton, London.

Gibson, E. (1983). Body talk. . .anorexia nervosa. . .a plea for a more humane approach. *Nursing Times*, 16 February, Vol. 79, No. 7, p. 64.

Goffman, E. (1961). *Stigma.* Penguin, Harmondsworth.

Ho, E. (1985). Anorexia nervosa in pregnancy. *Nursing Mirror*, 24 April, Vol. 160, No. 17, pp. 40–42.

Hughes, J. (1986). *An Outline of Modern Psychiatry*, 2nd edition. John Wiley, Chicester.

Jones, S. L., Doheny, M. O., Jones, P. K. and Bradley, N. (1986). Binge eaters: A comparison of eating patterns of those who admit to bingeing and those who do not. *Journal of Advanced Nursing*, Vol. 11, No. 5, pp. 545–552.

Lyttle, J. (1986). *Mental Disorder: Its Care and Treatment*. Baillière Tindall, London and San Diego.

Melville, J. (1986). When you can't stop eating. *Self Health*, September, No. 12, pp. 13–14.

Orbach, S. (1979). *Fat is a Feminist Issue*. Hamlyn, London.

Orbach, S. (1986). *Hunger Strike*. Faber and Faber, London.

Palmer, R. L. (1980). *Anorexia Nervosa. A Guide for Sufferers and Their Families*. Penguin, Harmondsworth.

Potts, N. L. (1984). The secret pattern of binge/purge. *American Journal of Nursing*. January, Vol. 84, No. 1, pp. 32–35.

Price, B. (1986). Mirror, mirror on the wall. . . *Nursing Times*, 24 September, Vol. 82, No. 39, pp. 30–32.

Sanger, E. and Cassino, T. (1984). Avoiding the power struggle. *American Journal of Nursing*. January, Vol. 84, No. 1, pp. 31–33.

Sims, A. (1988). *Symptoms in the Mind*. Baillière Tindall, London and San Diego.

Slade, R. (1984). *The Anorexia Nervosa Reference Book*. Harper and Row, London.

Snaith, P. (1981). *Clinical Neurosis*. Oxford University Press, Oxford.

Thompson, S. (1979). Hungry for knowledge – not food. *Nursing Mirror*, 12 July, Vol. 75, No. 28, p. 29–32.

Torrance, C. and Milligan, S. (1985). Boning up on exercise. *Nursing Times*, 23 October, Vol. 81, No. 43, p. 38.

Trethowan, W. and Sims, A. (1983). *Psychiatry*, 5th edition. Baillière Tindall, London and San Diego.

Waskett, C. (1983). Disordered eating patterns. *Nursing Times*, 22 June, Vol. 79, No. 25, p. 72.

Waskett, C. (1986). A weight off your mind. *Nursing Times*, 26 March, Vol. 82, No. 13, pp. 48–49.

Wells, B. (1983). *Body and Personality*. Longman, London.

Willis, J. (1976). *Clinical Psychiatry*. Blackwell Scientific, Oxford.

Self-assessment Questions

SAQ 1. Describe four factors associated with the onset of eating problems.
SAQ 2. Outline six characteristics of anorexia nervosa.
SAQ 3. List six consequences of long-term malnutrition.
SAQ 4. Identify four characteristics of bulimia nervosa.

Unit 15.1: Written Test

Janet Seddon, aged 15, has been brought by her distraught parents to the health centre after they had suddenly discovered the extent of their daughter's self-induced weight loss. In the last 6 months she has lost 10 kg through dieting and now weights 43 kg. They had become suspicious at her evasiveness about her food intake and her obsession with privacy.

It was only by accident that they discovered her inducing vomiting after a meal and physical examination showed her to be far thinner than they had realized.

The GP has referred Janet to you for a mental health assessment.

1. What observations and information would confirm that Janet's eating behaviour was anorexic in origin?
2. What factors in Janet's upbringing and home life may have led to the development of anorexia?
3. What are the physical signs and symptoms of prolonged malnutrition?

Care and Treatment of the Person with an Eating Problem

Unit Objectives

At the end of this Unit the learner should be able to:

1. Describe how sufferers and their families attempt to cope with an eating problem.
2. Identify the support required for the person and their family in the community.
3. Outline the range of therapeutic interventions for helping the person with an eating problem, both in the community and in residential settings.

Care and Treatment

A wide range of therapeutic interventions may be used to help the person with an eating problem. The interventions are concerned with both the physical consequences of prolonged disordered eating patterns and the underlying psychological disorder. There is no specific treatment as such for anorexia or bulimia nervosa. A broad range of therapeutic approaches are used to promote insight in the sufferer and to enable them to readjust to normal eating patterns. The general approach should be towards an integrated and readily accessible service that is able to support the person and their family in the community and in residential care as required.

Therapeutic aims

1. To enable the person to re-establish healthy eating patterns.
2. To correct the physical consequences of prolonged disordered eating patterns.
3. To facilitate the development of the person's and their family's coping skills.

Family and Self-care

Research surveys appear to confirm that the prevalence of disordered eating patterns is far higher than had previously been recognized. These indicate that health care agencies are perhaps only dealing with some 50–80% of people with anorexia and a much smaller percentage of those with bulimic eating patterns. Other worrying statistics are the high percentages of young teenage girls who:

- express high levels of dissatisfaction with their body image;
- periodically use self-induced vomiting or laxatives to regulate their weight.

A significant number of people with anorexia are only brought into contact with health care agencies when the sufferer has lost a high percentage of their body weight. This would indicate that the person has successfully avoided detection and that other family members have failed to recognize the significance of the weight loss or changes in the person's behaviour.

Initially, the person's attempts to diet may be actively reinforced by other family members who may even have their own weight problems. The experience of weight loss is intensely rewarding and the feedback from this motivates the person to pursue their diet with even more vigour. The person's preoccupation with food and the vicarious pleasure they get from watching others eat often means that other family members actually put weight on as they eat meals cooked by the anorexic. The person's sudden interest in cooking and the energy put into housework may be viewed as positive changes and of much help to the family.

To continue their dieting beyond what would be regarded as safe limits, the person has to adopt strategies to avoid detection and to facilitate further weight loss. The emotional strains and behavioural changes that this requires are often in retrospect the first signs identified by the family that something is wrong. However, the awareness that the person somehow seems vaguely "different", "irritable" or "stressed" may be mistaken for normal adolescent phases. Some anorexics, especially those who live alone, are able to avoid detection completely and to maintain a precarious balance between the need to survive and the perceived need to minimize their intake. Self-descriptions by anorexics who live this way indicate a life-style dominated by stress, guilt, the fear of detection and the constant struggle to contain their hunger.

Detection by family members of excessive weight loss may lead to a tense situation at home. The person may be forced by concerned relatives to attend meals, eat all their food and to submit to regular weighing. These are all situations that the person loathes and fears. Some families would not perceive the disordered eating pattern as a problem requiring medical intervention and would only seek outside help if their own actions were unsuccessful. A number of people, either on their own or with their family's help, make a spontaneous return to "normal" eating patterns.

Those with a bulimic eating pattern are often more successful at avoiding detection as their body weight may remain stable. Others may notice that the person seems "changed" or "different". The person's behaviour may only come to light through accidental detection by a family member, financial problems through spending large amounts on food, or disruption to family or working life. If detected, others may force the person to change their behaviour or to seek help. Sufferers may seek help themselves if the strain becomes intolerable or if they are alerted by a television programme or article about bulimia. Nonetheless, many people maintain a pattern of "binge and purge" for many years.

Detection and recognition of their difficulties may come as a profound relief to the person who may be finding the constant secrecy, guilt and shame an intolerable burden. Approaches may be made to their GP for some of the physical consequences of disordered eating without the underlying problems being identified.

Initially, the person and their family can be helped considerably in coping with their eating problems by:

1. Accurate information about eating disorders and their effects.
2. Involvement in the care and treatment process.
3. The opportunity to talk freely about their problems.
4. Reassurance that effective intervention is possible.
5. The address of a local contact support group.
6. Developing the person's and family's coping skills.
7. Reviewing their life-style and expectations to promote their mental health.

Community Care

Most people with eating problems do not approach mental health care services. They attempt in their own way to deal with the problems they experience. Clinical opinion is divided, but it is possible to treat and care successfully for the person at home. This will depend primarily upon the degree of weight loss and the role of the family in the development of the eating disorder. The aims of community care are:

1. To support the person and their family.
2. To monitor the person's mental and physical health.
3. To implement community-based therapeutic programmes.

The services available include:

1. The community mental health centre: with community psychiatric nurses, social workers, psychologists, occupational therapists and consultant psychiatrists working as a team to offer skills-based therapeutic interventions.

2. General practitioners.
3. Teachers and educational psychologists: if the person is attending school.
4. Voluntary agencies: Anorexic Aid, MIND, Samaritans.

Residential care

The reasons for admission to residential care for treatment include:

1. Lack of adequate support in the community.
2. The need for intensive care if the person is severely emaciated or has harmful physical consequences arising from prolonged disordered eating.
3. The need to remove the person from an environment that is causing excessive stress and is actively reinforcing the eating disorder.
4. Detailed assessment and the need for specific types of therapy.

Therapeutic Interventions

Psychotherapeutic interventions

1. *Skilled nursing care*: one of the most important therapeutic factors.
2. *Individual counselling and psychotherapy*: to increase insight, promote self-esteem and to facilitate psychosocial development. To promote body image awareness and the need for ordered eating patterns.
3. *Group therapy*: to increase insight and self-awareness.To share personal experiences, to provide opportunities for social learning and to work together to find solutions for their problems. To facilitate psychosocial development and body image awareness.
4. *Cognitive therapy*: to promote insight. To facilitate psychosocial development. To promote body image awareness and the need for ordered eating patterns.
5. *Family therapy*: to enable the family to be more supportive and to communicate more effectively. To resolve underlying conflicts and to facilitate the personal growth of family members. To explore expectations of parenthood and the relationship between family members.
6. *Couple therapy*: to enable the couple to be more supportive and to communicate more effectively. To help the couple find ways of coping with stress and to adopt a more healthy life-style.
7. *Assertiveness training*: to raise confidence and self-esteem. To facilitate communication and the expression of emotions.
8. *Health education*: nutritional advice and information, anatomy and physiology, psychosexual development, coping methods for stress, healthy relationships.
9. *Occupational therapy*: to develop life skills and diversional activities.

10. *Art therapy and psychodrama*: to help express and release feelings. To promote insight and self-awareness.
11. *Recreational and social activities*: to provide positively reinforcing experiences. To develop social and personal awareness.
12. *Voluntary organizations*: MIND, Anorexic Aid, Samaritans.
13. *Behavioural psychotherapy*: a programme based upon progressive weight gain and operant conditioning is often used in the treatment of anorexia. This approach is generally used in association with a broad range of other psychotherapeutic interventions and currently offers the most successful outcomes (see below).

Behavioural psychotherapy

Initially, a detailed assessment is made of the person's disordered eating habits and associated environmental factors. Potential positive reinforcers are also identified. This information is used to construct a programme of rewards related to the steady gaining and maintenance of weight. The person is required to reach and to maintain their "target weight". This is calculated from standard height/body build weight charts. At first, the prospect of regaining what seems an excessive weight that has taken them so much effort and suffering to lose seems terrifying. They require much support and reassurance throughout the programme to overcome their resistance and to promote compliance.

The rate of weight gain is carefully controlled to enable the person to make a gradual readjustment to normal eating habits and to consolidate their body image. The actual rate of weight gain will depend upon the person's needs and the treatment programme but is usually in the region of 0.5–1.5 kg per week. Even this limited weight gain is likely to make them feel large and conspicuous.

During the period of the programme the person is expected to eat all of the food that they are presented with. This may at times prove very difficult with much hostility, resentment and resistance from the person. Constant and vigilant observation is required to prevent the person using avoidance strategies, e.g. putting the food into bins, throwing it out of the window, self-induced vomiting or laxative abuse.

The carers will require much tact, patience, persistence and tolerance to ensure that food is eaten. Prompting and active encouragement will have to be given to provide positive feedback and also reassurance. For some people, the physical experience of eating a meal and not vomiting may prove uncomfortable and stressful. Some will eat readily with the intention of dieting again as soon as they are discharged from care.

A record is kept of all the food and fluid that the person consumes. Relatives are not allowed to bring in any extra food and are advised to avoid talking about food. The diet used will depend upon the therapists preferred approach and the seriousness of the person's physical condition. The person may be required to commence the programme on a formula food or on a normal diet that is calculated to permit steady weight gain.

In the early stages of therapy the person is only permitted a limited range of privileges and activities. As they gain weight they are also given more freedom and control. Many programmes start with bed rest to prevent overactivity and to ensure maximum observation.

The person is weighed regularly under standardized conditions.Care has to be taken to prevent "water loading" (drinking excessive amounts of fluids to distort the weighing) or the hiding of heavy objects in their clothing. Other observations that may be necessary include blood pressure and checking for diarrhoea or constipation.

If the person loses weight at any stage of the programme then they revert to the privileges and restrictions associated with their current weight. They have then to re-work their way through the programme. An example of a behavioural programme might appear as in Exhibit 15.2.1.

Exhibit 15.2.1 A behavioural programme in a residential setting

Weight on admission: 42 kg   Target weight: 51 kg

1. 42 kg: Complete bed rest. Parents visit 1 hour twice a week
2. 43 kg: Complete bed rest. Parents visit 1 hour four times a week
3. 44 kg: Up in ward in night clothes for 2 hours a day, otherwise bed rest. Parents and other visitors visit 1 hour four times a week
4. 45 kg: Up in ward 4 hours a day, required to stay in ward. Free visiting
5. 46 kg: Up in ward 4 hours a day, dressed and allowed off ward for 2 hours a day to take part in occupational therapy etc.
6. 47 kg: Dressed and nursed on ward 6 hours a day, dressed and off ward 2 hours a day, otherwise bed rest
7. 48 kg: Dressed all day, morning off the ward, afternoon on ward, evening social activities in the hospital
8. 49 kg: As above and allowed off ward/hospital with relatives for two afternoons/evenings a week
9. 50 kg: Dressed and off ward all day, allowed out with relatives and friends three afternoons/evenings a week
10. 51 kg: Takes active part in hospital programme, serves self with food under supervision
11. 51 kg: Maintain weight for 1 week as above and serves self with food without supervision
12. 51 kg: Maintain weight for 2 more weeks then consider for discharge

Other psychotherapeutic interventions would run in parallel with this programme. Community-based programmes can be designed and the relatives instructed how to implement and monitor this approach with support from the community mental health team.

If the person and family can afford it, the purchase of some well-fitting clothes also help to emphasize body shape and outline. They can give visual and tactile feedback to the person and help to promote satisfaction with their body image.

Physical treatment interventions

Chemotherapy

1. Benzodiazepine anxiolytics: if anxiety is a prominent feature. Effective in about 15% of people. For short period only.
2. Chlorpromazine: useful in reducing anxiety and in encouraging eating in about 25–33% of people. For short period only. Side-effects and possibility of epileptic fits limit its use.
3. Antidepressants: tricyclics effective in reducing anxiety and for antidepressant effects if depression is a prominent feature. For short-term use only.
4. Night sedation: if sleep disturbance is present. For short-term use at start of treatment only.
5. Medication may be prescribed for nutritional deficits, consequences of prolonged disordered eating, constipation or diarrhoea.
6. Modified insulin therapy: to promote rest and weight gain. Rarely used.

Electroconvulsive therapy (ECT)

Rarely used unless severe depression is present in a person who is grossly emaciated. The primary objective is to overcome the person's resistance to eating.

Psychosurgery

Rarely used unless person is highly obsessional, chronically tense and has failed to respond to other treatments for many years.

Outcomes

Most people with an anorexic eating pattern respond to therapeutic intervention and regain weight. However, relapse is not uncommon and it is important to provide adequate follow-up and support. Mild cases might recover within 1 year. It may take some 3–5 years for full resolution of the person's difficulties. By this time, approximately 60–70% of people are able to maintain a satisfactory weight. Many of the remainder make an intermediate adjustment and have periodic difficulties for which they may require help. Some 4–10% of sufferers still die from anorexia.

Leaving home, sexual relationships and marriage (60% within 10 years of regained weight) tends to be associated with positive outcomes. Many sufferers report favourably on the support given from voluntary support groups for anorexia.

The outcomes in bulimia are less well-documented. Some sufferers make a spontaneous recovery. Others continue for many years, successfully evading detection but suffering constant stress and guilt. If the person seeks help then most can be positively enabled to regain control of their eating behaviour.

Unit Instructions

When you have researched the suggested references, have mastered the Unit Objectives and successfully answered the Self-assessment Questions, proceed with the Unit Written Test.

Suggested References

Abraham, S. and Llewellyn-Jones, D. (1984). *Eating Disorders: The Facts*. Oxford University Press, Oxford.

Aniskowitz, S. (1984). Anorexia nervosa. *Nursing Mirror*, 11 April, Vol. 158, No. 15, pp. 42–43.

Beard, P. (1984). A cry for help. *Nursing Mirror*, 5 September, Vol. 159, No. 8, pp. 27–28.

Bhanji, S. (1980). Anorexia nervosa: Two schools of thought. *Nursing Times*, 21 February, Vol. 76, No. 8, pp. 323–324.

Chudley, P. (1986). An unhealthy obsession. *Nursing Times*, 26 March, Vol. 82, No. 13, pp. 50–52.

Crisp, A. H. (1980). *Anorexia Nervosa: Let Me Be*. Academic Press/Grune and Stratton, London and San Diego.

Dally, P. (1981). Treatment of anorexia nervosa. *British Journal of Hospital Medicine*, May, pp. 434–440.

Dally, P. and Gomez, J. (1979). *Anorexia Nervosa*. Heinemann Medical, London.

Dexter, J. M. (1980). Anorexia nervosa. *Nursing Times*, 21 February, Vol. 76, No. 8, pp. 325–327.

Gibbs, A. (1986). *Understanding Mental Health*. Consumer's Association/Hodder and Stoughton, London.

Gibson, E. (1983). Body talk. . .anorexia nervosa. . .a plea for a more humane approach. *Nursing Times*, 16 February, Vol. 79, No. 7, p. 64.

Ho, E. (1985). Anorexia nervosa in pregnancy. *Nursing Mirror*, 24 April, Vol. 160, No. 17, pp. 40–42.

Hughes, J. (1986). *An Outline of Modern Psychiatry*, 2nd edition. John Wiley, Chichester.

Lyttle, J. (1986). *Mental Disorder: Its Care and Treatment*. Baillière Tindall, London and San Diego.

Melville, J. (1986). When you can't stop eating. *Self Health*, September, No. 12, pp. 13–14.

Palmer, R. L. (1980). *Anorexia Nervosa. A Guide for Sufferers and Their Families.* Penguin, Harmondsworth.

Potts, N. L. (1984). The secret pattern of binge/purge. *American Journal of Nursing,* January, Vol. 84, No. 1, pp. 32–35.

Sanger, E. and Cassino, T. (1984). Avoiding the power struggle. *American Journal of Nursing,* January, Vol. 84, No. 1, pp. 31–33.

Slade, R. (1984). *The Anorexia Nervosa Reference Book.* Harper and Row, London.

Snaith, P. (1981). *Clinical Neurosis.* Oxford University Press, Oxford.

Thompson, S. (1979). Hungry for knowledge – not food. *Nursing Mirror,* 12 July, Vol. 75, No. 28, pp. 29–32.

Trethowan, W. and Sims, A. (1983). *Psychiatry,* 5th edition. Baillière Tindall, London and San Diego.

Waskett, C. (1983). Disordered eating patterns. *Nursing Times,* 22 June, Vol. 79, No. 25, p. 72.

Willis, J. (1976). *Clinical Psychiatry.* Blackwell Scientific, Oxford.

Self-assessment Questions

SAQ 5. Outline four ways that family members may react to the detection of an eating disorder in one of their members.

SAQ 6. Identify four community agencies that can help the person with an eating disorder.

SAQ 7. Describe the relationship between weight gain and access to privileges in a behavioural programme for anorexia.

SAQ 8. List four medications and describe their role in the treatment of anorexia.

Unit 15.2: Written Test

Stephanie Johnson, aged 16, has been admitted for treatment of an anorexic eating problem. She is severely emaciated yet still seems determined to lose weight. Her parents are shocked and guilty at her condition and are concerned that she will now miss her "O" level exams. On admission her weight was 42 kg. For her height, age and body build she should be 52 kg.

1. Stephanie's parents are concerned about the behavioural programme that has been suggested as they do not see how it can really help. What information do you think they will need in order to reassure them?
2. The care team has to agree jointly a behavioural programme linked to progressive weight gain. Briefly demonstrate your understanding of this approach by constructing a programme for Stephanie from her current weight to her target weight.
3. What other psychotherapeutic interventions are necessary to promote insight and the person's acceptance of their body image?

Nursing Care of the Person with an Anorectic Eating Pattern

Unit Objectives

At the end of this Unit the learner should be able to:

1. Identify the nursing care needs of the person with an anorectic eating pattern.
2. Plan an individualized care programme.
3. Select appropriate nursing care interventions for the person's needs.
4. Describe possible evaluation criteria for specific needs.

Mental Health Nursing Care

Each person's care needs are unique and have to be assessed individually. A range of potential care needs have been selected to illustrate some of the problems that the person with an anorectic eating pattern may experience and the potential nursing interventions that may help them.

For the person with an anorectic eating disorder these may include the need to:

A. Feel secure and free from threat.
B. Promote their insight and self-awareness.
C. Re-establish healthy and ordered eating patterns.
D. Facilitate the development of the person's and family's coping skills.

A. Feel Secure and Free From Threat

Associated problems/personal difficulties

Person may feel insecure and threatened as a result of:

1. Inadequate knowledge of their care and treatment programme.
2. Feelings of guilt and low self-esteem.

3. Fear of regaining weight.
4. Stress that their eating behaviour causes in their relationships.
5. Ambivalence about re-establishing healthy dietary pattern.
6. Mistrust of the intent of carers.

Assessment

1. Person's description of their anxieties and worries.
2. Information from relatives and friends.
3. Nurse's observations of the person's:

   (a) Response to questioning: topics avoided, incomplete replies, irritation, defensiveness.
   (b) Understanding: questions asked and statements made in relation to their health and treatment programme.
   (c) Emotional reactions: appropriateness in terms of degree of weight loss, indifference, lack of concern, edginess, tension, anxiety.
   (d) Verbal and non-verbal behaviour indicating anxiety: posture, gestures, tone of voice, eye movements, agitation, restlessness, tearfulness.
   (e) Relationships with others: accepting, clinging, hostile, rejecting, supportive.

4. Identification of potential stressors in the person's relationships, life-style and expectations.
5. Support network available to the person and family.
6. Potential risk of self-harm.

Desired outcomes

1. Person and family's understanding of their health care needs are increased.
2. Person demonstrates trust in carers.
3. Person is more relaxed and feels free from threat.

Nursing Intervention	Rationale
1. Initiate a therapeutic relationship. Spend time with them. Be available and approachable. Demonstrate active listening. Use touch where appropriate	Interventions more likely to be successful in an atmosphere of trust and cooperation. Also shows sense of worth and acceptance which helps to increase feelings of security and safety

Nursing intervention	*Rationale*
2. Role model calm behaviour. Adopt a non-threatening, open posture and tone of voice	Can have a powerful calming influence. Person is likely to reflect this behaviour and to feel more at ease
3. Approach unhurriedly. Demonstrate calmness. Do not rush the person. Be aware of your own reactions and experience of stress. Be patient and aware of your own feelings of frustration in dealing with the person	Anxiety in the carer communicates itself to the person. Caring can be a stressful experience at times. This may unconsciously influence your interactions with others. The person may be very demanding and resistant. Find ways of coping with your own stress
4. Arrange for your own clinical supervision	Supervision is an effective way of providing professional support and development
5. Reassure the person of non-harmful intent. Reassure about the need for slow weight gain that will be regulated and controlled (see **C.**)	Person is terrified by what they expect to be rapid and excessive weight gain. This makes them feel very threatened and vulnerable
6. Adopt a non-judgemental and non-critical approach	Being non-judgemental helps a person to deal with any guilt. Reduces feelings of anxiety
7. Provide clear and understandable information about their treatment, health care and the roles of different health care workers. Encourage questions. Ask for feedback on their understanding. Clarify any misunderstandings	A lot of anxiety is associated with fear of the unknown. People have a right to information about their health care. The nurse is in an ideal position to use this process to facilitate the development of the person's understanding about their health care needs
8. Enlist the person's cooperation in the planning of their health care	People are more likely to cooperate if they are well-informed and involved in the decision-making process. It also increases feelings of personal control

Nursing intervention	*Rationale*
9. Explain all actions in advance	Interventions less likely to be perceived as threatening if anticipated
10. Ensure that significant personal items are available	Familiar objects help to increase feelings of security
11. Encourage the person to express their feelings about their eating difficulties	Being identified as anorexic is a very stigmatizing process. The person feels guilty and bewildered. There is also a sense of loss over the change of role and self-identity
12. Encourage the person to talk about their stressful feelings. Encourage them to express their feelings in a more appropriate way. Minimize opportunities for self-harm (see Unit 7.4)	Venting their feelings in this way may reduce some of the necessity for communicating through disordered eating or self-harm. Person may feel trapped and desperate and feel unable to communicate in any way. Also risk of self-harm from low self-esteem, guilt and helplessness
13. Provide feedback to the person on their behaviour and use it as a learning situation	Provides an opportunity for health education in the appropriate expression of emotional stress. Promotes insight
14. Facilitate the development of the person's ability to communicate and relate to others	Helps the person to express and thereby release feelings of anxiety and tension
15. Encourage the person to rest or relax if they appear to be under stress. Provide feedback on their behaviour	Person may not be aware of the effect of anxiety on their behaviour
16. Teach the person appropriate relaxation skills and techniques (see Unit 6.3)	Reduces stress and tension. Increases feelings of personal control
17. Promote the person's self-esteem (see Unit 7.4)	Feelings of guilt and low self-esteem are central to the anorexic's life experience. Need to develop a

Nursing intervention	Rationale
	positive self-image and feelings of control for successful therapeutic progress. Also helps to reduce the risk of self-harm
18. Observe for signs of physical exhaustion	Person may attempt surreptitious exercise to encourage weight loss
19. Observe for signs of self-induced vomiting or purging with laxatives	May put person at risk of dehydration or metabolic upset. Person needs to be aware that others are concerned for their welfare and will intervene if necessary
20. Observe for signs of impending fits. Protect person's safety	Some 10% of anorexics experience epileptiform type fits. These appear to be related to prolonged malnutrition and metabolic disturbances. The risk decreases and is removed as the person regains weight and stabilizes at their target weight

Evaluation

1. Person and family demonstrate understanding of the health care programme.
2. Person demonstrates trust in the carers.
3. Person displays relaxed verbal and non-verbal behaviour.
4. Person remains safe within the care environment.

B. Promote Their Insight and Self-awareness

Associated problems/personal difficulties

Person may need to increase their insight and self-awareness as a result of:

1. Refusing to accept that their eating pattern is potentially harmful.
2. Difficulty in understanding why others react adversely to their eating behaviour.
3. Attempting to cope and communicate through a disordered eating pattern.

4. Failing to recognize their underlying motivation in following a disordered pattern of eating.
5. Misperception of their body image.

Assessment

1. Person's perception of their behaviour and motivation.
2. Information from relatives and friends.
3. Nurse's observations of the person's:

   (a) Responses to questioning about their motivation for weight loss.
   (b) Perception of their body image.
   (c) Inappropriate use of defence mechanisms.
   (d) Ability to recognize and accept the harmful consequences of their eating patterns.
   (e) Ability to communicate and express their feelings.
   (f) Relationships with family members: conflict, supportive, dependent, restrictive.
   (g) Identified needs for social and personal development.

4. History of the eating disorder: commencement, precipitants, strategies adopted, degree of weight loss.

Desired outcomes

1. Person is able to accept the need to adopt a healthier eating pattern.
2. Person is able to recognize that the eating disorder represents a maladaptive way of coping and communicating.
3. Person is able to communicate directly their needs to others.
4. Person is able to develop their ability to relate confidently to others.

Nursing intervention	Rationale
1. Initiate therapeutic relationship. Be available and approachable. Demonstrate active listening	Interventions more likely to be successful in an atmosphere of trust and cooperation
2. Offer reassurance. Demonstrate acceptance. Demonstrate non-judgemental and non-	To minimize anxiety and create the conditions for behavioural and cognitive change. Effective learning can only take place if the person feels secure

Nursing intervention	*Rationale*
critical approach. Promote feelings of security (see **A.**)	
3. Explore with the person the effects of their behaviour on their own and their family's life	Person may not be fully aware of how their behaviour is disrupting their life and relationships
4. Explore with the person reasons for criticisms by others. Explore with the person reasons for criticisms of others	Person may not be aware of why others may perceive them in a negative way. This also influences how they perceive others
5. Offer feedback on the person's behaviour and use it as a learning situation	Person may not be fully aware of how much their eating behaviour is dominating their life
6. Explore person's expectations and self-imposed standards. Identify criteria used to evaluate self and others	Many people with an eating disorder have very high and unattainable expectations that create stress and a sense of failure. This creates a great pressure on them to attain these unrealistic standards
7. Assist the person to acknowledge the influence of their expectations and personal standards on their behaviour. Explore alternative ways of evaluating their self-worth. Explore alternative expectations	Anorexics feel that restricting their diet is the only area of their life in which they can have a sense of mastery and control. The person needs to be helped to reshape their beliefs about themself and to develop more valid and realistic expectations
8. Offer alternative interpretations of life experiences that person uses to devalue themselves	Person needs to develop a more realistic image of themselves
9. Help person to develop more attainable expectations and standards. Encourage acceptance	The development of more realistic expectations is an important part in the person's long-term recovery. Tend to interpret responses by others as negative and threatening

Nursing intervention	*Rationale*
of self-limitations. Encourage honesty in presenting self. Support a realistic assessment of their life circumstances. Encourage awareness of positive responses from others	
10. Explore previous achievements and successes. Identify and work with their strengths and resources	May have positive assets that can be utilized in developing the way they relate to others
11. Teach the person how to keep a log or diary of their eating behaviour and feelings throughout the day	Self-recording promotes insight and helps to reduce the frequency of anxious thoughts. Helps to promote a sense of mastery and self-control. Also provides useful data for the therapist
12. Assist the person to identify specific factors associated with their eating patterns	Person may not be aware of the way that environmental factors are influencing their diet
13. Encourage the person to modify environmental factors, where possible, that are contributing to the maintenance of their eating disorder	Modification of contributing environmental factors may help to reduce stimuli that maintain the eating disorder
14. Role model social and communication skills	Modelling by nurses has a powerful influence on the people in their care
15. Explain the principles of assertiveness and social skills training	Social skills and assertiveness training help to develop communication and emotional expression skills
16. Identify situations with the person in which they experience a relationship or a communication difficulty	Many people with mental health problems are either lacking in social skills or have problems relating to others
17. Role play with feedback these situations with the	Social skills and assertiveness training help people to develop their communication and relationship skills.

Nursing intervention	*Rationale*
person. Give demonstration and guidance as required. Provide information on the nature of human interaction and the expression of feeling. Encourage gradual mastery. Provide opportunities to rehearse social skills. Promote self-evaluation of social competence. Identify real-life opportunities to practise social skills. Set specific assignments. Monitor and evaluate progress with person	It is a structured approach in which specific skills are: • identified and defined; • divided into their constituent elements; • the elements are practised with feedback in role play until competence is achieved; • the entire skill is practised with feedback until competence is achieved; • the skill is transferred to real-life situations
18. Provide feedback on the development of social skills. Give positive reinforcement. Encourage the transfer of newly learned skills to real-life situations	Improved social skills also improve self-esteem, confidence and the ability to communicate. Enhances feelings of personal control
19. Describe behaviour patterns indicating emotional maturity	Person's social understanding may be limited
20. Provide opportunities for the person to express themselves openly and honestly	Helps to relieve tension and to demonstrate acceptance. It also provides the opportunity for them to practise talking about their emotions which they may have had difficulty with in the past. May also reduce the need for the physical expression of anger and frustration through vomiting or self-harm
21. Facilitate the development of emotional and behavioural coping skills/strategies	Need to develop and use effective ways of coping with stress. May be possible to make life-style changes that promote mental health.

Nursing intervention	*Rationale*
22. Encourage the use of appropriate coping mechanisms in relation to stress-provoking situations	Limited coping skills increase their potential to react anxiously
23. Promote their autonomy and self-esteem	Self-belief in the person's own value and feelings of control and mastery increase confidence in dealing with others. More likely to relate to others in a "healthy" way and be committed to change
24. Encourage them to pay attention to their hygiene and appearance	Appearance and hygiene are two important factors in self-esteem. Feeling clean and looking presentable help to improve the person's self-image and the way they appear to others
25. Provide factual information about the incidence and nature of eating disorders in the community	Providing accurate information can help to promote insight and understanding. Reassuring to find that not "unique". Person may feel guilty and stigmatized about receiving care and treatment. This can be damaging to their self-esteem
26. Engage in physical activity as a precursor to verbal interaction, e.g. games, activities, drama, music. Organize social and recreational activities	Sometimes it is easier for people to relate as part of an activity or game, or afterwards
27. Identify options for work and leisure activities. Encourage personal interests	Relieves boredom and helps to raise self-esteem if meaningfully employed
28. Encourage social interaction with others. Organize group activities	Social activities can be very rewarding and also provide group dynamics that the person may find therapeutic
29. Promote contact with relatives and personal friends. Increase opportunities for group interaction	Helps to overcome feelings of isolation and rejection. Still valued by others

Nursing intervention	*Rationale*
30. Organize experiential exercises, e.g. drama, role-play and games, in which the person relates to others in an unstructured way and can express themselves freely	Structured and spontaneous experiential exercises can provide powerful feedback and personal learning opportunities. Specific exercises can be used to promote insight and body awareness

Evaluation

1. Person demonstrates a commitment towards regaining positive control of their diet.
2. Person acknowledges the harmful effects of disordered eating patterns.
3. Increase in the frequency of positive personal statements.
4. Person demonstrates more assertive verbal and non-verbal communications.
5. Person directly expresses their needs to others.

C. Re-establish Healthy and Ordered Eating Patterns

Associated problems/personal difficulties

Person with anorexia needs to re-establish healthy and ordered eating patterns due to:

1. The life-threatening consequences of prolonged malnutrition.
2. The risks of metabolic disorder and other harmful consequences of self-induced vomiting.
3. Chronic and long-term abuse of laxatives.
4. The deleterious physical consequences of long-term malnutrition.
5. The damage done to the person's self-esteem.
6. The stress experienced in maintaining their deceptive strategies.
7. The stress caused to family relationships by their eating pattern.
8. The misperception of their body image.
9. Inaccurate nutritional and physiological knowledge.

Assessment

1. Person's perception of their nutritional intake and needs.
2. Information from family members about the person's nutritional intake and strategies used by the person to control their intake.
3. Nurse's observations of:

   (a) The cognitive and behavioural strategies used by the person to control their intake of food: avoiding meals, cutting food into small pieces, excessive chewing, distractions used when hungry.
   (b) The strategies used by the person to increase their rate of weight loss: self-induced vomiting, laxative abuse, over-exercise. Frequency, timing, methods and history of strategies used.
   (c) The strategies used by the person to avoid detection and to disguise their weight loss: loose clothing, excessive concerns with privacy, change in activities and hobbies.
   (d) The person's emotional reactions to weight loss: guilt, anxiety, depression, helplessness.
   (e) The person's physical condition: current weight, weight at which began weight loss strategies, ideal or "target" weight for their body size and height. Physical consequences of prolonged malnutrition. Identified physical health deficits.
   (f) The person's perceptions of their body image: accuracy, distortions, desired body shape.
   (g) The person's knowledge and understanding of body physiology and nutritional needs.
   (h) The person's reactions to intervention by others to increase their nutritional intake and limit weight loss strategies.

4. Psychosocial environment: presence of identifiable triggering cues. Reactions of others to person's weight loss strategies. Potential reinforcers of anorexic behaviour. Presence of potential stress in person's environment or life-style.
5. The person's awareness and willingness to accept that their eating pattern is potentially harmful.

Desired outcomes

1. Person is able to follow planned nutritional programme.
2. Strategies to increase weight loss are halted.
3. Person is able to come to terms with their body image.
4. Person's knowledge of nutritional and physical development is enhanced.
5. Person accepts the need to re-adopt healthy eating patterns.
6. Person is able to identify accurately their nutritional needs.
7. Person independently maintains an adequate nutritional intake.

Nursing Intervention	*Rationale*
1. Initiate therapeutic relationship. Involve them in the care planning process	Interventions more likely to succeed in an atmosphere of trust and cooperation
2. Be available and approachable. Offer reassurance. Demonstrate acceptance. Demonstrate non-judgemental approach. Promote feelings of security and safety (see **A.**) Promote self-esteem	Helps to promote calm and to create the conditions for behavioural change. The person is very sensitive to implied criticism. Improving self-esteem helps to improve their self-image in relationships with others. Raising self-esteem also increases their commitment to regain personal control of disordered eating
3. Provide reassurance about potential for positive change and for regaining control of their eating behaviour	Person may feel that their situation is hopeless after their own long-term inability to follow ordered eating patterns
4. Observe their behaviour and relationships to identify factors that contribute to disordered eating	Can be used to identify any environmental factors that may be amenable to modification
5. Assist the person to identify any environmental factors related to their disordered eating	Person may not be aware of the way that environmental factors are influencing their eating behaviour
6. Encourage the person to modify environmental factors where possible that are contributing to disordered eating	Modification of contributing environmental factors may help to reduce stimuli that elicit disordered eating
7. Negatively reinforce maladaptive behaviour and cognitions. Positively reinforce healthy behaviour	Helps to decrease frequency of maladaptive behaviour

Nursing intervention	*Rationale*
8. Teach family members the skills of giving reinforcement and of communicating directly	Family members may be inadvertently contributing to the maintenance of disordered eating patterns. Family patterns of communication may be ambivalent and unclear
9. Explain to the person and family the reasons for structured programme of weight gain and progressive relaxation of restrictions	Person needs to understand the principle behind the approach and their own role. Increases feelings of personal responsibility and mutual cooperation
10. Explain the term "target weight". Specify that all of the food presented to the person must be eaten. Specify the stages of weight gain in the programme and the associated privileges. Reassure the person that the rate of weight gain will be moderated to stay within agreed weekly limits	Initially the carers have to set and maintain limits which can gradually be transferred to the person as they demonstrate compliance. Encouraging personal responsibility helps to raise self-esteem and to promote insight. Shows that others are concerned for their welfare. Person fears very rapid weight gain. Reassured by steady controlled weight gain
11. Explain the value of slow weight gain	This also gives time to adjust to their new body image. Diet will be determined by person's physical condition, present weight and desired target weight
12. Document in detail the stages of the programme	Programme needs to be written in detail to facilitate consistency by care team
13. Explain that written stages are readily accessible to carers. Give a copy to the person and their family	Helps to promote insight, compliance and responsibility
14. Ensure that all care workers are consistent in their approach to maintaining the programme. Refer detailed requests to key worker	Need to ensure consistency in the programme for it to be effective. Person will readily manipulate carers if they identify inconsistency

Nursing intervention	*Rationale*
15. Initiate therapeutic programme at agreed time and ensure compliance	Programme needs to be implemented consistently to be effective
16. Ensure that relatives are not present at meal-times. Ensure that relatives do not bring in either extra food or supplies of laxatives	In situations where family members are actively involved in the dynamics of the eating disorder it is better that they are excluded. May bring in food or laxatives that disrupt the intended programme
17. Present food attractively. Observe constantly at meal-times. Ensure that all the food is eaten as required	Food is then more likely to be eaten and to be appealing. May attempt to dispose of food surreptitiously. May try to negotiate with carers on only eating a portion of the meal
18. Encourage person to eat if appears reluctant. Use prompting and persuasion as required	May need encouragement from others to complete meals
19. Give positive reinforcement to self-initiated eating	Person needs rewarding for desired behaviour
20. Do not rush at meal-times. Be patient. Keep calm and relaxed	Person may eat very slowly or move food around plate to try and make carers lose interest in what she is eating. Needs to accept that carers will persist in their efforts to ensure adequate nutrition
21. Provide reassurance during mealtimes	Person may feel very anxious at having to eat a full meal when they may not have done so for a long time. The amount of food to them probably seems enormous. Takes time to readjust dietary and eating habits
22. Reassure and explain about any feelings of abdominal discomfort	Person may be so used to vomiting or purging that the presence of a meal in the stomach feels uncomfortable, possibly painful. Will take time to readjust to new physical sensations
23. Record details of all food that is eaten	Need to ensure that food is eaten and to correlate diet with weight gain

Nursing intervention	*Rationale*
24. Ensure that person takes a minimum of 2 litres of fluid a day. Record fluid intake	To avoid risk of dehydration, weight gain and the intake of nutrition should provide a good indication of the person's improving mental state
25. Observe closely after meal-times. Engage in diversionary therapeutic or social activities after eating	To reduce potential for strategies to eliminate food, e.g. vomiting, laxatives, excessive exercise
26. Intervene physically to prevent vomiting if discovered. Observe for smell of vomit on breath. Observe for marks and grazes on knuckles	Person may be able to vomit very readily and without signs of distress. Marks on hands come from pushing fingers down throat to induce vomiting
27. Promote oral hygiene	Prolonged self-induced vomiting is harmful to teeth enamel
28. Observe for signs of constipation or diarrhoea. Ensure that laxatives are not being abused by person. Provide extra roughage if required to diet	May be a consequence of prolonged laxative abuse and insufficient bulk in the diet
29. Reassure the person about anxieties associated with return to normal excretion. Explain the physiology of excretion to the person if they lack understanding	May take some weeks for normal faecal excretion to become re-established. In the short term this may cause some concern and distress to the person. Needs time to readjust to the physical sensations associated with normal excretion. May have distorted perceptions and understanding of how their body works
30. Promote feelings of physical comfort	Prolonged malnutrition may result in general physical discomfort and feelings of cold
31. Permit a limited amount of exercise and physical activity	Physical activity in anorexia is effective in reducing the risk of osteoporosis. However, it should not be of such a degree that it contributes to weight loss
32. Weigh person at predetermined times under agreed standard	Weighing needs to be done consistently to promote accuracy and to minimize the stress for the person if they know

Nursing intervention	Rationale
conditions. Ensure that weight readings are not being distorted by weights or water loading	how it is to be done. Person may attempt to distort the accuracy of the weighing
33. Reassure the person if they appear anxious during weighing	Likely to find weighing very stressful
34. Tell person how much they weigh. Display on chart	Person's weight is of great concern to them. Visual indication of weight gain may be positively reinforcing
35. Explain the outcomes of their weight in relation to their therapeutic programme. Ensure that alterations in status and privileges are identified with weight gain/loss	Need to clearly establish and link any weight gain with positive outcomes. Likewise with weight loss
36. Positively reinforce progressive weight gain and compliance with programme	To promote compliance
37. Be non-judgemental if person is discovered to be adopting strategies to avoid weight gain. Explain and enforce any consequences of avoidance strategies	Person feels very guilty about their deceptions but often is unable to think of any alternative. Fearful of the outcome of detection, they are reassured by non-judgemental consequences
38. Gradually increase incentives and rewards to person in line with programme compliance	Person needs to be made clear of the relationship between compliance and weight gain
39. Gradually return control of their diet and activities to the person. Reinforce compliance with programme	Person is given increasing responsibility for their own diet and behaviour. The autonomy helps to raise self-esteem and feelings of trust
40. Periodically review the programme with the care team	Need to monitor programme in relation to the person's progress

Nursing intervention	*Rationale*
41. Review with the person to promote learning	Promotes compliance and awareness
42. Explore with the person their understanding of diet and nutrition. Clarify any misconceptions about nutrition. Provide accurate information as required. Provide written information if available. Discuss the necessary elements of a healthy diet	May have distorted or inaccurate perceptions of food and nutrition. May need to re-educate the person in the principles of a healthy diet
43. Explain the principles of body growth and the development of secondary sexual characteristics	Many eating disorders appear to have their origin around the time of puberty. This is believed to be significant in the aetiology of anorexia as an attempt to arrest sexual development
44. Explore the person's perception of their body image. Identify the criteria they use for the evaluation of own body size and that of others. Compare the person's perceived body image with their actual size	Successful recovery is dependent upon the person developing a more realistic perception and acceptance of their own body size and shape. They tend to grossly over-exaggerate their own body size and yet may be able to make reasonable assessments of other people's body size
45. Offer reality-based external perceptions of their body size and shape. Explore the person's dissatisfaction with their body image. Discuss issues in relation to people's satisfaction and dissatisfaction with their physical size and shape	Need to facilitate the development of reality-based body perceptions. May find it useful to base discussions upon pictures of people or to work on person's reflection in mirrors or to use video feedback. Person may not realize that this type of dissatisfaction is common in people. Helps them to feel less isolated and unique
46. Provide accurate information on the physiology of physical	May have distorted and inaccurate expectations on what their body shape should be. Helps to develop

Nursing intervention	*Rationale*
growth and development	expectations based upon the reality of physical shapes and their variety in real people
47. Provide positive reinforcement for weight gain on person's body shape and size	To promote compliance with therapeutic programme and to enhance self-esteem
48. Reinforce the positive physical and mental health aspects of being at target weight	Need to provide external reinforcement until the person is able to internalize own appropriate body image and to gain reinforcement from maintaining normal body weight
49. Encourage the person to wear clothes that emphasize their body shape and outline	People with eating disorders frequently wear loose clothes to disguise body outline from others and themselves. Well-fitting clothes help to emphasize their body image and to provide visual and tactile feedback
50. Review programme when person has maintained target weight for set time and is complying with programme without prompting	By this stage the first part of the programme is complete – the restoration and maintenance of their weight. This therapeutic success now needs to be followed by longer-term and intense therapies to promote insight, coping and family relationships

Evaluation

1. Person steadily gains weight in line with therapeutic programme.
2. Person complies with the therapeutic programme.
3. Person can make positive statements about their body image.
4. Person can identify accurately the nutritional requirements for a healthy diet.
5. Person can describe the physiological processes of growth and psychosexual development.

D. Facilitate the Development of the Person's and Family's Coping Skills

Associated problems/personal difficulties

The presence of an eating disorder may show that:

1. Person is attempting to cope and communicate through a disordered eating pattern.
2. Family members may find it difficult to offer emotional support to each other.
3. Existing methods of coping may be limited.
4. Current life-styles, expectations and relationships may be potential sources of stress.
5. The person and their family may lack information about the resources available to help them.
6. There may be feelings of guilt in relation to their problems and asking for help.
7. Person and family may have difficulty understanding and coping with the outcomes of the eating disorder.

Assessment

1. Person and their family's perception of the current situation.
2. Coping methods being used by the person and their family and their effectiveness.
3. Accuracy of the knowledge and information given by the person and their family.
4. Statements of guilt.
5. Identification of stress and conflict within life-style and relationships.
6. Awareness of resources available to them.
7. Previous experience, if any, of dealing with similar problems.
8. Support network available to the person and their family.

Desired outcomes

1. Person and family able to make an informed choice about the resources they require.
2. Person and family able to cope better with the problems experienced.

Nursing Intervention	Rationale
1. Initiate therapeutic relationship	Interventions more likely to be successful in an atmosphere of trust and cooperation

Nursing intervention	*Rationale*
2. Advise that seeking help and recognition of problems are a positive step towards finding solutions	Many people feel that seeking help is a sign of weakness and failure. Also helps to reduce guilt
3. Encourage questions. Provide accurate information	May have inaccurate knowledge and expectations. Helps to promote understanding and reduce anxieties
4. Identify appropriate health care resources	Need to know what resources are available to them
5. Advise that highly emotional situations be avoided at first	May be pent-up feelings and stresses that need to be worked through and released in a controlled way. Sudden discharge of emotion may also increase the severity of the person's symptoms
6. Advise against early and unrealistic correction of problems	Under stress it is sometimes easier to make short-term compromises that only store up future problems. It takes time to help the family to work out what is best for them. Longstanding problems will also take time to resolve
7. Reassure that there are ways of improving the situation	Person's family may feel that the situation is hopeless
8. Reassure that it is possible to regain lost weight and to stabilize eating habits. Advise against recrimination and focussing on past problems	Person may feel trapped in maladaptive eating patterns. Need to focus on the present and future and to deal with anger and guilt in a more productive way
9. Advise on the need for acceptance and mutual support within their relationships	Family needs to come to terms with their situation. They are each other's primary source of support which will need to be utilized to cope effectively
10. Explain the need to identify and recognize potentially stressful situations	Stress can precipitate or exacerbate eating disorders.
11. Teach methods for achieving relaxation. Teach how to use problem-solving methods for coping with difficulties	In order to cope effectively the family needs to be taught ways of making the necessary long-term adjustments Mental health problems tend to be long-term in nature.

Nursing intervention	*Rationale*
12. Assist the family to learn new coping skills. Facilitate the development of communication within the family. Encourage the setting of realistic goals	Most of the education needs to be directed towards teaching effective coping methods. These include the way that the family members communicate, their expectations and the way that emotional support is given
13. Encourage the setting of progressive goals in small stages	The re-learning needs to be done in a gradual way in which the family provides the main support and reinforcement
14. Advise the family on how to give feedback and support to one another	Relationships may be based on negative rather than positive feedback. May not be offering effective support within their pattern of relationships
15. Teach family members how to reinforce healthy eating patterns	Family members may be inadvertently contributing to the maintenance of eating disorder
16. Encourage the use of newly acquired coping skills. Give feedback to the person and family	Skills need to be used in order to become part of everyday life
17. Teach the person and family how to recognize signs of impending recurrence of eating disorder and the actions to take	Family and person will be the main monitors of the person's mental health
18. Teach the family and person to recognize the limits of their ability to cope and when it is advisable to seek help	The family should not overburden itself, as this can damage relationships and its longer-term ability to cope
19. Put family in contact with self-help and voluntary group	Self-help groups able to offer effective and understanding practical help

Evaluation

1. Person and family identify and select resources they require.
2. Person and family able to give accurate information about their health care needs.
3. Person and family demonstrate use of improved coping methods.

Unit Instructions

When you have researched the suggested references, have mastered the Unit Objectives and successfully answered the Self-assessment Questions, proceed with the Unit Written Test.

Suggested References

Adams, C. G. and Macione, A. (Eds) (1983). *Handbook of Psychiatric/Mental Health Nursing*. John Wiley/Fleschner, New York.

Aniskowitz, S. (1984). Anorexia nervosa. *Nursing Mirror*, 11 April, Vol. 158, No. 15, pp. 42–43.

Barker, P. J. (1982). *Behaviour Therapy Nursing*. Croom Helm, London.

Barker, P. J. (1985). *Patient Assessment in Psychiatric Nursing*. Croom Helm, London.

Bauer, B. B. and Hill, S. S. (1986). *Essentials of Mental Health Care Planning and Interventions*. W. B. Saunders, Philadelphia.

Beard, P. (1984). A cry for help. *Nursing Mirror*, 5 September, Vol. 159, No.8, pp. 27–28.

Campbell, C. (1978). *Nursing Diagnosis and Intervention in Nursing Practice*. John Wiley, New York.

Chambers, K. and Yong, C. (1985). Management of the child with severe anorexia nervosa. A multi-disciplinary approach. *Nursing*, August, Vol. 2, No. 4, pp. 1198–1200.

Darcy, P. T. (1985). *Mental Health Nursing Source Book*. Baillière Tindall, London and San Diego.

Dexter, G. and Wash, M. (1986). *Psychiatric Nursing Skills: A Patient-centred Approach*. Croom Helm, London.

Dexter, J. M. (1980). Anorexia nervosa. *Nursing Times*, 21 February, Vol. 76, No. 8, pp. 325–327.

Dickson, A. (1982). *A Woman in Your Own Right. Assertiveness and You*. Quartet Books, London.

Goldberg, D. and Huxley, P. (1980). *Mental Illness in the Community*. Tavistock, London.

Ho, E. (1985). Anorexia nervosa in pregnancy. *Nursing Mirror*, 24 April, Vol. 160, No. 17, pp. 40–42.

Irving, S. (1983). *Basic Psychiatric Nursing*, 3rd edition. W. B. Saunders, Philadelphia.

Lancaster, J. (1980). *Adult Psychiatric Nursing*. Henry Kimpton, London.

Lyttle, J. (1986). *Mental Disorder: Its Care and Treatment*. Baillière Tindall, London and San Diego.

McFarland, G. and Wasli, E. (1986). *Nursing Diagnoses and Process in Psychiatric Mental Health Nursing*. J. B. Lippincott, Philadelphia.

Martin, P. (1987). *Psychiatric Nursing: A Therapeutic Approach*. Macmillan, London.

Pelletier, L. (Ed.) (1987). *Psychiatric Nursing Case Studies, Nursing Diagnoses and Care Plans*. Springhouse Corporation, Springhouse, Pennsylvania.

Pope, B. (1986). *Social Skills Training for Psychiatric Nurse*. Harper and Row, London.

Potts, N. L. (1984). The secret pattern of binge/purge. *American Journal of Nursing*, January, Vol. 84, No. 1, pp. 32–35.

Priestley, P., McGuire, J., Flegg, D., Hemsley, V. and Welham, D. (1978). *Social Skills and Personal Problem Solving*. Tavistock, London.

Robinson, L. (1983). *Psychiatric Nursing as a Human Experience*, 3rd edition. W. B. Saunders, Philadelphia.

Sanger, E. and Cassino, T. (1984). Avoiding the power struggle. *American Journal of Nursing*, January, Vol. 84, No. 1, pp. 31–33.

Simmons, S. and Brooker, C. (1986). *Community Psychiatric Nursing: A Social Perspective*. Heinemann Nursing, London.

Sugden, J., Bessant, A., Eastland, M. and Field, R. (1986). *A Handbook for Psychiatric Nurses*. Harper and Row, London.

Thompson, S. (1979). Hungry for knowledge – not food. *Nursing Mirror*, 12 July, Vol. 75, No. 28, pp. 29–32.

Ward, M. F. (1985). *The Nursing Process in Psychiatry*. Churchill Livingstone, Edinburgh.

Self-assessment Questions

SAQ 9. List four interventions that can promote security in the person with an anorexic eating disorder.

SAQ 10. Identify four areas of observation that need to be maintained while caring for a person with an anorexic eating disorder

SAQ 11. Describe six interventions that can help the person re-establish a healthy eating pattern.

SAQ 12. Outline four ways of promoting the person's acceptance of their body image.

Unit 15.3: Written Test

Joan Stevens, aged 17, has been discovered by her parents to have been stringently dieting and inducing vomiting in order to become "slim". At the commencement of her diet she was 58 kg. She is now 43 kg. She is 5 feet 6 inches tall and for her build should weigh in the region of 51–54 kg. She is convinced that she is grossly overweight and perceives her body size as being "huge". Although she feels guilty about having deceived her family she cannot really accept that there is anything harmful in her behaviour.

It has been decided that as her family appear very cooperative, Joan will initially be given intensive support at home. This will involve a CPN visiting at least twice a day for a minimum of 30 minutes. Other random visits may be made.

1. Describe how you would explain the programme of progressive weight gain and privileges to Joan and her family.
2. How can you help Joan to develop a more realistic assessment of her body image?
3. What particular problems might you anticipate in attempting to support Joan in her home as against admitting her to hospital?

TOPIC 16

Personality Disorders

At the end of this Topic the learner should aim to:

1. Describe behaviour patterns indicative of an underlying personality disorder.
2. Outline the range of care and therapeutic interventions used for people with personality disorders.
3. Identify potential care needs and interventions for the person with a personality disorder.

The Nature of Personality Disorders: Recognition and Therapeutic Interventions

---

Unit Objectives

At the end of this Unit the learner should be able to:

1. Describe the characteristic features of a personality disorder.
2. Define the term "psychopathic disorder".
3. Outline possible factors contributing towards the development of a personality disorder.
4. Identify the range of therapeutic interventions for people with personality disorders.

The Nature of Personality Disorders

The definition and classification of personality disorders is one of the most contentious and controversial areas of mental health practice. The primary issue is one of whether the individual is "mentally ill" and "requires treatment", or whether their behaviour is at the boundaries of what is normally considered desirable and acceptable. In this context, there are patterns of social behaviour and personal responsibility which are assumed to equate both with mental health and with individual morality. Characteristically, the person labelled as having a "personality disorder" is viewed by others as behaving in an irresponsible and antisocial way that transgresses these boundaries. This pattern of non-conforming behaviour identifies the person as belonging to a "deviant" sub-group or sub-culture. Their subsequent life experiences may determine whether they follow a path labelled as "criminal" or "sick". The distinction can be a very fine one.

The person with a personality disorder would rarely perceive themselves as suffering from a mental health problem. Their main problems would be in relation to conflict with others who sought to impose boundaries on the person's behaviour, or in terms of the sanctions that were applied to them. As most of the conflict is in terms of relationships, responsibility and a difficulty in conforming, the term "sociopath" is sometimes applied to them. Whether they actually lack insight into their behaviour is more problematic.

Some people with a personality disorder are very readily able to identify what other people need and want and are able to respond accordingly, manipulating with ease.

Characteristic Features of People with Personality Disorders

1. *Difficulty in conforming to social expectations*: Their behaviour is often a source of conflict with others. They might appear irresponsible, self-centred, demanding or insensitive. They care little for the views of others and will do whatever is necessary to meet their own needs, irrespective of the distress or harm it might cause. Aspects of their behaviour may seem shocking or offensive to others.
2. *Learns little from experience*: Repeated negative outcomes do not appear to modify their behaviour. Deeply ingrained maladaptive patterns of behaviour are pursued even though they may have socially and self-damaging consequences.
3. *Lack of remorse or guilt for their actions*: This apparent lack of conscience may make others view them as "cruel" or "wicked". Expressions of remorse may be used to manipulate people or be viewed by others as shallow and insincere. Often they find it hard to understand why others are distressed by their behaviour and to reject any notion of personal responsibility.
4. *An inability to delay gratification*: Thinks only of short-term needs and acts just for the moment. Does not think through the possible longer-term outcomes of their behaviour. Hence, is liable to be impulsive and impatient.

The Clinical classification of Personality Disorders

Personality disorders are categorized according to which behavioural and emotional traits are most prominent. The personality disorder may co-exist with other mental health problems. Classifications include:

1. *Paranoid*: suspicious, ideas of self-reference, very touchy, quarrelsome, blames others, "chip on their shoulder", may come to conflict with others.
2. *Affective*: may be characterized by a depressive personality, i.e. gloomy, pessimistic and negative. Can present as a cheerful, humorous and optimistic personality, i.e. "likeable rogue".
3. *Obsessional or anankastic*: perfectionist, stubborn, meticulous and inflexible. Extremely conscientious. Timid and cautious, self-critical, self doubt and underlying anxiety, inability to relax.
4. *Histrionic*: egocentric, excitable, shallow emotional life, attention seeking. High degree of dependency, but is unable to sustain long-term relationships. Exaggerated emotional responses and over-dramatization.
5. *Schizoid*: detached, cold, indifferent, solitary. Indifferent to others.

Withdrawn and solitary, needing little social contact. May seem odd or bizarre to others.

6. *Asthenic*: succumbs to prevailing influences. Easily led. Very compliant. Very dependent on others.

7. *Psychopathic*: ruthless and manipulative. Selfish and egocentric. Pursues own objectives. Indifferent to the suffering they might cause. Cold, detached and aloof from others. Low tolerance to stress, liable to react aggressively if confronted. Impulsive in pursuit of short-term needs. Often in conflict with others and with authority. The 1983 Mental Health Act defines a psychopathic disorder as a "Persistent disorder of personality (whether or not accompanied by subnormality of intelligence) which results in abnormally aggressive or seriously irresponsible conduct on the part of the person concerned."

Origins of Personality Disorders

The research evidence on the development of personality disorders is very inconclusive. A number of theories have been proposed that have subsequently been disputed. Possible factors may include:

1. *Early life experiences and upbringing*

   - Emotional and maternal deprivation as an infant.
   - Victim of child abuse and family violence.
   - Large family size. Low family income. Adverse home conditions.
   - Parental role models who are violent to one another.
   - Parents who fail to set or enforce limits on behaviour.
   - Parental criminality.
   - Peer group models who use and reinforce violent behaviour.

2. *Psychological*

   - Psychoanalytic: poorly formed superego (conscience) which is unable to moderate any strong instinctual desires (id).
   - Inability to delay gratification.
   - Need for high stimulation.

3. *Physical*

   - EEG abnormalities: a diffuse and non-specific reading that is somewhat similar to patterns in infancy. However, similar patterns are also seen in an equivalent number of non-psychopathic, normal people.
   - "XXY" chromosome: originally thought to be significant as more common in male prisoners. Subsequent research showed that most people with a personality disorder have normal chromosomes and that most people with XXY chromosomes are not psychopaths.
   - Organic brain damage: behaviour patterns similar to those seen in

personality disorders may be seen after trauma to the brain or following infection, e.g. meningitis, encephalitis.

Therapeutic Interventions for the Person with a Personality Disorder

There is no specific therapy for personality disorders. A wide range of therapeutic interventions may be used to promote insight and awareness in the person and to improve the way they relate to others. The general approach should be towards an integrated and amenable service that is able to support the person and their family in the community or in residential care, as required. In particular, carers will need to be firm, consistent, accepting and non-judgemental.

Therapeutic aims

1. To promote insight into their behaviour.
2. To facilitate the development of the person's coping and life skills.
3. To minimize potential conflict with others.

Family and Self-care

The incidence of psychopathic disorder in the population is estimated to be 0.25%. It is virtually impossible, given the loose definitions that are used, to identify the incidence of other types of personality disorder. It would seem, though, that there are considerable numbers of people whose behaviour would fall within the classification of "personality disorder". Most of these people would not nececessarily regard themselves as having a mental health problem.

Their life-style and relationships may seem to others to be aimless and irresponsible. To themselves, and those that accept them, it would be the rest of society who is at fault in trying to impose "unreasonable" limitations and make life hard for them. Some people might be completely rejected by their family as "black sheep" for their irresponsible, selfish and manipulative behaviour. Other families, who might tolerate or reinforce such behaviour, may provide support and non-judgemental acceptance to the person.

The person with a personality disorder might seek treatment as a means of dealing with short-term difficulties and as a way of legitimizing their behaviour. A number of others may be sent for treatment as a consequence of aggressive or criminal actions.

They can be very demanding clients to work with therapeutically, and are very resistive to change.

Residential and Community Care

Therapeutic approaches may be based either in a community or residential setting. The residential setting, depending upon the person's needs and the resources available, may be in a:

1. Regional secure unit or special hospital: where therapeutic programmes and assessment can be conducted in a secure environment with access to specialist forensic services. The person would normally be admitted under the 1983 Mental Health Act or be referred by the Courts to such a treatment centre.
2. Therapeutic community: a specialist setting where the residents are actively involved in all aspects of daily living and decision making. Social barriers between staff and residents are minimized and open and honest communication is encouraged. Residents have to negotiate with others and to learn to accept responsibility for their own actions. Members are confronted by the group if their behaviour causes conflict or is disapproved of. The resident group is able to both enforce social sanctions against individuals and to reward members whose behaviour is for the benefit of the community. The social experiences of communication, acceptance, confrontation and responsibility are believed to promote self-awareness, self-esteem and to develop relationship skills. There are few therapeutic communities in existence within the National Health Service. The therapeutic outcomes of such an approach have proved difficult to validate.
3. Psychiatric hospital or unit.

Community care may involve the members of the community mental health team depending upon their skills and the client's needs. There may also be liaison with probation and aftercare services if the person is referred by the courts or is on a probation order. Regional secure units and special hospitals may also offer community support programmes for recently discharged residents.

Psychotherapeutic Interventions

The therapeutic interventions are not specific to the treatment of personality disorders. They may, however, facilitate the ability of the person to relate to others in a more helpful and constructive way.

1. Behavioural psychotherapy

   - Operant conditioning: in which the person is positively reinforced for desirable behaviour. This may take the form of social rewards or of tokens that can be exchanged for privileges or goods.
   - Social skills training: to improve the person's ability to relate and communicate with others.
   - Assertiveness training: to enable the person to differentiate between

aggressive, manipulative behaviour and assertive, confident behaviour.

2. Group therapy: to promote insight and interpersonal perception. Participants would be encouraged to accept responsibility for their actions and to confront others who deny any responsibility.
3. Individual counselling and psychotherapy: to promote insight.
4. Occupational therapy: to develop life skills.
5. Art therapy and psychodrama: to help promote emotional expression and the release of feelings.
6. Recreational and social activities: to provide diversional activities, provide positively reinforcing situations and opportunities to practise social skills.
7. Problem solving and coping skills: to increase the range of options open to the person so that they can relate more effectively and use more constructive strategies.
8. Health education: on relationships, the expression of feelings, dealing with stress.

Unit Instructions

When you have researched the suggested references, have mastered the Unit Objectives and successfully answered the Self-assessment Questions, proceed with the Unit Written Test.

Suggested References

Altschul, A. and McGovern, M. (1985). *Psychiatric Nursing*, 6th edition. Baillière Tindall, London and San Diego.

Bandura, A. (1977). *Social Learning Theory*. Prentice-Hall, Englewood Cliffs.

Bolton, R. (1979). *People Skills*. Prentice-Hall, Englewood Cliffs.

Cadbury, S., Jones, E. and Lee, R. (1983). A secure unit is born. *Nursing Mirror*, 14 September, Vol. 157, No. 11, pp. 30–33.

Darcy, P. T. (1984). *Theory and Practice of Psychiatric Care*. Hodder and Stoughton, London.

Davis, D. R. (1984). *An Introduction to Psychopathology*, 4th edition. Oxford University Press, Oxford.

Dickson, A. (1982). A Woman In Your Own Right: Assertiveness and You. Quartet, London.

Dietrich, G. (1976). Nurses in the therapeutic community. *Journal of Advanced Nursing*, Vol. 1, No. 2 pp. 139–154.

Fottrell, E. (1981). Violent behaviour by psychiatric patients. *British Journal of Hospital Medicine*, January, Vol. 25, No. 1, pp. 28–38.

Gibbs, A. (1986). *Understanding Mental Health*. Consumers Association/Hodder and Stoughton, London.

Hardiman, F. (1985). Safe and secure. *Nursing Times*, 20 March, Vol. 181, No. 12, pp. 51–52.

Hendry, M. (1983). Nursing behind bars. *Nursing Mirror*, 2 March, Vol. 156, No. 9, pp. 16–18.

Hood, M. (1985). New horizons. *Nursing Times*, 20 March, Vol. 81, No. 12, pp. 53–54.

Hopson, B. and Scally, M. (1981). *Life Skills Teaching*. McGraw-Hill, London.

Hughes, J. (1986). *An Outline of Modern Psychiatry*, 2nd edition. John Wiley, New York.

Irving, S. (1983). *Basic Psychiatric Nursing*, 3rd edition. W. B. Saunders, Philadelphia.

Jansen, E. (Ed.) (1980). *The Therapeutic Community*. Croom Helm, London.

Lancaster, J. (1980). *Adult Psychiatric Nursing*. Henry Kimpton, London.

Lee, A. (1981). Nursing in the special hospitals. *Nursing*, October, Vol. 1, No. 30, pp. 1305–1306.

Lindsay, M. (1982). A critical review of the validity of the therapeutic community. *Nursing Times*, 22 September, Vol. 78, No. 27, pp. 105–107, Occasional Papers.

Loo, A. (1984). Assessing mentally disordered offenders. *Nursing Times*, 2 May, Vol. 80, No. 18, pp. 44–46.

Lyttle, J. (1986). *Mental Disorder: Its Care and Treatment*. Baillière Tindall, London and San Diego.

Martin, P. (1987). *Care of the Mentally Ill*, 2nd edition. Macmillan, London.

Nelson-Jones, R. (1984). *Personal Responsibility Counselling and Therapy*. Harper and Row, London.

Orme, J. E. (1984). *Abnormal and Clinical Psychology: An Introductory Text*. Croom Helm, London.

Pope, B. (1986). *Social Skills Training for Psychiatric Nurses*. Harper and Row, London.

Priestley, P., McGuire, J., Flegg, D., Hemsley, V. and Welham, D. (1978). *Social Skills and Personal Problem Solving*. Tavistock, London.

Reid, A., Lea, J. and Wallace, D. (1982). Rehabilitation in Elton Ward, an interim regional secure unit. *Nursing Times*, 17 March, Vol. 78, No. 8, pp. 29–32. Occasional Papers.

Robinson, L. (1983). *Psychiatric Nursing as a Human Experience*, 3rd edition. W. B. Saunders, Philadelphia.

Rowden, R. (1983). A unit for the future. *Nursing Times*, 20 July, Vol. 79, No. 29, pp. 10–11.

Sims, A. (1988). *Symptoms in the Mind*. Baillière Tindall, London and San Diego.

Smith, M. J. (1975). *When I Say No, I Feel Guilty*. Bantam, New York.

Trethowan, W. and Sims, A. (1983). *Psychiatry*, 5th edition. Baillière Tindall, London and San Diego.

Trower, P., Bryant, B., and Argyle, M. (1978). *Social Skills and Mental Health*. Methuen, London.

Wandless, D. (1983). Distribution of resources. *Nursing Mirror*, 2 March, Vol. 156, No. 9, pp. 22–25.

Wilkinson, J. and Canter, S. (1982). *Social Skills Training Manual*. John Wiley, Chichester.

Willis, J. (1976). *Clinical Psychiatry*. Blackwell Scientific, Oxford.

Self-assessment Questions

SAQ 1. Outline four characteristic features of a personality disorder.
SAQ 2. List and describe four types of personality disorder.
SAQ 3. Identify four factors in a person's upbringing that may contribute towards the development of a personality disorder.
SAQ 4. State four therapeutic interventions that may be of value in the care of a person with a personality disorder.

Unit 16.1: Written Test

David Jones, aged 28, was admitted yesterday following an attempted overdose. His subsequent behaviour, however, indicated that he was not clinically depressed. He quickly settled into the unit and was soon taking advantage of less assertive residents. Later that day the police contacted the unit, wishing to interview David in connection with threatening behaviour and criminal damage during an incident several days ago. They had had some difficulty in locating David who had been effectively evading them.

1. What aspects of David's behaviour and emotions would indicate that his life-style originated from a personality disorder rather than criminal intent?
2. What therapeutic approaches might be useful in promoting insight and enabling David to take responsibility for his actions?

Nursing Care of the Person with a Personality Disorder

Unit Objectives

1. Identify the nursing care needs of the person with a personality disorder.
2. Plan an individualized care programme.
3. Select appropriate nursing care interventions for the person's needs.
4. Describe possible evaluation criteria for specific needs.

Mental Health Nursing Care

Each person's care needs are unique and have to be assessed individually. For the client with a personality disorder a wide range of potential needs may be identified depending upon their background and the nature of their current difficulties. It is also possible that the person may have other superimposed mental health problems. A range of potential care needs have been selected to illustrate some of the problems that the person may experience and the potential nursing interventions that may help them.

For the client with a personality disorder these may include the needs to:

A. Promote their social and interpersonal awareness.
B. Develop behavioural self-control.
C. Feel secure and free from threat.
D. Facilitate the development of the person's and family's coping skills.

A. Promote their Social and Interpersonal Awareness

Associated problems/personal difficulties

Person may need to increase their social and interpersonal awareness due to:

1. Repeated conflicts with others.
2. Mistrust of others.
3. Use of manipulation and other maladaptive strategies to achieve personal goals.
4. Difficulty in understanding why others might react adversely.
5. Behaviour that is perceived as threatening or socially damaging by others.
6. Low tolerance to frustration and inability to delay needs gratification.

Assessment

1. Person's perception of their own behaviour and the way they relate to others.
2. Information from relatives and friends.
3. Nurse's observations of the person's:

   (a) Understanding and awareness of their health care needs.
   (b) Interaction with others: threatening, manipulative, aggressive, appropriate, inappropriate.
   (c) Expectations of others: realistic, unrealistic, distorted.
   (d) Personal expectations: realistic, unrealistic, attainable, non-attainable.
   (e) Consistency or inconsistency of behaviour.

4. Nature of person's current relationships: positive, negative, demanding, supportive, rewarding.
5. Past social history: key events and the person's reactions and perceptions of them.
6. Psychosocial environment: presence of identifiable triggering cues, reactions of others to person's behaviour, potential reinforcers of inappropriate behaviour. Presence of potential stresses in person's environment or lifestyle.

Desired outcomes

1. Person able to begin to trust others.
2. Person able to use more constructive ways of relating to others.
3. Person becomes more aware of the needs of others.

Nursing Intervention	*Rationale*
1. Initiate therapeutic relationship. Involve them in the care	Interventions more likely to succeed in an atmosphere of trust and cooperation. Helps to reduce tension

Nursing intervention	*Rationale*
planning process. Demonstrate active listening. Be available and approachable. Offer reassurance. Demonstrate acceptance. Demonstrate non-judgemental responses	and to create the conditions for behavioural change. Person is very sensitive to implied criticism
2. Promote feelings of security and safety (see **C.**)	Person needs to feel safe and to trust carers for effective personal growth
3. Model skilled social and communication skills	Modelling by nurses has a powerful influence on the people in their care
4. Promote their autonomy and self-esteem	Self-belief in the person's own value and feelings of control and mastery increase confidence in dealing with others. More likely to relate to others in a "healthy" way
5. Positively reinforce healthy behaviour and responses. Negatively reinforce maladaptive behaviour	Positive reinforcement of healthy behaviour is likely to increase its occurrence
6. Provide feedback on the person's behaviour and use it as a learning situation. Offer feedback on the person's emotional expression	Person may not be aware of how others perceive them or on the appropriateness of their behaviour. Also provides an opportunity for health education in the appropriate expression of feelings and relating to others. Promotes insight
7. Explore with the person the effects of their behaviour and emotions upon others	Person may not be aware of how their behaviour and emotional reactions affect others
8. Explore with the person reasons for criticisms by others. Explore with the person reasons for criticisms of others	Person may not be aware of why others perceive them in a negative way. This also influences how they perceive others
9. Explore with the person reasons for recurring problems	Person may not realize that their longstanding problems have a common origin

Nursing intervention	*Rationale*
10. Encourage the use of appropriate coping mechanisms for anger and frustration (see **D**.)	Need to develop and use effective ways of coping with frustration and anger
11. Encourage acceptance of self-limitations. Encourage honesty in presenting self. Support a realistic assessment of their life circumstances	Person needs to develop a more realistic image of themselves. May have felt the need to distort their self-presentation in order to protect their self-esteem. Many have very unrealistic expectations that cause frustration and resentment
12. Explore criticism of others. Identify criteria used to evaluate self and others. Assist the person to acknowledge the influence of this criteria on their self-esteem and the way they relate. Explore alternative ways of evaluating their self-worth and expectations. Promote a realistic assessment of situations. Encourage acceptance of self-limitations. Offer alternative interpretations of life experiences that person uses to devalue themselves. Encourage awareness of positive responses from others	Person may have unrealistic expectations which make them feel deprived and frustrated. May perceive others as having benefits denied to them, which causes resentment. Person may have created a "script" for themselves in which they need to relate in a manipulative way to meet their needs. The person needs to be helped to reshape their beliefs about themself and to develop more valid and realistic expectations. Tend to interpret responses by others as negative and threatening
13. Explore previous achievements and successes. Identify and work with their strengths and resources	May have positive assets that can be utilized in developing the way they relate to others

Nursing intervention	*Rationale*
14. Identify situations with the person in which they experience a relationship or a communication difficulty	Many people with mental health problems are either lacking in social skills or have problems relating to others
15. Role play with feedback these situations with the person. Give demonstration and guidance as required. Provide information on the nature of human interaction and expression of feeling. Encourage gradual mastery. Provide opportunities to rehearse social skills. Promote self-evaluation of social competence. Identify real-life opportunities to practise social skills. Set specific assignments. Monitor and evaluate with person	Social skills and assertiveness training help people to develop their communication and relationship skills. It is a structured approach in which specific skills are: ● identified and defined; ● divided into their constituent elements; ● the elements are practised with feedback in role-play until competence is achieved; ● the entire skill is practised with feedback until competence is achieved; ● the skill is transferred to real-life situations.
16. Describe behaviour patterns indicating emotional maturity. Provide opportunities for the person to express themselves openly and honestly	Person's social understanding may be limited. Helps to relieve tension and to demonstrate acceptance. It also provides the opportunity for them to practise talking about their emotions which they may have had difficulty with in the past. May also reduce the need for the physical expression of anger and frustration
17. Engage in physical activity as a precursor to verbal interaction, e.g. games, activities, drama, music. Organize social and recreational activities	Sometimes it is easier for people to relate as part of an activity or game, or afterwards

Nursing intervention	Rationale
18. Identify options for work and leisure activities. Encourage personal interests	Relieves boredom and helps to raise self-esteem if meaningfully employed
19. Encourage social interaction with others. Organize group activities	Social activities can be very rewarding and also provide group dynamics that the person may find therapeutic
20. Promote contact with relatives and personal friends. Increase opportunities for group interaction	Helps to overcome feelings of isolation and rejection. Still valued by others
21. Organize experiential exercises, e.g. drama, role-play, games, in which the person relates to others in an unstructured way and an express themselves freely	Structured and spontaneous experiential exercises can provide powerful feedback and personal learning opportunities. Specific exercises can be used to promote insight

Evaluation

1. Person demonstrates trust in carers and others.
2. Person observed to relate with others in a constructive and non-manipulative way.
3. Person demonstrates an awareness of the needs of others.

B. Develop Behavioural Self-control

Associated problems/personal difficulties

Person may need to develop behavioural self-control as a result of:

1. Short-term impulsiveness at the expense of negative longer-term consequences.
2. Difficulty in complying or conforming with social expectations.
3. Behaviour that is perceived by others as threatening.
4. Repeated conflicts with others.
5. Difficulty in managing own aggressive feelings constructively.

Assessment

1. Person's perception of their own behaviour patterns.
2. Information from relatives and friends.
3. Nurse's observation of other person's:

   (a) Response to questioning about their behaviour.
   (b) Interaction with others: frequency, duration, nature, content.
   (c) Coping strategies for stress and frustration: effective, ineffective, behavioural, cognitive, emotional.
   (d) Reaction to imposed limits by others: tolerance for frustration, willingness to negotiate, delay or compromise.

4. Relationship between environmental factors and maladaptive behaviour: - triggering cues, reaction of others, potential reinforcers.
5. Potential risk factors in the way they interact with others.
6. Person's perceived objectives for personal growth.
7. Presence of potential stresses in person's life-style or environment: noise, conflicts, alcohol, drugs, poor accommodation, unemployment.

Desired outcomes

1. Person able to develop behavioural self control and to delay gratification.
2. Episodes of conflict with others decrease.
3. Person learns to manage feelings of frustration and aggression constructively.
4. Person does not put themselves, or others, at risk as a consequence of their impulsiveness.

Nursing intervention	Rationale
1. Initiate therapeutic relationship. Involve the person in the care planning process	Interventions more likely to be successful in an atmosphere of trust and cooperation
2. Be available and approachable. Demonstrate non-judgemental responses. Demonstrate acceptance. Promote feelings of security and freedom from threat (see **C**.)	Need to develop trust in order to work effectively with client and to create the conditions for behavioural change. If the person feels insecure they will tend to be defensive and distrustful

Nursing intervention	*Rationale*
3. Observe their behaviour to identify factors that contribute to hostile behaviour	Can be used to identify any environmental factors that may be amenable to modification
4. Assist the person to identify any environmental factors related to frustration and hostility	Person may not be aware of the way that environmental factors are influencing their behaviour
5. Encourage the person to modify environmental factors where possible that are contributing to problems with others	Modification of contributing environmental factors may help to reduce stimuli that elicit anger and frustration
6. Identify potential reinforcers in the person's environment	Helps to promote adaptive behaviour
7. Positively reinforce healthy, constructive behaviour. Negatively reinforce manipulative and angry behaviour	Person needs to experience positive outcomes for desired behaviour
8. Teach family members the skills of giving reinforcement. Teach family members how to identify desirable behaviours	Family members may be inadvertently contributing to the maintenance of maladaptive behaviour
9. Model constructive responses for person in situations where they are manipulative or hostile	Modelling can be a powerful influence for positive behaviour change. People tend to reflect the behaviour of those around them
10. Identify situations with the person in which they experience difficulty in communicating or relating to others	Many people with mental health problems are either lacking in social skills or have problems relating to others
11. Role play, with feedback, these situations with the person. Give demonstration and guidance as required	Social skills and assertiveness training help to develop communication and emotional expression skills

Nursing intervention	*Rationale*
12. Teach the skills and principles of assertiveness. Encourage the person to discriminate between aggressive and assertive behaviour	Increases personal control that can be expressed in a more effective way. Increases confidence, self-esteem and the ability to communicate more effectively
13. Establish a hierarchy of situations in which the person experiences frustration or reacts aggressively. Teach the person the skills of behavioural and emotional control. Work through hierarchy of situations, substituting alternative coping behaviour. Encourage person to practise newly learned behaviour in safe settings. Encourage person to transfer learning to real-life situations. Provide on-going positive reinforcement. Monitor person's success in using newly acquired skills	A "systematic desensitization" approach has been used with effect in modifying habitually aggressive behaviour. Person gradually acquires new behavioural skills. Can also use imagery in the early stages of therapy before transferring to real-life practice and situations. Needs to be able to use behavioural control in real life for approach to be fully effective. Practice needs to be continued and developed to establish new habitual responses that are adaptive and non-threatening
14. Offer feedback on the person's behaviour and use it as a learning situation	Person may not be aware of how others perceive them
15. Explore with the person the effects of their behaviour upon others	Person may not be aware of how their behaviour affects others
16. Explore with the person the effects of their behaviour on their own and their family's life	Person may not be fully aware of how their behaviour is disrupting their life and relationships

Nursing intervention	*Rationale*
17. Advise person if their behaviour is perceived as threatening to others	May not realize that their behaviour causes others to behave aggressively towards them
18. Protect others who may find their behaviour threatening. Encourage respect for the rights of others	Others may react defensively to threatening behaviour which may elicit a stronger aggressive response
19. Inform the person as to what he can realistically expect from the staff and others	Promotes insight and reinforces social awareness
20. Meet reasonable demands. Keep promises that you make	Shows respect for the person
21. Explain the reasons for setting limits on their behaviour to the person. Negotiate contractual boundaries of person's behaviour. Specify the boundaries of acceptable behaviour. Clearly set limits on behaviour that is: • threatening to others, • manipulative. Record these in detail. Ensure that written limits are readily accessible to carers. Give a copy to the person and their family	The person with a personal disorder often lacks internal controls. Initially the carers have to set and maintain limits. These can gradually be regained by the person as they demonstrate and maintain compliance with care programme. Encouraging personal responsibility helps to raise self-esteem and promotes insight. Setting limits also promotes personal security. Limits need to be based on the use of rational authority, professional knowledge and understanding
22. Inform the person of the consequences of exceeding defined behavioural limits. Promote compliance with set limits. Positively reinforce compliance with limits	Person needs to know how others will react and intervene

Nursing intervention	*Rationale*
23. Ensure that all care workers are consistent in their approach to person and in maintaining limits. Direct person to their key worker for detailed information	Need to ensure consistency. Person will readily manipulate carers if they identify inconsistency. Helps to ensure consistency
24. Observe person for signs of mounting frustration. Help person to identify source of frustration and anger. Encourage them to express their feelings. Listen. Explore alternative responses. Facilitate problem solving	Person may not be aware of factors that cause them to react this way. Promotes self-esteem. Helps to facilitate the release of frustration and tension in a constructive way
25. Advise them that they have choice. Promote responsibility for their own actions	Person needs to be aware that they have options over their behaviour
26. Explain ways of redirecting feelings. Suggest more appropriate ways of emotional expression. Explain the importance of remaining calm	Need to develop their skills of coping with stress and frustration constructively. Also helps to promote self-awareness. Prevention is the key approach in avoiding physical hostility
27. Explain the importance of self-control. Encourage acceptance of partial goal attainment. Facilitate their ability to cope with frustration. Encourage person to write out their feelings	May lack insight and awareness of the role of behavioural self-control in everyday life. May need to relearn to compromise goal attainment. A low tolerance for frustration is a key factor in conflict with others. Need to develop a more robust level of tolerance.
28. Inform the person when and how their behaviour is approaching set limits	Can be an effective channel for experiencing feelings and provide useful material

Nursing intervention	*Rationale*
29. Inform the person of the consequences of exceeding limits. Avoid triggering an angry response. Absorb criticism	Using reality confrontation may help to avoid the situation escalating. Skilful intervention can avert the situation getting out of hand
30. Adopt a non-threatening posture. Moderate voice tone and tempo. De-escalate with key word. Distract the person's attention. Divert to more constructive activities	Important for carers to keep own behaviour controlled which can have a powerful calming effect
31. Be firm and consistent. Be assertive	Nurses need to show that they are in control of the situation and that they will impose limits the person is unable to maintain
32. If feel threatened withdraw. Provide space around the person. Put a "barrier" between yourself and the person. Ensure that bystanders are removed. Call for assistance. Do not attempt lone intervention	Risk of adding stress to the situation and of intervening effectively. For protection and to slow them down. May help you feel more secure in coping. May feel "hemmed in" or crowded. Also potent safety of others. May put both the person and nurse at risk if attempt to intervene on your own
33. Co-ordinate interventions of care staff if intervention is necessary. Act quickly and decisively. Use minimum force. Hold non-vulnerable areas. Hold for minimum period. Keep talking to the person and try to calm them	Intervention should be directed towards safely limiting the person's disturbed behaviour. Staff needed to act promptly and as a team to minimize the possibility of risk to both parties
34. Use seclusion or time out if specified in limits or if others are at significant risk.	Seclusion may be an appropriate intervention in certain conditions. Needs to be used with extreme caution and with their therapeutic

Nursing intervention	*Rationale*
Comply with organizational rules for seclusion	objectives
35. Ensure that the person's physical and safety needs are maintained during seclusion. Use minimum period of seclusion	To avoid harm or injury
36. After situation explore with the person alternatives ways of behaving. Encourage them to learn from the experience	Need to demonstrate a relationship between their actions and the outcomes. Also, that they had a choice and would have behaved in other, more constructive ways
37. Document in detail the situation and behaviour that required intervention. Detail the interventions made. Document any injuries caused to the person or to staff	Each organization has its own requirements. Important that accurate records are kept for both review and for possible legal purposes
38. Review staff practices afterwards to evaluate interventions, care programme and operational policies. Avoid recrimination. Be non-judgemental	May be significant lessons to be learned from the situation. Needs to be done as soon as possible
39. Periodically review limits that are set with the person to promote learning. Increase personal responsibility in small stages. Encourage gradual mastery of situations. Reinforce initiatives taken by person. Respect personal decisions	These should balance the person's therapeutic progress. More likely to promote compliance. Gradually need to re-introduce personal control over behaviour and life circumstances

Nursing intervention	*Rationale*
40. Recognize the effects of the person's behaviour upon yourself. Arrange for own clinical supervision	Caring for a person with a personality disorder can be a very demanding and draining experience. Need to be alert to the risk of manipulation. Need to maintain own mental health and to review own clinical practice and to facilitate professional development
41. Organize experiential activities, e.g. drama, role-play, games, in which the person relates to others in an unstructured way and can express themselves freely	Structured and spontaneous experiential activities can provide powerful feedback and personal learning opportunities. Can be specifically used to develop communication skills and to promote insight

Evaluation

1. Person observed to deal constructively with situations that previously would have evoked frustration and anger.
2. Reduction in the frequency of conflict with others.
3. Behaviour consistently stays within stated limits.

C. Feel Secure and Free From Threat

Associated problems/personal difficulties

Person may feel insecure and threatened as a result of:

1. Inadequate knowledge and understanding of their care and treatment.
2. Feelings of mistrust towards others.
3. Behaviour that is perceived by others as aggressive or manipulative.
4. Stresses that their behaviour causes to close relationships.
5. Tension arising from enforced treatment (if under section).
6. Feelings of frustration if unable to gratify needs immediately.

Assessment

1. Person's description of their anxieties and concerns: feelings of threat, frustration, specific fears.

2. Information from relatives and friends.
3. Nurse's observations of the person's:

(a) Response to questioning about their current situation.
(b) Understanding and insight shown: questions asked and statements made in relation to their health needs and treatment programme, the concerns expressed.
(c) Emotional state: emotions displayed, edginess, irritability, hostility, anger, threats.
(d) Non-verbal behaviour indicating insecurity: posture, gestures, tone of voice, eye movements, restlessness, excessive smoking.
(e) Interaction pattern and behaviour with others: aggressive, dominating, threatening, passive, non-assertive, confident, uncertain.
(f) Verbal communication pattern: rate, tone of voice, speech errors, over-talkativeness.

4. Identification of potential stressors in the person's relationships, lifestyle, expectations and environment.
5. Support network available to the person: relationships with key people.

Desired outcomes

1. Person's and family's understanding of their health care needs is increased.
2. Person demonstrates a degree of trust in their care.
3. Personal feelings of frustration are minimized.

Nursing Intervention	Rationale
1. Initiate a therapeutic relationship. Use the person's preferred name. Spend time with them. Be available and approachable. Demonstrate active listening. Use touch	Interventions more likely to be successful in an atmosphere of trust and cooperation. Also shows sense of worth and acceptance which helps to increase feelings of security and safety
2. Non-judgemental and non-critical approach. Emphasize the person's value as an individual	Being non-judgemental helps to promote acceptance. Person may have a long history of rejection and criticism by others
3. Provide clear and understandable	A lot of insecurity is associated with fear of the unknown. People have a right

Nursing intervention	*Rationale*
information about their health care and the roles of different health care workers. Encourage questions. Ask for feedback on their understanding. Clarify any misunderstandings. Enlist the person's cooperation in the planning of their health care. Promote their autonomy and self-esteem	to information about their health care. The nurse is in an ideal position to use this process to facilitate the development of the person's understanding about their care needs. People are more likely to cooperate if they are well-informed and involved in the decision-making process. It also increases feelings of personal control.
4. Ensure that significant personal possessions are available. Personalize the person's intimate environment	Familiar objects help to increase feelings of security and self-esteem. Also promotes the potential for personal change
5. Explain all actions in advance. Reassure the person of non-harmful intent	Actions less likely to be perceived as threatening and avoids sudden surprises
6. Approach unhurriedly. Demonstrate calmness. Do not rush the person. Be aware of your own reactions and experiences of stress. Adopt a non-threatening, open posture and tone of voice. Keep calm	Stress in the carer communicates itself to the person. Caring can be a stressful experience at times. This may unconsciously influence your interactions with them. Need to demonstrate a confident and assertive manner to promote credibility with client and also not to appear threatening
7. Be patient and aware of your own feelings of frustration in dealing with the person. Take periodic breaks if possible. Arrange for own clinical supervision	The person may be very demanding and resistant to interventions. Find ways of coping with your own stress. Supervision is an effective way of providing support to the practitioner and of professional development. May also be necessary to help maintain objectivity in the face of manipulative demands
8. Refrain from unnecessary actions and procedures if the	These just increase the tension and are likely to be misinterpreted

Nursing intervention	*Rationale*
person appears disturbed or agitated	
9. Do not whisper to others in the presence of the person or express inappropriate emotions	This increases feelings of suspicion and threat
10. Remove distracting and stressful influences	People with a personal disorder often have a low tolerance for stress
11. Encourage the person to talk about their hostile feelings and difficulties. Encourage them to express their feelings in a more appropriate way	Venting their feelings in this way may remove the necessity for the physical expression of hostility and anger. Provides an opportunity for health education in the appropriate expression of anger and frustration. Helps to promote insight
12. Facilitate the development of the person's ability to communicate and relate to others. Promote insight into the way they relate to others (see **A.**)	Helps the person to express and thereby release feelings of hostility and tension. Increased interpersonal perception may reduce situations of conflict
13. Encourage appropriate diversional recreational and social activities	Helps to avoid boredom and to divert the person's thoughts away from stressful topics. Physical activity is also a beneficial channel for frustration and anger
14. Encourage the person to rest or relax if they appear to be under stress. Provide feedback on their behaviour	Person may not be aware of the effect of tension on their behaviour
15. Set limits on behaviour that is potentially harmful. Be consistent and firm. Enforce limits if behaviour exceeds predetermined boundaries	Person needs to be aware that others are concerned for their safety and that they will intervene if necessary

Evaluation

1. Person demonstrates trust in their care.
2. Situations of conflict are averted and minimized.
3. Person is able to cope with feelings of frustration and hostility constructively.

D. Facilitate the Development of the Person's and Family's Coping Skills

Associated problems/personal difficulties

The difficulties experienced by the client with a personality disorder may show that:

1. Existing methods of coping may be counterproductive and maladaptive.
2. Current life-style, expectations and relationships may be potential sources of stress.
3. The person and their family may lack information about the resources available to help them.
4. Family members may find it difficult to offer emotional support to each other.
5. Family members may find it difficult to impose limits on behaviour.
6. The person and family may reject outside help even though under stress.
7. There may be feelings of guilt in relation to their problems and asking for help.

Assessment

1. Person and family's perceptions of their current situation.
2. Existing coping methods used and their effectiveness.
3. Support available to the person and family.
4. Accuracy of the knowledge and information given by the person and their family.
5. Statements of guilt and stigma.
6. Awareness of resources available to them.
7. Previous experience, if any, of dealing with similar problems.

Desired outcomes

1. Person and family able to make an informed choice about the resources they require.
2. Person and family able to cope better with life and personal problems.

Nursing Intervention	Rationale
1. Initiate therapeutic relationship	Interventions more likely to be successful in an atmosphere of trust and cooperation
2. Advise that seeking help and recognition of problems are a positive step towards finding solutions	Many people feel that seeking help is a sign of weakness and failure. Also helps to reduce guilt
3. Encourage questions. Provide accurate information. Identify appropriate health care resources	May have inaccurate knowledge and expectations. Fear of the unknown. Need to know what resources are available to them
4. Discuss potential entitlement to financial benefits and allowances	May need and not be aware of the financial help available to them
5. Advise that highly emotional situations be avoided at first	May be pent-up feelings and stresses that need to be worked through and released in a controlled way. Sudden discharge of emotion may cause unnecessary and harmful conflict
6. Advise against early and unrealistic correction of problems	Under stress it is sometimes easier to make short-term adaptations that only store up future problems. It takes time to help the family to work out what is best for them
7. Reassure that there are ways of improving the situation	Family may feel that the situation is hopeless
8. Advise against recrimination and focussing on past problems	Need to focus on the present and to deal with anger and guilt in a more productive way
9. Advise on the need for acceptance and mutual support within their relationships	Family needs to come to terms with their situation. They are each other's primary source of support which will need to be utilized to cope effectively
10. Explain the need to identify and recognize potentially stressful situations	Mental health problems tend to be long-term in nature. In order to cope effectively the family needs to be taught ways of making the necessary long-term adjustments

Nursing intervention	*Rationale*
11. Teach methods for coping with frustration and anger. Teach how to use problem-solving methods for coping with difficulties. Assist the family to learn new coping skills. Encourage the setting of realistic goals and expectations	Much of the education needs to be directed towards learning new coping methods. These include the way that the members of the family communicate, their expectations and the way that emotional support is given
12. Advise the family on how to give feedback and support to one another	Existing patterns may be non-supportive and be reinforcing inappropriate behaviour
13. Encourage the setting of progressive goals in small stages	The re-learning needs to be done in a gradual way in which the family provides the main support and reinforcement. The person also has the maximum opportunity to experience success. This also helps to raise self-esteem
14. Recommend ways of setting behavioural limits. Explain the purpose of making a contract with the person	Living together is a process of negotiation. It is often useful for all concerned if the boundaries are firmly defined. Many families make implicit contracts that can be contractualized. These may be quite effective in some situations
15. Encourage the use of newly acquired coping skills	Skills need to be used in order to become part of everyday living
16. Review occupational/ unemployment stresses. Encourage the development of appropriate work/non-work coping strategies	Work and unemployment can be major sources of stress. As these represent a major part of life it is important that the person learns how to cope with these stresses constructively
17. Put family in contact with self-help and voluntary groups	Self-help groups able to offer effective and understanding practical help
18. Teach the family and person to recognize the limits of their ability to cope and when it is advisable to seek help	The family should not over-burden itself as this can damage relationships and its longer-term ability to cope

Evaluation

1. Person and family identify and select resources they require.
2. Person and family demonstrate use of improved coping methods.
3. Person and family able to give accurate information about their health care needs.

Unit Instructions

When you have researched the suggested references, have mastered the Unit Objectives and successfully answered the Self-assessment Questions, proceed with the Unit Written Test.

Suggested References

Adams, C. G. and Macione, A. (Eds) (1983). *Handbook of Psychiatric Mental Health Nursing*. John Wiley/Fleschner, New York.

Alchin, S. and Weatherhead, R. (1976). *Psychiatric Nursing: A Practical Approach*. McGraw Hill, Sydney.

Altschul, A. and McGovern, M. (1985). *Psychiatric Nursing*, 6th edition. Baillière Tindall, London and San Diego.

Barker, P. J. (1982). *Behaviour Therapy Nursing*. Croom Helm, London.

Barker, P. J. (1985). *Patient Assessment in Psychiatric Nursing*, Croom Helm, London.

Bauer, B. B. and Hill, S. S. (1986). *Essentials of Mental Health Care Planning and Interventions*. W. B. Saunders, Philadelphia.

Burrows, R. (1984). Nurses and violence. *Nursing Times*, 25 January, Vol. 180, No. 4, pp. 56–58.

Campbell, C. (1978). *Nursing Diagnosis and Intervention in Nursing Practice*. John Wiley, New York.

Campbell, W. and Mawson, D. (1978). Violence in a psychiatric unit. *Journal of Advanced Nursing*, Vol. 3, No. 1, pp. 55–64.

Campbell, W., Shepherd, H. and Falconer, F. (1982). The use of seclusion. *Nursing Times*, 27 October, Vol. 78, No. 43, pp. 1821–1825.

Casseem, M. (1984). Violence on the wards. *Nursing Mirror*, 23 May, Vol. 158, No. 21, pp. 14–16.

Cobb, J. P. and Gossop, M. R. (1976). Locked doors in the management of disturbed psychiatric patients. *Journal of Advanced Nursing*, Vol. 1, No. 6, pp. 469–480.

Coffey, M. P. (1976). The violent pattern. *Journal of Advanced Nursing*, Vol. 1, No. 5, pp. 341–350.

Darcy, P. T. (1984). *Theory and Practice of Psychiatric Care*. Hodder and Stoughton, London.

Darcy, P. T. (1985). *Mental Health Nursing Source Book*. Baillière Tindall, London and San Diego.

Department of Health and Social Security (1976). *The Management of Violent or Potentially Violent, Hospital Patients*. HC(76)11. HMSO, London.

Dexter, G. and Wash, M. (1986). *Psychiatric Nursing Skills: A Patient-centred Approach*. Croom Helm, London.

Dickson, A. (1982). *A Woman In Your Own Right: Assertiveness and You*. Quartet Books, London.

Hase, S. and Douglas, A. (1986). *Human Dynamics and Nursing*. Churchill Livingstone, Edinburgh.

Hodkinson, P., Hillis, T. and Russell, D. (1984). Assaults on staff in a psychiatric hospital. *Nursing Times*, 18 April, Vol. 80, No. 16, pp. 44–46.

Hopson, B. and Scally, M. (1981). *Life Skills Teaching*. McGraw-Hill, London.

Irving, S. (1983). *Basic Psychiatric Nursing*, 3rd edition. W. B. Saunders, Philadelphia.

Lancaster, J. (1980). *Adult Psychiatric Nursing*. Henry Kimpton, London.

Leiba, P. A. (1980). Management of violent patients. *Nursing Times*, 2 October, Vol. 76, No. 23, pp. 101–104. Occasional Papers.

Leopoldt, H. (1985). A secure and secluded spot. *Nursing Times*, 6 February, Vol. 81, No. 6, pp. 26–28.

Lyttle, J. (1986). *Mental Disorder: Its Care and Treatment*. Baillière Tindall, London and San Diego.

McFarland, G. and Wasli, E. (1986). *Nursing Diagnoses and Process in Psychiatric Mental Health Nursing*. J. B. Lippincott, Philadelphia.

Martin, P. (1987a). *Psychiatric Nursing: A Therapeutic Approach*. Macmillan, London.

Martin, P. (1987b). *Care of the Mentally Ill*. 2nd edition. Macmillan, London.

Moran, J. (1984). Response and responsibility. *Nursing Times*, 4 April, Vol. 80, No. 14, pp. 28–31.

Owens, R. G. and Ashcroft, J. B. (1985). *Violence: A Guide for the Caring Professions*. Croom Helm, London.

Pisarcik, G. (1981). Danger you are. . .facing the violent patient. *Nursing 81*, September, Vol. 11, No. 9, pp. 61–65.

Pope, B. (1986). *Social Skills Training for Psychiatric Nurses*. Harper and Row, London.

Priestley, P., McGuire, J., Flegg, D., Hemsley, V. and Welham, D. (1978). *Social Skills and Personal Problem Solving*. Tavistock, London.

Rix, G. (1985). Compassion is better than conflict, aggression in the mentally ill. *Nursing Times*, 18 September, Vol. 81, No. 38, Mental Health Nursing, pp. 53–55.

Robinson, L. (1983). *Psychiatric Nursing as a Human Experience*, 3rd edition. W. B. Saunders, Philadelphia.

Russell, D., Hodgkinson, P. and Hillis, T. (1986). Time out. *Nursing Times*, 26 February, Vol. 82, No. 9, pp. 47–49.

Smeaton, W. and Field, R. (1985). The nature and management of hostility. *Nursing*, March, Vol. 2, No. 35, pp. 1033–1038.

Smith, L. (1978). Limit-setting. *Nursing Times*, 29 June, Vol. 74, No. 26, pp. 1074–1075.

Sugden, J., Bessant, A., Eastland, M. and Field, R. (1986). *A Handbook for Psychiatric Nurses*. Harper and Row, London.

Tibbles, P. (1980). Managing violent behaviour in a psychiatric ward: a psychiatric approach. *Nursing Times*, 20 November, Vol. 76, No. 47, pp. 2046–2048.

Trower, P., Bryant, B. and Argyle, M. (1978). *Social Skills and Mental Health*. Methuen, London.

Warburton, J. A. (1985). Violence and the nurse. *Nursing*, February, Vol. 2, No. 34, pp. 1533–1534.

Ward, M. F. (1985). *The Nursing Process in Psychiatry*. Churchill Livingstone, Edinburgh.

Weaver, S. M., Broome, A. K. and Kat, B. J. (1978). Some patterns of disturbed behaviour in a closed ward environment. *Journal of Advanced Nursing*, Vol. 3, No. 3, pp. 251–263.

Wilkinson, J. and Canter, S. (1982). *Social Skills Training Manual*. John Wiley, Chichester.

Self-assessment Questions

SAQ 5. List four observations that would confirm that a person with a personality disorder was lacking in social awareness.

SAQ 6. Describe four intervention approaches that could be used to enhance the person's social awareness.

SAQ 7. Outline how the process of establishing and setting limits can be used to help the person develop internalized boundaries.

SAQ 8. Identify four ways in which the person and their family may need to develop their coping skills.

Unit 16.2: Written Test

Susan Carter, aged 28, has been referred by her GP to the community mental health team. She has a long and troubled social history. She was expelled from school for irresponsible and unruly behaviour. Her occupational history has been sporadic. Invariably she is sacked or forced to leave due to conflict with other workers and authority figures. On several occasions she has been in trouble with the police and has been fined for shoplifting and other minor offences related to abusive and threatening behaviour.

Her parents are very concerned about her as they feel that she has little future if she carries on in the same way. They find her difficult to control and appear ambivalent towards her. As they see it "she just doesn't seem to know what's right or wrong".

1. As the CPN who has been allocated Susan's case at the team meeting, what advice could you give her parents on setting and enforcing limits on Susan's behaviour?

2. Susan is bemused when she first meets you as she does not think that she has any problems – "I'm no nutter." How could you explain to her the benefits of working on both her self-image and the way that she relates to others?

Appendix 1

Notes on The Mental Health Act 1983 and The Mental Health (Scotland) Act 1984

In the course of the last 100 years, legislation has been in existence to protect people who, by virtue of their mental disorder, are deemed to be vulnerable to abuse from members of the public and from unscrupulous members of staff of the institutions in which they are being cared for.

At the end of the nineteenth century, the Lunacy Acts and the Mental Deficiency Acts were primarily designed to prevent compulsory detention in an 'asylum' of anyone who was not a danger to others or to him/herself as well as suffering from a mental disorder. Apart from the many sections of these Acts which regulated admission to institutions, discharge from and care while in an institution, the Acts made provision for 'The Board of Control', a watchdog body with the duty to exercise protective functions on behalf of the mentally disordered.

The way the Lunacy Acts operated made it difficult, however, for people to obtain care and treatment unless they were in danger or a danger to others. In the 1930s, new legislation, the Mental Treatment Acts, made it possible to admit mentally disordered people, now referred to as 'patients' to institutions, renamed 'hospitals', on a voluntary basis. The protection against abuse which the Acts afforded applied also to voluntary patients.

To become a voluntary patient it was necessary to sign an application and patients had to give notice in writing of their intention to discharge themselves.

It was necessary to ensure that patients really understood what they were doing, and a medical officer had to ascertain that the patient was indeed 'volitional'. Many patients, though perfectly willing to be in hospital, were deemed not to be suitable for voluntary status because they were not regarded as volitional. Demented patients, confused patients, severely depressed patients or schizophrenic patients who were very withdrawn, and severely mentally handicapped people had to be admitted under 'certificate' for this reason.

In the 1950s a Royal Commission recommended changes in legislation and in 1959 in England and Wales, 1960 in Scotland and 1961 in Northern

Ireland, new legislation—'The Mental Health Acts'—came into operation. The main principles on which the Acts were based were:

1. That patients suffering from mental disorder should as far as possible be treated, in or outside hospital, on the same basis as patients suffering from any other disorder. They should be able to enter any hospital capable of offering treatment. They should enter hospital or leave hospital with no more formality or restrictions than any other patients.
2. That, outside hospital, provisions shold be made for treatment and care comparable to those offered to people suffering from other disorders.
3. That hospitals which offered psychiatric treatment should be free to refuse admission if they felt unable to help the patient or for any other reason, just as other hospitals are.
4. That the provisions made for the fairly small number of patients who must be detained against their will should entail only a minimal amount of legal restriction.
5. In England and Wales, that special provisions for protection were no longer necessary.

In order to achieve these objectives, all previous legislation relating both to Mental Illness and what was formally known as Mental Deficiency was repealed. One Act replaced all former legislation and it covered disorders not formerly dealt with.

The term 'Mental Disorder' was used to cover all disorders dealt with under the Act. The definition in the Act of 'Mental Disorder' was: 'Mental illness, arrested or incomplete development, psychopathic disorder and any other disorder or disability of mind.' In Scotland the term 'Psychopathic Disorder' was not used.

There were four subdivisions of Mental Disorder recognized for the purpose of the compulsory provisions of the Act of 1959:

1. Mental illness
2. Severe subnormality
3. Subnormality
4. Psychopathic disorder

The Scottish Act did not define the categories. The term 'Mental Disorder' meant Mental Illness and Mental Defect. The latter term remained in use.

Admission without compulsion.

Patients in all four of these categories could be admitted to any hospital without compulsion or application. It was not necessary that the patient should be capable of expressing a wish to be admitted. As long as he was not actively unwilling to enter hospital his admission could be informal.

Compulsory admission.

In England and Wales and in Northern Ireland, for those patients who had to be admitted against their will, only the signatures of two specifically designated doctors were necessary. In Scotland, only emergency admissions were possible on the authority of medical officers. Within seven days an application to the Sheriff had to be made to obtain his authority for further compulsory detention.

In England and Wales and in Northern Ireland, no watchdog organization was appointed. When the Board of Control was dissolved in Scotland, the Mental Welfare Commission was appointed with the general brief of exercising protective functions. It had less power, however, than its predecessor, the Board of Control.

By the end of the 1970s it had become clear that the legislation of the 1960s had provided insufficient safeguards for patients. Following a review, a new Mental Health Act was passed in 1983 and a new Mental Health (Scotland) Act in 1984.

THE MENTAL HEALTH ACT 1983

Application of the Act

The Act concerns 'the reception, care and treatment of mentally disordered patients, the management of their property and other related matters'. The definition of Mental Disorder is a mental illness, arrested or incomplete development of mind, psychopathic disorder or any other disorder or disability of mind. For most purposes of the Act it is not enough for a patient to be suffering from one of the four specific categories of mental disorder set out in the Act:

1. Mental illness
2. Mental impairment
3. Severe mental impairment
4. Psychopathic disorder

It is important to note that no person shall be treated as suffering from mental disorder by reason of promiscuity or other immoral conduct, sexual deviancy, or dependence on alcohol or drugs.

The Scottish Act does not define the categories. The words Mental Subnormality and Mental Deficiency cease to have effect.

Admission without compulsion

Informal admission should be the normal mode of admission to hospital whenever a patient is willing to be admitted and be treated without the use of compulsory powers. It is not necessary that the patient should be capable of expressing a wish to be admitted. As long as he is not actively unwilling to enter hospital the admission can be informal. The majority of patients enter hospital as informal admissions.

Compulsory admission: England and Wales

Some patients suffering from mental disorder may have to be compulsorily admitted to and detained in hospital or received into guardianship. There are a number of different powers under which a patient may be compulsorily detained in hospital:

The emergency admission

An application may be made by an approved social worker or by the nearest relative of the patient in exceptional circumstances. The applicant must state that it is of urgent necessity that the patient should be admitted and detained for assessment, and that compliance with the normal procedures would involve undesirable delay. Only one medical recommendation is required, but the practitioner concerned must have seen the patient within the previous 24 hours. The application is effective for 72 hours.

Admission for assessment

Admission to and detention in hospital for assessment may be authorized where a patient is (a) suffering from mental disorder of a nature of degree which warrants the detention of the patient in hospital for assessment (or for assessment followed by medical treatment) for at least a limited period and (b) he ought to be so detained in the interests of his health or safety, or with a view to the protection of others. Detention is for up to 28 days. An application for admission must be made by either the patient's nearest relative or an approved social worker. An application for admission must be accompanied by written recommendations from two medical practitioners, one of whom must be approved as having special experience in the diagnosis and treatment of mental disorder.

Admission for treatment

The grounds for admission for treatment are first that the patient is suffering from one or more of the four forms of mental disorder as previously described. Secondly, the mental disorder must be of a nature or degree which makes it appropriate for the patient to receive medical treatment in hospital. Thirdly, for a patient suffering from psychopathic disorder or mental impairment there is an additional condition that medical treatment is likely to alleviate or prevent a deterioration in the patient's condition. Treatment need not be expected to cure the patient's disorder: medical treatment should enable the patient to cope more satisfactorily with his disorder or it should stop his condition from becoming worse. Fourthly, it must be necessary for the health or safety of the patient or for the protection of others that he should receive this treatment and it cannot be provided unless he is detained. Application for admission for treatment must be made by either an approved social worker or the patient's nearest relative. The person who is to be regarded as nearest relative is defined in the Act. This must be accompanied by written recommendations from two medical practitioners, one of whom must be approved as having special experience in diagnosis and treatment of mental disorder. Detention for treatment is for a maximum period of six months unless the order is renewed.

Patients already in hospital

A patient must be compulsorily detained for up to 72 hours if the doctor in charge of his treatment reports that an application for admission ought to be made. If the doctor is not obtainable, a first level nurse trained in nursing people suffering from mental illness or mental handicap may detain an informal patient on behalf of the managers for a period of up to six hours while a doctor is found. It must appear to the nurse that (a) the patient is suffering from mental disorder to such a degree that it is necessary for his health or safety, or for the protection of others, for him to be immediately restrained from leaving hospital and (b) it is not practicable to secure the immediate attendance of a doctor for the purpose of furnishing a report. The nurse must record these facts in writing.

Safeguards for patients and staff

Patients who feel they are wrongfully detained may apply to a *Mental Health Review Tribunal* to have their case considered. The tribunal has the power to discharge a patient from hospital. Patients admitted for assessment may apply within the first 14 days of detention. Patients admitted for treatment may apply within the first six months of detention, and again within six months if the detention order is renewed. In addition, a *Mental Health Act Commission* will ensure that hospitals have adopted and are following proper procedures for using the powers of detention. The Commission will also assist in giving staff guidance on good practice, which will be included in a Code of Practice. The Mental Health Act Commission is a new body. It has evolved a structure in which it will operate in independent groups from several regional offices.

Patients' information

The hospital managers must provide certain information to detained patients and their nearest relatives. This is to ensure that the detained patient understands the nature of his detention and his right to apply to a Mental Health Review Tribunal. They must also inform the person with whom the patient had last been living.

Consent to treatment

Compulsory detention does not mean that the patient may be automatically compelled to accept treatment. There are safeguards to ensure that either a second opinion or consent to treatment or both are obtained in the case of certain forms of treatment.

Treatment requiring consent and a second opinion

This section of the Act applies to the following forms of treatment where outcome is irreversible.

1. Psychosurgery—any surgical operation for destroying brain tissues or the function of the brain
2. Surgical implantation of hormones. The Mental Health Act Commission must be notified to consider the validity of the patient's consent. They will jointly issue a certificate but, before doing so, the medical member will consult with a nurse and one other professional who have been concerned with the patient's treatment.

Treatment requiring consent or a second opinion

This section of the Act applies to the following forms of treatment.

1. The administration of medicine if three months or more have elapsed since medicine was first administered during that period of detention
2. Electroconvulsive therapy

If the patient does not consent to a treatment, the Mental Health Act Commission must be consulted for a second opinion. In addition the medical member will consult with a nurse and one other professional and the responsible medical officer before giving a second opinion.

Urgent treatment

Special conditions are set out for treating patients in an emergency but they exclude those treatments mentioned above. Such treatments will be necessary to save the patient's life, to prevent serious deterioration of his condition, to alleviate serious suffering by the patient or to prevent the patient from behaving violently or being a danger to himself or to others. In cases where treatment is not immediately necessary or it is proposed to continue treatment after the initial urgent administration, it will be necessary to contact the Mental Health Act Commission.

Withdrawing consent

If a patient withdraws his consent to any treatment, the treatment must not be given or must cease to be given immediately.

Powers of the Court and the Home Secretary

In certain circumstances patients may be admitted to and detained in hospital on the order of a Court, or may be transferred to hospital from penal institutions on the direction of the Home Secretary. The courts also have the powers: to remand to hospital for a medical report; to remand to hospital for treatment; and to obtain interim hospital orders.

Patients' property may be protected by the 'Court of Protection'.

Application of the Mental Health (Scotland) Act 1984

Unlike the Mental Health Act Commission in England and Wales, *The Mental Welfare Commission* in Scotland is not new. Under the 1984 Act it has increased duties and increased power. It is concerned with exercising 'protective function in respect of mentally disordered persons who may be incapable of adequately protecting their persons or their interests', whether they are compulsorily detained or not, and wherever they are, whether in hospital or in the community. (The Mental Health Act Commission in England and Wales is concerned only with detained patients.)

In Scotland there is no Mental Health Review Tribunal. Detained patients may appeal for discharge either to the Sheriff or to the Mental Welfare Commission, which has the power to order the discharge of a patient against medical advice.

The Mental Welfare Commission has the duty to bring to the attention of the managers any matter which they consider appropriate to secure the welfare of any patient by:

1. Preventing ill treatment
2. Remedying any deficiency in care or treatment
3. Preventing or redressing loss or damage to his property

Curator bonis

The Mental Welfare Commission has the power to petition for the appointment of a *curator bonis* to administer a patient's property and affairs.

The duties of the Mental Welfare Commission to visit, interview and examine patients who are compulsorily detained and to visit patients on leave of absence, and the power to hold enquiries and require persons to give evidence, are laid down in the Act.

Compulsory detention of patients

Provisions for Emergency Admission are similar to those in England and Wales. The term 'short-term detention' for a period of detention up to 28 days and 'long-term detention' for a period of detention beyond that. Short- and long-term detention must be authorized by the Sheriff.

Nurses have the power to detain a patient for only two hours.

The Mental Welfare Commission is informed at specified intervals of the movements in and out of hospital, of renewal of authority to detain a patient and of matters concerning guardianship.

Safeguards concerning consent to treatment are similar to those which apply in England and Wales.

Patients may be detained in hospital on the order of a court, under the Criminal Procedure (Scotland) Act 1975. The Secretary of State is empowered to make an order restricting discharge.

Reproduced with kind permission from "Psychiatric Nursing", Altschal & McGovern, Baillière Tindall.

Appendix 2

Useful Addresses

Age Concern England
Bernard Sunley House
60 Pitcairn Road
Mitcham
Surrey CR4 3LL
(01) 640 5431

Age Concern Northern Ireland
128 Great Victoria Street
Belfast BT2 7BG
(0232) 245729

Age Concern Scotland
33 Castle Street
Edinburgh EH2 3DW
(031) 225 5000

Age Concern Wales
1 Park Grove
Cardiff CF1 3BJ
(0222) 371566

Alateen
61 Dover Street
London SE1 4YF
(01) 403 0888

Alcohol Concern
305 Gray's Inn Road
London WC1X 8QF
(01) 833 3471

Alcohol Counselling Service
34 Electric Lane
London SW9 8JT
(01) 737 3579

Alcoholics Anonymous
PO Box 514
11 Redcliffe Gardens
London SW10 9BQ
(01) 352 9779

Alzheimer's Disease Society
3rd Floor Bank Buildings
Fulham Broadway
London SW6 1EP
(01) 381 3177

Anorexia Anonymous
24 Westmoreland Road
London SW13 9RY
(01) 748 3994

Anorexic Aid
The Priory Centre
11 Priory Road
High Wycombe
Bucks HP13 6SL
(0494) 21431

Anorexic Family Aid
National Information Centre
Sackville Place
44 Magdalen Street
Norwich
Norfolk NR3 1JE
(0603) 621414

Association for Post-Natal Illness
Institute of Obstetrics and
    Gynaecology
Queen Charlotte's Maternity
    Hospital
Goldhawk Road
London W6 0X9
(01) 748 4666

Association of Carers
Medway Homes
Balfour Road
Rochester
Kent ME4 6QU
(0634) 813981

Association of Self-Help and
    Community Groups
7 Chesham Terrace
London W13 9HX
(01) 579 5589

British Association for
    Counselling
37a Sheep Street, Rugby
Warwickshire CV21 3BX
(0788) 78328

College of Health
18 Victoria Park Square
London E2 9PF
(01) 980 6263

Cruse
Cruse House
126 Sheen Road
Richmond
Surrey TW9 1UR
(01) 940 4818/9047

Depressives Anonymous,
    Fellowship of
36 Chestnut Avenue
Beverley
North Humberside HU17 9QU
(0482) 860619

Depressives Associated
PO Box 5, Castletown
Portland
Dorset DT5 1BQ

Distance Learning Centre
Polytechnic of the South Bank
Manor House
58 Clapham Common North Side
London SW4 9R2

The English National Board for
    Nursing, Midwifery and Health
    Visiting
23 Portland Place
London W1N 3AF
(01) 637 7181

Families Anonymous
88 Caledonian Road
London N7
(01) 278 8805

Gamblers Anonymous
17/23 Blantyre Street
Cheyne Walk
London SW10 0DT
(01) 352 3060

Good Practices in Mental Health
380–384 Harrow Road
London W9 2HU
(01) 289 2034

Health Service Commissioner for
    England
Church House
Great Smith Street
London SW1P 3BW
(01) 212 7676

Health Service Commissioner for
    Scotland
2nd Floor, 11 Melville Crescent
Edinburgh EH3 7LU
(031) 225 7465

Health Service Commissioner for
    Wales
4th Floor
Pearl Assurance House
Greyfriars Road
Cardiff CF1 3AG
(0222) 394621

The Institute for the Study of
    Drug Dependence
1–4 Hatton Place
Hatton Garden
London EC1N 8ND

Manic Depression Fellowship
51 Sheen Road
Richmond, Surrey
(01) 940 6235

Mental After-care Association
110 Jermyn Street
London SW1 6HB

Mental Health Act Commission
Floor 2, Hepburn House
Marsham Street
London SW1 4HW
(01) 211 8061

Mental Health Foundation
8 Hallam Street
London W1N 6DH
(01) 580 0145

Mental Health Review Tribunals
write to the address nearest the
    hospital:
Room 1516 Euston Tower
286 Euston Road
London NW1 3DN
(01) 388 1188 (ext 787)

3rd Floor Cressington House
249 St Mary's Road
Garston
Liverpool L19 0NF
(051) 494 0095

Spur A, Block 5
Government Buildings
Chalfont Drive
Western Boulevard
Nottingham NG8 3RZ
(0602) 294222

2nd Floor, New Crown Buildings
Cathays Park
Cardiff CF1 3NQ
(0222) 823398/825111

Mental Welfare Commission for
    Scotland
22 Melville Street
Edinburgh EH3 7NS
(031) 225 7034

Mind
22 Harley Street
London W1N 2ED
(01) 637 0741

Narcotics Anonymous
PO Box 246
c/o 47 Milman Street
London SW10
(01) 351 6794

The National Board for Nursing,
    Midwifery and Health Visiting
    for Northern Ireland
RAC House
79 Chichester Street
Belfast BT1 4JE
(0232) 238152

The National Board for Nursing,
    Midwifery and Health Visiting
    for Scotland
22 Queen Street
Edinburgh EH2 1JX
(031) 226 7371

National Council for Carers and
    their Elderly Dependants
29 Chilworth Mews
London W2 3RG
(01) 262 1451

National Council for the Divorced
    and Separated
13 High Street
Little Shelford
Cambridge CB2 5ES
(0623) 648297

National Drinkwatchers Network
200 Seagrave Road
London SW6 1RQ
(01) 381 3157

National Marriage Guidance
    Council (Relate)
Herbert Gray College
Little Church Street
Rugby
Warwickshire

National Schizophrenic Fellowship
78 Victoria Road
Surbiton
Surrey
KT6 4NS
(01) 390 3651

National Schizophrenia Fellowship
(Northern Ireland)
Room 6, Bryson House
Bedford Street
Belfast
BT2 7FE
(0232) 248006

National Schizophrenia Fellowship
(Scotland)
40 Shandwick Place
Edinburgh EH2 4RT
(031) 226 2025

Northern Ireland Agoraphobic
Society
Beacon House
84 University Street
Belfast BT7 1HE
(0232) 228474

Northern Ireland Association for
Mental Health
Beacon House
84 University Street
Belfast BT7 1HE
(0232) 228474

Northern Ireland Council on
Alcoholism
36/40 Victoria Street
Belfast

Northern Ireland Mental Health
Review Tribunal
Mental Health Branch
Room 3C Dundonald House
Stormont Estate
Belfast BT4 3FF
(0232) 650111

Northern Schizophrenia
Fellowship
38 Collingwood Buildings
Collingwood Street
Newcastle-upon-Tyne
Tyne & Wear NE1 1JH
(0632) 614343

Open Door Association
447 Pensby Road
Heswall, Wirral
Merseyside L61 2PQ
(051) 648 2022

The Open University
Department of Health and Social
Welfare
Walton Hall
Milton Keynes MK 7 6AA

Phobics Society
4 Cheltenham Road
Chorlton-cum-Hardy
Manchester M21 1QN
(061) 881 1937

The Richmond Fellowship
8 Addison Road
London W14 8DL
(01) 603 6373

Royal College of Nursing of the
United Kingdom
20 Cavendish Square
London W1M 0AB
(01) 409 3333

Samaritans
3 Hornton Place
London W8
(01) 283 3400

Schizophrenia Association of
Great Britain
Bryn Hyfryd
The Crescent, Bangor
Gwynedd LL57 2AG
(0248) 354048

Scottish Association for Mental
  Health
40 Shandwick Place
Edinburgh EH2 4RT
(031) 225 4446

Scottish Council for Alcoholism
147 Blythswood Street
Glasgow G2 4EN

Solvent Abuse
Department M50
13–39 Standard Road
London NW10

South Wales Association for the
  Prevention of Addiction
111 Cowbridge Road East
Cardiff CF1 9AG
(0222) 26113

Support for Relatives of the
  Elderly Mentally Infirm
SREMI Office
St Martin's Hospital
Midford Road
Bath BA2 5RP
(0225) 834152

Tranx
17 Peel Road
Harrow
Middlesex HA3 7QX
(01) 427 2065

The Welsh National Board for
  Nursing, Midwifery and Health
  Visiting
13th Floor
Pearl Assurance House
Greyfriars Road
Cardiff CF1 3AG
(0222) 395535

Women's Health Concern
Ground Floor
17 Earls Terrace
London W8 6LP
(01) 602 6669

Women's Health Information
  Centre
52 Featherstone Street
London EC1Y 8RT
(01) 251 6580

Women's Information Referral
  and Enquiry Service
PO Box 20
Oxford
(0865) 240991

Women's Therapy Centre
6 Manor Gardens
London N7 6LA
(01) 263 6200

Index